CLINICIAN'S POCKET DRUG REFERENCE 2012

D1242272

CLINICIAN'S POCKET DRUG REFERENCE 2012

Tenth Anniversary Edition

EDITORS

Leonard G. Gomella, MD, FACS
Steven A. Haist, MD, MS, FACP
Aimee G. Adams, PharmD

www.eDrugbook.com
www.thescutmonkey.com

McGraw Hill **Medical**

New York   Chicago   San Francisco   Lisbon
London   Madrid   Mexico City   Milan   New Delhi
San Juan   Seoul   Singapore   Sydney   Toronto

Clinician's Pocket Drug Reference 2012

Copyright © 2012 by Leonard G. Gomella. Published by The McGraw-Hill Companies, Inc. All rights reserved. Printed in Canada. Except as permitted under the United States Copyright Act of 1976, no part of this publication may be reproduced or distributed in any form or by any means, or stored in a data base or retrieval system, without the prior written permission of the publisher.

1 2 3 4 5 6 7 8 9 0   QLM/QLM   15 14 13 12 11

ISBN 978-0-07-178162-6
MHID 0-07-178162-5
ISSN 1540-6725

Notice

Medicine is an ever-changing science. As new research and clinical experience broaden our knowledge, changes in treatment and drug therapy are required. The authors and the publisher of this work have checked with sources that are believed to be reliable in their efforts to provide information that is complete and generally in accord with the standards accepted at the time of publication. However, in view of the possibility of human error or changes in medical sciences, neither the authors nor the publisher nor any other party who has been involved in the preparation or publication of this work warrants that the information contained herein is in every respect accurate or complete, and they disclaim all responsibility for any errors or omissions or for the results obtained from use of the information contained in this work. Readers are encouraged to confirm the information contained herein with other sources. For example and in particular, readers are advised to check the product information sheet included in the package of each drug they plan to administer to be certain that the information contained in this work is accurate and that changes have not been made in the recommended dose or in the contraindications for administration. This recommendation is of particular importance in connection with new or infrequently used drugs.

The book was set in Times by Cenveo Publisher Services.
The editors were Joseph Morita and Harriet Lebowitz.
The production supervisor was Sherri Souffrance.
Project management was provided by Cenveo Publisher Services.
Quad/Graphics Leominster was printer and binder.

This book is printed on acid-free paper.

CONTENTS

v

GENERIC AND SELECTED BRAND DRUG DATA   **33**
NATURAL AND HERBAL AGENTS   **276**
TABLES   **281**

TIPS FOR SAFE PRESCRIPTION WRITING
    Inside Front Cover

EMERGENCY CARDIAC CARE MEDICATIONS
    Back Page and Inside Back Cover

Leonard G. Gomella, MD, FACS
The Bernard W. Godwin, Jr., Professor
Chairman, Department of Urology
Jefferson Medical College
Associate Director of Clinical Affairs
Kimmel Cancer Center
Thomas Jefferson University
Philadelphia, Pennsylvania

Steven A. Haist, MD, MS, FACP
Clinical Professor
Department of Medicine
Drexel University College of Medicine,
Philadelphia, Pennsylvania

Aimee G. Adams, PharmD
Clinical Pharmacist Specialist, Ambulatory Care
Adjunct Assistant Professor
College of Pharmacy and Department of Internal Medicine
University of Kentucky HealthCare
Lexington, Kentucky

EDITORIAL BOARD

PREFACE

We are pleased to present the 10th edition of the *Clinician's Pocket Drug Reference*. This edition represents the 10th anniversary, with the first edition as a free-standing publication released in 2002. This book is based on the drug presentation style originally used in 1983 in the *Clinician's Pocket Reference*, popularly known as the *Scut Monkey Book*. Our goal is to identify the most frequently used and clinically important medications, including branded, generic, OTC, and herbal products. The book now lists over 1400 generic products, with the true number approaching 4000 when specific brand names are considered.

Our style of presentation includes key "must know" facts of commonly used medications, essential for both the student and practicing clinician. The inclusion of common uses of medications rather than just the official FDA-labeled indications is based on supporting publications and community standards of care. All uses have been reviewed by our editors and editorial board and are designed to represent a cross-section of practices across the United States.

The limitation of difficult-to-read package inserts was formally acknowledged by the US Food and Drug Administration in 2001. Today, all newly approved medications provide a more user-friendly package insert. But these simplified versions do not accompany some similarly approved generic or "competing" products, or many older medications.

It is essential that students and residents in training learn more than the name and dose of medications they prescribe. Side effects, significant warnings, and contraindications are associated with prescription medications. Although, ideally, healthcare providers should be fully familiar with the package inserts of medications prescribed, the high number of prescriptions makes this expectation unreasonable. Reference sources such as the *Physicians' Desk Reference* and drug manufacturers' Web sites make package inserts readily available. Likewise, encyclopedic information, occasionally needed in unique clinical situations, can be found on many sites. However, resources that sort out the most common and essential facts are sometimes lacking. Newly released medications often have a prominent presence and easy access to all their FDA-approved data on the Web, but often not for older medications, OTC products, or generic medications. We strive to provide the reader access to not only dosing but these clinically significant facts and key data, whether for brand-name drugs, generics, or those available over the counter.

The editorial board and contributors have analyzed the information on these common medications and have made this key prescribing information available in this pocket-sized book. This information is intended for use by healthcare professionals who are already familiar with these commonly prescribed medications.

For 2012, we have added almost 100 new drugs and new formulations, and incorporated dozens of changes in other medications based on recent FDA actions. These include deletions of discontinued brand names and compounds and multiple black box updates. Subtle changes in formatting and presentation style have allowed us to keep the print version book portable yet maintain key information. Emergency cardiac care (ECC) guidelines for commonly used medications in the adult and pediatric patient have been updated, based on the latest recommendations from the American Heart Association (*Circulation.* 2010;122[18 suppl 3]:S639—available online at: http://circ.ahajournals.org/content/vol122/18_suppl_3/). The ECC emergency common medication summary for adults is also provided in table form on the back inside cover of the book, for quick reference.

Versions of this book are being constantly released, produced in a variety of electronic or eBook formats. Visit www.eDrugbook.com for links to some of the electronic versions currently available. This Web site has enhanced content features, such as a comprehensive listing of "look alike–sound alike" medications that can contribute to prescribing errors, as well as other useful information related to prescribing.

Nursing versions of this book (*Nurse's Pocket Drug Guide*), with a section of customized nursing interventions, is available and updated annually. An EMS guide based on this book (*EMS Pocket Drug Guide*), with enhanced content specifically for the field provider and emergency medical practitioner, is also available. Information and links for these related publications are also available at www.eDrugbook.com.

We express special thanks to our spouses and families for their support of this book and the Scut Monkey project (www.thescutmonkey.com). The Scut Monkey project, launched in 1979, is designed to provide new medical students and other health professionals with the basic tools needed when entering the world of hands-on patient care.

The contributions of the members of the editorial board, and Harriet Lebowitz and Joe Morita at McGraw-Hill, are gratefully acknowledged. As a reader, your comments and suggestions are always welcome. Improvements to this and all our books would be impossible without the interest and continued feedback from our readers. We hope this book will help you learn some of the key elements in prescribing medications and allow you to care for your patients in the best way possible.

Leonard G. Gomella, MD, FACS
Philadelphia, Pennsylvania
Leonard.Gomella@jefferson.edu

Steven A. Haist, MD, MS, FACP
Philadelphia, Pennsylvania

Aimee G. Adams, PharmD
Lexington, Kentucky

MEDICATION KEY

Medications are listed by prescribing class and the individual medications are then listed in alphabetical order by generic name. Some of the more commonly recognized trade names are listed for each medication (in parentheses after the generic name) or if available without prescription, noted as **OTC** (over-the-counter).

Generic Drug Name (Selected Common Brand Names) [Controlled Substance] BOX: Summarized/paraphrased versions of the "Black Box" precautions deemed necessary by the FDA. These are significant precautions, warnings, and contraindications concerning the individual medication. **Uses:** This includes both FDA-labeled indications bracketed by ** and other "off-label" uses of the medication. Because many medications are used to treat various conditions based on the medical literature and not listed in their package insert, we list common uses of the medication in addition the official "labeled indications" (FDA approved) based on input from our editorial board **Acts:** How the drug works. This information is helpful in comparing classes of drugs and understanding side effects and contraindications. *Spectrum:* Specifies activity against selected microbes for antimicrobials **Dose: Adults.** Where no specific pediatric dose is given, the implication is that this drug is not commonly used or indicated in that age group. At the end of the dosing line, important dosing modifications may be noted (i.e., take with food, avoid antacids, etc.) **Peds.** If appropriate dosing for children and infants is included with age ranges as needed **W/P (Warnings and Precautions):** [pregnancy/fetal risk categories, breast-feeding (as noted below)] Warnings and precautions concerning the use of the drug in specific settings **CI:** Contraindications **Disp:** Common dosing forms **SE:** Common or significant side effects **Notes:** Other key useful information about the drug.

CONTROLLED SUBSTANCE CLASSIFICATION

Medications under the control of the US Drug Enforcement Agency (DEA) (Schedules I–V controlled substances) are indicated by the symbol [C]. Most medications are "uncontrolled" and do not require a DEA prescriber number on the prescription. The following is a general description for the schedules of DEA-controlled substances:

Schedule (C-I) I: All nonresearch use forbidden (e.g., heroin, LSD, mescaline).
Schedule (C-II) II: High addictive potential; medical use accepted. No telephone call-in prescriptions; no refills. Some states require special prescription form (e.g., cocaine, morphine, methadone).
Schedule (C-III) III: Low to moderate risk of physical dependence, high risk of psychological dependence; prescription must be rewritten after 6 months or 5 refills (e.g., acetaminophen plus codeine).
Schedule (C-IV) IV: Limited potential for dependence; prescription rules same as for schedule III (e.g., benzodiazepines, propoxyphene).
Schedule (C-V) V: Very limited abuse potential; prescribing regulations often same as for uncontrolled medications; some states have additional restrictions.

FDA FETAL RISK CATEGORIES
Category A: Adequate studies in pregnant women have not demonstrated a risk to the fetus in the first trimester of pregnancy; there is no evidence of risk in the last two trimesters.
Category B: Animal studies have not demonstrated a risk to the fetus, but no adequate studies have been done in pregnant women.

or

Animal studies have shown an adverse effect, but adequate studies in pregnant women have not demonstrated a risk to the fetus during the first trimester of pregnancy, and there is no evidence of risk in the last two trimesters.
Category C: Animal studies have shown an adverse effect on the fetus, but no adequate studies have been done in humans. The benefits from the use of the drug in pregnant women may be acceptable despite its potential risks.

or

No animal reproduction studies and no adequate studies in humans have been done.
Category D: There is evidence of human fetal risk, but the potential benefits from the use of the drug in pregnant women may be acceptable despite its potential risks.
Category X: Studies in animals or humans or adverse reaction reports, or both, have demonstrated fetal abnormalities. The risk of use in pregnant women clearly outweighs any possible benefit.
Category ?: No data available (not a formal FDA classification; included to provide complete dataset).

BREAST-FEEDING CLASSIFICATION
No formally recognized classification exists for drugs and breast-feeding. This shorthand was developed for the *Clinician's Pocket Drug Reference.*
+   Compatible with breast-feeding
M   Monitor patient or use with caution
±   Excreted, or likely excreted, with unknown effects or at unknown concentrations
?/–   Unknown excretion, but effects likely to be of concern
–   Contraindicated in breast-feeding
?   No data available

ABBREVIATIONS

Δ: change
?: possible or uncertain
✓: check, follow, or monitor
↓: decrease/decreased
↑: increase/increased
≠: not equal to; not equivalent to
Ab: antibody, abortion
ABG: arterial blood gas
Abd: abdominal
ABMT: autologous bone marrow transplantation
ac: before meals (*ante cibum*)
ACE: angiotensin-converting enzyme
ACH: acetylcholine
ACIP: American College of International Physicians
ACLS: advanced cardiac life support
ACS: acute coronary syndrome, American Cancer Society, American College of Surgeons
ACT: activated coagulation time
Acts: Action(s)
ADH: antidiuretic hormone
ADHD: attention-deficit hyperactivity disorder
ADR: adverse drug reaction
ADT: androgen deprivation therapy
AF: atrial fibrillation
AHA: American Heart Association
AKA: also known as
ALL: acute lymphocytic leukemia
ALT: alanine aminotransferase
AMI: acute myocardial infarction
AML: acute myelogenous leukemia
amp: ampule
ANA: antinuclear antibody

ANC: absolute neutrophil count
APACHE: acute physiology and chronic health evaluation
APAP: acetaminophen [*N*-acetyl-*p*-aminophenol]
aPTT: activated partial thromboplastin time
ARB: angiotensin II receptor blocker
ARDS: adult respiratory distress syndrome
ARF: acute renal failure
AS: aortic stenosis
ASA: aspirin (acetylsalicylic acid)
ASAP: as soon as possible
AST: aspartate aminotransferase
ATP: adenosine triphosphate
AUB: abnormal uterine/vaginal bleeding
AUC: area under the curve
AV: atrioventricular
AVM: arteriovenous malformation
BBB: bundle branch block
BCL: B-cell lymphoma
BPM: beats per minute
bid: twice daily
bili: bilirubin
BM: bone marrow, bowel movement
↓BM: bone marrow suppression, myelosuppression
BMD: bone mineral density
BMT: bone marrow transplantation
BOO: bladder outlet obstruction
BP: blood pressure
↓BP: hypotension
↑BP: hypertension
BPH: benign prostatic hyperplasia

BSA: body surface area
BUN: blood urea nitrogen
Ca: calcium
CA: cancer
CABG: coronary artery bypass graft
CAD: coronary artery disease
CAP: community-acquired
  pneumonia
caps: capsule
cardiotox: cardiotoxicity
CBC: complete blood count
CCB: calcium channel blocker
CDC: Centers for Disease Control
  and Prevention
CF: cystic fibrosis
CFCs: chlorofluorocarbons
CFU: colony forming units
CHD: coronary heart disease
CHF: congestive heart failure
CI: contraindicated
CIDP: chronic inflammatory
  polyneuropathy
CK: creatinine kinase
CLL: chronic lymphocytic leukemia
CML: chronic myelogenous leukemia
CMV: cytomegalovirus
CNS: central nervous system
combo: combination
comp: complicated
conc: concentration
cont: continuous
COPD: chronic obstructive
  pulmonary disease
COX: cyclooxygenase
CP: chest pain
CPP: central precocious puberty
CR: controlled release
CrCl: creatinine clearance
CRF: chronic renal failure
CRPC: castrate-resistant prostate
  cancer
CSF: cerebrospinal fluid

CV: cardiovascular
CVA: cerebrovascular accident,
  costovertebral angle
CVH: common variable
  hypergammaglobulinemia
CXR: chest x-ray
CYP: cytochrome P450 enzyme
÷: divided
D: diarrhea
d: day
DA: dopamine
DBP: diastolic blood pressure
D/C: discontinue
DDP-4: dipeptidyl peptidase-4
derm: dermatologic
D_5LR: 5% dextrose in lactated Ringer
  solution
D_5NS: 5% dextrose in normal saline
D_5W: 5% dextrose in water
DHT: dihydrotestosterone
DI: diabetes insipidus
DIC: disseminated intravascular
  coagulation
Disp: dispensed as; how the drug is
  supplied
DKA: diabetic ketoacidosis
dL: deciliter
DM: diabetes mellitus
DMARD: disease-modifying
  antirheumatic drug; drugs in
  randomized trials to decrease
  erosions and joint space narrowing
  in rheumatoid arthritis (e.g.,
  D-penicillamine, methotrexate,
  azathioprine)
DN: diabetic nephropathy
DOT: directly observed therapy (used
  for TB treatment)
DR: delayed release
d/t: due to
DVT: deep venous thrombosis
Dz: disease

EC: enteric coated
ECC: emergency cardiac care
ECG: electrocardiogram
ED: erectile dysfunction
EGFR: epidermal growth factor receptor
EIB: exercise induced bronchoconstriction
ELISA: enzyme-linked immunosorbent assay
EL.U.: ELISA
EMG: electromyelogram
EMIT: enzyme-multiplied immunoassay test
epi: epinephrine
EPS: extrapyramidal symptoms (tardive dyskinesia, tremors and rigidity, restlessness [akathisia], muscle contractions [dystonia], changes in breathing and heart rate)
ER: extended release
ESA: erythropoiesis-stimulating agents
ESR: erythrocyte sedimentation rate
ESRD: end-stage renal disease
ET: endotracheal
EtOH: ethanol
extrav: extravasation
fam: family
FAP: familial adenomatous polyposis
Fe: iron
FSH: follicle-stimulating hormone
5-FU: fluorouracil
Fxn: function
g: gram
GABA: gamma-aminobutyric acid
GBM: glioblastoma multiforme
GC: gonorrhea
G-CSF: granulocyte colony-stimulating factor
gen: generation

GERD: gastroesophageal reflux disease
GF: growth factor
GFR: glomerular filtration rate
GHB: gamma-hydroxybutyrate
GI: gastrointestinal
GIST: gastrointestinal stromal tumor
GM-CSF: granulocyte-macrophage colony-stimulating factor
GnRH: gonadotropin-releasing hormone
G6PD: glucose-6-phosphate dehydrogenase
gtt: drop, drops (*gutta*)
GU: genitourinary
GVHD: graft-versus-host disease
h: hour(s)
H1N1: swine flu strain
HA: headache
HAE: hereditary angioedema
HBsAg: hepatitis B surface antigen
HBV: hepatitis B virus
HCL: hairy cell leukemia
HCM: hypercalcemia of malignancy
Hct: hematocrit
HCTZ: hydrochlorothiazide
HD: hemodialysis
HDL-C: high density lipoprotein cholesterol
hep: hepatitis
hepatotox: hepatotoxicity
HFA: hydrofluroalkane chemicals; propellant replacing CFCs in inhalers
Hgb: hemoglobin
HGH: human growth hormone
HIT: heparin-induced thrombocytopenia
HITTS: heparin-induced thrombosis-thrombocytopenia syndrome
HIV: human immunodeficiency virus
HMG-CoA: hydroxymethylglutaryl coenzyme A

HP: high potency
HPV: human papillomavirus
HR: heart rate
↑HR: increased heart rate (tachycardia)
hs: at bedtime (*hora somni*)
HSV: herpes simplex virus
5-HT: 5-hydroxytryptamine
HTN: hypertension
Hx: history of
IBD: irritable bowel disease
IBS: irritable bowel syndrome
IBW: ideal body weight
ICP: intracranial pressure
IFIS: intraoperative floppy iris syndrome
Ig: immunoglobulin
IGF: insulin-like growth factor
IHSS: idiopathic hypertropic subaortic stenosis
IL: interleukin
IM: intramuscular
impair: impairment
in: inches
Inf: infusion
Infxn: infection
Inh: inhalation
INH: isoniazid
inhib: inhibitor(s)
Inj: injection
INR: international normalized ratio
Insuff: insufficiency
Int: international
Intravag: intravaginal
IO: intraosseous
IOP: intraocular pressure
IR: immediate release
ISA: intrinsic sympathomimetic activity
IT: intrathecal
ITP: idiopathic thrombocytopenic purpura

Int units: international units
IUD: intrauterine device
IV: intravenous
JME: juvenile myoclonic epilepsy
JRA: juvenile rheumatoid arthritis (SJIA now preferred)
jt: joint
K: klebsiella
K^+: potassium
L&D: labor and delivery
LA: long-acting
LABA: long-acting beta$_2$-adrenergic agonists
LAIV: live attenuated influenza vaccine
LDL: low-density lipoprotein
LFT: liver function test
LH: luteinizing hormone
LHRH: luteinizing hormone-releasing hormone
liq: liquid(s)
LMW: low molecular weight
LP: lumbar puncture
LR: lactated ringers
LVD: left ventricular dysfunction
LVEF: left ventricular ejection fraction
LVSD: left ventricular systolic dysfunction
lytes: electrolytes
MAC: *Mycobacterium avium* complex
maint: maintenance dose/drug
MAO/MAOI: monoamine oxidase/ inhibitor
max: maximum
mcg: microgram(s)
mcL: microliter(s)
MDD: major depressive disorder
MDI: multidose inhaler
MDS: myelodysplasia syndrome
meds: medicines
mEq: milliequivalent
met: metastatic

mg: milligram(s)

Mg^{2+}: magnesium

$MgOH_2$: magnesium hydroxide

MI: myocardial infarction, mitral insufficiency

mill: million

min: minute(s)

mL: milliliter(s)

mo: month(s)

MoAb: monoclonal antibody

mod: moderate

MRSA: methicillin-resistant *Staphylococcus aureus*

MS: multiple sclerosis, musculoskeletal

msec: millisecond(s)

MSSA: methicillin-sensitive *Staphylococcus aureus*

MTC: medullary thyroid cancer

MTT: monotetrazolium

MTX: methotrexate

MyG: myasthenia gravis

N: nausea

NA: narrow angle

NAG: narrow angle glaucoma

NCI: National Cancer Institute

nephrotox: nephrotoxicity

neurotox: neurotoxicity

ng: nanogram(s)

NG: nasogastric

NHL: non-Hodgkin lymphoma

NIAON: nonischemic arterial optic neuritis

nl: normal

NO: nitric oxide

NPO: nothing by mouth (*nil per os*)

NRTI: nucleoside reverse transcriptase inhibitor

NS: normal saline

NSAID: nonsteroidal anti-inflammatory drug

NSCLC: non-small cell lung cancer

NSTEMI: non-ST elevation myocardial infarction

N/V: nausea and vomiting

N/V/D: nausea, vomiting, diarrhea

NYHA: New York Heart Association

OA: osteoarthritis

OAB: overactive bladder

obst: obstruction

OCD: obsessive compulsive disease

OCP: oral contraceptive pill

OD: overdose

ODT: orally disintegrating tablets

OK: recommended

oint: ointment

op: operative

ophthal: ophthalmic

OSAHS: obstructive sleep apnea/hypopnea syndrome

OTC: over the counter

ototox: ototoxicity

oz: ounces

PAT: paroxysmal atrial tachycardia

pc: after eating (*post cibum*)

PCa: cancer of the prostate

PCI: percutaneous coronary intervention

PCN: penicillin

PCP: *Pneumocystis jiroveci* (formerly *carinii*) pneumonia

PCWP: pulmonary capillary wedge pressure

PDE5: phosphodiesterase type 5

PDGF: platelet-derived growth factor

PE: pulmonary embolus, physical examination, pleural effusion

PEA: pulseless electrical activity

PEG: polyethylene glycol

PFT: pulmonary function test

pg: picogram(s)

PGE-1: prostaglandin E-1

PGTC: primary generalized tonic-clonic (PGTC)

Ph: Philadelphia chromosome
Pheo: pheochromocytoma
photosens: photosensitivity
PI: product insert (package label)
PID: pelvic inflammatory disease
PKU: phenylketonuria
plt: platelet
PMDD: premenstrual dysphoric disorder
PML: progressive multifocal leukoencephalopathy
PMS: premenstrual syndrome
PO: by mouth (*per os*)
PPD: purified protein derivative
PPI: proton pump inhibitor
PR: by rectum
PRG: pregnancy
PRN: as often as needed (*pro re nata*)
PSA: prostate-specific antigen
PSVT: paroxysmal supraventricular tachycardia
pt: patient
PT: prothrombin time
PTCA: percutaneous transluminal coronary angioplasty
PTH: parathyroid hormone
PTSD: post-traumatic stress disorder
PTT: partial thromboplastin time
PUD: peptic ulcer disease
pulm: pulmonary
PVC: premature ventricular contraction
PVD: peripheral vascular disease
PWP: pulmonary wedge pressure
Px: prevention
pyelo: pyelonephritis
q: every (*quaque*)
q_h: every _ hours
q day: every day
qh: every hour
qhs: every hour of sleep
(before bedtime)
qid: four times a day (*quater in die*)
q other day: every other day
QRS: electrocardiogram complex
QT: time from the start of QRS complex to the end of T wave on an electrocardiogram
RA: rheumatoid arthritis
RAS: renin-angiotensin system
RBC: red blood cell(s) (count)
RCC: renal cell carcinoma
RDA: recommended dietary allowance
RDS: respiratory distress syndrome
rec: recommends
REMS: risk evaluation and mitigation strategy; FDA plan to help ensure that the drug's benefits outweigh its risks. As part of that plan, the company must conduct educational outreach
resp: respiratory
RHuAb: recombinant human antibody
RIA: radioimmune assay
RLS: restless leg syndrome
R/O, r/o: rule out
RR: respiratory rate
RSI: rapid sequence intubation
RSV: respiratory syncytial virus
RT: reverse transcriptase
RTA: renal tubular acidosis
Rx: prescription or therapy
Rxn: reaction
s: second(s)
SAD: social anxiety disorder or seasonal affective disorder
SAE: serious adverse event
SBE: subacute bacterial endocarditis
SBP: systolic blood pressure
SCLC: small cell lung cancer
SCr: serum creatinine
SDV: single-dose vial
SE: side effect(s)

SIADH: syndrome of inappropriate antidiuretic hormone
sig: significant
SIRS: systemic inflammatory response syndrome/capillary leak syndrome
SJIA: systemic juvenile idiopathic arthritis
SJS: Stevens-Johnson syndrome
SL: sublingual
SLE: systemic lupus erythematosus
SLUDGE: mnemonic for: Salivation, Lacrimation, Urination, Diaphoresis, GI motility, Emesis
SMX: sulfmethoxazole
SNRIs: serotonin-norepinephrine reuptake inhibitors
SOB: shortness of breath
soln: solution
sp: species
SPAG: small particle aerosol generator
SQ: subcutaneous
SR: sustained release
SSRI: selective serotonin reuptake inhibitor
SSS: sick sinus syndrome
S/Sxs: signs & symptoms
stat: immediately (*statim*)
STD: sexually transmitted disease
STEMI: ST elevation myocardial infarction
supl: supplement
supp: suppository
susp: suspension
SVT: supraventricular tachycardia
SWFI: sterile water for injection
SWSD: shift work sleep disorder
synth: synthesis
Sx: symptom
Sz: seizure
tab/tabs: tablet/tablets
TB: tuberculosis

TCA: tricyclic antidepressant
TFT: thyroid function test
TIA: transient ischemic attack
TID: three times a day (*ter in die*)
TIV: trivalent influenza vaccine
TKI: tyrosine kinase inhibitors
TMP: trimethoprim
TMP-SMX: trimethoprim-sulfamethoxazole
TNF: tumor necrosis factor
tox: toxicity
TOUCH: Tysabri Outreach Unified Commitment to Health
TPA: tissue plasminogen activator
TRALI: transfusion-related acute lung injury
TSH: thyroid-stimulating hormone
tri: trimester
TTP: thrombotic thrombocytopenic purpura
TTS: transdermal therapeutic system
Tx: treatment
UC: ulcerative colitis
UGT: uridine 5′ diphosphoglucuronosyl transferase
ULN: upper limits of normal
uncomp: uncomplicated
URI: upper respiratory infection
US: United States
UTI: urinary tract infection
V: vomiting
VAERS: Vaccine Adverse Events Reporting System
Vag: vaginal
VEGF: vascular endothelial growth factor
VF: ventricular fibrillation
vit: vitamin
VLDL: very low density lipoprotein
VOD: venoocclusive disease
vol: volume

VPA: valproic acid
VRE: vancomycin-resistant
   Enterococcus
VT: ventricular tachycardia
WBC: white blood cell(s) (count)
W/P: warnings and precautions
Wgt: weight

WHI: Women's Health Initiative
wk: week(s)
WNL: within normal limits
WPW: Wolff–Parkinson–White
   syndrome
XR: extended release
ZE: Zollinger–Ellison (syndrome)

CLASSIFICATION (Generic and common brand names)

ALLERGY

Antihistamines

Azelastine (Astelin, Optivar)
Cetirizine (Zyrtec, Zyrtec-D)
Chlorpheniramine (Chlor-Trimeton)

Clemastine fumarate (Tavist)
Cyproheptadine (Periactin)
Desloratadine (Clarinex)
Diphenhydramine (Benadryl)

Fexofenadine (Allegra)
Hydroxyzine (Atarax, Vistaril)
Levocetirizine (Xyzal)
Loratadine (Alavert, Claritin)

Miscellaneous Antiallergy Agents

Budesonide (Rhinocort, Pulmicort)
Cromolyn Sodium (Intal, NasalCrom, Opticrom)

Montelukast (Singulair)
Phenylephrine, oral (Sudafed PE, SudoGest PE, Nasop,

Lusonal, AH-Chew D, Sudafed PE Quick Dissolve)

ANTIDOTES

Acetylcysteine (Acetadote, Mucomyst)
Amifostine (Ethyol)
Atropine, systemic (AtroPen Auto-Injector)
Atropine/pralidoxime (DuoDote Auto-Injector)
Charcoal, activated (SuperChar, Actidose, Liqui-Char)
Deferasirox (Exjade)

Dexrazoxane (Totect, Zinecard)
Digoxin immune Fab (Digibind, DigiFab)
Flumazenil (Romazicon)
Hydroxocobalamin (Cyanokit)
Iodine [potassium iodide] (Lugol's Solution, SSKI, Thyro-Block, ThyroSafe, ThyroShield) [OTC]

Ipecac syrup [OTC]
Mesna (Mesnex)
Methylene Blue (Urolene Blue, Various)
Naloxone (generic)
Physostigmine (Antilirium)
Succimer (Chemet)

ANTIMICROBIAL AGENTS

Antibiotics

AMINOGLYCOSIDES

Amikacin (Amikin)
Gentamicin (Garamycin, G-Mycitin)
Neomycin sulfate (Neo-Fradin, generic)
Streptomycin
Tobramycin (Nebcin)

CARBAPENEMS

Doripenem (Doribax)
Ertapenem (Invanz)
Imipenem-Cilastatin (Primaxin)
Meropenem (Merrem)

CEPHALOSPORINS, FIRST-GENERATION

Cefadroxil (Duricef, Ultracef)
Cefazolin (Ancef, Kefzol)
Cephalexin (Keflex, Panixine DisperDose)
Cephradine (Velosef)

CEPHALOSPORINS, SECOND-GENERATION

Cefaclor (Ceclor, Raniclor)
Cefotetan (Cefotan)
Cefoxitin (Mefoxin)
Cefprozil (Cefzil)
Cefuroxime (Ceftin [oral], Zinacef [parenteral])

CEPHALOSPORINS, THIRD-GENERATION

Cefdinir (Omnicef)
Cefditoren (Spectracef)
Cefixime (Suprax)
Cefoperazone (Cefobid)
Cefotaxime (Claforan)
Cefpodoxime (Vantin)
Ceftazidime (Fortaz, Ceptaz, Tazidime, Tazicef)
Ceftibuten (Cedax)
Ceftizoxime (Cefizox)
Ceftriaxone (Rocephin)

CEPHALOSPORINS, FOURTH-GENERATION

Cefepime (Maxipime)

CEPHALOSPORINS, UNCLASSIFIED ("FIFTH-GENERATION")

Ceftaroline (Teflaro)

FLUOROQUINOLONES

Ciprofloxacin (Cipro, Cipro XR, Proquin XR)
Gemifloxacin (Factive)
Levofloxacin (Levaquin, generic)
Moxifloxacin (Avelox)
Norfloxacin (Noroxin Oral, Chibroxin Ophthalmic)
Ofloxacin (Floxin)

MACROLIDES

Azithromycin (Zithromax)
Clarithromycin (Biaxin, Biaxin XL)

Erythromycin (E-Mycin, E.E.S., Ery-Tab, EryPed, Ilotycin)

Erythromycin/sulfisoxazole (Eryzole, Pediazole)

KETOLIDE

Telithromycin (Ketek)

PENICILLINS

Amoxicillin (Amoxil, Polymox)
Amoxicillin and clavulanate potassium (Augmentin, Augmentin ES-600, Augmentin XR)
Ampicillin (Amcill, Omnipen)
Ampicillin/sulbactam (Unasyn)

Dicloxacillin (Dynapen, Dycill)
Nafcillin (Nallpen, Unipen)
Oxacillin (Bactocill, Prostaphlin)
Penicillin G, aqueous (potassium or sodium) (Pfizerpen, Pentids)
Penicillin G benzathine (Bicillin)

Penicillin G procaine (Wycillin, others)
Penicillin V (Pen-Vee K, Veetids, others)
Piperacillin (Pipracil)
Piperacillin/tazobactam (Zosyn)
Ticarcillin/clavulanate potassium (Timentin)

TETRACYCLINES

Doxycycline (Adoxa, Periostat, Oracea, Vibramycin, Vibra-Tabs)

Minocycline (Dynacin, Minocin, Solodyn)
Tetracycline (Achromycin V, Sumycin)

Tigecycline (Tygacil)

Miscellaneous Antibiotic Agents

Aztreonam (Azactam)
Clindamycin (Cleocin, Cleocin T, others)
Fosfomycin (Monurol)
Linezolid (Zyvox)
Metronidazole (Flagyl, MetroGel)
Mupirocin (Bactroban, Bactroban Nasal)

Neomycin topical (*See* bacitracin/neomycin/polymyxin B, topical [Neosporin ointment]; bacitracin/neomycin/polymyxin B/hydrocortisone, topical [Cortisporin]; bacitracin/neomycin/polymyxin B/lidocaine, topical [Clomycin])

Nitrofurantoin (Furadantin, Macrodantin, Macrobid)
Quinupristin/dalfopristin (Synercid)
Rifaximin (Xifaxan)
Retapamulin (Altabax)
Telavancin (Vibativ)

Trimethoprim (Primsol, Proloprim)
Trimethoprim (TMP)/ sulfamethoxazole

(SMX) [Co-trimoxazole, TMP/SMX] (Bactrim, Septra)

Vancomycin (Vancocin, Vancoled)

Antifungals

Amphotericin B (Amphocin, Fungizone)
Amphotericin B cholesteryl (Amphotec)
Amphotericin B lipid complex (Abelcet)
Amphotericin B liposomal (AmBisome)
Anidulafungin (Eraxis)
Caspofungin (Cancidas)
Clotrimazole (Lotrimin, Mycelex, others) [OTC]

Clotrimazole/ betamethasone (Lotrisone)
Econazole (Spectazole)
Fluconazole (Diflucan)
Itraconazole (Sporanox)
Ketoconazole, oral (Nizoral)
Ketoconazole, topical (Extina, Kuric, Xolegel, Nizoral A-D shampoo) [shampoo OTC]

Miconazole (Monistat 1 combination pack, Monistat 3, Monistat 7) [OTC], (Monistat-Derm)
Miconazole, buccal (Oravig)
Nystatin (Mycostatin)
Oxiconazole (Oxistat)
Posaconazole (Noxafil)
Sertaconazole (Ertaczo)
Terbinafine (Lamisil, Lamisil AT [OTC])
Triamcinolone/nystatin (Mycolog-II)
Voriconazole (Vfend)

Antimycobacterials

Dapsone, oral
Ethambutol (Myambutol)

Isoniazid (INH)
Pyrazinamide (generic)
Rifabutin (Mycobutin)

Rifampin (Rifadin)
Rifapentine (Priftin)
Streptomycin

Antiparasitics

Benzyl alcohol (Ulesfia)

Lindane (Kwell, others)

Spinosad (Natroba)

Antiprotozoals

Artemether/ lumefantrine (Coartem)

Atovaquone (Mepron)
Atovaquone/proguanil (Malarone)

Nitazoxanide (Alinia)
Tinidazole (Tindamax)

Antiretrovirals

Abacavir (Ziagen)
Daptomycin (Cubicin)
Darunavir (Prezista)
Delavirdine (Rescriptor)
Didanosine [ddI] (Videx)
Efavirenz (Sustiva)
Efavirenz/emtricitabine/
tenofovir (Atripla)
Etravirine (Intelence)
Fosamprenavir (Lexiva)
Indinavir (Crixivan)

Lamivudine (Epivir,
Epivir-HBV, 3TC
[many combo
regimens])
Lopinavir/ritonavir
(Kaletra)
Maraviroc (Selzentry)
Nelfinavir (Viracept)
Nevirapine (Viramune)
Raltegravir (Isentress)
Ritonavir (Norvir)

Saquinavir (Fortovase,
Invirase)
Stavudine (Zerit)
Tenofovir (Viread)
Tenofovir/emtricitabine
(Truvada)
Zidovudine (Retrovir)
Zidovudine/lamivudine
(Combivir)

Antivirals

Acyclovir (Zovirax)
Adefovir (Hepsera)
Amantadine (Symmetrel)
Atazanavir (Reyataz)
Boceprevir (Victrelis)
Cidofovir (Vistide)
Emtricitabine (Emtriva)
Enfuvirtide (Fuzeon)
Famciclovir (Famvir)

Foscarnet (Foscavir)
Ganciclovir (Cytovene,
Vitrasert)
Oseltamivir (Tamiflu)
Palivizumab (Synagis)
Peginterferon alfa-2b
(PegIntron)
Penciclovir (Denavir)

Ribavirin (Virazole,
Copegus, Rebetol)
Rimantadine
(Flumadine)
Telbivudine (Tyzeka)
Valacyclovir (Valtrex)
Valganciclovir (Valcyte)
Zanamivir (Relenza)

Miscellaneous Antiviral Agents

Daptomycin (Cubicin)
Pentamidine (Pentam 300,
NebuPent)

Trimetrexate
(NeuTrexin)

ANTINEOPLASTIC AGENTS

Alkylating Agents

Altretamine (Hexalen)
Bendamustine (Treanda)
Busulfan (Myleran,
Busulfex)
Carboplatin (Paraplatin)

Cisplatin (Platinol,
Platinol-AQ)
Oxaliplatin (Eloxatin)
Procarbazine (Matulane)
Tapentadol (Nucynta)

Thiotriethylene-
phosphoramide
(Thiotepa, Thioplex,
Tespa, TSPA)

NITROGEN MUSTARDS

Chlorambucil (Leukeran)

Cyclophosphamide (Cytoxan, Neosar)

Ifosfamide (Ifex, Holoxan)

Mechlorethamine (Mustargen)

Melphalan [L-PAM] (Alkeran)

NITROSOUREAS

Carmustine [BCNU] (BiCNU, Gliadel)

Streptozocin (Zanosar)

Antibiotics

Bleomycin sulfate (Blenoxane)

Dactinomycin (Cosmegen)

Daunorubicin (Daunomycin, Cerubidine)

Doxorubicin (Adriamycin, Rubex)

Epirubicin (Ellence)

Idarubicin (Idamycin)

Mitomycin (Mutamycin)

Antimetabolites

Clofarabine (Clolar)

Cytarabine [Ara-C] (Cytosar-U)

Cytarabine liposome (DepoCyt)

Floxuridine (FUDR)

Fludarabine phosphate (Flamp, Fludara)

Fluorouracil [5-FU] (Adrucil)

Fluorouracil, topical [5-FU] (Efudex)

Gemcitabine (Gemzar)

Mercaptopurine [6-MP] (Purinethol)

Methotrexate (Rheumatrex Dose Pack, Trexall)

Nelarabine (Arranon)

Pemetrexed (Alimta)

Pralatrexate (Folotyn)

Romidepsin (Istodax)

6-Thioguanine [6-TG] (Tabloid)

Hormones

Anastrozole (Arimidex)

Bicalutamide (Casodex)

Degarelix (Firmagon)

Estramustine phosphate (Emcyt)

Exemestane (Aromasin)

Flutamide (Eulexin)

Fulvestrant (Faslodex)

Goserelin (Zoladex)

Leuprolide (Lupron, Lupron Depot, Lupron Depot-Ped, Viadur, Eligard)

Megestrol acetate (Megace, Megace ES)

Nilutamide (Nilandron)

Tamoxifen

Triptorelin (Trelstar 3.75, Trelstar 11.25, Trelstar 22.5)

Mitotic Inhibitors (Vinca Alkaloids)

Etoposide [VP-16]
(VePesid, Toposar)
Vinblastine (Velban,
Velbe)

Vincristine (Oncovin,
Vincasar PFS)
Vinorelbine (Navelbine)

Monoclonal Antibodies

Alemtuzumab (Campath)
Bevacizumab (Avastin)
Cetuximab (Erbitux)
Erlotinib (Tarceva)

Gemtuzumab
ozogamicin
(Mylotarg)
Ipilimumab (Yervoy)

Lapatinib (Tykerb)
Ofatumumab (Arzerra)
Panitumumab (Vectibix)
Trastuzumab (Herceptin)

Proteasome Inhibitor

Bortezomib (Velcade)

Taxanes

Cabazitaxel (Jevtana)
Docetaxel (Taxotere)

Paclitaxel (Taxol,
Abraxane)

Tyrosine Kinase Inhibitors (TKI)

Dasatinib (Sprycel)
Everolimus (Afinitor)
Gefitinib (Iressa)
Imatinib (Gleevec)

Nilotinib (Tasigna)
Pazopanib hydrochloride
(Votrient)

Sorafenib (Nexavar)
Sunitinib (Sutent)
Temsirolimus (Torisel)

Miscellaneous Antineoplastic Agents

Abiraterone (Zytiga)
Aldesleukin
[Interleukin-2, IL-2]
(Proleukin)
Aminoglutethimide
(Cytadren)
L-Asparaginase (Elspar,
Oncaspar)
BCG [Bacillus Calmette-
Guérin] (TheraCys,
Tice BCG)
Cladribine (Leustatin)

Dacarbazine (DTIC)
Eribulin (Halaven)
Hydroxyurea (Hydrea,
Droxia)
Irinotecan (Camptosar)
Ixabepilone (Ixempra
Kit)
Letrozole (Femara)
Leucovorin
(Wellcovorin)
Mitoxantrone
(Novantrone)

Panitumumab (Vectibix)
Pemetrexed (Alimta)
Rasburicase (Elitek)
Sipuleucel-T (Provenge)
Thalidomide (Thalomid)
Topotecan (Hycamtin)
Tretinoin, topical
[retinoic acid]
(Retin-A, Avita,
Renova, Retin-A
Micro)

CARDIOVASCULAR (CV) AGENTS

Aldosterone Antagonists

Eplerenone (Inspra)   Spironolactone
                             (Aldactone)

Alpha₁-Adrenergic Blockers

Doxazosin (Cardura,   Prazosin (Minipress)
 Cardura XL)   Terazosin (Hytrin)

Angiotensin-Converting Enzyme (ACE) Inhibitors

Benazepril (Lotensin)   Lisinopril (Prinivil,   Quinapril (Accupril)
Captopril (Capoten,   Zestril)   Ramipril (Altace)
 others)   Moexipril (Univasc)   Trandolapril (Mavik)
Enalapril (Vasotec)   Perindopril erbumine
Fosinopril (Monopril)   (Aceon)

Angiotensin II Receptor Antagonists/Blockers

Amlodipine/olmesartan   Candesartan (Atacand)   Telmisartan (Micardis)
 (Azor)   Eprosartan (Teveten)   Valsartan (Diovan)
Amlodipine/valsartan   Irbesartan (Avapro)
 (Exforge)   Losartan (Cozaar)

Antiarrhythmic Agents

Adenosine (Adenocard)   Dronedarone (Multaq)   Procainamide (Pronestyl,
Amiodarone (Cordarone,   Dofetilide (Tikosyn)   Pronestyl-SR,
 Nexterone, Pacerone)   Esmolol (Brevibloc)   Procanbid)
Atropine, systemic   Flecainide (Tambocor)   Propafenone (Rythmol)
 (AtroPen Auto-Injector)   Ibutilide (Corvert)   Quinidine (Quinidex,
Digoxin (Digitek,   Lidocaine, systemic   Quinaglute)
 Lanoxin, Lanoxicaps)   (Xylocaine, others)   Sotalol (Betapace,
Disopyramide (Norpace,   Mexiletine (Mexitil)   Betapace AF)
 Norpace CR)

Beta-Adrenergic Blockers

Acebutolol (Sectral)   Betaxolol (Kerlone)   Labetalol (Trandate,
Atenolol (Tenormin)   Bisoprolol (Zebeta)   Normodyne)
Atenolol/chlorthalidone   Carvedilol (Coreg,   Metoprolol succinate
 (Tenoretic)   Coreg CR)   (Toprol XL)

Metoprolol tartrate (Lopressor)
Nadolol (Corgard)
Nebivolol (Bystolic)
Penbutolol (Levatol)
Pindolol (Visken)
Propranolol (Inderal)
Timolol (Blocadren)

Calcium Channel Antagonists/Blockers (CCBs)

Amlodipine (Norvasc)
Amlodipine/olmesartan (Azor)
Amlodipine/valsartan (Exforge)
Clevidipine (Cleviprex)
Diltiazem (Cardizem, Cardizem CD,
Cardizem LA, Cardizem SR, Cartia XT, Dilacor XR, Diltia XT, Taztia XT, Tiamate, Tiazac)
Felodipine (Plendil)
Isradipine (DynaCirc)
Nicardipine (Cardene)
Nifedipine (Procardia, Procardia XL, Adalat CC)
Nimodipine (Nimotop)
Nisoldipine (Sular)
Verapamil (Calan, Covera-HS, Isoptin, Verelan)

Centrally Acting Antihypertensive Agents

Clonidine, oral (Catapres)
Clonidine, oral, extended-release (Kapvay)
Clonidine, transdermal (Catapres-TTS)
Guanfacine (Tenex)
Methyldopa (Aldomet)

Combination Antihypertensive Agents

Aliskiren/amlodipine (Tekamlo)
Aliskiren/amlodipine/hydrochlorothiazide (Amturnide)
Aliskiren/valsartan (Valturna)
Amlodipine/valsartan/hydrochlorothiazide (Exforge HCT)
Lisinopril/hydrochlorothiazide (Prinzide, Zestoretic, generic)
Olmesartan, olmesartan/hydrochlorothiazide (Benicar, Benicar HCT)
Olmesartan/amlodipine/hydrochlorothiazide (Tribenzor)
Telmisartan/amlodipine (Twynsta)

Diuretics

Acetazolamide (Diamox)
Amiloride (Midamor)
Bumetanide (Bumex)
Chlorothiazide (Diuril)
Chlorthalidone (Hygroton, others)
Furosemide (Lasix)
Hydrochlorothiazide (HydroDIURIL, Esidrix, others)
Hydrochlorothiazide/amiloride (Moduretic)
Hydrochlorothiazide/spironolactone (Aldactazide)
Hydrochlorothiazide/triamterene (Dyazide, Maxzide)
Indapamide (Lozol)
Mannitol (various)
Metolazone (Zaroxolyn)
Spironolactone (Aldactone)
Torsemide (Demadex)
Triamterene (Dyrenium)

Inotropic/Pressor Agents

Digoxin (Digitek, Lanoxin, Lanoxicaps)
Dobutamine (Dobutrex)
Dopamine (Intropin)
Epinephrine (Adrenalin, Sus-Phrine, EpiPen, EpiPen Jr, others)

Inamrinone [amrinone] (Inocor)
Isoproterenol (Isuprel)
Midodrine (Proamatine)
Milrinone (Primacor)
Nesiritide (Natrecor)

Norepinephrine (Levophed)
Phenylephrine, systemic (Neo-Synephrine)

Lipid-Lowering Agents

Colesevelam (WelChol)
Colestipol (Colestid)
Cholestyramine (Questran, Questran Light, Prevalite)
Ezetimibe (Zetia)

Fenofibrate (TriCor, Antara, Lofibra, Lipofen, Triglide)
Fenofibric acid (Trilipix)
Gemfibrozil (Lopid)
Niacin [nicotinic acid] (Niaspan, Slo-Niacin,

Niacor, Nicolar) [OTC forms]
Niacin/lovastatin (Advicor)
Niacin/simvastatin (Simcor)
Omega-3 fatty acid [fish oil] (Lovaza)

Statins

Atorvastatin (Lipitor)
Fluvastatin (Lescol)
Lovastatin (Mevacor, Altoprev)

Pitavastatin (Livalo)
Pravastatin (Pravachol)

Rosuvastatin (Crestor)
Simvastatin (Zocor)

Lipid-Lowering/Antihypertensive Combinations

Amlodipine/atorvastatin (Caduet)

Vasodilators

Alprostadil [prostaglandin E_1] (Prostin VR)
Epoprostenol (Flolan)
Fenoldopam (Corlopam)
Hydralazine (Apresoline, others)
Iloprost (Ventavis)
Isosorbide dinitrate (Isordil, Sorbitrate, Dilatrate-SR)

Isosorbide mononitrate (Ismo, Imdur)
Minoxidil, oral
Nitroglycerin (Nitrostat, Nitrolingual, Nitro-Bid Ointment, Nitro-Bid IV, Nitrodisc, Transderm-Nitro, NitroMist, others)

Nitroprusside (Nipride, Nitropress)
Tolazoline (Priscoline)
Treprostinil sodium (Remodulin, Tyvaso)

Miscellaneous Cardiovascular Agents

Aliskiren (Tekturna)
Aliskiren/
  hydrochlorothiazide
  (Tekturna HCT)

Ambrisentan (Letairis)
Conivaptan (Vaprisol)
Dabigatran (Pradaxa)
Prasugrel (Effient)

Ranolazine (Ranexa)
Sildenafil (Viagra,
  Revatio)

CENTRAL NERVOUS SYSTEM (CNS) AGENTS

Alzheimer Agents

Donepezil (Aricept)
Galantamine (Razadyne,
  Razadyne ER)

Memantine (Namenda,
  Namenda XR)
Rivastigmine (Exelon)

Rivastigmine transdermal
  (Exelon Patch)
Tacrine (Cognex)

Antianxiety Agents

Alprazolam (Xanax,
  Niravam)
Buspirone (BuSpar)
Chlordiazepoxide
  (Librium, Mitran,
  Libritabs)

Diazepam (Diastat,
  Valium)
Doxepin (Sinequan,
  Adapin)
Hydroxyzine (Atarax,
  Vistaril)

Lorazepam (Ativan,
  others)
Meprobamate (various)
Oxazepam

Anticonvulsants

Carbamazepine (Tegretol
  XR, Carbatrol, Epitol,
  Equetro)
Clonazepam (Klonopin)
Diazepam (Diastat,
  Valium)
Ethosuximide (Zarontin)
Fosphenytoin (Cerebyx)
Gabapentin (Neurontin)
Lacosamide (Vimpat)
Lamotrigine (Lamictal)

Lamotrigine, extended-
  release (Lamictal XR)
Levetiracetam (Keppra)
Lorazepam (Ativan,
  others)
Magnesium sulfate
  (various)
Oxcarbazepine
  (Trileptal)
Pentobarbital (Nembutal,
  others)

Phenobarbital
Phenytoin (Dilantin)
Rufinamide (Banzel)
Tiagabine (Gabitril)
Topiramate (Topamax)
Valproic acid (Depakene,
  Depakote)
Vigabatrin (Sabril)
Zonisamide (Zonegran)

Antidepressants

SELECTIVE SEROTONIN REUPTAKE INHIBITORS (SSRIS)

Citalopram (Celexa)
Escitalopram (Lexapro)

Fluoxetine (Prozac,
  Sarafem)
Fluvoxamine (Luvox)

Paroxetine (Paxil, Paxil
  CR, Pexeva)
Sertraline (Zoloft)

SEROTONIN-NOREPINEPHRINE REUPTAKE INHIBITORS (SNRIS)

Desvenlafaxine (Pristiq)   Venlafaxine (Effexor,
Duloxetine (Cymbalta)   Effexor XR)

TRICYCLIC ANTIDEPRESSANTS (TCAS)

Amitriptyline (Elavil)   Doxepin (Adapin)   Nortriptyline (Pamelor)
Desipramine (Norpramin)   Imipramine (Tofranil)

MONOAMINE OXIDASE INHIBITORS (MAOIS)

Phenelzine (Nardil)   Selegiline transdermal   Tranylcypromine
                               (Emsam)   (Parnate)

MISCELLANEOUS ANTIDEPRESSANTS

Bupropion hydrobromide   SR, Wellbutrin XL,   Nefazodone (Serzone)
   (Aplenzin)   Zyban)   Trazodone (Desyrel,
Bupropion hydrochloride   Milnacipran (Savella)   Oleptro)
   (Wellbutrin, Wellbutrin Mirtazapine (Remeron,   Vilazodone (Viibryd)
                               Remeron SolTab)

Antiparkinson Agents

Amantadine (Symmetrel)   Entacapone (Comtan)   Ropinirole (Requip,
Apomorphine (Apokyn)   Pramipexole (Mirapex,   Requip XL)
Benztropine (Cogentin)   Mirapex ER)   Selegiline (Eldepryl,
Bromocriptine (Parlodel)   Rasagiline (Azilect)   Zelapar)
Carbidopa/levodopa   Rivastigmine transdermal Tolcapone (Tasmar)
   (Parcopa, Sinemet)   (Exelon Patch)   Trihexyphenidyl

Antipsychotics

Aripiprazole (Abilify,   Lithium carbonate   Olanzapine, LA
   Abilify Discmelt)   (Eskalith, Lithobid,   parenteral (Zyprexa
Asenapine (Saphris)   others)   Relprevv)
Chlorpromazine   Lurasidone   Paliperidone (Invega,
   (Thorazine)   (Latuda)   Invega Sustenna)
Clozapine (Clozaril,   Molindone   Perphenazine (Trilafon)
   FazaClo)   (Moban)   Pimozide (Orap)
Haloperidol(Haldol)   Olanzapine (Zyprexa,   Prochlorperazine
Iloperidone (Fanapt)   Zyprexa Zydis)   (Compazine)

Quetiapine (Seroquel, Seroquel XR)
Risperidone, oral (Risperdal, Risperdal Consta, Risperdal M-Tab)

Risperidone, parenteral (Risperdal Consta)
Thioridazine (Mellaril)
Thiothixene (Navane)
Trifluoperazine (Stelazine)

Ziprasidone (Geodon)

Sedative Hypnotics

Chloral hydrate (Aquachloral Supprettes)
Dexmedetomidine (Precedex)
Diphenhydramine (Benadryl [OTC])
Doxepin (Silenor)
Estazolam (ProSom)
Eszopiclone (Lunesta)

Etomidate (Amidate)
Flurazepam (Dalmane)
Hydroxyzine (Atarax, Vistaril)
Midazolam (various)
Pentobarbital (Nembutal, others)
Phenobarbital
Propofol (Diprivan)
Ramelteon (Rozerem)

Secobarbital (Seconal)
Temazepam (Restoril)
Thiopental sodium (Pentothal)
Triazolam (Halcion)
Zaleplon (Sonata)
Zolpidem (Ambien IR, Ambien CR, Edluar, ZolpiMist)

Stimulants

Armodafinil (Nuvigil)
Atomoxetine (Strattera)
Dexmethylphenidate (Focalin, Focalin XR)
Dextroamphetamine (Dexedrine)

Guanfacine (Intuniv)
Lisdexamfetamine (Vyvanse)
Methylphenidate, oral (Concerta, Metadate CD, Methylin, Ritalin,

Ritalin LA, Ritalin SR, others)
Methylphenidate, transdermal (Daytrana)
Modafinil (Provigil)

Miscellaneous CNS Agents

Clomipramine (Anafranil)
Clonidine, oral, extended-release (Kapvay)
Dalfampridine (Ampyra)
Fingolimod (Gilenya)

Interferon beta-1a (Rebif)
Meclizine (Antivert) (Bonine, Dramamine OTC)
Natalizumab (Tysabri)
Nimodipine (Nimotop)

Rizatriptan (Maxalt, Maxalt-MLT)
Sodium oxybate (Xyrem)
Tetrabenazine (Xenazine)

DERMATOLOGIC AGENTS

Acitretin (Soriatane)

Acyclovir (Zovirax)

Adapalene (Differin)

Adapalene/benzoyl peroxide (Epiduo Gel)

Alefacept (Amevive)

Anthralin (Anthra-Derm)

Amphotericin B (Amphocin, Fungizone)

Bacitracin, topical (Baciguent)

Bacitracin/polymyxin B, topical (Polysporin)

Bacitracin/neomycin/ polymyxin B, topical (Neosporin ointment)

Bacitracin/neomycin/ polymyxin B/ hydrocortisone, topical (Cortisporin)

Bacitracin/neomycin/ polymyxin B/lidocaine, topical (Clomycin)

Botulinum Toxin Type A [abobotulinumtoxinA)] (Dysport)

Botulinum Toxin Type A [onabotulinumtoxinA] (Botox, Botox Cosmetic)

Calcipotriene (Dovonex)

Calcitriol ointment (Vectical)

Capsaicin (Capsin, Zostrix, others)

Ciclopirox (Loprox, Penlac)

Ciprofloxacin (Cipro, Cipro XR, Proquin XR)

Clindamycin (Cleocin, Cleocin T, others)

Clindamycin/tretinoin (Veltin Gel)

Clotrimazole/ betamethasone (Lotrisone)

Dapsone, topical (Aczone)

Dibucaine (Nupercainal)

Diclofenac, topical (Solaraze)

Doxepin, topical (Zonalon, Prudoxin)

Econazole (Spectazole)

Erythromycin, topical (A/T/S, Eryderm, Erycette, T-Stat)

Erythromycin/benzoyl peroxide (Benzamycin)

Finasteride (Propecia)

Fluorouracil, topical [5-FU] (Efudex)

Gentamicin, topical (Garamycin, G-Mycitin)

Imiquimod 5% cream (Aldara)

Isotretinoin [13-*cis*-retinoic acid] (Accutane, Amnesteem, Claravis, Sotret)

Ketoconazole (Nizoral)

Kunecatechins [sinecatechins] (Veregen)

Lactic acid/ammonium hydroxide [ammonium lactate] (Lac-Hydrin)

Lindane (Kwell, others)

Metronidazole (Flagyl, MetroGel)

Miconazole (Monistat 1 Combination Pack, Monistat 3, Monistat 7) [OTC], (Monistat-Derm)

Miconazole/zinc oxide/ petrolatum (Vusion)

Minocycline (Dynacin, Minocin, Solodyn)

Minoxidil, topical (Theroxidil, Rogaine) [OTC]

Mupirocin (Bactroban, Bactroban Nasal)

Naftifine (Naftin)

Nystatin (Mycostatin)

Oxiconazole (Oxistat)

Penciclovir (Denavir)

Permethrin (Nix, Elimite)

Pimecrolimus (Elidel)

Podophyllin (Podocon-25, Condylox Gel 0.5%, Condylox)

Pramoxine (Anusol Ointment, ProctoFoam NS)

Pramoxine/ hydrocortisone (Enzone, Proctofoam-HC)

Selenium sulfide (Exsel Shampoo, Selsun Blue shampoo, Selsun shampoo)

Silver sulfadiazine (Silvadene, others)
Steroids, topical (See Table 3, page 284)
Tacrolimus [FK506] (Prograf, Protopic)

Tazarotene (Tazorac, Avage)
Terbinafine (Lamisil, Lamisil AT [OTC])
Tolnaftate (Tinactin, others [OTC])

Tretinoin, topical [retinoic acid] (Avita, Retin-A, Retin-A Micro, Renova)
Ustekinumab (Stelara)
Vorinostat (Zolinza)

DIETARY SUPPLEMENTS

Calcium acetate (Calphron, Phos-Ex, PhosLo)
Calcium glubionate (Neo-Calglucon)
Calcium salts [chloride, gluconate, gluceptate]
Cholecalciferol [vitamin D_3] (Delta-D)
Cyanocobalamin [vitamin B_{12}] (Nascobal)
Ferric gluconate complex (Ferrlecit)

Ferrous gluconate (Fergon [OTC], others)
Ferrous sulfate
Ferumoxytol (Feraheme)
Fish oil (Lovaza, others [OTC])
Folic acid
Iron dextran (Dexferrum, INFeD)
Iron sucrose (Venofer)
Magnesium oxide (Mag-Ox 400, others [OTC])
Magnesium sulfate (various)

Multivitamins, oral [OTC] (See Table 12, page 304)
Phytonadione [vitamin K] (AquaMEPHYTON, others)
Potassium supplements (See Table 6, page 296)
Pyridoxine [vitamin B_6]
Sodium bicarbonate [$NaHCO_3$]
Thiamine [vitamin B_1]

EAR (OTIC) AGENTS

Acetic acid/aluminum acetate, otic (Domeboro Otic)
Benzocaine/antipyrine (Auralgan)
Ciprofloxacin, otic (Cetraxal)
Ciprofloxacin/ dexamethasone, otic (Ciprodex)
Ciprofloxacin/ hydrocortisone, otic (Cipro HC Otic)

Neomycin/colistin/ hydrocortisone (Cortisporin-TC Otic Drops)
Neomycin/colistin/ hydrocortisone/ thonzonium (Cortisporin-TC Otic Suspension)
Ofloxacin otic (Floxin Otic, Floxin Otic Singles)

Polymyxin B/ hydrocortisone (Otobiotic Otic)
Sulfacetamide/ prednisolone (Blephamide, others)
Triethanolamine (Cerumenex [OTC])

ENDOCRINE SYSTEM AGENTS

Antidiabetic Agents

Acarbose (Precose)
Bromocriptine mesylate
  (Cycloset)
Chlorpropamide
  (Diabinese)
Exenatide (Byetta)
Glimepiride
  (Amaryl)
Glimepiride/pioglitazone
  (Duetact)
Glipizide (Glucotrol,
  Glucotrol XL)

Glyburide (DiaBeta,
  Micronase, Glynase)
Glyburide/metformin
  (Glucovance)
Insulins, injectable (*See*
  Table 4, page 287)
Liraglutide recombinant
  (Victoza)
Metformin (Glucophage,
  Glucophage XR)
Miglitol (Glyset)
Nateglinide (Starlix)

Pioglitazone (Actos)
Pioglitazone/metformin
  (ACTO*plus* met)
Repaglinide (Prandin)
Repaglinide/metformin
  (PrandiMet)
Rosiglitazone (Avandia)
Sitagliptin/metformin
  (Janumet)
Tolazamide (Tolinase)
Tolbutamide (Orinase)

DIPEPTIDYL PEPTIDASE-4 (DPP-4) INHIBITORS

Linagliptin (Tradjenta)
Saxagliptin (Onglyza)

Saxagliptin/metformin
  (Kombiglyze XR)
Sitagliptin (Januvia)

Sitagliptin/metformin
  (Janumet)

Hormone and Synthetic Substitutes

Calcitonin (Fortical,
  Miacalcin)
Calcitriol (Rocaltrol,
  Calcijex)
Cortisone, systemic and
  topical (*See* Table 2,
  page 283, and Table 3,
  page 284)
Desmopressin (DDAVP,
  Stimate)
Dexamethasone,
  systemic and topical
  (Decadron)

Fludrocortisone
  (Florinef)
Fluoxymesterone
  (Halotestin, Androxy)
Glucagon
Hydrocortisone, topical
  and systemic (Cortef,
  Solu-Cortef)
Methylprednisolone
  (Solu-Medrol)
Prednisolone
Prednisone

Testosterone (AndroGel
  1%, AndroGel 1.62%
  Androderm, Axiron,
  Fortesta, Striant,
  Testim, Testopel)
Vasopressin [antidiuretic
  hormone, ADH]
  (Pitressin)

Hypercalcemia/Osteoporosis Agents

Alendronate (Fosamax, Fosamax Plus D)
Denosumab (Prolia, Xgeva)
Etidronate (Didronel)
Gallium nitrate (Ganite)

Ibandronate (Boniva)
Pamidronate (Aredia)
Raloxifene (Evista)
Risedronate (Actonel, Actonel with calcium)

Risedronate, delayed-release (Atelvia)
Teriparatide (Forteo)
Zoledronic acid (Zometa, Reclast)

Obesity

Orlistat (Xenical, Alli [OTC])

Thyroid/Antithyroid

Levothyroxine (Synthroid, Levoxyl, others)
Liothyronine [T$_3$] (Cytomel, Triostat)

Methimazole (Tapazole)
Potassium iodide (Lugol's Solution, Iosat, SSKI, Thyro-Block,

ThyroSafe, ThyroShield) [OTC]
Propylthiouracil [PTU]

Miscellaneous Endocrine Agents

Cinacalcet (Sensipar)
Demeclocycline (Declomycin)

Diazoxide (Proglycem)
Somatropin (Serostim)

Tesamorelin (Egrifta)

EYE (OPHTHALMIC) AGENTS

Glaucoma Agents

Acetazolamide (Diamox)
Apraclonidine (Iopidine)
Betaxolol, ophthalmic (Betoptic)
Brimonidine (Alphagan P)
Brimonidine/timolol (Combigan)

Brinzolamide (Azopt)
Carteolol, ophthalmic (Ocupress)
Dipivefrin (Propine)
Dorzolamide (Trusopt)
Dorzolamide/timolol (Cosopt)

Echothiophate iodide, ophthalmic (Phospholine Iodide)
Latanoprost (Xalatan)
Levobunolol (AK-Beta, Betagan)
Timolol, ophthalmic (Timoptic)

Ophthalmic Antibiotics

Azithromycin, ophthalmic, 1% (AzaSite)

Bacitracin, ophthalmic (AK-Tracin Ophthalmic)

Bacitracin/polymyxin B, ophthalmic (AK-Poly-Bac Ophthalmic, Polysporin Ophthalmic)

Bacitracin/neomycin/polymyxin B (AK-Spore Ophthalmic, Neosporin Ophthalmic)

Bacitracin/neomycin/polymyxin B/hydrocortisone (AK-Spore HC Ophthalmic, Cortisporin Ophthalmic)

Besifloxacin (Besivance)

Ciprofloxacin, ophthalmic (Ciloxan)

Erythromycin, ophthalmic (Ilotycin)

Gentamicin, ophthalmic (Garamycin, Genoptic, Gentacidin, Gentak, others)

Gentamicin/prednisolone, ophthalmic (Pred-G Ophthalmic)

Levofloxacin, ophthalmic (Quixin, Iquix)

Moxifloxacin, ophthalmic (Vigamox)

Neomycin/polymyxin B/hydrocortisone (Cortisporin Ophthalmic, Cortisporin Otic)

Neomycin/dexamethasone (AK-Neo-Dex Ophthalmic, NeoDecadron Ophthalmic)

Neomycin/polymyxin B/dexamethasone, ophthalmic (Maxitrol)

Neomycin/polymyxin B/prednisolone (Poly-Pred Ophthalmic)

Norfloxacin, ophthalmic (Chibroxin)

Ofloxacin, ophthalmic (Ocuflox)

Silver nitrate (Dey-Drop, others)

Sulfacetamide, ophthalmic (Bleph-10, Cetamide, Sodium Sulamyd)

Sulfacetamide/prednisolone, ophthalmic (Blephamide, others)

Tobramycin, ophthalmic (AKTob, Tobrex)

Tobramycin/dexamethasone, ophthalmic (TobraDex)

Trifluridine, ophthalmic (Viroptic)

Miscellaneous Ophthalmic Agents

Alcaftadine, ophthalmic (Lastacaft)

Artificial tears (Tears Naturale [OTC])

Atropine (Isopto Atropine, generic)

Bepotastine besilate (Bepreve)

Cromolyn sodium (Opticrom)

Cyclopentolate (Cyclogyl, Cyclate)

Cyclopentolate/phenylephrine (Cyclomydril)

Cyclosporine (Restasis)

Dexamethasone (AK-Dex Ophthalmic, Decadron Ophthalmic)

Diclofenac (Voltaren)

Emedastine (Emadine)

Epinastine (Elestat)

Ganciclovir, ophthalmic gel (Zirgan)

Ketotifen (Alaway, Zaditor) [OTC]

Ketorolac (Acular, Acular LS, Acular PF)

Levocabastine (Livostin)

Lodoxamide (Alomide)

Naphazoline (Albalon, Naphcon, others)

Naphazoline/
  pheniramine
  (Naphcon-A,
  Visine-A)
Nepafenac
  (Nevanac)

Olopatadine (Patanol,
  Pataday)
Pemirolast (Alamast)
Phenylephrine
  (Neo-Synephrine
  Ophthalmic,

AK-Dilate, Zincfrin
  [OTC]
Ranibizumab (Lucentis)
Rimexolone (Vexol)
Scopolamine, ophthalmic

GASTROINTESTINAL (GI) AGENTS

Antacids

Alginic acid/aluminum
  hydroxide/magnesium
  trisilicate (Gaviscon)
  [OTC]
Aluminum hydroxide
  (Amphojel,
  AlternaGEL,
  Dermagran) [OTC]
Aluminum hydroxide/
  magnesium carbonate
  (Gaviscon Extra
  Strength Liquid) [OTC]

Aluminum hydroxide/
  magnesium hydroxide
  (Maalox, Mylanta
  Ultimate Strength)
Aluminum hydroxide/
  magnesium hydroxide/
  simethicone (Mylanta
  Regular Strength,
  Maalox Advanced)
  [OTC]

Aluminum hydroxide/
  magnesium trisilicate
  (Gaviscon Regular
  Strength) [OTC]
Calcium carbonate
  (Tums, Alka-Mints)
  [OTC]
Magaldrate (Riopan
  Plus) [OTC]
Simethicone (Mylicon,
  others) [OTC]

Antidiarrheals

Bismuth subsalicylate
  (Pepto-Bismol) [OTC]
Diphenoxylate/atropine
  (Lomotil, Lonox)
Lactobacillus (Lactinex
  Granules) [OTC]

Loperamide (Diamode,
  Imodium) [OTC]
Octreotide (Sandostatin,
  Sandostatin LAR)

Paregoric [camphorated
  tincture of opium]
Rifaximin (Xifaxan,
  Xifaxan 550)

Antiemetics

Aprepitant (Emend)
Chlorpromazine
  (Thorazine)
Dimenhydrinate
  (Dramamine, others)
  [OTC]
Dolasetron (Anzemet)
Dronabinol (Marinol)
Droperidol (Inapsine)

Fosaprepitant (Emend,
  Injection)
Granisetron (Kytril)
Meclizine (Antivert,
  Bonine, Dramamine
  [OTC])
Metoclopramide
  (Reglan, Clopra,
  Octamide)

Nabilone (Cesamet)
Ondansetron (Zofran,
  Zofran ODT)
Ondansetron, oral
  soluble film
  (Zuplenz)
Palonosetron (Aloxi)
Prochlorperazine
  (Compazine)

Promethazine (Phenergan)
Scopolamine (Scopace, Transderm Scop)

Thiethylperazine (Torecan)

Trimethobenzamide (Tigan)

Antiulcer Agents

Bismuth subcitrate/ metronidazole/ tetracycline (Pylera)
Cimetidine (Tagamet, Tagamet HB 200 [OTC])
Dexlansoprazole (Dexilant, Kapidex)
Esomeprazole (Nexium)
Famotidine (Pepcid, Pepcid AC [OTC])

Lansoprazole (Prevacid, Prevacid IV)
Nizatidine (Axid, Axid AR [OTC])
Omeprazole (Prilosec, Prilosec [OTC])
Omeprazole/sodium bicarbonate (Zegerid, Zegerid [OTC])

Omeprazole/sodium bicarbonate/ magnesium hydroxide (Zegerid with Magnesium Hydroxide)
Pantoprazole (Protonix)
Rabeprazole (AcipHex)
Ranitidine (Zantac, Zantac [OTC])
Sucralfate (Carafate)

Cathartics/Laxatives

Bisacodyl (Dulcolax [OTC])
Docusate calcium (Surfak)
Docusate potassium (Dialose)
Docusate sodium (DOSS, Colace)
Glycerin suppository
Lactulose (Constulose, Generlac, Chronulac, Cephulac, Enulose, others)

Magnesium citrate (Citroma, others) [OTC]
Magnesium hydroxide (Milk of Magnesia) [OTC]
Mineral oil [OTC]
Mineral oil enema (Fleet Mineral Oil) [OTC]
Polyethylene glycol-electrolyte solution [PEG-ES] (GoLYTELY, CoLyte)

Polyethylene glycol [PEG] 3350 (MiraLAX [OTC])
Psyllium (Metamucil, Serutan, Effer-Syllium)
Sodium phosphate (Visicol)
Sorbitol (generic)

Enzymes

Pancrelipase (Pancrease, Cotazym, Creon, Ultrase)

Miscellaneous GI Agents

Alosetron (Lotronex)
Alvimopan (Entereg)
Budesonide, oral (Entocort EC)
Balsalazide (Colazal)
Certolizumab pegol (Cimzia)
Dexpanthenol (Ilopan-Choline [Oral], Ilopan)
Dibucaine (Nupercainal)
Dicyclomine (Bentyl)
Fidaxomicin (Dificid)
Hydrocortisone, rectal (Anusol-HC Suppository, Cortifoam Rectal, Proctocort, others)
Hyoscyamine (Anaspaz, Cystospaz, Levsin, others)
Hyoscyamine/atropine/scopolamine/

phenobarbital (Donnatal, others)
Infliximab (Remicade)
Lubiprostone (Amitiza)
Mesalamine (Apriso, Asacol, Canasa, Lialda, Pentasa, Rowasa)
Methylnaltrexone bromide (Relistor)
Metoclopramide (Reglan, Clopra, Octamide)
Mineral oil/pramoxine HCl/zinc oxide (Tucks Ointment) [OTC]
Misoprostol (Cytotec)
Neomycin sulfate (Neo-Fradin, generic)
Olsalazine (Dipentum)
Oxandrolone (Oxandrin)

Pramoxine (Anusol Ointment, ProctoFoam NS, others)
Pramoxine/hydrocortisone (Enzone, Proctofoam-HC)
Propantheline (Pro-Banthine)
Starch, topical, rectal (Tucks Suppositories) [OTC]
Sulfasalazine (Azulfidine, Azulfidine EN)
Vasopressin [antidiuretic hormone (ADH)] (Pitressin)
Witch hazel (Tucks Pads, others [OTC])

HEMATOLOGIC AGENTS

Anticoagulants

Antithrombin, recombinant (ATryn)
Argatroban (Acova)
Bivalirudin (Angiomax)
Dalteparin (Fragmin)

Desirudin (Iprivask)
Enoxaparin (Lovenox)
Fondaparinux (Arixtra)
Heparin
Lepirudin (Refludan)

Protamine (generic)
Tinzaparin (Innohep)
Warfarin (Coumadin)

Antiplatelet Agents

Abciximab (ReoPro)
Aspirin (Bayer, Ecotrin, St. Joseph's) [OTC]
Clopidogrel (Plavix)

Dipyridamole (Persantine)
Dipyridamole/aspirin (Aggrenox)
Eptifibatide (Integrilin)

Prasugrel (Effient)
Rivaroxaban (Xarelto)
Ticagrelor (Brilinta)
Ticlopidine (Ticlid)
Tirofiban (Aggrastat)

Antithrombotic Agents

Alteplase, recombinant [tPA] (Activase)
Aminocaproic acid (Amicar)

Anistreplase (Eminase)
Dextran 40 (Gentran 40, Rheomacrodex)
Reteplase (Retavase)

Streptokinase (Streptase, Kabikinase)
Tenecteplase (TNKase)
Urokinase (Abbokinase)

Hematinic Agents

Darbepoetin alfa (Aranesp)
Eltrombopag (Promacta)
Epoetin alfa [erythropoietin (EPO)] (Epogen, Procrit)

Filgrastim [G-CSF] (Neupogen)
Iron dextran (Dexferrum, INFeD)
Iron sucrose (Venofer)
Oprelvekin (Neumega)

Pegfilgrastim (Neulasta)
Plerixafor (Mozobil)
Romiplostim (Nplate)
Sargramostim [GM-CSF] (Leukine)

Volume Expanders

Albumin (Albuminar, Albutein, Buminate)
Dextran 40 (Gentran 40, Rheomacrodex)

Hetastarch (Hespan)
Plasma protein fraction (Plasmanate, others)

Miscellaneous Hematologic Agents

Antihemophilic factor VIII (Monoclate-P)
Antihemophilic factor [recombinant] (Xyntha)

Decitabine (Dacogen)
Desmopressin (DDAVP, Stimate)
Fibrinogen concentrate [human] (RiaSTAP)

Lenalidomide (Revlimid)
Pentoxifylline (Trental)

IMMUNE SYSTEM AGENTS

Immunomodulators

Interferon alfa-2b (Intron A)
Interferon alfacon-1 (Infergen)
Interferon beta-1a (Rebif)

Interferon beta-1b (Betaseron, Extavia)
Interferon gamma-1b (Actimmune)
Natalizumab (Tysabri)

Peginterferon alfa-2b [pegylated interferon] (PegIntron)
Peginterferon alfa-2a [pegylated interferon] (Pegasys)

Immunomodulators: Disease-Modifying Antirheumatic Drugs (DMARDs)

Abatacept (Orencia)
Adalimumab (Humira)
Anakinra (Kineret)

Certolizumab pegol
(Cimzia)
Etanercept (Enbrel)

Golimumab (Simponi)
Infliximab (Remicade)
Tocilizumab (Actemra)

Immunosuppressive Agents

Azathioprine (Imuran)
Basiliximab
(Simulect)
Belatacept (Nulojix)
Cyclosporine
(Sandimmune,
Gengraf, Neoral)
Daclizumab (Zenapax)
Everolimus (Zortress)

Lymphocyte immune
globulin
[antithymocyte
globulin (ATG)]
(Atgam)
Muromonab-CD3
(Orthoclone OKT3)
Mycophenolic acid
(Myfortic)

Mycophenolate mofetil
(CellCept)
Sirolimus [rapamycin]
(Rapamune)
Steroids, systemic (*See*
Table 2, page 283)
Tacrolimus [FK506]
(Prograf, Protopic)

MUSCULOSKELETAL AGENTS

Antigout Agents

Allopurinol (Zyloprim,
Lopurin, Aloprim)
Colchicine

Febuxostat (Uloric)
Pegloticase
(Krystexxa)

Probenecid (Benemid,
others)
Sulfinpyrazone

Muscle Relaxants

Baclofen (Lioresal
Intrathecal, generic)
Carisoprodol (Soma)
Chlorzoxazone (Paraflex,
Parafon Forte DSC,
others)

Cyclobenzaprine
(Flexeril)
Cyclobenzaprine,
extended-release
(Amrix)
Dantrolene (Dantrium)

Diazepam (Diastat,
Valium)
Metaxalone (Skelaxin)
Methocarbamol
(Robaxin)
Orphenadrine (Norflex)

Neuromuscular Blockers

Atracurium (Tracrium)
Botulinum toxin type A
[incobotulinumtoxinA]
(Xeomin)
Botulinum toxin type A
[onabotulinumtoxinA]

(Botox, Botox
Cosmetic)
Botulinum toxin type B
[rimabotulinumtoxinB]
(Myobloc)
Pancuronium (Pavulon)

Rocuronium (Zemuron)
Succinylcholine
(Anectine, Quelicin,
Sucostrin, others)
Vecuronium (Norcuron)

Miscellaneous Musculoskeletal Agents

Edrophonium (Tensilon, Reversol)
Leflunomide (Arava)
Methotrexate (Rheumatrex Dose Pack, Trexall)
Sulfasalazine (Azulfidine, Azulfidine EN)
Tizanidine (Zanaflex)

OB/GYN AGENTS

Contraceptives

Copper intrauterine device (IUD) (ParaGard T 380A)
Estradiol cypionate/ medroxyprogesterone acetate (Lunelle)
Ethinyl estradiol/ norelgestromin (Ortho Evra)
Etonogestrel, implant (Implanon)
Etonogestrel/ethinyl estradiol, vaginal insert (NuvaRing)
Levonorgestrel intrauterine device (IUD) (Mirena)
Medroxyprogesterone (Provera, Depo-Provera, Depo-Sub Q Provera)
Oral contraceptives (See page XXX, and Table 5, page XXX)

Emergency Contraceptives

Levonorgestrel (Plan B One-Step, Next Choice)
Ulipristal acetate (Ella)

Estrogen Supplementation

ESTROGEN ONLY

Estradiol, oral (Delestrogen, Estrace, Femtrace, others)
Estradiol, gel (Divigel, Elestrin)
Estradiol, spray (Evamist)
Estradiol, transdermal (Estraderm, Climara, Vivelle-Dot)
Estradiol, vaginal (Estring, Femring, Vagifem)
Estrogen, conjugated (Premarin)
Estrogen, conjugated-synthetic (Cenestin, Enjuvia)
Esterified estrogens (Estratab, Menest)
Ethinyl estradiol (Estinyl, Feminone)

COMBINATION ESTROGEN/PROGESTIN

Esterified estrogens/
methyltestosterone
(Estratest, Estratest
HS, Syntest DS,
Syntest HS)
Estrogen, conjugated/
medroxyprogesterone
(Prempro,
Premphase)

Estrogen, conjugated/
methyl progesterone
(Premarin with methyl
progesterone)
Estrogen, conjugated/
methyltestosterone
(Premarin with
methyltestosterone)

Estradiol/levonorgestrel,
transdermal (Climara
Pro)
Estradiol/
medroxyprogesterone
(Lunelle)
Ethinyl estradiol/
norethindrone
(FemHRT, Activela)

Vaginal Preparations

Amino-Cerv pH 5.5
Cream
Miconazole (Monistat 1
combination pack,

Monistat 3,
Monistat 7) [OTC],
(Monistat-Derm)

Nystatin (Mycostatin)
Terconazole (Terazol 7)
Tioconazole (Vagistat)

Miscellaneous OB/GYN Agents

Clomiphene (Clomid)
Dinoprostone (Cervidil
Vaginal Insert,
Prepidil Gel,
Prostin E2)
Gonadorelin (Factrel)
Leuprolide (Lupron)
Lutropin alfa
(Luveris)

Tranexamic acid
(Lysteda)
Magnesium sulfate
(various)
Medroxyprogesterone
(Provera,
Depo-Provera,
Depo-Sub
Q Provera)

Methylergonovine
(Methergine)
Mifepristone [RU 486]
(Mifeprex)
Oxytocin (Pitocin)
Terbutaline (Brethine,
Bricanyl)
Tranexamic acid
(Lysteda)

PAIN MEDICATIONS

Local/Topical
(*See also* Local Anesthetics Table 1, page 282)

Benzocaine (Americaine,
Lanacaine, Hurricane,
various [OTC])
Benzocaine/antipyrine
(Auralgan)
Bupivacaine (Marcaine)
Capsaicin (Capsin,
Zostrix, others) [OTC]

Cocaine
Dibucaine (Nupercainal)
Lidocaine, lidocaine/
epinephrine
(Anestacon Topical,
Xylocaine, Xylocaine
Viscous, Xylocaine
MPF, others)

Lidocaine, powder
intradermal
injection system
(Zingo)
Lidocaine/prilocaine
(EMLA, LMX)
Mepivacaine
(Carbocaine)

Procaine
(Novocaine)

Pramoxine (Anusol
Ointment, ProctoFoam
NSothers)

Migraine Headache

Acetaminophen/
butalbital, with and
without caffeine
(Fioricet, Medigesic,
Repan, Sedapap-10,
Two-Dyne, Triaprin,
Axocet, Phrenilin
Forte)
Almotriptan (Axert)

Aspirin/butalbital
compound (Fiorinal)
Aspirin/butalbital/
caffeine/codeine
(Fiorinal with
Codeine)
Eletriptan (Relpax)
Frovatriptan (Frova)
Naratriptan (Amerge)

Sumatriptan (Alsuma,
Imitrex Injection,
Imitrex Nasal Spray,
Imitrex Oral)
Sumatriptan/naproxen
sodium (Treximet)
Sumatriptan needleless
system (Sumavel
DosePro)
Zolmitriptan (Zomig)

Narcotic Analgesics

Acetaminophen/codeine
(Tylenol 2, 3, 4)
Alfentanil (Alfenta)
Aspirin/codeine
(Empirin 2, 3, 4)
Buprenorphine
(Buprenex)
Buprenorphine/naloxone
(Suboxone)
Buprenorphine,
transdermal (Butrans)
Butorphanol (Stadol)
Codeine
Fentanyl (Sublimaze)
Fentanyl, iontophoretic
transdermal system
(Ionsys)
Fentanyl, transdermal
(Duragesic)
Fentanyl, transmucosal
(Abstral, Actiq,
Fentora, Onsolis)
Hydrocodone/
acetaminophen

(Lorcet, Vicodin,
Hycet, others)
Hydrocodone/aspirin
(Lortab ASA,
others)
Hydrocodone/ibuprofen
(Vicoprofen)
Hydromorphone
(Dilaudid,
Dilaudid-HP)
Hydromorphone,
extended-release
(Exalgo)
Levorphanol
(Levo-Dromoran)
Meperidine (Demerol,
Meperitab)
Methadone (Dolophine,
Methadose)
Morphine (Avinza XR,
Astramorph/PF,
Duramorph,
Infumorph, MS
Contin, Kadian SR,

Oramorph SR,
Roxanol)
Morphine/naltrexone
(Embeda)
Morphine, liposomal
(DepoDur)
Nalbuphine
(Nubain)
Oxycodone [Dihydro
hydroxycodeinone]
(OxyContin,
Roxicodone)
Oxycodone/
acetaminophen
(Percocet, Tylox)
Oxycodone/aspirin
(Percodan)
Oxycodone/ibuprofen
(Combunox)
Oxymorphone (Opana,
Opana ER)
Pentazocine (Talwin,
Talwin Compound,
Talwin NX)

Nonnarcotic Analgesics

Acetaminophen [N-acetyl-p-aminophenol (APAP)] (Acephen, Tylenol, other generic)

Acetaminophen/ butalbital/± caffeine

(Fioricet, Medigesic, Repan, Sedapap-10, Two-Dyne, Triapin, Axocet, Phrenilin Forte)

Aspirin (Bayer, Ecotrin, St. Joseph's) [OTC]

Tramadol (Ultram, Ultram ER)

Tramadol/acetaminophen (Ultracet)

Nonsteroidal Anti-inflammatory Agents (NSAIDs)

Celecoxib (Celebrex)

Diclofenac/misoprostol (Arthrotec)

Diclofenac, oral (Cataflam, Voltaren, Voltaren-XR)

Diclofenac, topical (Flector Patch, Pennsaid, Voltaren gel)

Diflunisal (Dolobid)

Etodolac

Fenoprofen (Nalfon)

Flurbiprofen (Ansaid, Ocufen)

Ibuprofen, oral (Motrin, Rufen, Advil)

Ibuprofen, parenteral (Caldolor)

Indomethacin (Indocin)

Ketoprofen (Orudis, Oruvail)

Ketorolac (Toradol)

Ketorolac, nasal (Sprix)

Meloxicam (Mobic)

Nabumetone (Relafen)

Naproxen (Aleve [OTC], Anaprox, Naprosyn)

Naproxen/esomeprazole (Vimovo)

Oxaprozin (Daypro, Daypro ALTA)

Piroxicam (Feldene)

Sulindac (Clinoril)

Tolmetin (Tolectin)

Miscellaneous Pain Medications

Amitriptyline (Elavil)

Imipramine (Tofranil)

Pregabalin (Lyrica)

Tapentadol (Nucynta)

Tramadol (Ultram, Ultram ER)

Ziconotide (Prialt)

RESPIRATORY AGENTS

Antitussives, Decongestants, and Expectorants

Acetylcysteine (Acetadote, Mucomyst)

Benzonatate (Tessalon Perles)

Codeine

Dextromethorphan (Benylin DM, Delsym, Mediquell, PediaCare 1, others) [OTC]

Guaifenesin (Robitussin, others)

Guaifenesin/codeine (Robitussin AC, Brontex, others)

Guaifenesin/
dextromethorphan
(many OTC bands)
Hydrocodone/
guaifenesin
(Hycotuss
Expectorant)
Hydrocodone/
homatropine

(Hycodan, Hydromet,
others)
Hydrocodone/
pseudoephedrine
(Detussin, Histussin
D, others)
Hydrocodone/
chlorpheniramine/
phenylephrine/

acetaminophen/
caffeine (Hycomine
compound)
Potassium iodide
(Lugol's Solution,
SSKI)
Pseudoephedrine
(Sudafed, Novafed,
Afrinol, others) [OTC]

Bronchodilators

Albuterol (Proventil,
Ventolin, Volmax)
Albuterol/ipratropium
(Combivent, DuoNeb)
Aminophylline
Arformoterol (Brovana)
Ephedrine
Epinephrine (Adrenalin,
Sus-Phrine, EpiPen,
EpiPen Jr, others)

Formoterol fumarate
(Foradil, Performist)
Indacaterol (Arcapta
Neohaler)
Isoproterenol (Isuprel)
Levalbuterol (Xopenex,
Xopenex HFA)
Metaproterenol
(Alupent, Metaprel)
Pirbuterol (Maxair)

Salmeterol (Serevent,
Serevent Diskus)
Terbutaline (Brethine,
Bricanyl)
Theophylline (Theo24,
Theochron)

Respiratory Inhalants

Acetylcysteine
(Acetadote, Mucomyst)
Beclomethasone
(QVAR)
Beclomethasone, nasal
(Beconase AQ)
Beractant (Survanta)
Budesonide (Rhinocort
Aqua, Pulmicort)
Budesonide/formoterol
(Symbicort)
Calfactant (Infasurf)
Ciclesonide, inhaled
(Alvesco)
Ciclesonide, nasal
(Omnaris)
Cromolyn sodium (Intal,
NasalCrom, Opticrom,
others)

Dexamethasone, nasal
(Dexacort Phosphate
Turbinaire)
Flunisolide (AeroBid,
Aerospan, Nasarel)
Fluticasone furoate,
nasal (Veramyst)
Fluticasone propionate,
nasal (Flonase)
Fluticasone propionate,
inhaled (Flovent HFA,
Flovent Diskus)
Fluticasone propionate/
salmeterol xinafoate
(Advair Diskus,
Advair HFA)
Formoterol fumarate
(Foradil Aerolizer,
Perforomist)

Ipratropium (Atrovent
HFA, Atrovent Nasal)
Mometasone/formoterol
(Dulera)
Mometasone, inhaled
(Asmanex Twisthaler)
Mometasone, nasal
(Nasonex)
Olopatadine, nasal
(Patanase)
Phenylepherine, nasal
(Neo-Synephrine
Nasal [OTC])
Tiotropium (Spiriva)
Triamcinolone
(Azmacort)

Miscellaneous Respiratory Agents

Alpha$_1$-protease inhibitor (Prolastin)
Aztreonam, inhaled
Dornase alfa (Pulmozyme, DNase)

Montelukast (Singulair)
Omalizumab (Xolair)
Tadalafil (Adcirca)
Zafirlukast (Accolate)

Zileuton (Zyflo, Zyflo CR)

UROGENITAL SYSTEM AGENTS

Erectile Dysfunction

Alprostadil, intracavernosal (Caverject, Edex)
Alprostadil, urethral suppository (Muse)

Sildenafil (Viagra, Revatio)
Tadalafil (Cialis)
Vardenafil (Levitra, Stayxn)

Yohimbine (Yocon, Yohimex)

Bladder Agents

Belladonna/opium, suppositories (B & O Supprettes)
Bethanechol (Duvoid, Urecholine, others)
Botulinum Toxin Type A [onabotulinumtoxin A] (Botox)
Butabarbital/ hyoscyamine/ phenazopyridine (Pyridium Plus)
Darifenacin (Enablex)
Fesoterodine fumarate (Toviaz)

Flavoxate (Urispas)
Hyoscyamine (Anaspaz, Cystospaz, Levsin)
Hyoscyamine/atropine/ scopolamine/ phenobarbital (Donnatal, others)
Methenamine hippurate (Hiprex)
Methenamine mandelate (Uroquid-Acid No. 2)
Oxybutynin (Ditropan, Ditropan XL)
Oxybutynin transdermal system (Oxytrol)

Oxybutynin, topical (Gelnique)
Phenazopyridine (Pyridium, Azo-Standard, Urogesic, many others)
Solifenacin (VESIcare)
Tolterodine (Detrol, Detrol LA)
Trospium chloride (Sanctura, Sanctura XR)

Urolithiasis

Potassium citrate (Urocit-K)
Potassium citrate/citric acid (Polycitra-K)

Sodium citrate/citric acid (Bicitra, Oracit)

Trimethoprim (Trimpex, Proloprim)

Benign Prostatic Hyperplasia

Alfuzosin (Uroxatral)

Doxazosin (Cardura, Cardura XL)

Dutasteride (Avodart)

Dutasteride/tamsulosin (Jalyn)

Finasteride (Proscar, generic)

Silodosin (Rapaflo)

Tamsulosin (Flomax, generic)

Terazosin (Hytrin)

Miscellaneous Urology Agents

Ammonium aluminum sulfate (Alum [OTC])

Methenamine, phenyl salicylate, methylene blue, benzoic acid, hyoscyamine (Prosed)

Dimethyl sulfoxide [DMSO] (Rimso-50)

Neomycin/polymyxin bladder irrigant [Neosporin GU Irrigant]

Nitrofurantoin (Furadantin, Macrodantin, Macrobid)

Pentosan polysulfate sodium (Elmiron)

VACCINES/SERUMS/TOXOIDS

Cytomegalovirus immune globulin [CMV-IG IV] (CytoGam)

Diphtheria/tetanus toxoids [Td] (Decavac, for >7y)

Diphtheria/tetanus toxoids [DT] (generic only, for <7y)

Diphtheria/tetanus toxoids/acellular pertussis, adsorbed [DTaP; for <7y] (Daptacel, Infanrix, Tripedia)

Diphtheria/tetanus toxoids/acellular pertussis, adsorbed [Tdap; for >10-11y] (Boosters: Adacel, Boostrix)

Diphtheria/tetanus toxoids/acellular pertussis adsorbed/

inactivated poliovirus vaccine [IPV]/ Haemophilus B conjugate vaccine combined (Pentacel)

Diphtheria/tetanus toxoids/acellular pertussis, adsorbed, hepatitis B [recombinant], and inactivated poliovirus vaccine [IPV] combined (Pediarix)

Haemophilus B conjugate vaccine (ActHIB, HibTITER, PedvaxHIB, Prohibit, TriHIBit, others)

Hepatitis A [inactivated] and hepatitis B [recombinant] vaccine (Twinrix)

Hepatitis A vaccine (Havrix, Vaqta)

Hepatitis B immune globulin (HyperHep B, HepaGam B, Nabi-HB, H-BIG)

Hepatitis B vaccine (Engerix-B, Recombivax HB)

Human papillomavirus recombinant vaccine (Cervarix [Types 16, 18], Gardasil [Types 6, 11, 16, 18])

Immune globulin, IV (Gamimune N, Gammaplex, Gammar IV, Sandoglobulin, others)

Immune globulin, subcutaneous (Hizentra)

Influenza vaccine, inactivated, trivalent [TIV] for 2011-2012 season (Afluria, Fluarix, FluLaval, Fluvirin, Fluzone, Fluzone High Dose, Fluzone Intradermal)

Influenza virus vaccine, live, intranasal [LAIV] (FluMist)

Measles/mumps/rubella vaccine, live [MMR] (M-M-R II)

Measles/mumps/rubella/ varicella virus vaccine, live [MMRV] (ProQuad)

Meningococcal conjugate vaccine [quadrivalent, MCV4] (Menactra, Menveo)

Meningococcal polysaccharide vaccine [MPSV4] (Menomune A/C/Y/ W-135)

Pneumococcal 13-valent conjugate vaccine (Prevnar 13)

Pneumococcal vaccine, polyvalent (Pneumovax-23)

Rotavirus vaccine, live, oral, monovalent (Rotarix)

Rotavirus vaccine, live, oral, pentavalent (RotaTeq)

Smallpox vaccine (Dryvax)

Tetanus immune globulin

Tetanus toxoid (TT)

Varicella immune globulin (VarZIG)

Varicella virus vaccine (Varivax)

Zoster vaccine, live (Zostavax)

WOUND CARE

Becaplermin (Regranex Gel)

Silver nitrate (Dey-Drop, others)

MISCELLANEOUS THERAPEUTIC AGENTS

Acamprosate (Campral)

Alglucosidase alfa (Myozyme)

C1 esterase inhibitor [human] (Berinert, Cinryze)

Cilostazol (Pletal)

Dextrose 50%/25%

Drotrecogin alfa (Xigris)

Ecallantide (Kalbitor)

Eculizumab (Soliris)

Lanthanum carbonate (Fosrenol)

Megestrol acetate (Megace, Megace-ES)

Mecasermin (Increlex, Iplex)

Methylene blue (Urolene Blue, various)

Naltrexone (Depade, ReVia, Vivitrol)

Nicotine, gum (Nicorette, others)

Nicotine, nasal spray (Nicotrol NS)

Nicotine, transdermal (Habitrol, NicoDerm CQ [OTC], others)

Palifermin (Kepivance)

Potassium iodide (Lugol's Solution, SSKI, Thyro-Block, ThyroSafe, ThyroShield) [OTC]

Sevelamer hydrochloride (Renagel)

Sevelamer carbonate (Renvela)

Sodium polystyrene sulfonate (Kayexalate)

Talc (Sterile Talc Powder)

Varenicline (Chantix)

NATURAL AND HERBAL AGENTS

Black cohosh

Chamomile

Cranberry (*Vaccinium macrocarpon*)

Dong quai (*Angelica polymorpha, sinensis*)

Echinacea (*Echinacea purpurea*)

Ephedra/ma huang

Evening primrose oil

Feverfew (*Tanacetum parthenium*)

Fish oil supplements (omega-3 polyunsaturated fatty acid)

Garlic (*Allium sativum*)

Ginger (*Zingiber officinale*)

Ginkgo biloba

Ginseng

Glucosamine sulfate (chitosamine) and chondroitin sulfate

Kava kava (kava kava root extract, *Piper methysticum*)

Melatonin

Milk thistle (*Silybum marianum*)

Red yeast rice

Resveratrol

Saw palmetto (*Serenoa repens*)

St John's wort (*Hypericum perforatum*)

Valerian (*Valeriana officinalis*)

Yohimbine (*Pausinystalia yohimbe*) (Yocon, Yohimex)

GENERIC AND SELECTED BRAND DRUG DATA

Abacavir (Ziagen) **BOX:** Allergy (fever, rash, fatigue, GI, resp) reported; stop drug immediately & do not rechallenge; lactic acidosis & hepatomegaly/steatosis reported **Uses:** *HIV Infxn in combo w/ other antiretrovirals* **Acts:** NRTI **Dose:** *Adults.* 300 mg PO bid or 600 mg PO daily *Peds.* 8 mg/kg bid/300 mg bid max **W/P:** [C, −] CDC rec: HIV-infected mothers not breast-feed (transmission risk) **Disp:** Tabs 300 mg; soln 20 mg/mL **CI:** Mod–severe hepatic impair **SE:** See Box, ↑ LFTs, fat redistribution, N, V, HA, chills **Notes:** Many drug interactions; HLA-B*5701 ↑ risk for fatal hypersens Rxn, genetic screen before use

Abatacept (Orencia) **Uses:** *Mod/severe RA w/ inadequate response to one or more DMARDs, juvenile idiopathic arthritis* **Acts:** Selective costimulation modulator, ↓ T-cell activation **Dose:** *Adults.* Initial 500 mg (< 60 kg), 750 mg (60–100 kg); 1 g (> 100 kg) IV over 30 min; repeat at 2 and 4 wk, then q4wk *Peds 6–17 y.* 10 mg/kg (< 75 kg), 750 mg (75–100 kg), IV × 1 wk 0, 2, 4, then q4wk (> 100 kg, adult dose) **W/P:** [C; ?/−] w/ TNF blockers; COPD; Hx predisposition to Infxn; w/ immunosuppressants **CI:** w/ Live vaccines w/in 3 mo of D/C abatacept **Disp:** IV powder 250 mg/10 mL **SE:** HA, URI, N, nasopharyngitis, Infxn, malignancy, Inf Rxns/hypersens (dizziness, HA, HTN), COPD exacerbations, cough, dyspnea **Notes:** Screen for TB before use

Abciximab (ReoPro) **Uses:** *Prevent acute ischemic comps in PTCA*, MI **Acts:** ↓ Plt aggregation (glycoprotein IIb/IIIa inhib) **Dose:** *ECC 2010.* ACS with immediate PCI: 0.25 mg/kg IV bolus 10–60 min before PCI, then 0.125 mcg/kg/min IV for 12 h; w/ heparin. ACS w/ planned PCI w/in 24 h: 0.25 mg/kg IV bolus, then 10 mcg/min IV over 18–24 h concluding 1 h post PCI; *PCI:* 0.25 mg/kg bolus 10–60 min pre-PTCA, then 0.125 mcg/kg/min (max = 10 mcg/min) cont inf for 12 h **W/P:** [C, ?/−] **CI:** Active/recent (w/in 6 wk) internal hemorrhage, CVA w/in 2 y or CVA w/ sig neuro deficit, bleeding diathesis or PO anticoagulants w/in 7 d (unless PT < 1.2 × control), ↓ plt (< 100,000 cells/mcL), recent trauma or major surgery (w/in 6 wk), CNS tumor, AVM, aneurysm, severe uncontrolled HTN, vasculitis, dextran use w/ PTCA, murine protein allergy, w/ other glycoprotein IIb/IIIa inhib **Disp:** Inj 2 mg/mL **SE:** ↓ BP, CP, allergic Rxns, bleeding, ↓ plt **Notes:** Use w/ heparin/ASA

Abiraterone (Zytiga) **Uses:** *Castrate-resistant metastatic PCa s/p docetaxel* **Acts:** CYP17 inhibitor; ↓ testosterone **Dose:** 1000 mg PO qd w/ 5 mg prednisone bid; w/o food 2 h AC and 1 h PC; w/ hepatic impair **W/P:** [X, N/A] w/ severe CHF, monitor for adrenocortical insuff/excess, w/ CYP2D6 inhib/CYP3A4 inhib or inducers **CI:** PRG **Disp:** Tabs 250 mg **SE:** ↑ LFTs, joint swell, ↓ K+, edema, muscle pain, hot flush, D, UTI, cough, ↑ BP, ↑ URI, urinary frequency, dyspepsia **Notes:** ✓ LFTs; CYP17 inhib may ↑ mineralocorticoid SEs; prednisone ↓ ACTH limiting SEs

Acamprosate (Campral) **Uses:** *Maintain abstinence from EtOH* **Acts:** ↓ Glutamatergic transmission; modulates neuronal hyperexcitability; related to GABA **Dose:** 666 mg PO tid; CrCl 30–50 mL/min: 333 mg PO tid **W/P:** [C; ?/–] **CI:** CrCl < 30 mL/min **Disp:** Tabs 333 mg EC **SE:** N/D, depression, anxiety, insomnia **Notes:** Does not eliminate EtOH withdrawal Sx; continue even if relapse occurs

Acarbose (Precose) **Uses:** *Type 2 DM* **Acts:** α-Glucosidase inhib; delays carbohydrate digestion to ↓ glucose **Dose:** 25–100 mg PO tid w/ 1st bite each meal; 50 mg tid (< 60 kg); 100 mg tid (> 60 kg); usual maint 50–100 mg PO tid **W/P:** [B, ?] w/ CrCl < 25 mL/min; can affect digoxin levels **CI:** IBD, colonic ulceration, partial intestinal obst; cirrhosis **Disp:** Tabs 25, 50, 100 mg **SE:** Abd pain, D, flatulence, ↑ LFTs, hypersens Rxn **Notes:** OK w/ sulfonylureas; ✓ LFTs q3mo for 1st y

Acebutolol (Sectral) **Uses:** *HTN, arrhythmias* chronic stable angina **Acts:** Blocks β-adrenergic receptors, β₁, & ISA **Dose:** *HTN:* 400–800 mg/d 2 ÷ doses *Arrhythmia:* 400–1200 mg/d 2 ÷ doses; ↓ w/ CrCl < 50 mL/min or elderly; elderly initial 200–400 mg/d; max 800 mg/d **W/P:** [B, D in 2nd & 3rd tri, +] Can exacerbate ischemic heart Dz, do not D/C abruptly **CI:** 2nd-, 3rd-degree heart block **Disp:** Caps 200, 400 mg **SE:** Fatigue, HA, dizziness, ↓ HR

Acetaminophen [APAP, N-acetyl-p-Aminophenol] (Acephen, Tylenol, Other Generic) [OTC] **Uses:** *Mild–mod pain, HA, fever* **Acts:** Nonnarcotic analgesic; ↓ CNS synth of prostaglandins & hypothalamic heat-regulating center **Dose:** *Adults.* 650 mg PO or PR q4–6h or 1000 mg PO q6h; max 4 g/24 h *Peds < 12 y.* 10–15 mg/kg/dose PO or PR q4–6h; max 5 doses/24 h. Administer q6h if CrCl 10–50 mL/min & q8h if CrCl < 10 mL/min **W/P:** [B, +] w/ hepatic/renal impair in elderly & w/ EtOH use (> 3 drinks/day) w/ > 4 g/d; EtOH liver Dz, G6PD deficiency; w/ warfarin **CI:** Hypersens **Disp:** Tabs melt away/ dissolving 80, 160 mg; tabs: 325, 500, 650 mg; chew tabs 80, 160 mg; gel caps 500 mg liq 100 mg/mL, 160 mg/5 mL, 325 mg/5 mL, 500 mg/15 mL, 80 mg/ 0.8 mL; *Acephen* supp 80, 120, 125, 325, 650 mg **SE:** hepatotoxic; OD hepatotoxic at 10 g; 15 g can be lethal; Rx w/ *N*-acetylcysteine **Notes:** No anti-inflammatory or plt-inhibiting action; avoid EtOH risk of liver injury primarily occurs when patients take multiple products containing acetaminophen at one time and exceed the current max dose of 4,000 milligrams within a 24-hour period; consider max dose of 3 g daily for long-term therapy (> 2 weeks); FDA has requested that all APAP-containing meds be max of 325 mg to limit toxicity

Acetaminophen + Butalbital ± Caffeine (Fioricet, Medigesic, Repan, Sedapap-10, Two-Dyne, Triaprin, Axocet, Phrenilin Forte) [C-III] **Uses:** *Tension HA*, mild pain **Acts:** Nonnarcotic analgesic w/ barbiturate **Dose:** 1–2 tabs or caps PO q4–6h PRN; ↓ in renal/hepatic impair; 4 g/24 h APAP max **W/P:** [C, D, +] Alcoholic liver Dz, G6PD deficiency **CI:** Hypersens **Disp:** Caps *Dolgic Plus:* butalbital 50 mg, caffeine 40 mg, APAP

750 mg; Caps *Medigesic, Repan, Two-Dyne:* butalbital 50 mg, caffeine 40 mg, APAP 325 mg; Caps *Axocet, Phrenilin Forte:* butalbital 50 mg + APAP 650 mg; Caps *Esgic-Plus, Zebutal:* butalbital 50 mg, caffeine 40 mg, APAP 500 mg; Liq. *Dolgic LQ:* butalbital 50 mg, caffeine 40 mg, APAP 325 mg/15 mL. Tabs *Medigesic, Fioricet, Repan:* butalbital 50 mg, caffeine 40 mg, APAP 325 mg; *Phrenilin:* butalbital 50 mg + APAP 325 mg; *Sedapap-10:* butalbital 50 mg + APAP 650 mg **SE:** Drowsiness, dizziness, "hangover" effect, N/V **Notes:** Butalbital habit forming; avoid EtOH; see Acetaminophen note page 34

Acetaminophen + Codeine (Tylenol No. 2, 3, No. 4) [C-III, C-V]
Uses: *Mild–mod pain (No. 2–3); mod–severe pain (No. 4)* **Acts:** Combined APAP & narcotic analgesic **Dose:** *Adults.* 1–2 tabs q4–6h PRN or 30–60 mg/ codeine q4–6h based on codeine content (max dose APAP = 4 g/d). *Peds.* APAP 10–15 mg/kg/dose; codeine 0.5–1 mg/kg dose q4–6h (guide: 3–6 y, 5 mL/dose; 7–12 y, 10 mL/dose) max 2.6 g/d if < 12 y; ↓ in renal/hepatic impair **W/P:** [C, +] Alcoholic liver Dz; G6PD deficiency **CI:** Hypersens **Disp:** Tabs 300 mg APAP + codeine(No. 2 = 15 mg, No. 3 = 30 mg, No. 4 = 60 mg); caps 325 mg APAP + codeine; susp (C-V) APAP 120 mg + codeine 12 mg/5 mL **SE:** Drowsiness, dizziness, N/V **Notes:** See Acetaminophen note page 34

Acetazolamide (Diamox)
Uses: *Diuresis, drug and CHF edema, glaucoma, prevent high-altitude sickness, refractory epilepsy*, metabolic alkalosis **Acts:** Carbonic anhydrase inhib; ↓ renal excretion of hydrogen & ↑ renal excretion of Na^+, K^+, HCO_3^-, & H_2O **Dose:** *Adults. Diuretic:* 250–375 mg IV or PO q24h *Glaucoma:* 250–1000 mg PO q24h in ÷ doses *Epilepsy:* 8–30 mg/kg/d PO in ÷ doses *Altitude sickness:* 250 mg PO q8–12h or SR 500 mg PO q12–24h start 24–48 h before & 48 h after highest ascent *Metabolic alkalosis:* 250 mg IV q6h × 4 or 500 mg IV × 1 *Peds. Epilepsy:* 8–30 mg/kg/24 h PO in ÷ doses; max 1 g/d *Diuretic:* 5 mg/kg/24 h PO or IV *Alkalinization of urine:* 5 mg/kg/dose PO bid-tid *Glaucoma:* 8–30 mg/kg/24 h PO in ÷ doses; max 1 g/d; ↓ dose w/ CrCl 10–50 mL/min; avoid if CrCl < 10 mL/min **W/P:** [C, +] **CI:** Renal/hepatic/adrenal failure, sulfa allergy, hyperchloremic acidosis **Disp:** Tabs 125, 250 mg; ER caps 500 mg; Inj 500 mg/vial, powder for recons **SE:** Malaise, metallic taste, drowsiness, photosens, hyperglycemia **Notes:** Follow Na^+ & K^+; watch for metabolic acidosis; ✓ CBC & plts; SR forms not for epilepsy

Acetic Acid & Aluminum Acetate (Otic Domeboro)
Uses: *Otitis externa* **Acts:** Anti-infective **Dose:** 4–6 gtt in ear(s) q2–3h **W/P:** [C, ?] **CI:** Perforated tympanic membranes **Disp:** 2% otic soln **SE:** Local irritation

Acetylcysteine (Acetadote, Mucomyst)
Uses: *Mucolytic, antidote to APAP hepatotox/OD*, adjuvant Rx chronic bronchopulmonary Dzs & CF* prevent contrast-induced renal dysfunction **Acts:** Splits mucoprotein disulfide linkages; restores glutathione in APAP OD to protect liver **Dose:** *Adults & Peds. Nebulizer:* 3–5 mL of 20% soln diluted w/ equal vol of H_2O or NS tid-qid *Antidote:* PO or NG: 140 mg/kg load, then 70 mg/kg q4h × 17 doses (dilute 1:3 in carbonated

beverage or OJ), repeat if emesis w/in 1 h of dosing *Acetadote:* 150 mg/kg IV over 60 min, then 50 mg/kg over 4 h, then 100 mg/kg over 16 h *Prevent renal dysfunction:* 600–1200 mg PO bid × 2 d **W/P:** [B, ?] **Disp:** Soln, inhaled and oral 10%, 20%; Acetadote IV soln 20% **SE:** Bronchospasm (inhaled), N/V, drowsiness, anaphylactoid Rxns w/ IV **Notes:** Activated charcoal adsorbs PO acetylcysteine for APAP ingestion; start Rx for APAP OD w/in 6–8 h

Acitretin (Soriatane)   BOX: Not to be used by females who are PRG or who intend to become PRG during/for 3 y following drug D/C; no EtOH during/2 mo following D/C; no blood donation for 3 y following D/C; hepatotoxic **Uses:** *Severe psoriasis*; other keratinization Dz (lichen planus, etc) **Acts:** Retinoid-like activity **Dose:** 25–50 mg/d PO, w/ main meal; ↑ if no response by 4 wk to 75 mg/d **W/P:** [X, –] Renal/hepatic impair; in women of reproductive potential **CI:** See Box; ↑ serum lipids; w/ MTX or tetracyclines **Disp:** Caps 10, 25 mg **SE:** Hyperesthesia, cheilitis, skin peeling, alopecia, pruritus, rash, arthralgia, GI upset, photosenes, thrombocytopenia, ↑ triglycerides, ↑ Na⁺, K⁺, PO₄⁻² **Notes:** ↓ LFTs/lytes/lipids; response takes up to 2–3 mo; informed consent & FDA guide w/ each Rx required

Acyclovir (Zovirax)   Uses: *Herpes simplex* (HSV) (genital/mucocutaneous, encephalitis, keratitis), *Varicella zoster*, *Herpes zoster* (shingles) Infxns* **Acts:** Interferes w/ viral DNA synth **Dose:** *Adults.* Dose on IBW if obese (> 125% IBW) PO: *Initial genital HSV:* 200 mg PO q4h while awake (5 caps/d) × 10 d or 400 mg PO tid × 7–10 d *Chronic HSV suppression:* 400 mg PO bid *Intermittent HSV Rx:* As initial, except Rx × 5 d, or 800 mg PO bid, at prodrome *Topical: Initial herpes genitalis:* Apply q3h (6×/d) for 7 d *HSV encephalitis:* 10 mg/kg IV q8h × 10 d *Herpes zoster:* 800 mg PO 5×/d for 7–10 d *IV:* 5–10 mg/kg/dose IV q8h *Peds. Genital HSV:* **3 mo–2 y:** 15 mg/kg/d IV ÷ q8h × 5–7 d, 60 mg/kg/d max *2–12 y:* 1200 mg/d PO ÷ q8h × 7–10 d > *12 y:* 1000–1200 mg PO ÷ q8h × 7–10 d *HSV encephalitis:* **3 mo–12 y:** 60 mg/kg/d IV ÷ q8h × 10 d > *12 y:* 30 mg/kg/d IV ÷ q8h × 10 d *Chickenpox:* ≥2 y: 20 mg/kg/dose PO qid × 5 d *Shingles: < 12 y:* 30 mg/kg/d PO or 1500 mg/ m²/d IV ÷ q8h × 7–10 d; ↓ w/ CrCl < 50 mL/min **W/P:** [B, +] **CI:** Component hypersens **Disp:** Caps 200 mg; tabs 400, 800 mg; susp 200 mg/5 mL; Inj 500 & 1000 mg/vial; Inj soln 25 mg/mL, 50 mg/mL oint 5% and cream 5% **SE:** Dizziness, lethargy, malaise, confusion, rash, IV site inflammation; transient ↑ Cr/BUN **Notes:** PO better than topical for herpes genitalis

Adalimumab (Humira)   BOX: Cases of TB have been observed; ✓ TB skin test prior to use; hep B reactivation possible, invasive fungal, and other opportunistic Infxns reported; lymphoma/other cancer possible in children/adolescents **Uses:** *Mod–severe RA w/ an inadequate response to one or more DMARDs, psoriatic arthritis (PA), juvenile idiopathic arthritis (JIA), plaque psoriasis, ankylosing spondylitis (AS), Crohn Dz* **Acts:** TNF-α inhib **Dose:** *RA, PA, AS:* 40 mg SQ q other wk; may ↑ 40 mg qwk if not on MTX. JIA 15–30 kg 20 mg q other wk *Crohn Dz:* 160 mg d 1, 80 mg 2 wk later, then 2 wk later start maint 40 mg q other wk **W/P:** [B, ?/–] See Box; do not use w/ live vaccines **CI:** None **Disp:** Prefilled 0.4 mL

(20 mg) & 0.8 mL (40 mg) syringe **SE:** Inj site Rxns, anaphylaxis, cytopenias, demyelinating Dz, new onset psoriasis **Notes:** Refrigerate prefilled syringe, rotate Inj sites, OK w/ other DMARDs

Adapalene (Differin) Uses: *Acne vulgaris* **Acts:** Retinoid-like, modulates cell differentiation/keratinization/inflammation **Dose:** *Adults & Peds > 12 y.* Apply 1×/d to clean/dry skin **W/P:** [C, ?/–] products w/ sulfur/resorcinol/salicylic acid ↑ irritation **Disp:** Top lotion, gel, cream 0.1%; gel 0.3% **SE:** Skin redness, dryness, burning, stinging, scaling, itching, sunburn **Notes:** Avoid exposure to sunlight/ sunlamps; wear sunscreen

Adapalene & Benzoyl Peroxide (Epiduo Gel) Uses: *Acne vulgaris* **Action:** Retinoid-like, modulates cell differentiation, keratinization, and inflammation w/ antibacterial **Dose:** *Adults & Peds > 12 y.* Apply 1 × daily to clean/dry skin **W/P:** [C, ?] Bleaching effects, photosensitivity **CI:** Component sensitivity **Disp:** Topical gel: adapalene 0.1% and benzoyl peroxide 2.5% (45g) **SE:** Local irritation, dryness **Notes:** Vit A may ↑ SE

Adefovir (Hepsera) **BOX:** Acute exacerbations of hep seen after D/C Rx (monitor LFTs); nephrotoxic w/ underlying renal impair w/ chronic use (monitor renal Fxn); HIV resistance/untreated may emerge; lactic acidosis & severe hepatomegaly w/ steatosis reported Uses: *Chronic active hep B* **Acts:** Nucleotide analog **Dose:** CrCl > 50 mL/min: 10 mg PO daily; CrCl 20–49 mL/min: 10 mg PO q48h; CrCl 10–19 mL/min: 10 mg PO q72h; HD: 10 mg PO q7d postdialysis; adjust w/ CrCl < 50 mL/min **W/P:** [C, –] **Disp:** Tabs 10 mg **SE:** Asthenia, HA, Abd pain; see Box **Notes:** ✓ HIV status before use

Adenosine (Adenocard) Uses: *PSVT*; including w/ WPW **Acts:** Class IV antiarrhythmic; slows AV node conduction **Dose:** *Adults. ECC 2010.* 6-mg rapid IV push, then 20-mL NS bolus. Elevate extremity; repeat 12 mg in 1–2 min PRN *Peds. ECC 2010. Symptomatic SVT:* 0.1 mg/kg rapid IV/IO push (max dose 6 mg); can follow with 0.2 mg/kg rapid IV/IO push (max dose 12 mg); follow each dose with 10 mL NS flush **W/P:** [C, ?] Hx bronchospasm **CI:** 2nd-/3rd-degree AV block or SSS (w/o pacemaker); A flutter, AF, V tachycardia, recent MI or CNS bleed **Disp:** Inj 3 mg/mL **SE:** Facial flushing, HA, dyspnea, chest pressure, ↓ BP **Notes:** Doses > 12 mg not OK; can cause momentary asystole w/ use; caffeine, theophylline antagonize effects

Albumin (Albuminar, Buminate, Albutein) Uses: *Plasma vol expansion for shock* (e.g., burns, hemorrhage) **Acts:** Maintain plasma colloid oncotic pressure **Dose:** *Adults.* Initial 25 g IV; then based on response; 250 g/48 h max *Peds.* 0.5–1 g/kg/dose; Inf at 0.05–0.1 g/min; max 6 g/kg/d **W/P:** [C, ?] Severe anemia; cardiac, renal, or hepatic Insuff d/t protein load & hypervolemia **CI:** CHF, severe anemia **Disp:** Soln 5%, 25% **SE:** Chills, fever, CHF, tachycardia, ↓ BP, hypervolemia **Notes:** Contains 130–160 mEq Na⁺/L; may cause pulm edema

Albuterol (Proventil, Ventolin, Volmax) Uses: *Asthma, COPD, prevent exercise-induced bronchospasm* **Acts:** β-Adrenergic sympathomimetic bronchodilator; relaxes bronchial smooth muscle **Dose: *Adults. Inhaler:*** 2 Inh q4–6h PRN; 1 Rotacaps inhaled q4–6h *PO:* 2–4 mg PO tid-qid *Nebulizer:* 1.25–5 mg (0.25–1 mL of 0.5% soln in 2–3 mL of NS) tid-qid *Prevent exercise-induced asthma:* 2 puffs 5–30 min prior to activity ***Peds. Inhaler:*** 2 Inh q4–6h *PO:* 0.1–0.2 mg/kg/dose PO; max 2–4 mg PO tid *Nebulizer:* 0.05 mg/kg (max 2.5 mg) in 2–3 mL of NS tid-qid *2–6 y.* 12 mg/d max, 6–12 y 24 mg/d max **W/P:** [C, +] **Disp:** Tabs 2, 4 mg; XR tabs 4, 8 mg; syrup 2 mg/5 mL; 90 mcg/dose metered-dose inhaler; soln for nebulizer 0.083, 0.5% **SE:** Palpitations, tachycardia, nervousness, GI upset

Albuterol & Ipratropium (Combivent, DuoNeb) **Uses:** *COPD* **Acts:** Combo of β-adrenergic bronchodilator & quaternary anticholinergic **Dose:** 2 Inh qid; nebulizer 3 mL q6h; max 12 Inh/24 h or 3 mL q4h **W/P:** [C, +] **CI:** Peanut/soybean allergy **Disp:** Metered-dose inhaler, 18 mcg ipratropium & 103 mcg albuterol/puff (contains ozone-depleting CFCs; will be gradually removed from US market); nebulization soln (DuoNeb) ipratropium 0.5 mg & albuterol 2.5 mg/3 mL 0.042%, 0.21% **SE:** Palpitations, tachycardia, nervousness, GI upset, dizziness, blurred vision

Alcaftadine (Lastacaft) **Uses:** *Allergic conjunctivitis* **Acts:** Histamine H₁-receptor antag **Dose:** 1 gtt in eye(s) daily **W/P:** [B, ?] **Disp:** Ophth sol 0.25% **SE:** Eye irritation **Notes:** Remove contacts before use

Aldesleukin [IL-2] (Proleukin) **BOX:** High dose associated w/ capillary leak synd w/ hypotension and ↓ organ perfusion; ↑ Infxn d/t poor neutrophil activity; D/C w/ mod-severe lethargy, may progress to coma **Uses:** *Met RCC & melanoma* **Acts:** Acts via IL-2 receptor; many immunomodulatory effects **Dose:** 600,000 Int Units/kg q8h × 14 doses days 1–5 and days 15–19 of 28-d cycle (FDA-approved dose/schedule for RCC); other schedules (e.g., "high dose" 24 × 10⁶ Int Units/m² IV q8h on days 1–5 & 12–16) **W/P:** [C, ?/–] **CI:** Organ allografts **Disp:** Powder for recons 22 × 10⁶ Int Units, when reconstituted 18 mill Int Units/mL = 1.1 mg/mL **SE:** Flu-like synd (malaise, fever, chills), N/V/D, ↑ bili; capillary leak synd; ↓ BP, tachycardia, pulm & edema, fluid retention, & wgt gain; renal & mild hematologic tox (↓ Hgb, plt, WBC), eosinophilia; cardiac tox (ischemia, atrial arrhythmias); neurotox (CNS depression, somnolence, delirium, rare coma); pruritic rashes, urticaria, & erythroderma common

Alefacept (Amevive) **BOX:** Monitor CD4 before each dose; w/hold if < 250; D/C if < 250 × 1 mo **Uses:** *Mod/severe chronic plaque psoriasis* **Acts:** Fusion protein inhib **Dose:** 7.5 mg IV or 15 mg IM once/wk × 12 wk **W/P:** [B, ?/–] PRG registry; associated w/ serious Infxn **CI:** Lymphoma/eny, HIV **Disp:** 15-mg powder for recons **SE:** Pharyngitis, myalgia, Inj site Rxn, malignancy, Infxn **Notes:** IV/IM different formulations; may repeat course 12 wk later if CD4 OK

Alemtuzumab (Campath) **BOX:** Serious, including fatal, cytopenias, Inf Rxns, and Infxns can occur; limit dose to 30 mg (single) & 90 mg (weekly), higher doses ↑ risk of pancytopenia; ↑ dose gradually & monitor during Inf, D/C for Grade 3 or 4 Inf Rxns; give prophylaxis for PCP & herpes virus Infxn **Uses:** *B-cell

CLL* **Acts:** CD52-directed cytolytic ab **Dose:** *Adults.* ↑ dose to 30 mg/d IV 3×/wk for 12 wk (see label for escalation strategy); infuse over 2 h; premedicate w/ oral antihistamine & APAP **W/P:** [C, –] Do not give live vaccines; D/C for autoimmune/severe hematologic Rxns **Disp:** Inj **SE:** Cytopenias, Infxns, Inf Rxns, N/V/D, insomnia, anxiety **Notes:** ✓ CBC & plt weekly & CD4 counts after Rx until > 200 cells/μL

Alendronate (Fosamax, Fosamax Plus D) **Uses:** *Rx & prevent osteoporosis male & postmenopausal female, Rx steroid-induced osteoporosis, Paget Dz* **Acts:** ↓ nl & abnormal bone resorption, ↓ osteoclast action **Dose:** *Osteoporosis:* Rx: 10 mg/d PO or 70 mg qwk; *Postmenopausal:* Rx: 5 mg/d PO, 10 mg/d postmenopausal not on estrogen *Prevention:* 5 mg/d PO or 35 mg qwk *Paget Dz:* 40 mg/d PO **W/P:** [C, ?] Not OK if CrCl < 35 mL/min, w/ NSAID use **CI:** Esophageal anomalies, inability to sit/stand upright for 30 min, ↓ Ca²⁺ **Disp:** Tabs 5, 10, 35, 40, 70 mg, soln 70 mg/75 mL *Fosamax plus D:* Alendronate 70 mg w/ cholecalciferol (vit D₃) 2800 or 5600 Int Units **SE:** Abd pain, acid regurgitation, constipation, D/N, dyspepsia, musculoskeletal pain, jaw osteonecrosis (w/ dental procedures, chemo) **Notes:** Take 1st thing in AM w/ H₂O (8 oz) > 30 min before 1st food/beverage of day; do not lie down for 30 min after. Use Ca²⁺ & vit D supl w/ regular tab; may ↑ atypical subtrochanteric femur fractures

Alfentanil (Alfenta) [C-II] **Uses:** *Adjunct in maint of anesthesia; analgesia* **Acts:** Short-acting narcotic analgesic **Dose:** *Adults & Peds > 12 y.* 3–75 mcg/kg (IBW) IV Inf; total depends on duration of procedure **W/P:** [C, +/–] ↑ ICP, resp depression **Disp:** Inj 500 mcg/mL **SE:** ↓ HR, ↓ BP arrhythmias, peripheral vasodilation, ↑ ICP, drowsiness, resp depression, N/V/constipation

Alfuzosin (Uroxatral) **Uses:** *symptomatic BPH* **Acts:** α-Blocker **Dose:** 10 mg PO daily immediately after the same meal **W/P:** [B, –]w/ any Hx ↓ BP; use w/ PDE5 inhibitors may ↓ BP; may ↑ QTc interval; IFIS during cataract surgery **CI:** w/ CYP3A4 inhib; mod–severe hepatic impair; protease inhibitors for HIV **Disp:** Tabs 10 mg ER **SE:** Postural ↓ BP, dizziness, HA, fatigue **Notes:** Do not cut or crush; ↓ ejaculatory disorders compared w/ similar drugs

Alginic Acid + Aluminum Hydroxide & Magnesium Trisilicate (Gaviscon) [OTC] **Uses:** *Heartburn*; hiatal hernia pain **Acts:** Protective layer blocks gastric acid **Dose:** Chew 2–4 tabs or 15–30 mL PO qid followed by H₂O **W/P:** [B, –] Avoid w/ renal impair or Na⁺-restricted diet **Disp:** Chew tabs, susp **SE:** D, constipation

Alglucosidase Alfa (Myozyme) **BOX:** Life-threatening anaphylactic Rxns seen w/ Inf; medical support measures should be immediately available **Uses:** *Rx Pompe DZ* **Acts:** Recombinant acid α-glucosidase; degrades glycogen in lysosomes **Dose:** *Peds 1 mo–3.5 y.* 20 mg/kg IV q2wk over 4 h (see PI) **W/P:** [B, ?/–] Illness at time of Inf may ↑ Inf Rxns **Disp:** Powder 50 mg/vial **SE:** Hypersens, fever, rash, D, V, gastroenteritis, pneumonia, URI, cough, resp distress/failure, Infxns, cardiac arrhythmia w/ general anesthesia, ↑/↓ HR, flushing, anemia

Aliskiren (Tekturna) **BOX:** May cause injury and death to a developing fetus; D/C immediately when PRG detected **Uses:** *HTN* **Acts:** 1st direct renin inhib **Dose:** 150–300 mg/d PO **W/P:** [C (1st tri), D (2nd & 3rd tri); ?] Avoid w/ CrCl < 30 mL/min; ketoconazole and other CYP3A4 inhib may ↑ aliskiren levels **CI:** Anuria, sulfur sensitivity **Disp:** Tabs 150, 300 mg **SE:** D, Abd pain, dyspepsia, GERD, cough, ↑ K+, angioedema, ↓ BP, dizziness

Aliskiren and Amlodipine (Tekamlo) **BOX:** May cause fetal injury & death; D/C immediately when PRG detected **Uses:** *HTN* **Acts:** Renin inhib w/ dihydropyridine CCB **Dose:** *Adult.* 150/5 mg PO 1×/d; max 300/10 mg/d); max effect in 2 wk **W/P:** [D, –] do not use w/ cyclosporine/itraconazole **Disp:** Tabs (aliskiren mg/amlodipine mg) 150/5, 150/10, 300/5, 300/10 **SE:** ↓ BP, ↑ K+, angioedema, peripheral edema, D, dizziness, angina, MI

Aliskiren, Amlodipine, Hydrochlorothiazide (Amturnide) **BOX:** May cause fetal injury & death; D/C immediately when PRG detected **Uses:** *HTN* **Acts:** Renin inhib, dihydropyridine CCB, & thiazide diuretic **Dose:** *Adult.* Titrate q2wk PRN to 300/10/25 mg PO max/d **W/P:** [D, –] Avoid w/ CrCl < 30 mL/min; do not use w/ cyclosporine/itraconazole; ↓ BP in salt/volume depleted pts; HCTZ may exacerbate/activate SLE; D/C if myopia or NAG **CI:** Anuria, sulfonamide allergy **Disp:** Tabs (aliskiren mg/amlodipine mg/HCTZ mg) 150/5/12.5, 300/5/12.5, 300/5/25, 300/10/12.5, 300/10/25 **SE:** ↓ BP, ↑ K+, hyperuricemia, angioedema, peripheral edema, D, HA, dizziness, angina, MI, nasopharyngitis

Aliskiren/Hydrochlorothiazide (Tekturna HCT) **BOX:** May cause injury and death to a developing fetus; D/C immediately when PRG detected **Uses:** *HTN, not primary Rx* **Acts:** Renin inhib w/ diuretic **Dose:** *Monotherapy failure:* 150 mg/12.5 mg PO q day; may ↑ to 150 mg/25 mg, 300 mg/12.5 mg q day after 2–4 wk *Max:* 300 mg/25 mg **W/P:** [D, ?] Avoid w/ CrCl ≤30 mL/min; avoid w/ CYP3A4 inhib (Li, ketoconazole, etc.) may ↑ aliskiren levels; ↓ BP in salt/volume depleted pts **Disp:** Tabs (aliskiren mg/HCTZ mg) 150/12.5, 150/25, 300/12.5, 300/25 **SE:** Dizziness, influenza, D, cough, vertigo, asthenia, arthralgia, angioedema

Aliskiren and Valsartan (Valturna) **BOX:** May cause fetal injury & death; D/C immediately when PRG detected **Uses:** *HTN* **Acts:** Renin inhib w/ ARB **Dose:** *Adult.* 150/160 mg PO once daily; Max 300/320 mg/d; max effect in 2 wk **W/P:** [D, –] w/ K+ sparing diuretics, K+ supls, salt substitutes; do not use w/ cyclosporine or itraconazole; ↓ BP in salt/volume depleted pts **Disp:** Tabs (aliskiren mg/valsartan mg) 150/160, 300/320 **SE:** ↓ BP, ↑ K+, angioedema, D, HA, dizziness, nasopharyngitis, fatigue, ↑ SCr

Allopurinol (Zyloprim, Lopurin, Aloprim) **Uses:** *Gout, hyperuricemia of malignancy, uric acid urolithiasis* **Acts:** Xanthine oxidase inhib; ↓ uric acid production **Dose:** *Adults. PO:* Initial 100 mg/d; usual 300 mg/d; max 800 mg/d; ÷ dose if > 300 mg/d *IV:* 200–400 mg/m^2/d (max 600 mg/24 h); (after meal w/ plenty of fluid) *Peds.* Only for hyperuricemia of malignancy if < 10 y: 10 mg/kg/24 h PO or 200 mg/m^2/d IV ÷ q6–8h; max 600 mg/24 h; ↓ in renal impair **W/P:** [C, M] **Disp:** Tabs 100, 300 mg; Inj 500 mg/30 mL (Aloprim) **SE:** Rash, N/V, renal impair, angioedema **Notes:** Aggravates acute gout; begin after acute attack resolves; IV dose of 6 mg/mL final conc as single daily Inf or ÷ 6-, 8-, or 12-h intervals

Almotriptan (Axert) **Uses:** *Rx acute migraine* **Acts:** Vascular serotonin receptor agonist **Dose:** *Adults.* PO: 6.25–12 mg PO, repeat in 2 h PRN; 2 dose/24 h max PO dose; max 12 or 24 mg/d; w/ hepatic/renal impair 6.25 mg single dose (max 12.5 mg/d) **W/P:** [C, ?/–] **CI:** Angina, ischemic heart Dz, coronary artery vasospasm, hemiplegic or basilar migraine, uncontrolled HTN, ergot use, MAOI use w/in 14 d **Disp:** Tabs 6.25, 12.5 mg **SE:** N, somnolence, paresthesias, HA, dry mouth, weakness, numbness, coronary vasospasm, HTN

Alosetron (Lotronex) **BOX:** Serious GI SEs, some fatal, including ischemic colitis reported. Prescribed only through participation in the prescribing program **Uses:** *Severe D/predominant IBS in women who fail conventional Rx* **Acts:** Selective 5-HT$_3$ receptor antagonist **Dose:** *Adults.* 0.5 mg PO bid; ↑ to 1 mg bid max after 4 wk; D/C after 8 wk not controlled **W/P:** [B, ?/–] **CI:** Hx chronic/severe constipation, GI obst, strictures, toxic megacolon, GI perforation, adhesions, ischemic/ulcerative colitis, Crohn Dz, diverticulitis, thrombophlebitis, hypercoagulability **Disp:** Tabs 0.5, 1 mg **SE:** Constipation, Abd pain, N **Notes:** D/C immediately if constipation or Sxs of ischemic colitis develop; informed consent prior to use

Alpha-1-Protease Inhibitor (Prolastin) **Uses:** *α$_1$-Antitrypsin deficiency*; panacinar emphysema **Acts:** Replace human α$_1$-protease inhib **Dose:** 60 mg/kg IV once/wk **W/P:** [C, ?] **CI:** Selective IgA deficiencies w/ IgA antibodies **Disp:** Inj 500 mg/20 mL, 1000 mg/40 mL powder for Inj **SE:** HA, MS discomfort, fever, dizziness, flu-like Sxs, allergic Rxns, ↑ AST/ALT

Alprazolam (Xanax, Niravam) [C-IV] **Uses:** *Anxiety & panic disorders*, anxiety w/ depression **Acts:** Benzodiazepine; antianxiety agent **Dose:** *Anxiety:* Initial, 0.25–0.5 mg tid; ↑ to 4 mg/d max ÷ doses *Panic:* Initial, 0.5 mg tid; may gradually ↑ to response; ↓ in elderly, debilitated, & hepatic impair **W/P:** [D, –] **CI:** NAG, concomitant itra-/ketoconazole **Disp:** Tabs 0.25, 0.5, 1, 2 mg; Xanax XR 0.5, 1, 2, 3 mg; Niravam (ODTs) 0.25, 0.5, 1, 2 mg; soln 1 mg/mL **SE:** Drowsiness, fatigue, irritability, memory impair, sexual dysfunction, paradoxical Rxns **Notes:** Avoid abrupt D/C after prolonged use

Alprostadil [Prostaglandin E$_1$] (Prostin VR) **BOX:** Apnea in up to 12% of neonates especially < 2 kg at birth **Uses:** *Conditions where ductus arteriosus flow must be maintained*, sustain pulm/systemic circulation until OR (e.g., pulm atresia/stenosis, transposition) **Acts:** Vasodilator (ductus arteriosus very sensitive), plt inhib **Dose:** 0.05 mcg/kg/min IV; ↓ to lowest *ECC 2010. Maintain patency of ductus:* 0.05–0.1 mcg/kg/min IV/IO inf; then maint 0.01–0.05 mcg/kg/min **W/P:** [X, –] **CI:** Neonatal resp distress synd **Disp:** Inj 500 mcg/mL **SE:** Cutaneous vasodilation, Sz-like activity, jitteriness, ↑ temp, ↓ Ca^{2+}, thrombocytopenia, ↓ BP; may cause apnea **Notes:** Keep intubation kit at bedside

Alprostadil, Intracavernosal (Caverject, Edex)   Uses: *ED* **Acts:** Relaxes smooth muscles, dilates cavernosal arteries, ↑ lacunar spaces w/ blood entrapment **Dose:** 2.5–60 mcg intracavernosal; titrate in office **W/P:** [X, –] **CI:** ↑ risk of priapism (e.g., sickle cell); penile deformities/implants; men in whom sexual activity inadvisable **Disp:** *Caverject:* 5-, 10-, 20-, 40-mcg powder for Inj vials ± diluent syringes 10-, 20-, 40-mcg amp *Caverject Impulse:* Self-contained syringe (29 gauge) 10 & 20 mcg *Edex:* 10-, 20-, 40-mcg cartridges **SE:** Local pain w/ Inj **Notes:** Counsel about priapism, penile fibrosis, & hematoma risks, titrate dose in office

Alprostadil, Urethral Suppository (Muse)   Uses: *ED* **Acts:** Urethral absorption; vasodilator, relaxes smooth muscle of corpus cavernosa **Dose:** 125–1000-mcg system 5–10 min prior to sex; repeat × 1/24 h; titrate in office **W/P:** [X, –] **CI:** ↑ Priapism risk (especially sickle cell, myeloma, leukemia) penile deformities/ implants; men in whom sex inadvisable **Disp:** 125, 250, 500, 1000 mcg w/ transurethral system **SE:** ↓ BP, dizziness, syncope, penile/testicular pain, urethral burning/ bleeding, priapism **Notes:** Titrate dose in office; duration 30–60 min

Alteplase, Recombinant [tPA] (Activase)   Uses: *AMI, PE, acute ischemic stroke, & CV cath occlusion* **Acts:** Thrombolytic; binds fibrin in thrombus, initiates fibrinolysis **Dose:** *ECC 2010. STEMI:* 15-mg bolus; then 0.75 mg/kg over 30 min (50 mg max); then 0.50 mg/kg over next 60 min (35 mg max; max total dose 100 mg) Acute ischemic stroke: 0.9 mg/kg IV (max 90 mg) over 60 min; give 10% of total dose over 1 min; remaining 90% over 1 h (or 3-h inf) Stroke: w/in 3 h of onset *S&S:* 0.09 mg/kg IV over 1 min, then 0.81 mg/kg; max 90 mg/h Inf over 60 min *(ECC 2005)* Cath occlusion: 10–29 kg 1 mg/mL; ≥30 kg 2 mg/mL **W/P:** [C, ?] **CI:** Active internal bleeding; uncontrolled HTN (SBP > 185 mm Hg, DBP > 110 mm Hg); recent (w/in 3 mo) CVA, GI bleed, trauma; intracranial or intraspinal surgery or Dzs (AVM/aneurysm/subarachnoid hemorrhage/neoplasm); prolonged cardiac massage; suspected aortic dissection, w/ anticoagulants or INR > 1.7, heparin w/in 48 h, plts < 100,000, Sz at the time of stroke **Disp:** Powder for Inj 2, 50, 100 mg **SE:** Bleeding, bruising (e.g., venipuncture sites), ↓ BP **Notes:** Give heparin to prevent reocclusion; in AMI, doses of > 150 mg associated w/ intracranial bleeding

Altretamine (Hexalen)   **BOX:** BM suppression, neurotox common **Uses:** *Epithelial ovarian CA* **Acts:** Unknown; ? cytotoxic/alkylating agent; ↓ nucleotide incorporation **Dose:** 260 mg/m²/d in 4 ÷ doses for 14–21 d of a 28-d Rx cycle; dose ↑ to 150 mg/m²/d × 14 d multiagent regimens (per protocols); after meals and hs **W/P:** [D, ?/–] **CI:** Preexisting BM depression or neurologic tox **Disp:** Gel caps 50 mg **SE:** N/V/D, cramps; neurotox (neuropathy, CNS depression); minimal myelosuppression **Notes:** ✓ CBC, routine neurologic exams

Alvimopan (Entereg)   **BOX:** For short-term hospital use only (max 15 doses) **Uses:** *↓ Time to GI recovery w/ bowel resection and primary anastomosis* **Action:** Opioid (μ) receptor antagonist; selectively binds GI receptors, antagonizes effects of opioids on GI motility/secretion **Dose:** 12 mg 30 min–5 h preop PO, then 12 mg bid up to 7 d; max 15 doses **W/P:** [B,±] Not rec in complete bowel obstruction surgery, hepatic/renal impair **CI:** Therapeutic opioids > 7 consecutive days prior **Disp:** Caps 12 mg **SE:** ↓ K⁺, dyspepsia, urinary retention, anemia, back pain **Notes:** Hospitals must be registered to use.

Aluminum Hydroxide (Amphojel, AlternaGEL, Dermagran) [OTC]
Uses: *Heartburn, upset or sour stomach, or acid indigestion*; supl to Rx of ↑PO_4^{2-}; *minor cuts, burns (Dermagran)* **Acts:** Neutralizes gastric acid; binds PO_4^{2-} **Dose:** *Adults.* 10–30 mL or 300–1200 mg PO q4–6h *Peds.* 5–15 mL PO q4–6h or 50–150 mg/kg/24 h PO ÷ q4–6h (hyperphosphatemia) **W/P:** [C, ?] **Disp:** Tabs 300, 600 mg; susp 320, 600 mg/5 mL; oint 0.275% (*Dermagran*) **SE:** Constipation **Notes:** OK w/ renal failure; topical ointment for cuts/burns

Aluminum Hydroxide + Magnesium Carbonate (Gaviscon Extra Strength, Liquid) [OTC]
Uses: *Heartburn, acid indigestion* **Acts:** Neutralizes gastric acid **Dose:** *Adults.* 15–30 mL PO pc & hs; 2–4 chew tabs up to qid. *Peds.* 5–15 mL PO qid or PRN; **W/P:** [C, ?] ↑ Mg^{2+}; avoid w/in renal impair **Disp:** Liq w/ AlOH 95 mg/Mg carbonate 358 mg/15 mL; Extra Strength liq AlOH 254 mg/Mg carbonate 237 mg/15 mL; chew tabs AlOH 160 mg/Mg carbonate 105 mg **SE:** Constipation, D **Notes:** qid doses best pc & hs; may ↓ absorption of some drugs, take 2–3 h apart to ↓ effect

Aluminum Hydroxide + Magnesium Hydroxide (Maalox, Mylanta Ultimate Strength) [OTC]
Uses: *Hyperacidity* (peptic ulcer, hiatal hernia, etc) **Acts:** Neutralizes gastric acid **Dose:** *Adults.* 10–20 mL or 2–4 tabs PO qid or PRN *Peds.* 5–15 mL PO qid or PRN **W/P:** [C, ?] **Disp:** Chew tabs, susp **SE:** May ↑ Mg^{2+} w/ renal Insuff, constipation, D **Notes:** Doses qid best pc & hs

Aluminum Hydroxide + Magnesium Hydroxide & Simethicone (Mylanta Regular Strength, Maalox Advanced) [OTC]
Uses: *Hyperacidity w/ bloating* **Acts:** Neutralizes gastric acid & defoaming **Dose:** *Adults.* 10–20 mL or 2–4 tabs PO qid or PRN *Peds.* 5–15 mL PO qid or PRN; avoid in renal impair **W/P:** [C, ?] **Disp:** Tabs, susp, liq **SE:** ↑ Mg^{2+} in renal Insuff, D, constipation **Notes:** Mylanta II contains twice Al & Mg hydroxide of Mylanta; may affect absorption of some drugs

Aluminum Hydroxide + Magnesium Trisilicate (Gaviscon, Regular Strength) [OTC]
Uses: *Relief of heartburn, upset or sour stomach, or acid indigestion* **Acts:** Neutralizes gastric acid **Dose:** Chew 2–4 tabs qid; avoid in renal impair **W/P:** [C, ?] **CI:** Mg^{2+}, sensitivity **Disp:** AlOH 80 mg/Mg trisilicate 20 mg/tab **SE:** ↑ Mg^{2+} in renal Insuff, constipation, D **Notes:** May affect absorption of some drugs

Amantadine (Symmetrel)
Uses: *Rx/prophylaxis influenza A, Parkinsonism, & drug-induced EPS* d/t **Acts:** Prevents infectious viral nucleic acid release into host cell; releases dopamine and blocks reuptake of dopamine in presynaptic nerves **Dose:** *Adults. Influenza A:* 200 mg/d PO or 100 mg PO bid w/in 48 h of Sx *Parkinsonism:* 100 mg PO daily-bid *Peds 1–9 y.* 4.4–8.8 mg/kg/24 h to

150 mg/24 h max ÷ doses daily-bid **10–12 y.** 100–200 mg/d in 1–2 ÷ doses; ↓ in renal impair **W/P:** [C, M] **Disp:** Caps 100 mg; tabs 100 mg; soln 50 mg/5 mL **SE:** Orthostatic ↓ BP, edema, insomnia, depression, irritability, hallucinations, dream abnormalities, N/D, dry mouth **Notes:** Not for influenza use in US d/t resistance including H1N1

Ambrisentan (Letairis) **BOX:** May cause ↑ AST/ALT to > 3× ULN, LFTs monthly. CI in PRG; ✓ monthly PRG tests **Uses:** *Pulm arterial HTN* **Acts:** Endothelin receptor antagonist **Dose:** *Adults.* 5 mg PO/d, max 10 mg/d; not OK w/ hepatic impair **W/P:** [X, –] w/ Cyclosporine, strong CYP3A or 2C19 inhib, inducers of P-glycoprotein, CYPs and UGTs **CI:** PRG **Disp:** Tabs 5, 10 mg **SE:** Edema, nasal congestion, sinusitis, dyspnea, flushing, constipation, HA, palpitations, hepatotoxic **Notes:** Available only through the Letairis Education and Access Program (LEAP); D/C AST/ALT > 5× ULN or bili > 2× ULN or S/Sx of liver dysfunction; childbearing females must use 2 methods of contraception

Amifostine (Ethyol) **Uses:** *Xerostomia prophylaxis during RT (head, neck, etc) where parotid is in radiation field; ↓ renal tox w/ repeated cisplatin* **Acts:** Prodrug, dephosphorylated by alkaline phosphatase to active thiol metabolite; binds cisplatin metabolites **Dose:** 910 mg/m² IV 15-min IV Inf 30 min prechemotherapy **W/P:** [C, +/–] CV Dz **Disp:** 500-mg vials powder, reconstitute in NS **SE:** Transient ↓ BP (> 60%), N/V, flushing w/ hot or cold chills, dizziness, ↓ Ca²⁺, somnolence, sneezing **Notes:** Does not ↓ effectiveness of cyclophosphamide + cisplatin chemotherapy

Amikacin (Amikin) **Uses:** *Serious gram(–) bacterial Infxns* & mycobacteria **Acts:** Aminoglycoside; ↓ protein synth **Spectrum:** Good gram(–) bacterial coverage: *Pseudomonas* & *Mycobacterium* sp **Dose:** *Adults & Peds. Conventional:* 5–7.5 mg/kg/dose q8h; once daily; 15–20 mg/kg q24h; ↑ interval w/ renal impair *Neonates < 1200 g, 0–4 wk:* 7.5 mg/kg/dose q18h–24h *Age < 7 d, 1200–2000 g:* 7.5 mg/kg/dose q12h > 2000 g: 10 mg/kg/dose q12h *Age > 7 d, 1200–2000 g:* 7 mg/kg/dose q8h > 2000 g: 7.5–10 mg/kg/dose q8h **W/P:** [C, +/–] Avoid w/ diuretics **Disp:** Inj 50 & 250 mg/mL **SE:** Nephro-/oto-/neurotox, neuromuscular blockage, resp paralysis **Notes:** May be effective in gram(–) resistance to gentamicin & tobramycin; follow Cr; Levels: *Peak:* 30 min after Inf *Trough* < 0.5 h before next dose *Therapeutic: Peak* 20–30 mcg/mL, *Trough:* < 8 mcg/mL. *Toxic peak* > 35 mcg/mL; *half-life:* 2 h

Amiloride (Midamor) **Uses:** *HTN, CHF, & thiazide-induced ↓ K⁺* **Acts:** K⁺-sparing diuretic; interferes w/ K⁺/Na⁺ exchange in distal tubule **Dose:** *Adults.* 5–10 mg PO daily *Peds.* 0.625 mg/kg/d; ↓ w/ renal impair **W/P:** [B, ?] **CI:** ↑ K⁺, SCr > 1.5, BUN > 30, diabetic neuropathy, w/ other K⁺-sparing diuretics **Disp:** Tabs 5 mg **SE:** ↑ K⁺; HA, dizziness, dehydration, impotence **Notes:** ✓ K⁺

Aminocaproic Acid (Amicar) **Uses:** *Excessive bleeding from systemic hyperfibrinolysis & urinary fibrinolysis* **Acts:** ↓ Fibrinolysis; inhibits TPA, inhibits conversion of plasminogen to plasmin **Dose:** *Adults.* 5 g IV or PO (1st h) then

1–1.25 g/h IV or PO × 8 h or until bleeding controlled; 30 g/d max *Peds.* 100 mg/kg IV (1st h) then 1 g/m²/h; max 18 g/m²/d; ↓ w/ renal Insuff **W/P:** [C, ?] Not for upper urinary tract bleeding **CI:** DIC **Disp:** Tabs 500, syrup 250 mg/mL; Inj 250 mg/mL **SE:** ↓ BP, ↓ HR, dizziness, HA, fatigue, rash, GI disturbance, ↓ plt Fxn **Notes:** Administer × 8 h or until bleeding controlled

Amino-Cerv pH 5.5 Cream **Uses:** *Mild cervicitis*, postpartum cervicitis/ cervical tears, post-cauterization/cryosurgery/conization **Acts:** Hydrating agent; removes excess keratin in hyperkeratotic conditions **Dose:** 1 Applicator-full intra-vag hs × 2–4 wk **W/P:** [C, ?] w/ Viral skin Infxn **Disp:** Vag cream **SE:** Stinging, local irritation **Notes:** AKA carbamide or urea; contains 8.34% urea, 0.5% sodium propionate, 0.83% methionine, 0.35% cystine, 0.83% inositol, & benzalkonium chloride

Aminoglutethimide (Cytadren) **Uses:** *Cushing synd*, adrenocortical carcinoma, breast CA & PCa **Acts:** ↓ Adrenal steroidogenesis & conversion of androgens to estrogens; 1st gen aromatase inhib **Dose:** Initial 250 mg PO 4× d, titrate q1–2wk max 2 g/d; w/ hydrocortisone 20–40 mg/d; ↓ w/ renal Insuff **W/P:** [D, ?] **Disp:** Tabs 250 mg **SE:** Adrenal Insuff ("medical adrenalectomy"), hypothy-roidism, masculinization, ↓ BP, N/V, rare hepatotox, rash, myalgia, fever, drowsi-ness, lethargy, anorexia **Notes:** Give q6h to ↓ N

Aminophylline (Generic) **Uses:** *Asthma, COPD* & bronchospasm **Acts:** Relaxes smooth muscle (bronchi, pulm vessels); stimulates diaphragm **Dose:** *Adults. Acute asthma:* Load 6 mg/kg IV, then 0.4–0.9 mg/kg/h IV cont Inf, not > than 25 mg/min *Chronic asthma:* 24 mg/kg/24 h PO ÷ q6h *Peds.* Load 6 mg/kg IV, then 6 wk–6 mo 0.5 mg/kg/h, 6 mo–1 y 0.6–0.7 mg/kg/h, 1–9 y 1 mg/kg/h IV Inf; ↓ w/ hepatic Insuff & w/ some drugs (macrolide & quinolone antibiotics, cimetidine, propranolol) **W/P:** [C, +] Uncontrolled arrhythmias, HTN, Sz disorder, hyperthy-roidism, peptic ulcers **Disp:** Tabs 100, 200 mg; ER tabs 100, 200 mg, soln 105 mg/5 mL, Inj 25 mg/mL **SE:** N/V, irritability, tachycardia, ventricular arrhyth-mias, Szs **Notes:** Individualize dosage *Level:* 10 to 20 mcg/mL *Toxic:* > 20 mcg/ mL; aminophylline 85% theophylline; erratic rectal absorption

Amiodarone (Cordarone, Nexterone, Pacerone) **BOX:** Liver tox, exacerbation of arrhythmias and lung damage reported **Uses:** *Recurrent VF or unstable VT*, supraventricular arrhythmias, AF **Acts:** Class III antiarrhythmic (Table 9, p 301) **Dose:** *Adults. Ventricular arrhythmias:* IV: 15 mg/min × 10 min, then 1 mg/min × 6 h, maint 0.5-mg/min cont Inf or *PO:* Load: 800–1600 mg/d PO × 1–3 wk Maint: 600–800 mg/d PO for 1 mo, then 200–400 mg/d *Supraventricular arrhythmias: IV:* 300 mg IV over 1 h, then 20 mg/kg for 24 h, then 600 mg PO daily for 1 wk; maint 100–400 mg daily or *PO:* Load 600–800 mg/d PO for 1–4 wk *Maint:* Slow ↓ to 100–400 mg daily *ECC 2010. VF/VT cardiac arrest refractory to CPR, shock and pressor:* 300 mg IV/IO push; can give additional 150 mg IV/IO once; *Life-threatening arrhythmias:* Max dose: 2.2 g IV/24 h; rapid inf: 150 mg IV over first 10 min (15 mg/min); can repeat 150 mg IV q10 min PRN; slow inf: 360 mg

IV over 60 min (1 mg/min); maint: 540 mg IV over 18 h (0.5 mg/min) *Peds.* 10–15 mg/kg/24 h ÷ q12h PO for 7–10 d, then 5 mg/kg/24 h ÷ q12h or daily (infants require ↑ loading); *ECC 2010. Pulseless VT/Refractory VF:* 5 mg/kg IV/IO bolus, repeat PRN to 15 mg/kg (2.2 g in adolescents)/24 h; max single dose 300 mg; *Perfusing SVT/Ventricular arrhythmias:* 5 mg/kg IV/IO load over 20–60 min; repeat PRN to 15 mg/kg (2.2 g in adolescents)/24h **W/P:** [D, –] May require ↓ digoxin/warfarin dose, ↓ w/ liver insuff; many drug interactions **CI:** Sinus node dysfunction, 2nd-/3rd-degree AV block, sinus brady (w/o pacemaker), iodine sensitivity **Disp:** Tabs 100, 200, 400 mg; Inj 50 mg/mL **SE:** Pulm fibrosis, exacerbation of arrhythmias, ↑ QT interval; CHF, hypo-/hyperthyroidism, ↑ LFTs, liver failure, corneal microdeposits, optic neuropathy/neuritis, peripheral neuropathy, photosens; blue skin **Notes:** IV conc > 2.0 mg/mL central line only *Levels: Trough:* just before next dose *Therapeutic:* 1–2.5 mcg/mL *Toxic:* > 2.5 mcg/mL *1/2-life:* 30–100 h

Amitriptyline (Elavil)   BOX: Antidepressants may ↑ suicide risk; consider risks/benefits of use. Monitor pts closely **Uses:** *Depression (not bipolar depression)* peripheral neuropathy, chronic pain, tension HAs **Acts:** TCA; ↓ reuptake of serotonin & norepinephrine by presynaptic neurons **Dose:** *Adults.* Initial: 30–50 mg PO hs; may ↑ to 300 mg tis. *Peds.* Not OK < 12 y unless for chronic pain *Initial:* 0.1 mg/kg PO hs, ↑ over 2–3 wk to 0.5–2 mg/kg PO hs; taper to D/C **W/P:** CV Dz, Szs [D,+/–] NAG, hepatic impair **CI:** w/ MAOIs or w/in 14 d of use, during acute MI recovery **Disp:** Tabs 10, 25, 50, 75, 100, 150 mg; Inj 10 mg/mL **SE:** Strong anticholinergic SEs; OD may be fatal; urine retention, sedation, ECG changes, photosens **Notes:** Levels: *Therapeutic:* 120 to 150 ng/mL *Toxic:* > 500 ng/mL; levels may not correlate w/ effect

Amlodipine (Norvasc)   Uses: *HTN, stable or unstable angina* **Acts:** CCB; relaxes coronary vascular smooth muscle **Dose:** 2.5–10 mg/d PO; ↓ w/ hepatic impair **W/P:** [C, ?] **Disp:** Tabs 2.5, 5, 10 mg **SE:** Edema, HA, palpitations, flushing, dizziness **Notes:** Take w/o regard to meals

Amlodipine/Atorvastatin (Caduet)   Uses: *HTN, chronic stable/vasospastic angina, control cholesterol & triglycerides* **Acts:** CCB & HMG-CoA reductase inhib **Dose:** Amlodipine 2.5–10 mg w/ atorvastatin 10–80 mg PO daily **W/P:** [X, –] **CI:** Active liver Dz, ↑ LFTs **Disp:** Tabs amlodipine/atorvastatin: 2.5/10, 2.5/20, 2.5/40, 5/10, 5/20, 5/40, 5/80, 10/10, 10/20, 10/40, 10/80 mg **SE:** Edema, HA, palpitations, flushing, myopathy, arthralgia, myalgia, GI upset, liver failure **Notes:** ✓ LFTs; instruct pt to report muscle pain/weakness

Amlodipine/Olmesartan (Azor)   BOX: Use of renin-angiotensin agents in PRG can cause injury and death to fetus, D/C immediately when PRG detected **Uses:** *Hypertension* **Acts:** CCB w/ angiotensin II receptor blocker **Dose:** *Adults.* Initial 2 mg/20 mg, max 10 mg/40 mg q day **W/P:** [C 1st tri, D 2nd, 3rd tri, –] w/ K+ supl or K+-sparing diuretics, renal impair, RAS, severe CAD, AS **CI:** PRG **Disp:** Tabs amlodipine/olmesartan 5 mg/20 mg, 10/20, 5/40, 10/40 **SE:** Edema, vertigo, dizziness, ↓ BP

Amlodipine/Valsartan (Exforge) BOX: Use of renin-angiotensin agents in PRG can cause fetal injury and death, D/C immediately when PRG detected Uses: * ↑ BP not controlled on single med* Acts: CCB w/ angiotensin II receptor blocker Dose: *Adults.* Initial 5 mg/160 mg, may ↑ after 1–2 wk, max 10 mg/320 mg q day, start elderly at 1/2 initial dose W/P: [C 1st tri, D 2nd, 3rd tri, –] w/ K⁺ supl or K⁺-sparing diuretics, renal impair, RAS, severe CAD CI: PRG, Disp: Tabs amlodipine/valsartan 5/160, 10/160, 5/320, 10 mg/320 mg SE: Edema, vertigo, nasopharyngitis, URI, dizziness, ↓ BP

Amlodipine/Valsartan/HCTZ (Exforge HCT) BOX: Use of renin-angiotensin agents in PRG can cause fetal injury and death, D/C immediately when PRG detected Uses: *Hypertension* Acts: CCB, angiotensin II receptor blocker, & thiazide diuretic Dose: 1 tab 1 × daily, may ↑ dose after 2 wk; max dose 10/320/25 mg W/P: [D, –] w/ Severe hepatic or renal impair CI: Anuria, sulfonamide allergy Disp: Tabs amlodipine/valsartan/HCTZ: 5/160/12.5, 10/160/12.5, 5/160/25, 10/160/25, 10/320/25 mg SE: edema, dizziness, headache, fatigue, nasopharyngitis, dyspepsia, N, back pain, muscle spasm, ↓ BP

Ammonium Aluminum Sulfate [Alum] [OTC] Uses: *Hemorrhagic cystitis when saline bladder irrigation fails* Acts: Astringent Dose: 1–2% soln w/ constant NS bladder irrigation W/P: [+/–] Disp: Powder for recons SE: Encephalopathy possible; ✓ aluminum levels, especially w/ renal Insuff; can precipitate & occlude catheters Notes: Safe w/o anesthesia & w/ vesicoureteral reflux

Amoxicillin (Amoxil, Polymox) Uses: *Ear, nose, & throat, lower resp, skin, urinary tract Infxns from susceptible gram(+) bacteria* endocarditis prophylaxis, *H. pylori* eradication w/ other agents (gastric ulcers) Acts: β-Lactam antibiotic; ↓ cell wall synth Spectrum: Gram(+) (*Streptococcus* sp, *Enterococcus* sp); some gram(−) (*H. influenzae, E. coli, N. gonorrhoeae, H. pylori, & P. mirabilis*) Dose: *Adults.* 250–500 mg PO tid or 500–875 mg bid Peds. 25–100 mg/kg/24 h PO ÷ q8h, 200–400 mg PO bid (equivalent to 125–250 mg tid); ↓ in renal impair W/P: [B, +] Disp: Caps 250, 500 mg; chew tabs 125, 200, 250, 400 mg; susp 50 mg/mL, 125, 200, 250, & 400 mg/5 mL; tabs 500, 875 mg SE: D; rash Notes: Cross hypersens w/ PCN; many *E. coli* strains resistant; chew tabs contain phenylalanine

Amoxicillin & Clavulanic Acid (Augmentin, Augmentin 600 ES, Augmentin XR) Uses: *Ear, lower resp, sinus, urinary tract, skin Infxns caused by β-lactamase–producing H. influenzae, S. aureus, & E. coli* Acts: β-Lactam antibiotic w/ β-lactamase inhib Spectrum: Gram(+) same as amoxicillin alone, MSSA; gram(−) as w/ amoxicillin alone, β-lactamase–producing *H. influenzae, Klebsiella* sp, *M. catarrhalis* Dose: *Adults.* 250–500 mg PO q8h or 875 mg q12h; XR 2000 mg PO q12h Peds. 20–40 mg/kg/d as amoxicillin PO ÷ q8h or 45 mg/kg/d ÷ q12h; ↓ in renal impair; take w/ food W/P: [B, enters breast milk] Disp: Supplied (as amoxicillin/clavulanic): Tabs 250/125, 500/125, 875/125 mg; chew tabs 125/31.25, 200/28.5, 250/62.5, 400/57 mg; susp 125/31.25, 250/62.5,

200/28.5, 400/57 mg/5 mL; susp ES 600/42.9 mg/5 mL; XR tab 1000/62.5 mg **SE:** Abd discomfort, N/V/D, allergic Rxn, vaginitis **Notes:** Do not substitute two 250-mg tabs for one 500-mg tab (possible OD of clavulanic acid); max clavulanic acid 125 mg/dose

Amphotericin B (Amphocin, Fungizone)
Uses: *Severe, systemic fungal Infxns; oral & cutaneous candidiasis* **Acts:** Binds ergosterol in the fungal membrane to alter permeability **Dose:** **Adults & Peds.** *Test dose:* 1 mg IV adults or 0.1 mg/kg to 1 mg IV in children; then 0.25–1.5 mg/kg/24 h IV over 2–6 h (25–50 mg/d or q other day). Total varies w/ indication *PO:* 1 mL qid **W/P:** [B, ?] **Disp:** Powder (Inj) 50 mg/vial **SE:** ↓ K⁺/Mg²⁺ from renal wasting; anaphylaxis, HA, fever, chills, nephrotox, ↓ BP, anemia, rigors **Notes:** ✓ Cr/LFTs/K⁺/Mg²⁺; ↓ in renal impair; pretreatment w/ APAP & antihistamines (*Benadryl*) ↓ SE

Amphotericin B Cholesteryl (Amphotec)
Uses: *Aspergillosis if intolerant/refractory to conventional amphotericin B*, systemic candidiasis **Acts:** Binds ergosterol in fungal membrane, alters permeability **Dose:** **Adults & Peds.** *Test dose:* 1.6–8.3 mg, over 15–20 min, then 3–4 mg/kg/d; 1 mg/kg/h Inf, 7.5 mg/kg/d max; ↓ w/ renal Insuff **W/P:** [B, ?] **Disp:** Powder for Inj 50, 100 mg/vial **SE:** Anaphylaxis; fever, chills, HA, ↓ K⁺, ↓ Mg²⁺, nephrotox, ↓ BP, anemia **Notes:** Do not use in-line filter; ✓ LFTs/lytes

Amphotericin B Lipid Complex (Abelcet)
Uses: *Refractory invasive fungal Infxn in pts intolerant to conventional amphotericin B* **Acts:** Binds ergosterol in fungal membrane, alters permeability **Dose:** **Adults & Peds.** 5 mg/kg/d IV × 1 daily **W/P:** [B, ?] **Disp:** Inj 5 mg/mL **SE:** Anaphylaxis; fever, chills, HA, ↓ K⁺, ↓ Mg²⁺, nephrotox, ↓ BP, anemia **Notes:** Filter w/ 5-micron needle; do not mix in electrolyte containing solns; if Inf > 2 h, manually mix bag

Amphotericin B Liposomal (AmBisome)
Uses: *Refractory invasive fungal Infxn w/ intolerance to conventional amphotericin B; cryptococcal meningitis in HIV; empiric for febrile neutropenia; visceral leishmaniasis* **Acts:** Binds ergosterol in fungal membrane, alters membrane permeability **Dose:** **Adults & Peds.** 3–6 mg/kg/d, Inf 60–120 min; varies by indication; ↓ in renal Insuff **W/P:** [B, ?] **Disp:** Powder Inj 50 mg **SE:** Anaphylaxis, fever, chills, HA, ↓ K⁺, ↓ Mg²⁺ nephrotox, ↓ BP, anemia **Notes:** Do not use < 1-micron filter

Ampicillin (Amcill, Omnipen)
Uses: *Resp, GU, or GI tract Infxns, meningitis d/t gram(−) & (+) bacteria; SBE prophylaxis* **Acts:** β-Lactam antibiotic; ↓ cell wall synth **Spectrum:** Gram(+) (*Streptococcus* sp, *Staphylococcus* sp, *Listeria*); gram(−) (*Klebsiella* sp, *E. coli, H. influenzae, P. mirabilis, Shigella* sp, *Salmonella* sp) **Dose:** **Adults.** 500 mg–2 g IM or IV q6h or 250–500 mg PO q6h; varies by indication **Peds Neonates < 7 d.** 50–100 mg/kg/24 h ÷ q8h IM or IV **Term infants.** 75–150 mg/kg/24 h ÷ q6–8h IV or PO **Children > 1 mo.** 100–200 mg/kg/24 h ÷ q4–6h IM or IV; 50–100 mg/kg/24 h ÷ q6h PO up to 250 mg/dose **Meningitis:** 200–400 mg/kg/24 h ÷ q4–6h IV; ↓ w/ renal impair; take on empty stomach **W/P:** [B, M] Cross-hypersens w/ PCN **Disp:** Caps 250, 500 mg; susp 100 mg/mL

(reconstituted drops), 125 mg/5 mL, 250 mg/5 mL; powder (Inj) 125, 250, 500 mg, 1, 2, 10 g/vial **SE:** D, rash, allergic Rxn **Notes:** Many *E. coli* resistant

Ampicillin–Sulbactam (Unasyn) **Uses:** *Gynecologic, intra-Abd, skin Infxns d/t β-lactamase–producing S. aureus, Enterococcus, H. influenzae, P. mirabilis, & Bacteroides sp* **Acts:** β-Lactam antibiotic & β-lactamase inhib *Spectrum:* Gram(+) & (−) as for amp alone; also *Enterobacter, Acinetobacter, Bacteroides* **Dose:** **Adults.** 1.5–3 g IM or IV q6h **Peds.** 100–400 mg ampicillin/kg/d (150–300 mg Unasyn) q6h; ↓ w/ renal Insuff **W/P:** [B, M] **Disp:** Powder for Inj 1.5, 3 g/vial, 15 g bulk package **SE:** Allergic Rxns, rash, D, Inj site pain **Notes:** A 2:1 ratio ampicillin:sulbactam

Anakinra (Kineret) **BOX:** Associated w/ ↑ incidence of serious Infxn; D/C w/ serious Infxn **Uses:** *Reduce S/Sxs of mod/severe active RA, failed 1 or more DMARD* **Acts:** Human IL-1 receptor antagonist **Dose:** 100 mg SQ daily; w/ CrCl < 30 mL/min, q other day **W/P:** [B, ?] **CI:** *E. coli*-derived protein allergy, active Infxn, < 18 y **Disp:** 100-mg prefilled syringes; 100 mg (0.67 mL/vial) **SE:** ↓ WBC especially w/ TNF-blockers, Inj site Rxn (may last up to 28 d), Infxn, N/D, Abd pain, flu-like sx, HA

Anastrozole (Arimidex) **Uses:** *Breast CA: postmenopausal w/ metastatic breast CA, adjuvant Rx postmenopausal early hormone-receptor(+) breast CA* **Acts:** Selective nonsteroidal aromatase inhib, ↓ circulatory estradiol **Dose:** 1 mg/d **W/P:** [D, ?] **CI:** PRG **Disp:** Tabs 1 mg **SE:** May ↑ cholesterol; N/V/D, HTN, flushing, ↑ bone/tumor pain, HA, somnolence, mood disturbance, depression, rash **Notes:** No effect on adrenal steroids or aldosterone

Anidulafungin (Eraxis) **Uses:** *Candidemia, esophageal candidiasis, other Candida Infxn (peritonitis, intra-Abd abscess)* **Acts:** Echinocandin; ↓ cell wall synth *Spectrum: C. albicans, C. glabrata, C. parapsilosis, C. tropicalis* **Dose:** Candidemia, others: 200 mg IV × 1, then 100 mg IV daily [Tx ≥14 d after last (+)culture]; Esophageal candidiasis: 100 mg IV × 1, then 50 mg IV daily (Tx > 14 d and 7 d after resolution of Sx); 1.1 mg/min max Inf rate **W/P:** [C, ?/–] **CI:** Echinocandin hypersens **Disp:** Powder 50, 100 mg/vial **SE:** Histamine-mediated Inf Rxns (urticaria, flushing, ↓ BP, dyspnea, etc), fever, N/V/D, ↑ K⁺, HA, ↑ LFTs, hep, worsening hepatic failure **Notes:** ↓ Inf rate to < 1.1 mg/min w/ Inf Rxns

Anistreplase (Eminase) **Uses:** *AMI* **Acts:** Thrombolytic; activates conversion of plasminogen to plasmin, ↑ thrombolysis **Dose:** *ECC 2010.* **ACS:** 30 units IV over 2–5 min **W/P:** [C, ?] **CI:** Active internal bleeding, Hx CVA, recent (< 2 mo) intracranial or intraspinal surgery/trauma/neoplasm, AVM, aneurysm, bleeding diathesis, severe HTN **Disp:** 30 units/vial **SE:** Bleeding, ↓ BP, hematoma **Notes:** Ineffective if readministered > 5 d after the previous dose of anistreplase or streptokinase, or streptococcal Infxn (production of antistreptokinase Ab)

Anthralin (Anthra-Derm) **Uses:** *Psoriasis* **Acts:** Keratolytic **Dose:** Apply daily **W/P:** [C, ?] **CI:** Acutely inflamed psoriatic eruptions, erythroderma **Disp:** Cream, oint 0.1, 0.25, 0.4, 0.5, 1% **SE:** Irritation; hair/fingernails/skin discoloration

Antihemophilic Factor [AHF, Factor VIII] (Monoclate) Uses: *Classic hemophilia A, von Willebrand Dz* Acts: Provides factor VIII needed to convert prothrombin to thrombin Dose: *Adults & Peds.* 1 AHF unit/kg ↑ factor VIII level by 2 Int Unit/dL; units required = (wgt in kg) (desired factor VIII ↑ as % nl) × (0.5); prevent spontaneous hemorrhage = 5% nl; hemostasis after trauma/surgery = 30% nl; head injuries, major surgery, or bleeding = 80–100% nl W/P: [C, ?] Disp: ✓ each vial for units contained, powder for recons SE: Rash, fever, HA, chills, N/V Notes: Determine ✓ nl factor VIII before dosing

Antihemophilic Factor (Recombinant) (Xyntha) Uses: *Control/prevent bleeding & surgical prophylaxis in hemophilia A* Acts: ↑ Levels of factor VIII Dose: *Adults.* Required units = body wgt (kg) × desired factor VIII rise (Int Units/dL or % of nl) × 0.5 (Int Units/kg per Int Units/dL); frequency/duration determined by type of bleed (see PI) W/P: [C, ?/–] Severe hypersens Rxn possible CI: None Disp: Inj powder: 250, 500, 1000, 2000 Int Units SE: HA, fever, N/V/D, weakness, allergic Rxn Notes: Monitor for the development of factor VIII neutralizing antibodies

Antithrombin, Recombinant (Atryn) Uses: * Prevent peri-op/peri-partum thromboembolic events w/ hereditary antithrombin (AT) deficiency* Acts: Inhibits thrombin and factor Xa Dose: *Adults.* Based on pre-Rx AT level, BW (kg) and drug monitoring; see package. Goal AT levels 0.8–1.2 IU/mL W/P: [C, +/–] Hypersensitivity Rxns; ↑ effect of heparin/LMWH CI: Hypersens to goat/goat milk proteins Disp: Powder 1750 IU/vial SE: Bleeding, infusion site Rxn Notes: ✓aPTT and anti-factor Xa; monitor for bleeding or thrombosis

Antithymocyte Globulin (See Lymphocyte Immune Globulin, p 172)

Apomorphine (Apokyn) BOX: Do not administer IV Uses: *Acute, intermittent hypomobility ("off") episodes of Parkinson Dz* Acts: Dopamine agonist Dose: *Adults.* 0.2 mL SQ supervised test dose; if BP OK, initial 0.2 mL (2 mg) SQ during "off" periods; only 1 dose per "off" period; titrate dose; 0.6 mL (6 mg) max single doses; use w/ antiemetic; ↓ in renal impair W/P: [C, +/–] Avoid EtOH; antihypertensives, vasodilators, cardio-/cerebrovascular Dz, hepatic impair CI: 5-HT₃ antagonists, sulfite allergy Disp: Inj 10 mg/mL, 3-mL pen cartridges; 2-mL amp SE: Emesis, syncope, ↑ QT, orthostatic ↓ BP, somnolence, ischemia, Inj site Rxn, abuse potential, dyskinesia, fibrotic conditions, priapism, chest pain/angina, yawning, rhinorrhea Notes: Daytime somnolence may limit activities; trimethobenzamide 300 mg tid PO or other non–5-HT₃ antagonist antiemetic given 3 d prior to & up to 2 mo following initiation

Apraclonidine (Iopidine) Uses: *Glaucoma, intraocular HTN* Acts: α₂-Adrenergic agonist Dose: 1–2 gtt of 0.5% tid; 1 gtt of 1% before and after surgical procedure W/P: [C, ?] CI: w/in 14 d of or w/ MAOI Disp: 0.5, 1% soln SE: Ocular irritation, lethargy, xerostomia

Aprepitant (Emend, Oral) Uses: *Prevents N/V associated w/ emetogenic CA chemotherapy (e.g., cisplatin) (use in combo w/ other antiemetics)*, postop N/V Acts: Substance P/neurokinin 1 (NK₁) receptor antagonist Dose: 125 mg PO day 1, 1 h before chemotherapy, then 80 mg PO qam days 2 & 3; postop N/V: 40 mg w/in 3 h of induction W/P: [B, ?/–]; substrate & mod CYP3A4 inhib; CYP2C9 inducer (Table 10, p 301); ↓ Effect OCP and warfarin CI: Use w/ pimozide Disp: Caps 40, 80, 125 mg SE: Fatigue, asthenia, hiccups Notes: See also fosaprepitant (Emend, Injection)

Apriso (Salix) Uses: *Maintenance of UC remission* Acts: Locally acting aminosalicylate Dose: 1.5 g (0.375 g caps × 4) PO daily in am; not w/ antacids W/P: [B, ±] May cause renal impair, exacerbation of colitis CI: Hypersens to salicylates/aminosalicylates Disp: Caps ER 0.375 g SE: HA, N/D, Abd pain, nasopharyngitis, influenza, sinusitis, acute intolerance synd Notes: for PKU patients, product contains aspartame; monitor CBC, SCr

Arformoterol (Brovana) BOX: Long-acting β₂-adrenergic agonists may increase the risk of asthma-related death. Use only for pts not adequately controlled on other asthma-controller meds Uses: *Maint in COPD* Acts: Selective LA β₂-adrenergic agonist Dose: Adults. 15 mcg bid nebulization W/P: [C, ?] CI: Hypersens Disp: Soln 15 mcg/2 mL SE: Pain, back pain, CP, D, sinusitis, nervousness, palpitations, allergic Rxn Notes: Not for acute bronchospasm. Refrigerate, use immediately after opening

Argatroban (Acova) Uses: *Prevent/Tx thrombosis in HIT, PCI in pts w/ HIT risk* Acts: Anticoagulant, direct thrombin inhib Dose: 2 mcg/kg/min IV; adjust until aPTT 1.5–3 × baseline not to exceed 100 s; 10 mcg/kg/min max; ↓ w/ hepatic impair W/P: [B, ?] Avoid PO anticoagulants; ↑ bleeding risk; avoid use w/ thrombolytics CI: Overt major bleed Disp: Inj 100 mg/mL SE: AF, cardiac arrest, cerebrovascular disorder, ↓ BP, VT, N/V/D, sepsis, cough, renal tox, ↓ Hgb Note: Steady state in 1–3 h; ✓ aPTT w/ Inf start and after each dose change

Aripiprazole (Abilify, Abilify Discmelt) BOX: Increased mortality in elderly w/ dementia-related psychosis; ↑ suicidal thinking in children, adolescents, and young adults w/ MDD Uses: *Schizophrenia adults and peds 13–17 y, mania or mixed episodes associated w/ bipolar disorder, MDD in adults, agitation w/ schizophrenia* Acts: Dopamine & serotonin antagonist Dose: Adults. Schizophrenia: 10–15 mg PO/d Acute agitation: 9.75 mg/1.3 mL IM Bipolar: 15 mg/d; MDD adjunct w/ other antidepressants initial 2 mg/d, 10 mg/d OK Peds. Schizophrenia: 13–17 y: Start 2 mg/d, usual 10 mg/d; max 30 mg/d for all adult and peds uses; ↓ dose w/ CYP3A4/CYP2D6 inhib (Table 10, p 301); ↑ dose w/ CYP3A4 inducer W/P: [C, –] w/ Low WBC Disp: Tabs 2, 5, 10, 15, 20, 30 mg; Discmelt (disintegrating tabs 10, 15, 20, 30 mg), soln 1 mg/mL, Inj 7.5 mg/mL SE: Neuroleptic malignant synd, tardive dyskinesia, orthostatic ↓ BP, cognitive & motor impair, ↑ glucose, leukopenia, neutropenia, and agranulocytosis Notes: Discmelt contains phenylalanine; monitor CBC

Armodafinil (Nuvigil) Uses: *Narcolepsy, SWSD, and OSAHS* Acts: ?; binds dopamine receptor, ↓ dopamine reuptake Dose: *Adults. OSAHS/narcolepsy:* 150 or 250 mg PO daily in AM *SWSD:* 150 mg PO q day 1 h prior to start of shift; ↓ w/ hepatic impair; adjust w/ substrates for CYP3A4/5, CYP2C19 W/P: [C, ?] CI: Hypersens to modafinil/armodafinil Disp: Tabs 50, 150, 200 mg SE: HA, N, dizziness, insomnia, xerostomia, rash including SJS, angioedema, anaphylactoid Rxns, multiorgan hypersens Rxns

Artemether & Lumefantrine (Coartem) Uses: *Acute, uncomplicated malaria (P. falciparum)* Action: Antiprotozoal/Antimalarial Dose: *Adults > 16 y. 25–< 35 kg:* 3 tabs hour 0 & 8 day 1, then 3 tabs bid day 2 & 3 (18 tabs/course) ≥ 35 kg: 4 tabs hour 0 & 8 day 1, then 4 tabs bid day 2 & 3 (24 tabs/course) *Peds. 2 mo to < 16 y. 5–< 15 kg:* 1 tab at hour 0 & 8 day 1, then 1 tab bid day 2 & 3 (6 tabs/course) *15–< 25 kg:* 2 tabs hour 0 & 8 day 1, then 2 tabs bid day 2 & 3 (12 tabs/course) *25–< 35 kg:* 3 tabs at hour 0 & 8 day 1, then 3 tabs bid on day 2 & 3 (18 tabs/course) ≥ 35 kg: See Adult dose W/P: [C, ?] ↑ QT, hepatic/renal impair, CYP3A4 inhib CI: Component hypersens Disp: Tabs artemether 20 mg/lumefantrine 120 mg SE: Palp, HA, dizziness, chills, sleep disturb, fatigue, anorexia, N/V/D, Abd pain, weakness, arthralgia, myalgia, cough, splenomegaly, hepatomegaly, ↑ AST, ↑ QT Notes: Not rec w/ other agents that ↑ QT

Artificial Tears (Tears Naturale) [OTC] Uses: *Dry eyes* Acts: Ocular lubricant Dose: 1–2 gtt tid-qid Disp: OTC soln SE: mild stinging, temp blurred vision

L-Asparaginase (Elspar, Oncaspar) Uses: *ALL* (in combo w/ other agents) Acts: Protein synth inhib Dose: 500–20,000 Int Units/m²/d for 1–14 d (per protocols) W/P: [C, ?] CI: Active/Hx pancreatitis; Hx of allergic Rxn, thrombosis or hemorrhagic event w/ prior Rx w/ asparaginase Disp: Powder (Inj) 10,000 units/vial SE: Allergy 20–35% (urticaria to anaphylaxis); fever, chills, N/V, anorexia, Abd cramps, depression, agitation, Sz, pancreatitis, ↑ glucose or LFTs, coagulopathy Notes: Test dose OK, ✓ glucose, coagulation studies, LFTs

Asenapine Maleate (Saphris) BOX: ↑Mortality in elderly w/ dementia-related psychosis Uses: *Schizophrenia; manic/mixed bipolar disorder* Acts: Dopamine/serotonin antagonist Dose: *Adults. Schizophrenia:* 5 mg twice daily; *Bipolar disorder:* 10 mg twice daily W/P: [C, ?/–] Disp: SL Tabs 5, 10 mg SE: Dizziness, somnolence, akathisia, oral hypoesthesia, EPS, ↑ weight, ↑ glucose, ↓ BP, ↑ QT interval, hyperprolactinemia, ↓ WBC, neuroleptic malignant syndrome, severe allergic Rxns Notes: Do not swallow/crush/chew tab; avoid eating/drinking 10 min after dose

Aspirin (Bayer, Ecotrin, St. Joseph's) [OTC] Uses: *Angina, CABG, PTCA, carotid endarterectomy, ischemic stroke, TIA, ACS/MI, arthritis, pain*, HA, *fever*, inflammation, Kawasaki Dz Acts: Prostaglandin inhib by COX-2 inhib Dose: *Adults. Pain, fever:* 325–650 mg q4–6h PO or PR (4 g/d max) *RA:* 3–6 g/d PO in ÷ doses; *Plt inhib:* 81–325 mg PO daily; *Prevent MI:* 81 (preferred)–325 mg PO daily; *ECC 2010. ACS:* 160–325 mg nonenteric coated PO ASAP (chewing preferred at ACS onset) **Peds.** *Antipyretic:* 10–15 mg/kg/dose PO or PR q4–6h up to 80 mg/kg/24 h *RA:* 60–100 mg/kg/24 h PO ÷ q4–6h (levels 15–30 mg/dL); *Kawasaki Dz:* 80–100 mg/kg/d ÷ q6h, 3–5 mg/kg/d after fever resolves; for all uses 4 g/d max; avoid w/ CrCl < 10 mL/min, severe liver Dz **W/P:** [C, M] Related to Reye synd; avoid w/ viral illness in peds < 18 y **CI:** Allergy to ASA, chicken-pox/flu Sxs, synd of nasal polyps, angioedema, & bronchospasm to NSAIDs **Disp:** Tabs 325, 500 mg; chew tabs 81 mg; EC tabs 81, 162, 325, 500, 650, 975 mg; SR tabs 650, 800 mg; effervescent tabs 325, 500 mg; supp 125, 200, 300, 600 mg **SE:** GI upset, erosion, & bleeding **Notes:** D/C 1 wk preop; avoid/limit EtOH; Salicy-late levels: *Therapeutic:* 100–250 mcg/mL *Toxic:* > 300 mcg/mL

Aspirin & Butalbital Compound (Fiorinal) [C-III] Uses: *Tension HA*, pain **Acts:** Barbiturate w/ analgesic **Dose:** 1–2 PO q4h PRN, max 6 tabs/d; avoid w/ CrCl < 10 mL/min or severe liver Dz **W/P:** [C (D w/ prolonged use or high doses at term), ?] **CI:** ASA allergy, GI ulceration, bleeding disorder, porphy-ria, synd of nasal polyps, angioedema, & bronchospasm to NSAIDs **Disp:** Caps (*Fiorgen PF, Lanorinal*), Tabs (*Lanorinal*) ASA 325 mg/butalbital 50 mg/caffeine 40 mg **SE:** Drowsiness, dizziness, GI upset, ulceration, bleeding **Notes:** Butalbital habit-forming; D/C 1 wk prior to surgery, avoid or limit EtOH

Aspirin + Butalbital, Caffeine, & Codeine (Fiorinal + Codeine) [C-III] Uses: Mild *pain*, HA, especially tension HA w/ stress **Acts:** Sedative and narcotic analgesic **Dose:** 1–2 tabs/caps PO q4–6h PRN max 6/d **W/P:** [C, ?] **CI:** Allergy to ASA and codeine; synd of nasal polyps, angioedema, & bronchos-pasm to NSAIDs, bleeding diathesis, peptic ulcer or sig GI lesions, porphyria **Disp:** Caps/tabs contains 325 mg ASA, 40 mg caffeine, 50 mg butalbital, 30 mg codeine **SE:** Drowsiness, dizziness, GI upset, ulceration, bleeding **Notes:** D/C 1 wk prior to surgery, avoid/limit EtOH

Aspirin + Codeine (Empirin No. 3, 4) [C-III] Uses: Mild–*mod pain*, symptomatic nonproductive cough **Acts:** Combined effects of ASA & codeine **Dose:** *Adults.* 1–2 tabs PO q4–6h PRN *Peds.* ASA 10 mg/kg/dose; codeine 0.5–1 mg/kg/dose q4h **W/P:** [D, M] **CI:** Allergy to ASA/codeine, PUD, bleeding, anticoagulant Rx, children w/ chickenpox or flu Sxs, synd of nasal polyps, angioedema, & bronchospasm to NSAIDs **Disp:** Tabs 325 mg of ASA & codeine (codeine in No. 3 = 30 mg, No. 4 = 60 mg) **SE:** Drowsiness, dizziness, GI upset, ulceration, bleeding **Notes:** D/C 1 wk prior to surgery; avoid/limit EtOH

Atazanavir (Reyataz) BOX: Hyperbilirubinemia may require drug D/C Uses: *HIV-1 Infxn* **Acts:** Protease inhib **Dose:** Antiretroviral naïve 400 mg PO daily w/ food; experienced pts 300 mg w/ ritonavir 100 mg; when given w/ efa-virenz 600 mg, administer atazanavir 300 mg + ritonavir 100 mg once/d; separate doses from didanosine; ↓ w/ hepatic impair **W/P:** CDC rec: HIV-infected mothers not breast-feed [B, –]; ↑ levels of statins (avoid use) sildenafil, antiarrhythmics, warfarin, cyclosporine, TCAs; ↓ w/ St. John's wort, H$_2$-receptor antagonists; do not use w/salmeterol, colchicine (w/renal/hepatic failure); adjust dose w/ bosentan, tadalafil for PAH **CI:** w/ Midazolam, triazolam, ergots, pimozide, alpha 1-adreno-receptor antagonist (alfuzosin), PDE5 inhibitor sildenafil **Disp:** Caps 100, 150, 200, 300 mg **SE:** HA, N/V/D, rash, Abd pain, DM, photosens, ↑ PR interval **Notes:** May have less-adverse effect on cholesterol; if given w/ H_2 blocker, give together or at least 10 h after H_2; if given w/ proton pump inhib, separate by 12 h; concurrent use not OK in experienced pts

Atenolol (Tenormin) Uses: *HTN, angina, MI* Acts: selective β-adrenergic receptor blocker **Dose:** *HTN & angina:* 50–100 mg/d PO *ECC 2010. AMI:* 5 mg IV over 5 min; in 10 min, 5 mg slow IV; if tolerated in 10 min, start 50 mg PO, titrate; ↓ in renal impair **W/P:** [D, M] DM, bronchospasm; abrupt D/C can exacerbate angina & ↑ MI risk **CI:** ↓ HR, cardiogenic shock, cardiac failure, 2nd-/3rd-degree AV block, sinus node dysfunction, pulm edema **Disp:** Tabs 25, 50, 100 mg; Inj 5 mg/10 mL **SE:** ↓ HR, ↓ BP, 2nd-/3rd-degree AV block, dizziness, fatigue

Atenolol & Chlorthalidone (Tenoretic) Uses: *HTN* Acts: β-Adrenergic blockade w/ diuretic **Dose:** 50–100 mg/d PO based on atenolol; ↓ dose w/ CrCl < 35 mL/min **W/P:** [D, M] DM, bronchospasm **CI:** See Atenolol; anuria, sulfonamide cross-sensitivity **Disp:** *Tenoretic 50:* Atenolol 50 mg/chlorthalidone 25 mg *Tenoretic 100:* Atenolol 100 mg/chlorthalidone 25 mg **SE:** ↓ HR, ↓ BP, 2nd-/3rd-degree AV block, dizziness, fatigue, ↓ K^+, photosens

Atomoxetine (Strattera) BOX: Severe liver injury may rarely occur; DC w/ jaundice or ↑ LFTs, ↑ frequency of suicidal thinking; monitor closely Uses: *ADHD* Acts: Selective norepinephrine reuptake inhib **Dose:** *Adults & children > 70 kg:* 40 mg PO/d, after 3 d minimum, ↑ to 80–100 mg ÷ daily-bid *Peds < 70 kg.* 0.5 mg/kg × 3 d, then ↑ 1.2 mg/kg daily or bid (max 1.4 mg/kg or 100 mg); ↓ dose w/ hepatic Insuff or in combo w/ CYP2D6 inhib (Table 10, p 301) **W/P:** [C, ?/–] w/ Known structural cardiac anomalies, cardiac Hx **CI:** NAG, w/ or w/in 2 wk of D/C an MAOI **Disp:** Caps 5, 10, 18, 25, 40, 60, 80, 100 mg **SE:** HA, insomnia, dry mouth, Abd pain, N/V, anorexia ↑ BP, tachycardia, wgt loss, sexual dysfunction, jaundice, ↑ LFTs **Notes:** AHA rec: All children receiving stimulants for ADHD receive CV assessment before Rx initiated; D/C immediately w/ jaundice

Atorvastatin (Lipitor) Uses: *↑ Cholesterol & triglycerides* Acts: HMG-CoA reductase inhib **Dose:** Initial 10 mg/d, may ↑ to 80 mg/d w/o grapefruit **W/P:** [X, –] **CI:** Active liver Dz, unexplained ↑ LFTs **Disp:** Tabs 10, 20, 40, 80 mg **SE:** Myopathy, HA, arthralgia, myalgia, GI upset, chest pain, edema, insomnia dizziness, liver failure **Notes:** Monitor LFTs, instruct pt to report unusual muscle pain or weakness

Atovaquone (Mepron) Uses: *Rx & prevention PCP and Toxoplasma gondii encephalitis* Acts: ↓ Nucleic acid & ATP synth **Dose:** *Rx:* 750 mg PO bid for 21 d *Prevention:* 1500 mg PO once/d (w/ meals) **W/P:** [C, ?] **Disp:** Susp 750 mg/5 mL **SE:** Fever, HA, anxiety, insomnia, rash, N/V, cough

Atovaquone/Proguanil (Malarone) Uses: *Prevention or Rx P. falciparum malaria* Acts: Antimalarial **Dose:** *Adults. Prevention:* 1 tab PO 2 d before, during, & 7 d after leaving endemic region *Rx:* 4 tabs PO single dose daily × 3 d **Peds.** See PI **W/P:** [C, ?] **CI:** prophylactic use when CrCl < 30 mL/min **Disp:** Tabs atovaquone 250 mg/proguanil 100 mg; peds 62.5/25 mg **SE:** HA, fever, myalgia, N/V, ↑ LFTs

Atracurium (Tracrium) **Uses:** *Anesthesia adjunct to facilitate ET intubation* **Acts:** Nondepolarizing neuromuscular blocker **Dose:** *Adults & Peds > 2 y.* 0.4–0.5 mg/kg IV bolus, then 0.08–0.1 mg/kg q20–45min PRN **W/P:** [C, ?] **Disp:** Inj 10 mg/mL **SE:** Flushing **Notes:** Pt must be intubated & on controlled ventilation; use adequate amounts of sedation & analgesia

Atropine, Systemic (AtroPen Auto-Injector) **BOX:** Primary protection against exposure to chemical nerve agent and insecticide poisoning is the wearing of specially designed protective garments **Uses:** *Preanesthetic; symptomatic ↓ HR & asystole, AV block, organophosphate (insecticide) and acetylcholinesterase (nerve gas) inhib antidote; cycloplegic* **Acts:** Antimuscarinic; blocks acetylcholine at parasympathetic sites, cycloplegic **Dose:** *Adults. ECC 2010. Asystole or PEA:* Routine use for asystole or PEA no longer recommended; *Bradycardia:* 0.5 mg IV q3–5min as needed; max 3 mg or 0.04 mg/kg ET 2–3 mg in 10 mL NS *Preanesthetic:* 0.3–0.6 mg IM *Poisoning:* 1–2 mg IV bolus, repeat q3–5min PRN to reverse effects **Peds. ECC 2010.** *Symptomatic bradycardia:* 0.2 mg/kg IV/IO (min dose 0.1 mg, max single dose 0.5 mg); repeat PRN X1; max total dose 1 mg child, 3 mg adolescent; *Toxins/overdose (organophosphates):* < 12 y 0.02–0.05 mg/kg IV/IO; repeat PRN q20–30min; > 12 y 2 mg IV/IO, then 1–2 mg IV/IO PRN; *RSI:* 0.01–0.02 mg/kg IV/IO or 0.02 mg/kg IM (min dose 0.1 mg, max 0.5 mg) **W/P:** [C, +] **CI:** NAG, adhesions between iris and lens, tachycardia, GI obst, ileus, severe ulcerative colitis, obstructive uropathy, Mobitz II block **Disp:** Inj 0.05, 0.1, 0.3, 0.4, 0.5, 0.8, 1 mg/mL *AtroPen Auto-injector:* 0.25, 0.5, 1, 2 mg/dose; tabs 0.4 mg, MDI 0.36 mg/Inh **SE:** Flushing, mydriasis, tachycardia, dry mouth & nose, blurred vision, urinary retention, constipation, psychosis **Notes:** SLUDGE are Sx of organophosphate poisoning; *Auto-injector* limited distribution; see ophthal forms below

Atropine, Benzoic Acid, Hyoscyamine Sulfate, Methenamine, Methylene Blue, Phenyl Salicylate (Urised) Withdrawn from US market.

Atropine, Ophthalmic (Isopto Atropine, Generic) **Uses:** *Cycloplegic refraction, uveitis, amblyopia* **Acts:** Antimuscarinic; cycloplegic, dilates pupils **Dose:** *Adults.* *Refraction:* 1–2 gtt 1 h before *Uveitis:* 1–2 gtt daily-qid **Peds.** 1 gtt in nonamblyopic eye daily **W/P:** [C, +] **CI:** NAG, adhesions between iris and lens **Disp:** 2.5- & 15-mL bottle 1% ophthal soln, 1% oint **SE:** Local irritation, burning, blurred vision, light sensitivity **Notes:** Compress lacrimal sac 2–3 min after instillation; effects can last 1–2 wk

Atropine/Pralidoxime (DuoDote) **BOX:** For use by personnel w/ appropriate training; wear protective garments; do not rely solely on medication; evacuation and decontamination ASAP **Uses:** *Nerve agent (tabun, sarin, others),* insecticide poisoning* **Acts:** Atropine blocks effects of excess acetylcholine; pralidoxime reactivates acetylcholinesterase inactivated by poisoning **Dose:** 1 Inj midlateral thigh; 10–15 min for effect; w/ severe Sx, give 2 additional Inj; if alert/oriented no more doses **W/P:** [C, ?] **Disp:** Auto-injector 2.1 mg atropine/600 mg pralidoxime **SE:** Dry mouth, blurred vision, dry eyes, photophobia, confusion, HA, tachycardia, ↑ BP, flushing, urinary retention, constipation, Abd pain N, V, emesis **Notes:** See "SLUDGE" under Atropine, Systemic; limited distribution

Azathioprine (Imuran) **BOX:** May ↑ neoplasia w/ chronic use; mutagenic and hematologic tox possible **Uses:** *Adjunct to prevent renal transplant rejection, RA*, SLE, Crohn Dz, ulcerative colitis **Acts:** Immunosuppressive; antagonizes purine metabolism **Dose:** *Adults. Crohn and ulcerative colitis:* Start 50 mg/d, ↑ 25 mg/d q1–2wk, target dose 2–3 mg/kg/d *Adults & Peds. Renal transplant:* 3–5 mg/kg/d IV/PO single daily dose, taper by 0.5 mg/kg q4wk to lowest effective dose *RA:* 1 mg/kg/d once daily or ÷ bid × 6–8 wk, ↑ 0.5 mg/kg/d q4wk to 2.5 mg/kg/d; ↓ w/ renal Insuff **W/P:** [D, ?] **CI:** PRG **Disp:** Tabs 50, 75, 100 mg; powder for Inj 100 mg **SE:** GI intolerance, fever, chills, leukopenia, thrombocytopenia **Notes:** Handle Inj w/ cytotoxic precautions; interaction w/ allopurinol; do not administer live vaccines on drug; ✓ CBC and LFTs; dose per local transplant protocol, usually start 1–3 d pretransplant

Azelastine (Astelin, Astepro, Optivar) **Uses:** *Allergic rhinitis (rhinorrhea, sneezing, nasal pruritus), vasomotor rhinitis; allergic conjunctivitis* **Acts:** Histamine H_1-receptor antagonist **Dose:** *Adults & Peds > 12 y. Nasal:* 1–2 sprays/nostril bid *Ophth:* 1 gtt in each affected eye bid *Peds 5–11 y.* 1 spray/nostril 1× d **W/P:** [C, ?/–] **CI:** Component sensitivity **Disp:** Nasal 137 mcg/spray; ophthalmic soln 0.05% **SE:** Somnolence, bitter taste, HA, colds Sx (rhinitis, cough)

Azithromycin (Zithromax) **Uses:** *Community-acquired pneumonia, pharyngitis, otitis media, skin Infxns, nongonococcal (chlamydial) urethritis, chancroid & PID; Rx & prevention of MAC in HIV* **Acts:** Macrolide antibiotic; bacteriostatic; ↓ protein synth *Spectrum: Chlamydia, H. ducreyi, H. influenzae, Legionella, M. catarrhalis, M. pneumoniae, M. hominis, N. gonorrhoeae, S. aureus, S. agalactiae, S. pneumoniae, S. pyogenes* **Dose:** *Adults. Resp tract Infxns:* PO: Caps 500 mg day 1, then 250 mg/d PO × 4 d *Sinusitis:* 500 mg PO × 3 d *IV:* 500 mg × 2 d, then 500 mg PO × 7–10 d or 500 mg IV daily × 2 d, then 500 mg PO × 7–10 d *Nongonococcal urethritis:* 1 g PO × 1 *Gonorrhea, uncomplicated:* 2 g PO × 1 *Prevent MAC:* 1200 mg PO once/wk *Peds. Otitis media:* 10 mg/kg PO day 1, then 5 mg/kg/d days 2–5 *Pharyngitis:* 12 mg/kg/d PO × 5 d; take susp on empty stomach; tabs OK w/ or w/o food; ↓ w/ CrCl < 10 mL/mg **W/P:** [B, +] **Disp:** Tabs 250, 500, 600 mg; Z-Pack (5-d, 250 mg); Tri-Pack (500-mg tabs × 3); susp 1 g; single-dose packet (Zmax) ER susp (2 g); susp 100, 200 mg/5 mL; Inj powder 500 mg; 2.5 mL ophthal soln 1% **SE:** GI upset, metallic taste

Azithromycin Ophthalmic 1% (AzaSite) **Uses:** *Bacterial conjunctivitis* **Acts:** Bacteriostatic **Dose:** *Adults.* 1 gtt bid, q8–12 h × 2 d, then 1 gtt q day × 5 d *Peds*

≥ *1 y*. 1 gtt bid, q8–12h × 2 d, then 1 gtt q day × 5 d **W/P:** [B, +/−] **CI:** None **Disp:** 1% in 2.5-mL bottle **SE:** Irritation, burning, stinging, contact dermatitis, corneal erosion, dry eye, dysgeusia, nasal congestion, sinusitis, ocular discharge, keratitis

Aztreonam (Azactam) Uses: *Aerobic gram(−) UTIs, lower resp, intra-Abd, skin, gynecologic Infxns & septicemia* Acts: *Monobactam:* ↓ Cell wall synth *Spectrum:* Gram(−) (*Pseudomonas, E. coli, Klebsiella, H. influenzae, Serratia, Proteus, Enterobacter, Citrobacter*) Dose: **Adults.** 1–2 g IV/IM q6–12h *UTI:* 500–1 g IV q8–12h *Meningitis:* 2 g IV q6–8h **Peds.** *Premature:* 30 mg/kg/dose IV q12h *Term & children:* 30 mg/kg/dose q6–8h; ↓ in renal impair **W/P:** [B, +] **Disp:** Inj (soln), 1 g, 2 g/50 mL Inj powder for recons 500 mg 1 g, 2 g **SE:** N/V/D, rash, pain at Inj site Notes: No gram(+) or anaerobic activity; OK in PCN-allergic pts

Aztreonam, Inhaled (Cayston) Uses: *Improve respiratory Sx in CF pts with P. aeruginosa* Acts: Monobactam: ↓ cell wall synth Dose: **Adults & Peds ≥7 y.** One dose 3×/d × 28 d (space doses q4h) **W/P:** [B, +] w/ beta-lactam allergy **CI:** Allergy to aztreonam Disp: Lyophilized aztreonam w/ NaCl **SE:** Allergic Rxn, bronchospasm, cough, nasal congestion, wheezing, pharyngolaryngeal pain, V, abd pain, chest discomfort, pyrexia, rash Notes: Use immediately after reconstitution, use only w/ Altera Nebulizer System; bronchodilator prior to use

Bacitracin, Ophthalmic (AK-Tracin Ophthalmic); Bacitracin & Polymyxin B, Ophthalmic (AK-Poly-Bac Ophthalmic, Polysporin Ophthalmic); Bacitracin, Neomycin, & Polymyxin B, Ophthalmic (AK-Spore Ophthalmic, Neosporin Ophthalmic); Bacitracin, Neomycin, Polymyxin B, & Hydrocortisone, Ophthalmic (AK-Spore HC Ophthalmic, Cortisporin Ophthalmic) Uses: *Steroid-responsive inflammatory ocular conditions* Acts: Topical antibiotic w/ anti-inflammatory Dose: Apply q3–4h into conjunctival sac **W/P:** [C, ?] **CI:** Viral, mycobacterial, fungal eye Infxn Disp: See Bacitracin, Topical equivalents, next listing

Bacitracin, Topical (Baciguent); Bacitracin & Polymyxin B, Topical (Polysporin); Bacitracin, Neomycin, & Polymyxin B, Topical (Neosporin); Bacitracin, Neomycin, Polymyxin B, & Hydrocortisone, Topical (Cortisporin); Bacitracin, Neomycin, Polymyxin B, & Lidocaine, Topical (Clomycin) Uses: Prevent/Rx of *minor skin Infxns* Acts: Topical antibiotic w/ added components (anti-inflammatory & analgesic) Dose: Apply sparingly bid-qid **W/P:** [C, ?] Not for deep wounds, puncture, or animal bites Disp: Bacitracin 500 units/g oint; bacitracin 500 units/polymyxin B sulfate 10,000 units/g oint & powder; bacitracin 400 units/neomycin 3.5 mg/polymyxin B 5000 units/g oint; bacitracin 400 units/neomycin 3.5 mg/polymyxin B 5000 units/hydrocortisone 10 mg/g oint; Bacitracin 500 units/neomycin 3.5 mg/polymyxin B 5000 units/lidocaine 40 mg/g oint Notes: Ophthal, systemic, & irrigation forms available, not generally used d/t potential tox

Baclofen (Lioresal Intrathecal, Generic) BOX: IT abrupt discontinuation can lead to organ failure, rhabdomyolysis, and death Uses: *Spasticity d/t severe chronic disorders (e.g., MS, amyotrophic lateral sclerosis, or spinal cord lesions)*, trigeminal neuralgia, intractable hiccups **Acts:** Centrally acting skeletal muscle relaxant; ↓ transmission of monosynaptic & polysynaptic cord reflexes **Dose:** *Adults.* Initial, 5 mg PO tid; ↑ q3d to effect; max 80 mg/d *IT:* Via implantable pump (see PI) *Peds 2–7 y.* 10–15 mg/d ÷ q8h; titrate, max 40 mg/d > *8 y:* Max 60 mg/d *IT:* Via implantable pump (see PI); ↓ in renal impair; take w/ food or milk **W/P:** [C, +] Epilepsy, neuropsychological disturbances; **Disp:** Tabs 10, 20 mg; IT Inj 50 mcg/mL, 10 mg/20 mL, 10 mg/5 mL **SE:** Dizziness, drowsiness, insomnia, ataxia, weakness, ↓ BP

Balsalazide (Colazal) **Uses:** *Ulcerative colitis* **Acts:** 5-ASA derivative, anti-inflammatory, ↓ leukotriene synth **Dose:** 2.25 g (3 caps) tid × 8–12 wk **W/P:** [B, ?] Severe renal failure **CI:** Mesalamine or salicylate hypersens **Disp:** Caps 750 mg **SE:** Dizziness, HA, N, Abd pain, agranulocytosis, renal impair, allergic Rxns **Notes:** Daily dose of 6.75 g = 2.4 g mesalamine

Basiliximab (Simulect) **BOX:** Use only under the supervision of a physician experienced in immunosuppression Rx in an appropriate facility **Uses:** *Prevent acute transplant rejection* **Acts:** IL-2 receptor antagonists **Dose:** *Adults & Peds > 35 kg.* 20 mg IV 2 h before transplant, then 20 mg IV 4 d posttransplant. *Peds < 35 kg.* 10 mg 2 h prior to transplant; same dose IV 4 d posttransplant **W/P:** [B, ?/−] **CI:** Hypersens to murine proteins **Disp:** Inj powder 10, 20 mg **SE:** Edema, HTN, HA, dizziness, fever, pain, Infxn, GI effects, electrolyte disturbances **Notes:** A murine/human MoAb

BCG [Bacillus Calmette-Guérin] (TheraCys, Tice BCG) **BOX:** Contains live, attenuated mycobacteria; transmission risk; handle as biohazard; nosocomial Infxns reported in immunosuppressed; fatal Rxns reported **Uses:** *Bladder CA (superficial)*, TB prophylaxis: Routine US adult BCG immunization not recommended. Children who are PPD(−) & continually exposed to untreated/ineffectively treated adults or whose TB strain is INH/rifampin resistant. Healthcare workers in high-risk environments **Acts:** Attenuated live BCG culture, immunomodulator **Dose:** Bladder CA, 1 vial prepared & instilled in bladder for 2 h. Repeat once/wk × 6 wk; then 1 Tx at 3, 6, 12, 18, & 24 mo after **W/P:** [C, ?] Asthma w/ TB immunization **CI:** Immunosuppression, PRG, steroid use, febrile illness, UTI, gross hematuria, w/ traumatic catheterization **Disp:** Powder 81 mg (10.5 ± 8.7 × 10⁸ CFU/vial) (*TheraCys*), 50 mg (1–8 × 10⁸ CFU/vial) (*Tice BCG*) **SE:** Intravesical: Hematuria, urinary frequency, dysuria, bacterial UTI, rare BCG sepsis **Notes:** PPD is not CI in BCG vaccinated persons; intravesical use, dispose/void in toilet w/ chlorine bleach

Becaplermin (Regranex Gel) **BOX:** Increased mortality d/t malignancy reported; use w/ caution in known malignancy **Uses:** Local wound care adjunct w/ *diabetic foot ulcers*: **Acts:** Recombinant PDGF, enhances granulation tissue **Dose:** *Adults. Based on lesion:* Calculate the length of gel, measure the greatest length of ulcer by the greatest width; tube size and measured result determine the formula used in the calculation. Recalculate q1–2wk based on change in lesion size. *15-g tube:* [length × width] × 0.6 = length of gel (in inches) or for *2-g tube:* [length × width] × 1.3 = length of gel (in inches); rinse after 15 min; do not reapply w/in 24 h; repeat in 12 h *Peds.* See PI **W/P:** [C, ?] **CI:** Neoplasmatic site **Disp:** 0.01% gel in 2-, 15g tubes **SE:** Rash **Notes:** Use w/ good wound care; wound must be vascularized; reassess after 10 wk if ulcer not ↓ by 30% or not healed by 20 wk

Beclomethasone Nasal (Beconase AQ) **Uses:** *Allergic rhinitis* refractory to antihistamines & decongestants; *nasal polyps* **Acts:** Inhaled steroid **Dose:** *Adults & Peds. Aqueous inhaler:* 1–2 sprays/nostril bid **W/P:** [C, ?] **Disp:** Nasal metered-dose inhaler 42 mcg/spray **SE:** Local irritation, burning, epistaxis **Notes:** Effect in days to 2 wk

Beclomethasone (QVAR) **Uses:** Chronic *asthma* **Acts:** Inhaled corticosteroid **Dose:** *Adults & Peds 5–11 y.* 40–160 mcg 1–4 Inhs bid; initial 40–80 mcg Inh bid if on bronchodilators alone; 40–160 mcg w/ other inhaled steroids; 320 mcg bid max; taper to lowest effective dose bid; rinse mouth/throat after **W/P:** [C, ?] **CI:** Acute asthma **Disp:** PO metered-dose inhaler; 40, 80 mcg/Inh **SE:** HA, cough, hoarseness, oral candidiasis **Notes:** Not effective for acute asthma; effect in 1–2 days or as long as 2 wks; rinse mouth after use

Belatacept (Nulojix) **BOX:** may ↑ risk of post-transplant lymphoproliferative disorder (PTLD)mostly CNS; use in EBV seropositive pt only; for use by physicians experienced in immunosuppressive therapy; ↑ risk of malignancies; not for liver transplant **Uses:** *prevention rejection in kidney transplant* **Acts:** T-cell costimulation blocker **Dose:** Day 1 (transplant day, pre-op) & day 5 10 mg/kg; End of Wk 2 ,Wk 4, Wk 8, Wk 12 after transplant 10 mg/kg; Maint: End of Wk 16 after transplant 7 Q 4 wks 5 mg/kg **W/P:** [C, −] w/ CYP3A4 inhib/inducers, other anticoagulants or plt inhib; avoid w/CrCl < 30 or mod/severe hepatic impair mL/min **CI:** EBV seronegative or unknown EBV status **Disp:** Inj **SE:** anemia, N/V/D, UTI, edema, constipation, ↑ BP, pyrexia, graft dysfunction, cough, HA, ↑/↓ K⁺, ↓ WBC **Notes:** REMS; use in combo w/ basiliximab, mycophenolate mofetil (MMF), & steroids; PML with excess belatacept dosing

Belladonna & Opium Suppositories (B&O Supprettes) [C-II] **Uses:** *Bladder spasms; mod/severe pain* **Acts:** Antispasmodic, analgesic **Dose:** 1 supp PR q6h PRN; **W/P:** [C, ?] **CI:** Glaucoma, resp depression **Disp:** 15A = 30 mg opium/16.2 mg belladonna extract; 16A = 60 mg opium/16.2 mg belladonna extract **SE:** Anticholinergic (e.g., sedation, urinary retention, constipation)

Benazepril (Lotensin) **Uses:** *HTN*, DN, CHF **Acts:** ACE inhib **Dose:** 10–80 mg/d PO **W/P:** [C (1st tri), D (2nd & 3rd tri), +] **CI:** Angioedema, Hx edema, bilateral RAS **Disp:** Tabs 5, 10, 20, 40 mg **SE:** Symptomatic ↓ BP w/ diuretics; dizziness, HA, ↑ K⁺, nonproductive cough

Bendamustine (Treanda) **Uses:** *CLL* **Acts:** Mechlorethamine derivative; alkylating agent **Dose:** *Adults.* 100 mg/m² IV over 30 min days 1 & 2 of 28-d cycle, up to 6 cycles (w/ tox see PI for dose changes); do not use w/ CrCl < 40 mL/min, severe hepatic impair) **W/P:** [D, ?/–] do not use w/ CrCl < 40 mL/min, severe hepatic impair **CI:** Hypersens to bendamustine or mannitol **Disp:** Inj powder 100 mg **SE:** Pyrexia, N/V, dry mouth, fatigue, cough, stomatitis, rash, myelosuppression, Infxn, Inf Rxns & anaphylaxis, tumor lysis synd, skin Rxns **Notes:** Consider use of allopurinol to prevent tumor lysis synd

Benzocaine (Americaine, Hurricane Lanacane, Various [OTC])
Uses: *topical anesthetic, lubricant for ET tubes, catheters, etc; pain relief in external otitis, cerumen removal, skin conditions, sunburn, insect bites, mouth and gum irritation, hemorrhoids* **Acts:** topical local anesthetic **Dose:** *Adults & Peds > 1 year. Anesthetic lubricant:* apply evenly to tube/instrument; *Cerumen removal:* Instill 3×/d for 2–3 days; *Otic drops:* 4–5 gtt in external canal, insert cotton plug, repeat q1–2h PRN; other uses per manufacturer instructions **W/P:** [C, –] do not use on broken skin; see provider if condition does not respond; avoid in infants and those w/ pulmonary Dzs **Disp:** Many site-specific OTC forms creams, gels, liquids, sprays, 2–20% **SE:** itching, irritation, burning, edema, erythema, pruritus, rash, stinging, tenderness, urticaria; methemoglobinemia (infants or in COPD) **Notes:** Use minimum amount to obtain effect; methemoglobinemia S&Sxs: HA, light-headedness, SOB, anxiety, fatigue, pale, gray or blue colored skin, and tachycardia; treat w/ IV methylene blue

Benzocaine & Antipyrine (Auralgan) **Uses:** *Analgesia in severe otitis media* **Acts:** Anesthetic w/ local decongestant **Dose:** Fill ear, & insert a moist cotton plug; repeat 1–2 h PRN **W/P:** [C, ?] **CI:** w/ Perforated eardrum **Disp:** Soln 5.4% antipyrine, 1.4% benzocaine **SE:** Local irritation

Benzonatate (Tessalon Perles) **Uses:** Symptomatic relief of *cough* **Acts:** Anesthetizes the stretch receptors in the resp passages **Dose:** *Adults & Peds > 10 y.* 100 mg PO tid (max 600 mg/d) **W/P:** [C, ?] **Disp:** Caps 100, 200 mg **SE:** Sedation, dizziness, GI upset **Notes:** Do not chew or puncture the caps; deaths reported in peds < 10 y w/ ingestion

Benztropine (Cogentin) **Uses:** *Parkinsonism & drug-induced extrapyramidal disorders* **Acts:** Partially blocks striatal cholinergic receptors **Dose:** *Adults. Parkinsonism:* initial 0.5–1 mg PO/IM/IV qhs, ↑ q 5–6 d PRN by 0.5 mg, usual dose 1–2 mg, 6 mg/d max. *Extrapyramidal:* 1–4 mg PO/IV/IM q day-bid. *Acute Dystonia:* 1–2 mg IM/IV, then 1–2 mg PO bid. *Peds > 3 y.* 0.02–0.05 mg/kg/dose 1–2/d **W/P:** [C, ?] w/ Urinary Sxs, NAG, hot environments, CNS or mental disorders, other phenothiazines or TCA **CI:** < 3 y **Disp:** Tabs 0.5, 1, 2 mg; Inj 1 mg/mL **SE:** Anticholinergic (tachycardia, ileus, N/V, etc), anhidrosis, heat stroke **Notes:** Physostigmine 1–2 mg SQ/IV to reverse severe Sxs

Benzyl Alcohol (Ulesfia) **Uses:** *Head lice* **Action:** Pediculicide **Dose:** Apply volume for hair length to dry hair; saturate the scalp; leave on 10 min; rinse w/ water; repeat in 7 days; *Hair length 0–2 in:* 4–6 oz; *2–4 in:* 6–8 oz; *4–8 in:* 8–12 oz; *8–16 in:* 12–24 oz; *16–22 in:* 24–32 oz; *> 22 inches:* 32–48 oz **W/P:** [B, ?] Avoid eyes **CI:** none **Disp:** 5% lotion 4-, 8-oz bottles **SE:** Pruritus, erythema, irritation (local, eyes) **Notes:** Use fine-tooth/nit comb to remove nits and dead lice; no ovocidal activity.

Bepotastine Besilate (Bepreve) **Uses:** *Allergic conjunctivitis * **Acts:** H_1 receptor antagonist **Dose:** *Adults.* 1 gtt into affected eye(s) twice daily **W/P:** [C, ?/–] Do not use while wearing contacts **Disp:** Soln 1.5% **SE:** Mild taste, eye irritation, HA, nasopharyngitis

Beractant (Survanta) **Uses:** *Prevention & Rx RDS in premature infants* **Acts:** Replaces pulm surfactant **Dose:** 100 mg/kg via ET tube; repeat 3 × q6h PRN; max 4 doses/48 h **Disp:** Susp 25 mg of phospholipid/mL **SE:** Transient ↓ HR, desaturation, apnea **Notes:** Administer via 4-quadrant method

Besifloxacin (Besivance) **Uses:** *Bacterial conjunctivitis* **Action:** Inhibits DNA gyrase & topoisomerase IV. **Dose:** *Adults & Peds > 1 y.* 1 gtt into eye(s) TID 4–12 h apart × 7 d **W/P:** [C, ?] Remove contacts during Tx **CI:** None **Disp:** 0.6% susp **SE:** HA, redness, blurred vision, irritation

Betaxolol (Kerlone) **Uses:** *HTN* **Acts:** Competitively blocks β-adrenergic receptors, $β_1$ **W/P:** [C (1st tri), D (2nd or 3rd tri), +/–] **CI:** Sinus ↓ HR, AV conduction abnormalities, uncompensated cardiac failure **Dose:** 5–20 mg/d **Disp:** Tabs 10, 20 mg **SE:** Dizziness, HA, ↓ HR, edema, CHF

Betaxolol, Ophthalmic (Betoptic) **Uses:** Open-angle glaucoma **Acts:** Competitively blocks $β_1$-adrenergic receptors, **Dose:** 1–2 gtt bid **W/P:** [C (1st tri), D (2nd or 3rd tri), ?/–] **Disp:** Soln 0.5%; susp 0.25% **SE:** Local irritation, photophobia

Bethanechol (Duvoid, Urecholine, Others) **Uses:** *Acute post-op/postpartum nonobstructive urinary retention; neurogenic bladder w/ retention* **Acts:** Stimulates cholinergic smooth muscle in bladder & GI tract **Dose:** *Adults.* Initial 5–10 mg PO, then repeat qh until response or 50 mg, typical 10–50 mg tid-qid, 200 mg/d max tid-qid; 2.5–5 mg SQ tid-qid & PRN. *Peds.* 0.3–0.6 mg/kg/24 h PO ÷ tid-qid or 0.15–2 mg/kg/d SQ ÷ 3–4 doses; take on empty stomach **W/P:** [C, –] **CI:** BOO, PUD, epilepsy, hyperthyroidism, ↓ HR, COPD, AV conduction defects, Parkinsonism, ↓ BP, vasomotor instability **Disp:** Tabs 5, 10, 25, 50 mg; Inj 5 mg/mL **SE:** Abd cramps, D, salivation, ↓ BP **Notes:** Do not use IM/IV

Bevacizumab (Avastin) **BOX:** Associated w/ GI perforation, wound dehiscence, & fatal hemoptysis **Uses:** *Met colorectal CA w/5-FU, NSCLC w/ paclitaxel and carboplatin; glioblastoma; metastatic RCC w/ IFN-alpha* **Acts:** Vascular endothelial GF inhibitor **Dose:** *Adults. Colon:* 5 mg/kg or 10 mg/kg IV q14d; *NSCLC:* 15 mg/kg q21d; 1st dose over 90 min; 2nd over 60 min, 3rd over 30 min if tolerated; *RCC:* 10 mg/kg IV q2 wks w/ IFN-α alfa **W/P:** [C, –] Do not use w/in 28 d of surgery if time for separation of drug & anticipated surgical procedures is unknown; D/C w/ serious adverse effects **CI:** serious hemorrhage or hemoptysis **Disp:** 100 mg/4 mL, 400 mg/16 mL vials **SE:** Wound dehiscence, GI perforation, tracheoesophageal fistula, arterial thrombosis, hemoptysis, hemorrhage, HTN, proteinuria, CHF, Inf Rxns, D, leukopenia **Notes:** Monitor for ↑ BP & proteinuria

Bicalutamide (Casodex) Uses: *Advanced PCa w/ GnRH agonists ([e.g., leuprolide, goserelin])* CI: Women Disp: Caps 50 mg SE: Hot flashes, ↓ loss of libido, impotence, D/N/V, gynecomastia, & ↑ LFTs elevation Acts: Nonsteroidal antiandrogen Dose: 50 mg/d W/P: [X, ?]

Bicarbonate (See Sodium Bicarbonate, p 241)

Bisacodyl (Dulcolax) [OTC] Uses: *Constipation; pre-op bowel prep* Acts: Stimulates peristalsis Dose: Adults. 5–15 mg PO or 10 mg PR PRN. Peds: < 2 y. 5 mg PR PRN. > 2 y: 5 mg PO or 10 mg PR PRN (do not chew tabs or give w/ in 1 h of antacids or milk) W/P: [C, ?] CI: Acute abdomen, bowel obst, appendicitis, gastroenteritis Disp: EC tabs 5 mg; tabs 5 mg; supp 10 mg, enema soln 10 mg/30 mL SE: Abd cramps, proctitis, & inflammation w/ supps

Bismuth Subcitrate/Metronidazole/Tetracycline (Pylera) BOX: Metronidazole possibly carcinogenic (based on animal studies) Uses: *H. pylori Infxn w/ omeprazole* Acts: Eradicates H. pylori, see agents Dose: 3 caps qid w/ omeprazole 20 mg bid for × 10 d W/P: [D, –] CI: PRG, peds < 8 yrs (tetracycline during tooth development causes teeth discoloration), w/ renal/hepatic impair, component hypersens Disp: Caps w/ 140-mg bismuth subcitrate potassium, 125-mg metronidazole, & 125-mg tetracycline hydrochloride SE: Stool abnormality, D, dyspepsia, Abd pain, HA, flu-like synd, taste perversion, vaginitis, dizziness; see SE for each component

Bismuth Subsalicylate (Pepto-Bismol) [OTC] Uses: Indigestion, N, & *D*; combo for Rx of *H. pylori Infxn* Acts: Antisecretory & anti-inflammatory Dose: Adults. 2 tabs or 30 mL PO PRN (max 8 doses/24 h). Peds. (For all max 8 doses/24 h.) 3–6 y: 1/3 tab or 5 mL PO PRN. 6–9 y: 2/3 tab or 10 mL PO PRN. 9–12 y: 1 tab or 15 mL PO PRN W/P: [C, D (3rd tri), –] Avoid w/ renal failure; Hx severe GI bleed [D] CI: Influenza or chickenpox (↑ risk of Reye synd), ASA allergy (see aspirin) Disp: Chew tabs, caplets 262 mg; liq 262, 525 mg/15 mL; susp 262 mg/15 mL SE: May turn tongue & stools black

Bisoprolol (Zebeta) Uses: *HTN* Acts: Competitively blocks β_1-adrenergic receptors Dose: 2.5–10 mg/d (max dose 20 mg/d); ↓ w/ renal impair W/P: [C (D 2nd & 3rd tri), +/–] CI: Sinus bradycardia, AV conduction abnormalities, uncompensated cardiac failure Disp: Tabs 5, 10 mg SE: Fatigue, lethargy, HA, ↓ HR, edema, CHF Notes: Not dialyzed

Bivalirudin (Angiomax) Uses: *Anticoagulant w/ ASA in unstable angina undergoing PTCA, PCI, or in pts undergoing PCI w/ or at risk for HIT/HITTS* Acts: Anticoagulant, thrombin inhib Dose: 0.75 mg/kg IV bolus, then 1.75 mg/kg/h for duration of procedure and up to 4 h postprocedure. ✓ ACT 5 min after bolus, may repeat 0.3 mg/kg bolus if necessary (give w/ aspirin ASA 300–325 mg/d; start pre-PTCA) W/P: [B, ?] CI: Major bleeding Disp: Powder 250 mg for Inj SE: Bleeding, back pain, N, HA

Bleomycin Sulfate (Blenoxane) Uses: *Testis CA; Hodgkin Dz & NHLs; cutaneous lymphomas; & squamous cell CA (head & neck, larynx, cervix, skin,* penis); malignant pleural effusion sclerosing agent* **Acts:** Induces DNA breakage (scission) **Dose:** (per protocols); ↓ w/ renal impair **W/P:** [D, ?] **CI:** Severe pulm Dz (pulm fibrosis) **Dose:** Powder (Inj) 15, 30 units **SE:** Hyperpigmentation & allergy (rash to anaphylaxis); fever in 50%; lung tox (idiosyncratic & dose related); pneumonitis w/ fibrosis; Raynaud phenomenon, N/V **Notes:** Test dose 1 unit, especially in lymphoma pts; lung tox w/ total dose > 400 units or single dose > 30 units; avoid high FiO_2 in general anesthesia to ↓ tox

Boceprevir (Victrelis) **Uses:** *Chronic Hep C genotype 1 combo w/ peginterferon alpha and ribavirin* **Acts:** NS3/4A protease inhibitor **Dose:** 800 mg PO tid w/ food with peginterferon alpha (PegIntron) and ribavirin (Rebetol) (see individual products) **W/P:** [B but treat as X due to ribavirin use, ?/–]w/ CYP3A4/5 metabolized drugs; follow for ↓ Hct/WBC **CI:** PRG, same as for peginterferon alpha and ribavirin **Disp:** caps 200 mg **SE:** Fatigue, anemia, N, HA, dysgeusia **Notes:** Not a monotherapy; PRG test before

Bortezomib (Velcade) **BOX:** May worsen preexisting neuropathy **Uses:** *Rx multiple myeloma or mantel cell lymphoma w/ one failed previous Rx* **Acts:** Proteasome inhib **Dose:** 1.3 mg/m² bolus IV 2×/wk for 2 wk (days 1, 2, 8, 11), w/ 10-d rest period (=1 cycle); ↓ dose w/ hematologic tox, neuropathy **W/P:** [D, ?/–] w/ Drugs CYP450 metabolized (Table 10, p 301) **Disp:** 3.5-mg vial **SE:** Asthenia, GI upset, anorexia, dyspnea, HA, orthostatic ↓ BP, edema, insomnia, dizziness, rash, pyrexia, arthralgia, neuropathy

Botulinum Toxin Type A [abobotulinumtoxinA] (Dysport) **BOX:** Effects may spread beyond Tx area leading to swallowing and breathing difficulties (may be fatal); Sxs may occur hrs to wks after Inj **Uses:** *cervical dystonia (adults), glabellar lines (cosmetic)* **Acts:** Neurotoxin, ↓ ACH release from nerve endings, ↓ neuromuscular transmission **Dose:** *Cervical dystonia:* 500 units IM ÷ dose units into muscles; retreat no less than 12–16 wks PRN dose range 250–100 units based on response. *Glabellar lines:* 50 units ÷ in 10 units/Inj into muscles, repeat no less than q3mo **W/P:** [C, ?] sedentary pt to resume activity slowly after Inj; aminoglycosides and nondepolarizing muscle blockers may ↑↑ effects; do not exceed dosing **CI:** Hypersens to components (cow milk), infect at Inj site **Disp:** Inj **SE:** Anaphylaxis, erythema multiforme, dysphagia, dyspnea, syncope, HA, NAG, Inj site pain **Notes:** Botulinum toxin products not interchangeable

Botulinum Toxin Type A [incobotulinumtoxinA] (Xeomin) **BOX:** Effects may spread beyond Tx area leading to swallowing and breathing difficulties (may be fatal); Sxs may occur hrs to wks after Inj **Uses:** *cervical dystonia (adults), blepharospasm* **Acts:** Neurotoxin, ↓ ACH release from nerve endings, ↓ neuromuscular transmission **Dose:** *Cervical dystonia:* 120 units IM ÷ dose into muscles; *Blepharospasm:* 1.25–2.5 units IM/site; typical 5.6 units/Inj, 6 Inj/eye **W/P:** [C, ?] sedentary pt to resume activity slowly after Inj; aminoglycosides and nondepolarizing muscle blockers may ↑↑ effects; do not exceed dosing **CI:** Hypersens to components (cow milk), infect at Inj site **Disp:** Inj **SE:** *Cervical dystonia:*

Dysphagia, neck/musculoskeletal pain, muscle weakness, Inj site pain; *Blepharospasm:* Ptosis, dry eye/mouth, D, HA, visual impair, dyspnea, nasopharyngitis, URI *Notes:* Botulinum toxin products not interchangeable; for eye Inj, D/C if diplopia develops

Botulinum Toxin Type A [onabotulinumtoxinA] (Botox, Botox Cosmetic) BOX: Effects may spread beyond Tx leading to swallowing/breathing difficulties (may be fatal); Sxs may occur hrs to wks after Inj *Uses:* *Glabellar lines (cosmetic) < 65 y, blepharospasm, cervical dystonia, axillary hyperhidrosis, strabismus, chronic migraine, upper limb spasticity, incontinence in OAB due to neurologic Dz *Acts:* Neurotoxin, ↓ ACH release from nerve endings; denervates sweat glands/muscles *Dose:* **Adults.** *Glabellar lines (cosmetic):* 0.1 mL IM × 5 sites q3–4 mo; *Blepharospasm:* 1.25–2.5 units IM/site q3mo; max 200 units/30 d total; *Cervical dystonia:* 198–300 units IM ÷ < 100 units into muscle; *Hyperhidrosis:* 50 units intradermal/axilla ÷; *Strabismus:* 1.25–2.5 units IM/site q3mo; inject eye muscles w/ EMG guidance; *Chronic migraine:* 155 units total, 0.1 mL (5 unit) Inj ÷ into 7 head/neck muscles; *Upper limb spasticity:* Dose based on history; use EMG guidance **Peds.** *Blepharospasm:* > 12 y. Adult dose *Cervical dystonia:* > 16 y: 198–300 units IM ÷ among affected muscles; use < 100 units in sternocleidomastoid; *Strabismus:* > 12 y: 1.25–2.5 units IM/site q3mo; 25 units/site max; inject eye muscles w/ EMG guidance *W/P:* [C, ?] w/ neurologic Dz; do not exceed rec doses; sedentary pt to resume activity slowly after Inj; aminoglycosides and nondepolarizing muscle blockers may ↑↑ effects; Do not exceed dosing *CI:* Hypersens to components, infect at Inj site *Disp:* Inj powder, single-use vial (dilute w/ NS); *(Botox cosmetic)* 50, 100 units; *(Botox)* 100, 200 unit vials *SE:* Anaphylaxis, erythema multiforme, dysphagia, dyspnea, syncope, HA, NAG, Inj site pain *Notes:* Botulinum toxin products not interchangeable; do not exceed total dose of 360 units q12–16wks

Botulinum Toxin Type B [rimabotulinumtoxinB] (Myobloc) BOX: Effects may spread beyond Tx area leading to swallowing and breathing difficulties (may be fatal); Sxs may occur hrs to wks after Inj *Uses:* *cervical dystonia (adults)* *Acts:* Neurotoxin, ↓ ACH release from nerve endings, ↓ neuromuscular transmission *Dose:* *Cervical dystonia:* 2500–5000 units IM ÷ into units into muscles; lower dose if naïve *W/P:* [C, ?] sedentary pt to resume activity slowly after Inj; aminoglycosides and nondepolarizing muscle blockers may ↑↑ effects; do not exceed dosing *CI:* Hypersens to components, infect at Inj site *Inj SE:* Anaphylaxis, erythema multiforme, dysphagia, dyspnea, syncope, HA, NAG, Inj site pain *Notes:* Effect 12–16 wks w/5000–10000 units; botulinum toxin products not interchangeable

Brimonidine (Alphagan P) *Uses:* *Open-angle glaucoma, ocular HTN* *Acts:* α₂-Adrenergic agonist *Dose:* 1 gtt in eye(s) tid (wait 15 min to insert contacts) *W/P:* [B, ?] *CI:* MAOI Rx *Disp:* 0.15, 0.1% soln *SE:* Local irritation, HA, fatigue

Brimonidine/Timolol (Combigan) *Uses:* *↓ IOP in glaucoma or ocular HTN* *Acts:* Selective α₂-adrenergic agonist and nonselective β-adrenergic antagonist *Dose:* **Adults & Peds ≥ 2 y.** 1 gtt in eye bid *W/P:* [C, –] *CI:* Asthma, severe COPD, sinus brady, 2nd-/3rd-degree AV block, CHF cardiac failure, cardiogenic shock, component hypersens **Disp:** Soln: (2 mg/mL brimonidine, 5 mg/mL timolol) 5, 10, 15 mL **SE:** Allergic conjunctivitis, conjunctival folliculosis, conjunctival hyperemia, eye pruritus, ocular burning & stinging **Notes:** Instill other ophthal products 5 min apart

Brinzolamide (Azopt) Uses: *Open-angle glaucoma, ocular HTN* **Acts:** Carbonic anhydrase inhib **Dose:** 1 gtt in eye(s) tid **W/P:** [C, ?] **CI:** Sulfonamide allergy **Disp:** 1% susp **SE:** Blurred vision, dry eye, blepharitis, taste disturbance

Bromocriptine (Parlodel) Uses: *Parkinson Dz, hyperprolactinemia, acromegaly, pituitary tumors* **Acts:** Agonist to striatal dopamine receptors; ↓ prolactin secretion **Dose:** Initial, 1.25 mg PO bid; titrate to effect, w/ food **W/P:** [B, ?] **CI:** Severe ischemic heart Dz or PVD **Disp:** Tabs 2.5 mg; caps 5 mg **SE:** ↓ BP, Raynaud phenomenon, dizziness, N, GI upset, hallucinations

Bromocriptine Mesylate (Cycloset) Uses: *Improve glycemic control in adults w/ type 2 DM* **Acts:** Dopamine receptor agonist; ?? DM mechanism **Dose:** *Initial:* 0.8 mg PO daily, ↑ weekly by 1 tab; usual dose 1.6–4.8 mg 1×/d; w/in 2 hrs after waking w/ food **W/P:** [B, –] may cause orthostatic ↓ BP, psychotic disorders; not for type 1 DM or DKA; w/ strong inducers/inhib of CYP3A4, avoid w/ dopamine antagonists/receptor agonists **CI:** hypersens to ergots drugs, w/ syncopal migraine, nursing mothers **Disp:** Tabs 0.8 mg **SE:** N/V, fatigue, HA, dizziness, somnolence

Budesonide (Rhinocort Aqua, Pulmicort) Uses: *Allergic & nonallergic rhinitis, asthma* **Acts:** Steroid **Dose:** *Adults. Rhinocort Aqua:* 1–4 sprays/nostril/d; *Turbohaler:* 1–4 Inh bid; *Pulmicort Flexhaler:* 1–2 Inh bid *Peds. Rhinocort Aqua intranasal:* 1–2 sprays/nostril/d; *Pulmicort Turbuhaler:* 1–2 Inh bid; *Respules:* 0.25–0.5 mg daily or bid (rinse mouth after PO use) **W/P:** [B, ?/–] **CI:** w/ Acute asthma **Disp:** Metered-dose *Turbuhaler:* 200 mcg/Inh; *Flexhaler:* 90, 180 mcg/Inh; *Respules:* 0.25, 0.5,1 mg/2 mL; *Rhinocort Aqua:* 32 mcg/spray **SE:** HA, N, cough, hoarseness, *Candida* Infxn, epistaxis

Budesonide, Oral (Entocort EC) Uses: *Mild–mod Crohn Dz* **Acts:** Steroid, anti-inflammatory **Dose:** *Adults.* initial: 9 mg PO q A.M. to 8 wk max: maint 6 mg PO q A.M. taper by 3 mo; avoid grapefruit juice **CI:** Active TB and fungal Infxn **W/P:** [C, ?/–] DM, glaucoma, cataracts, HTN, CHF **Disp:** Caps 3 mg ER **SE:** HA, N, ↑ wgt, mood change, *Candida* Infxn, epistaxis **Notes:** Do not cut/crush/chew; taper on D/C

Budesonide/Formoterol (Symbicort) **BOX:** Long-acting β_2-adrenergic agonists may ↑ risk of asthma-related death. Use only for pts not adequately controlled on other meds Uses: *Rx of asthma, main in COPD (chronic bronchitis and emphysema)* **Acts:** Steroid w/ LA β_2-adrenergic agonist **Dose:** *Adults & Peds > 12 y.* 2 inh bid (use lowest effective dose), 640/18 mcg/d max **W/P:** [C, ?/–] **CI:** Status asthmaticus/acute asthma **Disp:** Inh (budesonide/formoterol): 80/4.5 mcg, 160/4.5 mcg **SE:** HA, GI discomfort, nasopharyngitis, palpitations, tremor, nervousness,

URI, paradoxical bronchospasm, hypokalemia, cataracts, glaucoma **Notes:** Not for acute bronchospasm; not for transferring pt from chronic systemic steroids; rinse & spit w/ water after each dose

Bumetanide (Bumex) **Uses:** *Edema from CHF, hepatic cirrhosis, & renal Dz* **Acts:** Loop diuretic; ↓ reabsorption of Na⁺ & Cl⁻, in ascending loop of Henle & the distal tubule **Dose:** *Adults.* 0.5–2 mg PO; 0.5–1 mg IV/IM q8–24h (max 10 mg/d). *Peds.* 0.015–0.1 mg/kg PO q6h–24h (max 10 mg/d) **W/P:** [D,?] **CI:** Anuria, hepatic coma, severe electrolyte depletion **Disp:** Tabs 0.5, 1, 2 mg; Inj 0.25 mg/mL **SE:** ↓ K⁺, ↓ Na⁺, ↑ Cr, ↑ uric acid, dizziness, ototox **Notes:** Monitor fluid & lytes

Bupivacaine (Marcaine) **BOX:** Administration only by clinicians experienced in local anesthesia d/t potential tox; avoid 0.75% for OB anesthesia d/t reports of cardiac arrest and death **Uses:** *Local, regional, & spinal anesthesia, local & regional analgesia* **Acts:** Local anesthetic **Dose:** *Adults & Peds.* Dose dependent on procedure (tissue vascularity, depth of anesthesia, etc) (Table 1, p 282) **W/P:** [C, ?] **CI:** Severe bleeding, ↓ BP, shock & arrhythmias, local Infxns at site, septicemia **Disp:** Inj 0.25, 0.5, 0.75% **SE:** ↓ BP, ↑ HR, dizziness, anxiety

Buprenorphine (Buprenex) [C-III] **Uses:** *Mod/severe pain* **Acts:** Opiate agonist-antagonist **Dose:** 0.3–0.6 mg IM or slow IV push q6h PRN **W/P:** [C, ?/–] **Disp:** 0.3 mg/mL **SE:** Sedation, ↓ BP, resp depression **Notes:** Withdrawal if opioid-dependent

Buprenorphine and Naloxone (Suboxone) [C-III] **Uses:** *Maint opioid withdrawal* **Acts:** Opioid agonist-antagonist + opioid antagonist **Dose:** 2/0.5–24/6 mg SL daily; ↑/↓ by 2/0.5 mg or 4/1 mg to effect of S/Sys **W/P:** [C, +/–] **CI:** Hypersens **Disp:** SL film buprenorphine/naloxone: 2/0.5, 8/2 mg **SE:** Oral hypoparesthesia, pain, constipation, diaphoresis **Notes:** Not for analgesia

Buprenorphine, Transdermal (Butrans) [C-III] **BOX:** Limit use to severe around-the-clock chronic pain; assess for opioid abuse/addiction before use; 20 mcg/h max due to ↑ QTc; avoid heat on patch, may result in OD **Uses:** *Mod/severe chronic pain requiring around-the-clock opioid analgesic* **Acts:** Opiate agonist-antagonist **Dose:** Wear patch ×7/d; if opioid naïve, start 5 mcg/h; see label for conversion from opioid; wait 72 h before Δ dose; wait 3 wks before using same application site **W/P:** [C, ?/–] **CI:** resp depression, severe asthma, ileus, component hypersens, short-term opioid need, post-op/mild/intermittent pain **Disp:** Transdermal patch 5, 10, 20 mcg/h **SE:** N/V, HA, site Rxns pruritus, dizziness, constipation, somnolence, dry mouth **Notes:** Taper on D/C

Bupropion (Aplenzin) **BOX:** ↑ suicide risk in pts < 24 y w/ major depressive/ other psychiatric disorders; not for peds use **Uses:** *Depression* **Acts:** Aminoketone, ? action **Dose:** *Adults.* 174 mg PO, q day q A.M., ↑ PRN to 348 mg q day on day 4 if tolerated, max 522 mg/d; see PI if switching from Wellbutrin; mild–mod hepatic/ renal impair ↓ frequency/dose; severe hepatic impair 174 mg max q other day **W/P:** [C, –] w/ Drugs that ↓ Sz threshold, ↑ w/ stimulants, CYP2D6-metabolized meds

(Table 10, p 301) **CI:** Sz disorder, bulimia, anorexia nervosa, w/in 14 d of MAOIs, other forms of bupropion, abrupt D/C of EtOH, or sedatives **Disp:** ER tab 174, 348, 522 mg **SE:** Dry mouth, N, Abd pain, insomnia, dizziness, pharyngitis, agitation, anxiety, tremor, palpitation, tremor, sweating, tinnitus, myalgia, anorexia, urinary frequency, rash **Notes:** Do not cut/crush/chew, avoid EtOH

Bupropion (Wellbutrin, Wellbutrin SR, Wellbutrin XL, Zyban)
BOX: All pts being treated w/ bupropion for smoking cessation Tx should be observed for neuropsychiatric S&Sxs (hostility, agitation, depressed mood, and suicide-related events; most during/after *Zyban*; Sxs may persist following D/C; Closely monitor for worsening depression or emergence of suicidality, increased suicidal behavior in young adults **Uses:** *Depression, smoking cessation adjunct*, ADHD **Acts:** Weak inhib of neuronal uptake of serotonin & norepinephrine; ↓ neuronal dopamine reuptake **Dose:** *Depression:* 100–450 mg/d ÷ bid-tid; SR 150–200 mg bid; XL 150–450 mg daily. *Smoking cessation (Zyban, Wellbutrin XR):* 150 mg/d × 3 d, then 150 mg bid × 8–12 wks, last dose before 6 P.M.; ↓ dose w/ renal/hepatic impair **W/P:** [C, ?/–] **CI:** Sz disorder, Hx anorexia nervosa or bulimia, MAOI w/ or w/in 14 d; abrupt D/C of EtOH or sedatives; inhibitors/inducers of CYP2B6 (Table 10, p 301); w/ritonavir and lopinavir/ritonavir **Disp:** Tabs 75, 100 mg; SR tabs 100, 150, 200 mg; XL tabs 150, 300 mg; Zyban 150 mg tabs **SE:** Szs, agitation, insomnia, HA, tachycardia, ↓ wgt **Notes:** Avoid EtOH & other CNS depressants, SR & XR do not cut/chew/crush, may ↑ adverse events including Szs

Buspirone (BuSpar)
BOX: Closely monitor for worsening depression or emergence of suicidality **Uses:** Short-term relief of *anxiety* **Acts:** Anti-anxiety; antagonizes CNS serotonin and dopamine receptors **Dose:** Initial: 7.5 mg PO bid; ↑ by 5 mg q2–3d to effect; usual 20–30 mg/d; max 60 mg/d **CI:** w/ MAOI **W/P:** [B, ?/–] Avoid w/ severe hepatic/renal Insuff **Disp:** Tabs ÷ dose 5, 10, 15, 30 mg **SE:** Drowsiness, dizziness, HA, N, EPS, serotonin synd, hostility, depression **Notes:** No abuse potential or physical/psychological dependence

Busulfan (Myleran, Busulfex)
BOX: Can cause severe bone marrow suppression **Uses:** *CML*, preparative regimens for allogeneic & ABMT in high doses **Acts:** Alkylating agent **Dose:** (per protocol) **W/P:** [D, ?] **Disp:** Tabs 2 mg, Inj 60 mg/10 mL **SE:** Bone marrow suppression, ↑ BP, pulm fibrosis, N (w/ high dose), gynecomastia, adrenal Insuff, skin hyperpigmentation

Butabarbital, Hyoscyamine Hydrobromide, Phenazopyridine (Pyridium Plus)
Uses: *Relieve urinary tract pain w/ UTI, procedures, trauma* **Acts:** Phenazopyridine (topical anesthetic), hyoscyamine (parasympatholytic, ↓ spasm), & butabarbital (sedative) **Dose:** 1 PO qid, pc & hs; w/ antibiotic for UTI, 2 d max **W/P:** [C, ?] **Disp:** Tab butabarbital/hyoscyamine/phenazopyridine, 15 mg/0.3 mg/150 mg **SE:** HA, rash, itching, GI distress, methemoglobinemia, hemolytic anemia, anaphylactoid-like Rxns, dry mouth, dizziness, drowsiness, blurred vision **Notes:** Colors urine orange, may tint skin, sclera; stains clothing/contacts

Butorphanol (Stadol) [C-IV] Uses: *Anesthesia adjunct, pain* & migraine HA Acts: Opiate agonist-antagonist w/ central analgesic actions Dose: 1–4 mg IM or IV q3–4h PRN. *Migraine:* 1 spray in 1 nostril, repeat × 1 60–90 min, then q3–4h;. ↓ in renal impair W/P: [C (D if high dose or prolonged use at term), +] Disp: Inj 1, 2 mg/mL; nasal 1 mg/spray (10 mg/mL) SE: Drowsiness, dizziness, nasal congestion Notes: May induce withdrawal in opioid dependency

C1 Esterase Inhibitor [Human] (Berinert, Cinryze) Uses: *Berinert:* Rx Acute abdominal or facial attacks of hereditary angioedema (HAE)*, *Cinryze:* Prophylaxis of HAE* Acts: ↓ complement system by ↓ factor XIIa and kallikrein activation Dose: *Adults & Adolescents. Berinert:* 20 units/kg IV × 1; *Cinryze:* 1000 units IV q3–4d W/P: [C, ?/–] Hypersens Rxns, monitor for thrombotic events, may contain infectious agents CI: Hypersen Rxns to C1 esterase inhibitor preparations Disp: 500 units/vial SE: HA, abd pain, N/V/D, muscle spasms, pain, subsequent HAE attack, anaphylaxis, thromboembolism

Cabazitaxel (Jevtana) BOX: Neutropenic deaths reported; ✓ CBCs, CI w/ ANC ≤ 1500 cells/mm³; severe hypersens (rash/erythema, ↓ BP, bronchospasm) may occur, CI/D drug & Tx; CI w/ Hx of hypersens to cabazitaxel or others formulated w/ polysorbate 80 Uses: *Hormone refractory metastatic PCa after taxotere* Acts: Microtubule inhib Dose: 25 mg/m² IV Inf (over 1 h) q3wk w/ prednisone 10 mg PO daily; premed w/ antihistamine, corticosteroid, H₂ antagonist; do not use w/ bili ≥ ULN, AST/ALT ≥ 1.5 × ULN W/P: [D, ?/–] w/ CYP3A inhib/inducers CI: See Box Disp: Inj SE: ↓ WBC, ↓ Hgb, ↓ plt, sepsis, N/V/D, constipation, abd/ back/jt pain, dysgeusia, fatigue, hematuria, neuropathy, anorexia, cough, dyspnea, alopecia, pyrexia, hypersens Rxn, renal failure Notes: Monitor closely pts > 65 y

Calcipotriene (Dovonex) Uses: *Plaque psoriasis* Acts: Keratolytic Dose: Apply bid W/P: [C, ?] CI: ↑ Ca²⁺; vit D tox; do not apply to face Disp: Cream; oint; soln 0.005% SE: Skin irritation, dermatitis

Calcitonin (Fortical, Miacalcin) Uses: *Miacalcin:* *Paget Dz, emergent Rx hypercalcemia, postmenopausal osteoporosis*; *Fortical:* *postmenopausal osteoporosis*; osteogenesis imperfecta Acts: Polypeptide hormone (salmon derived), inhibits osteoclasts Dose: *Paget Dz:* 100 units/d IM/SQ initial, 50 units/d or 50–100 units q1–3d maint. *Hypercalcemia:* 4 units/kg IM/SQ q12h; ↑ to 8 units/kg q12h, max q6h. *Osteoporosis:* 100 units/q other day IM/SQ; intranasal 200 units = 1 nasal spray/d W/P: [C, ?] Disp: *Fortical, Miacalcin* nasal spray 200 Int Units/activation; Inj, *Miacalcin* 200 units/mL (2 mL) SE: Facial flushing, N, Inj site edema, nasal irritation, polyuria, may ↑ granular casts in urine Notes: For nasal spray alternate nostrils daily; ensure adequate calcium and vit D intake; *Fortical* is rDNA derived from salmon

Calcitriol (Rocaltrol, Calcijex) Uses: *Predialysis reduction of ↑ PTH levels to treat bone Dz; ↑ Ca²⁺ on dialysis* Acts: 1,25-Dihydroxycholecalci-ferol (vit D analog);↑ Ca²⁺ and phosphorus absorption; ↑ bone mineralization Dose: *Adults. Renal failure:* 0.25 mcg/d PO, ↑ 0.25 mcg/d q4–6wk PRN; 0.5 mcg 3×/wk

IV; ↑ PRN *Hypoparathyroidism:* 0.5–2 mcg/d. **Peds.** *Renal failure:* 15 ng/kg/d, ↑ PRN; maint 30–60 ng/kg/d. *Hypoparathyroidism:* < *5 y:* 0.25–0.75 mcg/d. > *6 y:* 0.5–2 mcg/d **W/P:** [C, ?] ↑ Mg²⁺ possible w/ antacids **CI:** ↑ Ca²⁺; vit D tox **Disp:** Inj 1 mcg/mL (in 1 mL); caps 0.25, 0.5 mcg; soln 1 mcg/mL **SE:** ↑ Ca²⁺ possible **Notes:** ✓ to keep Ca²⁺ WNL; Use non–aluminum phosphate binders and low-phosphate diet to control serum phosphate

Calcitriol, Ointment (Vectical) **Uses:** *mild/moderate plaque psoriasis* **Acts:** Vitamin D₃ analog **Dose:** *Adults.* Apply to area BID; max 200 g/wk **W/P:** [C, ?/–] avoid excess sunlight **CI:** None **Disp:** Oint 3 mcg/g (5-, 100-g tube) **SE:** Hypercalcemia, hypercalciuria, nephrolithiasis, worsening psoriasis, pruritus, skin discomfort

Calcium Acetate (PhosLo) **Uses:** *ESRD-associated hyperphosphatemia* **Acts:** Ca²⁺ supl w/o aluminum to ↓ PO₄²⁻ absorption **Dose:** 2–4 tabs PO w/ meals **W/P:** [C, ?] **CI:** ↑ Ca²⁺ **Disp:** Gel-Cap 667 mg **SE:** Can ↑ Ca²⁺, hypophosphatemia, constipation **Notes:** Monitor Ca²⁺

Calcium Carbonate (Tums, Alka-Mints) [OTC] **Uses:** *Hyperacidity-associated w/ peptic ulcer Dz, hiatal hernia, etc* **Acts:** Neutralizes gastric acid **Dose:** 500 mg–2 g PO PRN, 7 g/d max; ↓ w/ renal impair **W/P:** [C, ?] **Disp:** Chew tabs 350, 420, 500, 550, 750, 850 mg; susp **SE:** ↑ Ca²⁺, ↓ PO₄²⁻, constipation

Calcium Glubionate (Neo-Calglucon) [OTC] **Uses:** *Rx & prevent calcium deficiency* **Acts:** Ca²⁺ supl **Dose:** *Adults.* 6–18 g/d ÷ doses. **Peds.** 600–2000 mg/kg/d ÷ qid (9 g/d max); ↓ in renal impair **W/P:** [C, ?] **CI:** ↑ Ca²⁺ **Disp:** OTC syrup 1.8 g/5 mL = elemental Ca 115 mg/5 mL **SE:** ↑ Ca²⁺, ↓ PO₄²⁻, constipation

Calcium Salts (Chloride, Gluconate, Gluceptate) **Uses:** *Ca²⁺ replacement*, VF, Ca²⁺ blocker tox (CCB), Mg²⁺ intoxication, tetany, *hyperphosphatemia in ESRD* **Acts:** Ca²⁺ supl/replacement **Dose:** *Adults. Replacement:* 1–2 g/d PO. *Tetany:* 1 g CaCl over 10–30 min; repeat in 6 h PRN; *ECC 2010. Hyperkalemia/ hypermagnesemia/CCB OD:* 500–1000 mg (5–10 mL of 10% soln) IV; repeat PRN; comparable dose of 10% calcium gluconate is 15–30 mL **Peds.** *Replacement:* 200–500 mg/kg/24 h PO or IV ÷ qid. *Tetany:* 10 mg/kg CaCl over 5–10 min; repeat in 6 h or use Inf (200 mg/kg/d max). *ECC 2010. Hypocalcemia/hyperkalemia/hypermagnesemia/CCB OD:* Calcium chloride or gluconate 20 mg/kg (0.2 mL/kg) slow IV/IO, repeat PRN; central venous route preferred *Adults & Peds.* ↓ Ca²⁺ d/t citrated blood Inf: 0.45 mEq Ca/100 mL of 10% citrated blood Inf (↓ in renal impair) **W/P:** [C, ?] **CI:** ↑ Ca²⁺ **Disp:** CaCl Inj 10% = 100 mg/mL = Ca 27.2 mg/mL = 10-mL amp; Ca gluconate Inj 10% = 100 mg/mL = Ca 9 mg/mL; tabs 500 mg = 45-mg Ca, 650 mg = 58.5-mg Ca, 975 mg = 87.75-mg Ca, 1 g = 90-mg Ca; Ca gluceptate Inj 220 mg/mL = 18-mg/mL Ca **SE:** ↓ HR, cardiac arrhythmias, ↑ Ca²⁺, constipation **Notes:** CaCl 270 mg (13.6 mEq) elemental Ca/g, & calcium gluconate 90 mg (4.5 mEq) Ca/g. RDA for Ca intake: *Peds < 6 mo.* 210 mg/d; *6 mo–1 y:* 270 mg/d; *1–3 y:* 500 mg/d; *4–9 y:* 800 mg/d; *10–18 y:* 1200 mg/d. *Adults.* 1000 mg/d; > *50 y:* 1200 mg/d

Calfactant (Infasurf) Uses: *Prevention & Rx of RSD in infants* Acts: Exogenous pulm surfactant Dose: 3 mL/kg instilled into lungs. Can repeat 3 total doses given 12 h apart Disp: Intratracheal susp 35 mg/mL SE: Monitor for cyanosis, airway obst, ↓ HR during administration

Candesartan (Atacand) Uses: *HTN*, DN, CHF Acts: Angiotensin II receptor antagonist Dose: 4–32 mg/d (usual 16 mg/d) W/P: [C (1st tri, D) (2nd & 3rd tri), –] CI: Primary hyperaldosteronism; bilateral RAS Disp: Tabs 4, 8, 16, 32 mg SE: Dizziness, HA, flushing, angioedema

Capsaicin (Capsin, Zostrix, Others) [OTC] Uses: Pain d/t *postherpetic neuralgia*, chronic neuralgia, *arthritis, diabetic neuropathy*, post-op pain, psoriasis, intractable pruritus Acts: Topical analgesic Dose: Apply tid-qid W/P: [C, ?] Disp: OTC creams; gel; lotions; roll-ons SE: Local irritation, neurotox, cough Note: Wk to onset of action

Captopril (Capoten, Others) Uses: *HTN, CHF, MI*, LVD, DN Acts: ACE inhib Dose: *Adults. HTN:* Initial, 25 mg PO bid-tid; ↑ to maint q1–2wk by 25-mg increments/dose (max 450 mg/d) to effect. *CHF:* Initial, 6.25–12.5 mg PO tid; titrate PRN *LVD:* 50 mg PO tid. *DN:* 25 mg PO tid. *Peds Infants < 2 mo.* 0.05–0.5 mg/kg/dose PO q8–24h. *Children:* Initial, 0.3–0.5 mg/kg/dose PO; ↑ to 6 mg/kg/d max in 2–4 ÷ doses; 1 h ac W/P: [C (1st tri); D (2nd & 3rd tri) +]; unknown effects in renal impair CI: Hx angioedema, bilateral RAS Disp: Tabs 12.5, 25, 50, 100 mg SE: Rash, proteinuria, cough, ↑ K⁺

Carbamazepine (Tegretol XR, Carbatrol, Epitol, Equetro) BOX: Aplastic anemia & agranulocytosis have been reported w/ carbamazepine; pts w/ Asian ancestry should be tested to determine potential for skin Rxns Uses: *Epilepsy, trigeminal neuralgia, acute mania w/ bipolar disorder (Equetro)* EtOH withdrawal Acts: Anticonvulsant Dose: *Adults. Initial:* 200 mg PO bid or 100 mg 4 ×/d as susp; ↑ by 200 mg/d; usual 800–1200 mg/d ÷ doses. *Acute Mania (Equetro):* 400 mg/d, ↑ bid, adjust by 200 mg/d to response 1600 mg/d max. *Peds < 6 y.* 5 mg/kg/d; ↑ to 10–20 mg/kg/d ÷ in 2–4 doses. *6–12 y:* Initial: 100 mg PO bid or 10 mg/kg/24 h PO ÷ daily-bid; ↑ to maint 20–30 mg/kg/24 h ÷ tid-qid; ↓ in renal impair; take w/ food W/P: [D, +] CI: MAOI use, Hx BM suppression Disp: Tabs 100, 200, 300, 400 mg; chew tabs 100 mg, 200 mg; XR tabs 100, 200,400 mg; *Equetro* Caps ER 100, 200, 300 mg; susp 100 mg/5 mL SE: Drowsiness, dizziness, blurred vision, N/V, rash, SJS/toxic epidermal necrolysis (TEN), ↓ Na⁺, leukopenia, agranulocytosis Notes: Monitor CBC & levels: *Trough:* Just before next dose; *Therapeutic: Peak:* 8–12 mcg/mL (monotherapy), 4–8 mcg/mL (polytherapy); *Toxic Trough:* > 15 mcg/mL; *1/2-life:* 15–20 h; generic products not interchangeable, many drug interactions, administer susp in 3–4 ÷ doses daily; skin tox (SJS/TEN) ↑ w/ HLA-B*1502 allele

Carbidopa/Levodopa (Sinemet, Parcopa) Uses: *Parkinson Dz* Acts: ↑ CNS dopamine levels Dose: 25/100 mg bid-qid; ↑ as needed (max 200/2000 mg/d) W/P: [C, ?] CI: NAG, suspicious skin lesion (may activate melanoma), melanoma, MAOI use **Disp:** Tabs (mg carbidopa/mg levodopa) 10/100, 25/100, 25/250; tabs SR (mg carbidopa/mg levodopa) 25/100, 50/200; ODT 10/100, 25/100, 25/250 **SE:** Psych disturbances, orthostatic ↓ BP, dyskinesias, cardiac arrhythmias

Carboplatin (Paraplatin) **BOX:** Administration only by physician experienced in cancer CA chemotherapy; BM suppression possible; anaphylaxis may occur **Uses:** *Ovarian*, lung, head & neck, testicular, urothelial, & brain CA, NHL & allogeneic & ABMT in high doses **Acts:** DNA cross-linker; forms DNA-platinum adducts **Dose:** 360 mg/m^2 (ovarian carcinoma); AUC dosing 4–8 mg/mL (Culvert formula: mg = AUC × [25 + calculated GFR]); adjust based on plt count, CrCl, & BSA (Egorin formula); up to 1500 mg/m^2 used in ABMT setting (per protocols) **W/P:** [D, ?] **CI:** Severe BM suppression, excessive bleeding **Disp:** Inj 50-, 150-, 450 -mg vial (10 mg/mL) **SE:** Anaphylaxis, ↓ BM, N/V/D, nephrotox, hematuria, neurotox, ↑ LFTs **Notes:** Physiologic dosing based on Culvert or Egorin formula allows ↑ doses w/ ↓ tox

Carisoprodol (Soma) **Uses:** *Adjunct to sleep & physical therapy to relieve painful musculoskeletal conditions* **Acts:** Centrally acting muscle relaxant **Dose:** 250–350 mg PO tid-qid **W/P:** [C, M] Tolerance may result; w/ renal/hepatic impair **CI:** Allergy to meprobamate; acute intermittent porphyria **Disp:** Tabs 250, 350 mg **SE:** CNS depression, drowsiness, dizziness, HA, tachycardia **Notes:** Avoid EtOH & other CNS depressants; available in combo w/ ASA or codeine.

Carmustine [BCNU] (BiCNU, Gliadel) **BOX:** BM suppression, dose-related pulm tox possible; administer under direct supervision of experienced physician **Uses:** *Primary or adjunct brain tumors, multiple myeloma, Hodgkin and non-Hodgkin lymphomas*, induction for allogeneic & ABMT (high dose)* surgery & RT adjunct high-grade glioma and recurrent glioblastoma (*Gliadel* implant)* **Acts:** Alkylating agent; nitrosourea forms DNA cross-links to inhibit DNA **Dose:** 150–200 mg/m^2 q6–8wk single or ÷ dose daily Inj over 2 d; 20–65 mg/m^2 q4–6wk; 300–900 mg/m^2 in BMT (per protocols); up to 8 implants in CNS op site; ↓ w/ hepatic & renal impair **W/P:** [D, ?] ↓ WBC, RBC, plt counts, renal/hepatic impair **CI:** ↓ BM, PRG **Disp:** Inj 100 mg/vial; *Gliadel* wafer 7.7 mg **SE:** ↓ BP, N/V, ↓ WBC & plt, phlebitis, facial flushing, hepatic/renal dysfunction, pulm fibrosis (may occur years after), optic neuroretinitis; heme tox may persist 4–6 wk after dose **Notes:** Do not give course more frequently than q6wk (cumulative tox); ✓ baseline PFTs, monitor pulm status

Carteolol (Ocupress, Carteolol Ophthalmic) **Uses:** *HTN, ↑ IOP pressure, chronic open-angle glaucoma* **Acts:** Blocks β-adrenergic receptors (β$_1$, β$_2$), mild ISA **Dose:** Ophthal 1 gtt in eye(s) bid **W/P:** [C, ?/–] Cardiac failure, asthma **CI:** Sinus bradycardia; heart block > 1st degree; bronchospasm **Disp:** Ophthal soln 1% **SE:** conjunctival hyperemia, anisocoria, keratitis, eye pain **Notes:** Oral forms no longer available in US

Carvedilol (Coreg, Coreg CR) **Uses:** *HTN, Mild to severe CHF, LVD post-MI* **Acts:** Blocks adrenergic receptors, β$_1$, β$_2$, α$_1$ **Dose:** *HTN:* 6.25–12.5 mg bid or CR 20–80 mg PO daily. *CHF:* 3.125–25 mg bid; w/ food to minimize ↓ BP **W/P:** [C (1st tri); D (2nd & 3rd tri), ?/–] asthma, DM **CI:** Decompensated CHF, 2nd-/3rd-degree heart block, SSS, severe ↓ HR w/o pacemaker, acute asthma, severe hepatic impair **Disp:** Tabs 3.125, 6.25, 12.5, 25 mg; CR Tabs 10, 20, 40, 80 mg **SE:** Dizziness, fatigue, hyperglycemia, may mask/potentiate hypoglycemia, ↓ HR, edema, hypercholesterolemia **Notes:** Do not D/C abruptly; ↑ digoxin levels

Caspofungin (Cancidas) Uses: *Invasive aspergillosis refractory/intolerant to standard Rx, esophageal candidiasis* **Acts:** Echinocandin; ↓ fungal cell wall synth; highest activity in regions of active cell growth **Dose:** 70 mg IV load day 1, 50 mg IV; slow Inf; ↓ in hepatic impair **W/P:** [C, ?/–] Do not use w/ cyclosporine; not studied as initial Rx **CI:** Allergy to any component **Disp:** Inj 50, 70 mg powder for recons **SE:** Fever, HA, N/V, thrombophlebitis at site, ↑ LFTs **Notes:** Monitor during Inf; limited experience beyond 2 wk of Rx

Cefaclor (Ceclor, Raniclor) Uses: *Bacterial Infxns of the upper & lower resp tract, skin, bone, urinary tract, Abd* **Acts:** 2nd-gen cephalosporin; ↓ cell wall synth. *Spectrum:* More gram(–) activity than 1st-gen cephalosporins; effective against gram(+) (*Streptococcus* sp, *S. aureus*); good gram(–) against *H. influenzae, E. coli, Klebsiella, Proteus* **Dose:** *Adults.* 250–500 mg PO tid; ER 375–500 mg bid. *Peds.* 20–40 mg/kg/d PO ÷ 8–12 h; ↓ renal impair **W/P:** [B, +] antacids ↓ absorption **CI:** Cephalosporin/PCN allergy **Disp:** Caps 250, 500 mg; Tabs ER 375, 500 mg; chew tabs (*Raniclor*) 250, 375 mg; susp 125, 187, 250, 375 mg/5 mL **SE:** N/D, rash, eosinophilia, ↑ LFTs, HA, rhinitis, vaginitis

Cefadroxil (Duricef) Uses: *Infxns skin, bone, upper & lower resp tract, urinary tract* **Acts:** 1st-gen cephalosporin; ↓ cell wall synth. *Spectrum:* Good gram(+) (group A β-hemolytic *Streptococcus, Staphylococcus*); gram(–) (*E. coli, Proteus, Klebsiella*) **Dose:** *Adults.* 1–2 g/d PO, 2 ÷ doses *Peds.* 30 mg/kg/d ÷ bid; ↓ in renal impair **W/P:** [B, +] CI: Cephalosporin/PCN allergy **Disp:** Caps 500 mg; tabs 1 g; susp, 250, 500 mg/5 mL **SE:** N/V/D, rash, eosinophilia, ↑ LFTs

Cefazolin (Ancef, Kefzol) Uses: *Infxns of skin, bone, upper & lower resp tract, urinary tract* **Acts:** 1st-gen cephalosporin; β-lactam ↓ cell wall synth. *Spectrum:* Good gram(+) bacilli & cocci, (*Streptococcus, Staphylococcus* [except *Enterococcus*]); some gram(–) (*E. coli, Proteus, Klebsiella*) **Dose:** *Adults.* 1–2 g IV q8h *Peds.* 25–100 mg/kg/d IV ÷ q6–8h; ↓ in renal impair **W/P:** [B, +] CI: Cephalosporin/PCN allergy **Disp:** Inj: 500 mg, 1, 10, 20 g **SE:** D, rash, eosinophilia, ↑ LFTs, Inj site pain **Notes:** Widely used for surgical prophylaxis

Cefdinir (Omnicef) Uses: * infxns of the resp tract, skin, bone, & urinary tract* **Acts:** 3rd-gen cephalosporin; ↓ cell wall synth *Spectrum:* Many gram (+) & (–) organisms; more active than cefaclor & cephalexin against *Streptococcus, Staphylococcus*; some anaerobes **Dose:** *Adults.* 300 mg PO bid or 600 mg/d PO. *Peds.* 7 mg/kg PO bid or 14 mg/kg/d PO; ↓ in renal impair **W/P:** [B, +] w/ PCN-sensitive pts, serum sickness-like Rxns reported **CI:** Hypersens to cephalosporins **Disp:** Caps 300 mg; susp 125, 250 mg/5 mL **SE:** Anaphylaxis, D, rare pseudomembranous colitis

Cefditoren (Spectracef) Uses: *Acute exacerbations of chronic bronchitis, pharyngitis, tonsillitis; skin Infxns* Acts: 3rd-gen cephalosporin; ↓ cell wall synth. *Spectrum:* Good gram(+) (*Streptococcus & Staphylococcus*); gram (−) (*H. influenzae & M. catarrhalis*) Dose: **Adults & Peds > 12 y.** Skin: 200 mg PO bid × 10 d. *Chronic bronchitis, pharyngitis, tonsillitis:* 400 mg PO bid × 10 d; avoid antacids w/ in 2 h; take w/ meals; ↓ in renal impair W/P: [B, ?] Renal/hepatic impair CI: Cephalosporin/PCN allergy, milk protein, or carnitine deficiency Disp: 200 mg tabs SE: HA, N/V/D, colitis, nephrotox, hepatic dysfunction, SJS, toxic epidermal necrolysis, allergic Rxns Notes: Causes renal excretion of carnitine; tabs contain milk protein

Cefepime (Maxipime) Uses: *Comp/uncomp UTI, pneumonia, empiric febrile neutropenia, skin/soft-tissue Infxns, comp intra-Abd Infxns* Acts: 4th-gen cephalosporin; ↓ cell wall synth. *Spectrum:* Gram(+) S. pneumoniae, S. aureus, gram(−) K. pneumoniae, E. coli, P. aeruginosa, & Enterobacter sp Dose: **Adults.** 1–2 g IV q8–12h. **Peds.** 50 mg/kg q8h for febrile neutropenia; 50 mg/kg bid for skin/soft-tissue Infxns; ↓ in renal impair W/P: [B, +] CI: Cephalosporin/PCN allergy Disp: Inj 500 mg, 1, 2 g SE: Rash, pruritus, N/V/D, fever, HA, (+) Coombs test w/o hemolysis Notes: Can give IM or IV; concern over ↑ death rates not confirmed by FDA

Cefixime (Suprax) Uses: *Resp tract, skin, bone, & urinary tract Infxns* Acts: 3rd-gen cephalosporin; ↓ cell wall synth. *Spectrum:* S. pneumoniae, S. pyogenes, H. influenzae, & enterobacteria Dose: **Adults.** 400 mg PO ÷ daily-bid. **Peds.** 8–20 mg/kg/d PO ÷ daily-bid; ↓ w/ renal impair W/P: [B, +] CI: Cephalosporin/PCN allergy Disp: Susp 100, 200 mg/5 mL SE: N/V/D, flatulence, & Abd pain Notes: ✓renal & hepatic Fxn; use susp for otitis media

Cefoperazone (Cefobid) Uses: *Rx Infxns of the resp, skin, urinary tract, sepsis* Acts: 3rd-gen cephalosporin; ↓ bacterial cell wall synth. *Spectrum:* gram(−) (e.g., E. coli, Klebsiella), P. aeruginosa but < ceftazidime; gram(+) variable against Streptococcus & Staphylococcus sp Dose: **Adults.** 2–4 g/d IM/IV ÷ q 8–12h (16 g/d max). **Peds.** (Not approved) 100–150 mg/kg/d IM/IV ÷ bid-tid (12 g/d max); ↓ in renal/hepatic impair W/P: [B, +] May ↑ bleeding risk CI: Cephalosporin/PCN allergy Disp: Powder for Inj 1, 2, 10 g SE: D, rash, eosinophilia, ↑ LFTs, hypoprothrombinemia, & bleeding (d/t MTT side chain) Notes: May interfere w/ warfarin; disulfiram-like Rxn

Cefotaxime (Claforan) Uses: *Infxns of lower resp tract, skin, bone & joint, urinary tract, meningitis, sepsis, PID, GC* Acts: 3rd-gen cephalosporin; ↓ cell wall synth. *Spectrum:* Most gram(−) (not Pseudomonas), some gram(+) cocci S. pneumoniae, S. aureus (penicillinase/nonpenicillinase producing), H. influenzae (including ampicillin-resistant), not Enterococcus; many PCN-resistant pneumococci Dose: **Adults.** Uncomplicated Infxn: 2 g IV/IM q12h; Mod–severe Infxn: 1–2 g IV/IM q 8–12 h; Severe/septicemia: 2 g IV/IM q4–8h; GC urethritis, cervicitis, rectal in female: 0.5 g IM × 1; rectal GC men 1 g IM × 1; **Peds.** 50–200 mg/kg/d

IV ÷ q6–8h; ↓ w/ renal/hepatic impair **W/P:** [B, +] Arrhythmia w/ rapid Inj; w/ colitis **CI:** Cephalosporin/PCN allergy **Disp:** Powder for Inj 500 mg, 1, 2, 10, 20 g, premixed Inf 20 mg/mL, 40 mg/mL **SE:** D, rash, pruritus, colitis, eosinophilia, ↑ transaminases

Cefotetan (Cefotan) Uses: *Infxns of the upper & lower resp tract, skin, bone, urinary tract, abd, & gynecologic system* **Acts:** 2nd-gen cephalosporin; ↓ cell wall synth **Spectrum:** Less active against gram(+) anaerobes including *B. fragilis*; gram(–), including *E. coli, Klebsiella, & Proteus* **Dose:** *Adults.* 1–3 g IV q12h. **Peds.** 20–40 mg/kg/d IV ÷ q12h (6 g/d max) ↓ w/ renal impair **W/P:** [B, +] May ↑ bleeding risk; w/ Hx of PCN allergies, w/ other nephrotoxic drugs **CI:** Cephalosporin/PCN allergy **Disp:** Powder for Inj 1, 2, 10 g **SE:** D, rash, eosinophilia, ↑ transaminases, hypoprothrombinemia, & bleeding (d/t MTT side chain) **Notes:** May interfere w/ warfarin

Cefoxitin (Mefoxin) Uses: *Infxns of the upper & lower resp tract, skin, bone, urinary tract, abd, & gynecologic system* **Acts:** 2nd-gen cephalosporin; ↓ cell wall synth. **Spectrum:** Good gram(–) against enteric bacilli (i.e., *E. coli, Klebsiella, & Proteus*); anaerobic: *B. fragilis* **Dose:** *Adults.* 1–2 g IV q6–8h. **Peds.** 80–160 mg/kg/d ÷ q4–6h (12 g/d max); ↓ w/ renal impair **W/P:** [B, +] **CI:** Cephalosporin/PCN allergy **Disp:** Powder for Inj 1, 2, 10 g **SE:** D, rash, eosinophilia, ↑ transaminases

Cefpodoxime (Vantin) Uses: *Rx resp, skin, & urinary tract Infxns* **Acts:** 3rd-gen cephalosporin; ↓ cell wall synth. **Spectrum:** *S. pneumoniae* or non-β-lactamase-producing *H. influenzae*; acute uncomplicated *N. gonorrhoeae*; some uncomplicated gram(–) (*E. coli, Klebsiella, Proteus*) **Dose:** *Adults.* 100–400 mg PO q12h. **Peds.** 10 mg/kg/d PO ÷ bid; ↓ in renal impair, w/ food **W/P:** [B, +] **CI:** Cephalosporin/PCN allergy **Disp:** Tabs 100, 200 mg; susp 50, 100 mg/5 mL **SE:** D, rash, HA, eosinophilia, ↑ transaminases **Notes:** Drug interactions w/ agents that ↑ gastric pH

Cefprozil (Cefzil) Uses: *Rx resp tract, skin, & urinary tract Infxns* **Acts:** 2nd-gen cephalosporin; ↓ cell wall synth. **Spectrum:** Active against MSSA, *Streptococcus*, & gram(–) bacilli (*E. coli, Klebsiella, P. mirabilis, H. influenzae, Moraxella*) **Dose:** *Adults.* 250–500 mg PO daily-bid. **Peds.** 7.5–15 mg/kg/d PO ÷ bid; ↓ in renal impair **W/P:** [B, +] **CI:** Cephalosporin/PCN allergy **Disp:** Tabs 250, 500 mg; susp 125, 250 mg/5 mL **SE:** D, dizziness, rash, eosinophilia, ↑ transaminases **Notes:** Use higher doses for otitis & pneumonia

Ceftaroline (Teflaro) Uses: *Tx skin/skin structure Infxn & CAP* **Acts:** Unclassified ("5th gen") cephalosporin; ↓ cell wall synthesis; **Spectrum:** Gram(+) *Staph aureus* (MSSA/MRSA), *Strep pyogenes, Strep agalactiae, Strep pneumoniae*; Gram(–) *E. coli, K. pneumoniae, K. oxytoca, H. influenzae* **Dose:** *Adults.* 600 mg IV q12h; CrCl 30–50 mL/min: 400 mg IV q12h; CrCl 15–29 mL/min: 300 mg IV q12h; CrCl < 15 mL/min: 200 mg IV q12h; inf over 1 h **W/P:** [B, ?/–] monitor for *C. difficile*-associated D **CI:** Cephalsporin sensitivity **Disp:** Inj **SE:** Hypersens Rxn, D/N, rash, constipation, ↓ K⁺, phlebitis, ↑ LFTs

Ceftazidime (Fortaz, Tazicef) Uses: *Rx resp tract, skin, bone, urinary tract Infxns, meningitis, & septicemia* **Acts:** 3rd-gen cephalosporin; ↓ cell wall synth. *Spectrum: P. aeruginosa* sp, good gram(–) activity **Dose: Adults.** 500–2 g IV/IM q8–12h. **Peds.** 30–50 mg/kg/dose IV q8h; ↓ in renal impair **W/P:** [B, +] PCN sensitivity **CI:** Cephalosporin/PCN allergy **Disp:** Powder for Inj 500 mg, 1, 2, 6 g **SE:** D, rash, eosinophilia, ↑ transaminases **Notes:** Use only for proven or strongly suspected Infxn to ↓ development of drug resistance

Ceftibuten (Cedax) Uses: *Rx resp tract, skin, urinary tract Infxns & otitis media* **Acts:** 3rd-gen cephalosporin; ↓ cell wall synth. *Spectrum: H. influenzae & M. catarrhalis;* weak against *S. pneumoniae* **Dose: Adults.** 400 mg/d PO. **Peds.** 9 mg/kg/d PO; ↓ in renal impair; take on empty stomach (susp) **W/P:** [B, +] **CI:** Cephalosporin/PCN allergy **Disp:** Caps 400 mg; susp 90 mg/5 mL **SE:** D, rash, eosinophilia, ↑ transaminases

Ceftizoxime (Cefizox) Uses: *Rx resp tract, skin, bone, & urinary tract Infxns, meningitis, septicemia* **Acts:** 3rd-gen cephalosporin; ↓ cell wall synth. *Spectrum:* Good gram(–) bacilli (not *Pseudomonas*), some gram(+) cocci (not *Enterococcus*), & some anaerobes **Dose: Adults.** 1–4 g IV q8–12h. **Peds.** 150–200 mg/kg/d IV ÷ q6–8h; ↓ in renal impair **W/P:** [B, +] **CI:** Cephalosporin/PCN allergy **Disp:** Inj 1, 2, 10 g **SE:** D, fever, rash, eosinophilia, thrombocytosis, ↑ transaminases

Ceftriaxone (Rocephin) **BOX:** Avoid in hyperbilirubinemic neonates or co-infusion w/ calcium-containing products Uses: *Resp tract (pneumonia), skin, bone, abd & urinary tract Infxns, meningitis, septicemia, GC, PID, peri-operative* **Acts:** 3rd-gen cephalosporin; ↓ cell wall synth. *Spectrum:* Mod gram(+); excellent β-lactamase producers **Dose: Adults.** 1–2 g IV/IM q12–24h. **Peds.** 50–100 mg/kg/d IV/IM ÷ q12–24h; ↓ w/ renal impair **W/P:** [B, +] **CI:** Cephalosporin allergy; hyperbilirubinemic neonates **Disp:** Powder for Inj 250 mg, 500 mg, 1, 2, 10 g; premixed 20, 40 mg/mL **SE:** D, rash, ↑ WBC, thrombocytosis, eosinophilia, ↑ LFTs

Cefuroxime (Ceftin [PO], Zinacef [Parenteral]) Uses: *Upper & lower resp tract, skin, urinary tract, abd, gynecologic Infxns* **Acts:** 2nd-gen cephalosporin; ↓ cell wall synth *Spectrum:* Staphylococci, group B streptococci, *H. influenzae, E. coli, Enterobacter, Salmonella, & Klebsiella* **Dose: Adults.** 750 mg–1.5 g IV q6h or 250–500 mg PO bid **Peds.** 75–150 mg/kg/d IV ÷ q8h or 20–30 mg/kg/d PO ÷ bid; ↓ w/ renal impair; take PO w/ food **W/P:** [B, +] **CI:** Cephalosporin/PCN allergy **Disp:** Tabs 250, 500 mg; susp 125, 250 mg/5 mL; powder for Inj 750 mg, 1.5, 7.5 g **SE:** D, rash, eosinophilia, ↑ LFTs **Notes:** Cefuroxime film-coated tabs & susp not bioequivalent; do not substitute on a mg/mg basis; IV crosses blood–brain barrier

Celecoxib (Celebrex) **BOX:** ↑ Risk of serious CV thrombotic events, MI, & stroke; can be fatal; ↑ risk of serious GI adverse events including bleeding, ulceration, & perforation of the stomach or intestines; can be fatal Uses: *OA, RA, ankylosing spondylitis, acute pain, primary dysmenorrhea, preventive in FAP* **Acts:** NSAID;

↓ COX-2 pathway **Dose:** 100–200 mg/d or bid; *FAP:* 400 mg PO bid; ↓ w/ hepatic impair; take w/ food/milk **W/P:** [C/D (3rd tri), ?] w/ Renal impair **CI:** Sulfonamide allergy, perioperative coronary artery bypass graft **Disp:** Caps 100, 200, 400 mg **SE:** See Box; GI upset, HTN, edema, renal failure, HA **Notes:** Watch for Sxs of GI bleed; no effect on plt/bleeding time; can affect drugs metabolized by P-450 pathway

Cephalexin (Keflex, Panixine DisperDose) **Uses:** *Skin, bone, upper/ lower resp tract (streptococcal pharyngitis), otitis media, uncomp cystitis Infxns* **Acts:** 1st-gen cephalosporin; ↓ cell wall synth. *Spectrum: Streptococcus (including β-hemolytic), Staphylococcus, E. coli, Proteus, & Klebsiella* **Dose:** *Adults & Peds > 15 y.* 250–1000 mg PO qid; Rx cystitis 7–14 d (4 g/d max). *Peds < 15 y.* 25–100 mg/kg/d PO ÷ bid-qid; ↓ in renal impair; on empty stomach **W/P:** [B, +] **CI:** Cephalosporin/PCN allergy **Disp:** Caps 250, 500 mg; *(Panixine DisperDose)* tabs for oral susp 100, 125, 250 mg; susp 125, 250 mg/5 mL **SE:** D, rash, eosinophilia, gastritis, dyspepsia, ↑ LFTs, *C. difficile* colitis, vaginitis

Cephradine (Velosef) **Uses:** *Resp, GU, GI, skin, soft-tissue, bone, & joint Infxns* **Acts:** 1st-gen cephalosporin; ↓ cell wall synth. *Spectrum:* Gram(+) bacilli & cocci (not *Enterococcus*); some gram(−) (*E. coli, Proteus, & Klebsiella*) **Dose:** *Adults.* 250–500 mg q6–12h (8 g/d max). *Peds > 9 mo.* 25–100 mg/kg/d ÷ bid-qid (4 g/d max); ↓ in renal impair **W/P:** [B, +] **CI:** Cephalosporin/PCN allergy **Disp:** Caps: 250, 500 mg; powder for susp 125, 250 mg/5 mL **SE:** Rash, eosinophilia, ↑ LFTs, N/V/D

Certolizumab Pegol (Cimzia) **BOX:** Serious Infxns (bacterial, fungal, TB, opportunistic) possible. D/C w/ severe Infxn/sepsis, test and monitor for TB w/ Tx; lymphoma/other CA possible in children/adolescents **Uses:** *Crohn Dz w/inadequate response to conventional Tx; moderate/severe RA* **Action:** TNF–α blocker **Dose:** *Crohn: Initial:* 400 mg SQ, repeat 2 & 4 wk after; *Maint:* 400 mg SQ q 4 wk. *RA: Initial:* 400 mg SQ, repeat 2 & 4 wk after; *Maint:* 200 mg SQ q other wk or 400 mg SQ q 4 wk. **W/P:** [B, ?] Infection, TB, autoimmune Dz, demyelinating CNS Dz, hepatitis B reactivation **CI:** None **Disp:** Inj, powder for reconstitution 200 mg; Inj, soln: 200 mg/mL (1 mL) **SE:** HA, N, upper respiratory Infxns, serious Infxns, TB, opportunistic Infxns, malignancies, demyelinating Dz, CHF, pancytopenia, lupus-like synd, new-onset psoriasis **Notes:** 400 mg dose is 2 inj of 200 mg each. Monitor for Infxn. Do not give live/attenuated vaccines during Rx; avoid use w/ anakinra

Cetirizine (Zyrtec, Zyrtec D) [OTC] **Uses:** *Allergic rhinitis & other allergic Sxs including urticaria* **Acts:** Nonsedating antihistamine; *Zyrtec D* contains decongestant **Dose:** *Adults & Children > 6 y:* 5–10 mg/d; *Zyrtec D* 5/120 mg PO bid whole *Peds 6–11 mo.* 2.5 mg daily. *12 mo–5 y:* 2.5 mg daily-bid; ↓ to q day in renal/ hepatic impair **W/P:** [C, ?/–] w/ HTN, BPH, rare CNS stimulation, DM, heart Dz **CI:** Allergy to cetirizine, hydroxyzine **Disp:** Tabs 5, 10 mg; chew tabs 5, 10 mg; syrup 5 mg/5 mL; *Zyrtec D:* Tabs 5/120 mg (cetirizine/pseudoephedrine) **SE:** HA, drowsiness, xerostomia **Notes:** Can cause sedation; swallow ER tabs whole

Cetuximab (Erbitux) **BOX:** Severe Inf Rxns including rapid onset of airway obst (bronchospasm, stridor, hoarseness), urticaria, & ↓ BP; permanent D/C required; ↑ risk sudden death and cardiopulmonary arrest **Uses:** *EGFR + metastatic colorectal CA w/ or w/o irinotecan, unresectable head/neck small cell carcinoma w/ RT; monotherapy in metastatic head/neck CA* **Acts:** Human/mouse recombinant MoAb; binds EGFR, ↓ tumor cell growth **Dose:** Per protocol; load 400 mg/m² IV over 2 h; 250 mg/m² given over 1h × 1 wk **W/P:** [C, −] **Disp:** Inj 100 mg/50 mL **SE:** Acneform rash, asthenia/malaise, N/V/D, Abd pain, alopecia, Inf Rxn, derm tox, interstitial lung Dz, fever, sepsis, dehydration, kidney failure, PE **Notes:** Assess tumor for EGFR before Rx; pretreatment w/ diphenhydramine; w/ mild SE ↓ Inf rate by 50%; limit sun exposure

Charcoal, Activated (SuperChar, Actidose, Liqui-Char) **Uses:** *Emergency poisoning by most drugs & chemicals (see CI)* **Acts:** Adsorbent detoxicant **Dose:** Give w/ 70% sorbitol (2 mL/kg); repeated use of sorbitol not OK **Adults.** *Acute intoxication:* 25–100 g/dose. *GI dialysis:* 20–50 g q6h for 1–2 d. **Peds** *1–12 y.* *Acute intoxication:* 1–2 g/kg/dose. *GI dialysis:* 5–10 g/dose q4–8h **W/P:** [C, ?] May cause V (hazardous w/ petroleum & caustic ingestions); do not mix w/ dairy **CI:** Not effective for cyanide, mineral acids, caustic alkalis, organic solvents, iron, EtOH, methanol poisoning, Li; do not use sorbitol in pts w/ fructose intolerance, intestinal obst, non-intact GI tracts **Disp:** Powder, liq, caps **SE:** Some liq dosage forms in sorbitol base (a cathartic); V/D, black stools, constipation **Notes:** Charcoal w/ sorbitol not OK in children < 1 y; monitor for ↓ K⁺ & Mg²⁺; protect airway in lethargic/comatose pts

Chloral Hydrate (Aquachloral, Supprettes) [C-IV] **Uses:** *Short-term nocturnal & pre-op sedation* **Acts:** Sedative hypnotic; active metabolite trichloroethanol **Dose:** **Adults.** *Hypnotic:* 500 mg–1 g PO or PR 30 min hs or before procedure. *Sedative:* 250 mg PO or PR tid. **Peds.** *Hypnotic:* 20–50 mg/kg/24 h PO or PR 30 min hs or before procedure. *Sedative:* 5–15 mg/kg/dose q8h; avoid w/ CrCl < 50 mL/min or severe hepatic impair **W/P:** [C, +] Porphyria & in neonates, long-term care facility residents **CI:** Allergy to components; severe renal, hepatic, or cardiac Dz **Disp:** Caps 500 mg; syrup 500 mg/5 mL; supp 325, 500 mg **SE:** GI irritation, drowsiness, ataxia, dizziness, nightmares, rash **Notes:** May accumulate; tolerance may develop > 2 wk; taper dose; mix syrup in H₂O or fruit juice; do not crush caps; avoid EtOH & CNS depressants

Chlorambucil (Leukeran) **BOX:** Myelosuppressive, carcinogenic, teratogenic, associated w/ infertility **Uses:** *CLL, Hodgkin Dz*, Waldenström macroglobulinemia **Acts:** Alkylating agent (nitrogen mustard) **Dose:** (per protocol) 0.1–0.2 mg/kg/d for 3–6 wk or 0.4 mg/kg/dose q2wk; ↓ w/ renal impair **W/P:** [D, ?] Sz disorder & BM suppression; affects human fertility **CI:** Previous resistance; alkylating agent allergy; w/ live vaccines **Disp:** Tabs 2 mg **SE:** ↓ BM, CNS stimulation, N/V, drug fever, rash, secondary leukemias, alveolar dysplasia, pulm fibrosis, hepatotoxic **Notes:** Monitor LFTs, CBC, plts, serum uric acid; ↓ dose if pt has received radiation

Chlordiazepoxide (Librium, Mitran, Libritabs) [C-IV] Uses: *Anxiety, tension, EtOH withdrawal*, & pre-op apprehension **Acts:** Benzodiazepine; antianxiety agent **Dose:** *Adults. Mild anxiety:* 5–10 mg PO tid-qid or PRN. *Severe anxiety:* 25–50 mg IM, IV, or PO q6–8h or PRN *Peds > 6 y.* 0.5 mg/kg/24 h PO or IM ÷ q6–8h; ↓ in renal impair, elderly **W/P:** [D, ?] Resp depression, CNS impair, Hx of drug dependence; avoid in hepatic impair **CI:** Preexisting CNS depression, NAG **Disp:** Caps 5, 10, 25 mg; Inj 100 mg **SE:** Drowsiness, CP, rash, fatigue, memory impair, xerostomia, wgt gain **Notes:** Erratic IM absorption

Chlorothiazide (Diuril) Uses: *HTN, edema* **Acts:** Thiazide diuretic **Dose:** *Adults.* 500 mg–1 g PO daily-bid; 100–1000 mg/d IV (for edema only). *Peds > 6 mo.* 10–20 mg/kg/24 h PO ÷ bid; 4 mg/kg/d IV; OK w/ food **W/P:** [D, +] **CI:** Sensitivity to thiazides/sulfonamides, anuria **Disp:** Tabs 250, 500 mg; susp 250 mg/5 mL; Inj 500 mg/vial **SE:** ↓ K+, Na+, dizziness, hyperglycemia, hyperuricemia, hyperlipidemia, photosens **Notes:** Do not use IM/SQ; take early in the day to avoid nocturia; use sunblock; monitor lytes

Chlorpheniramine (Chlor-Trimeton, Others) [OTC] BOX: OTC meds w/ chlorpheniramine should not be used in peds < 2 y Uses: *Allergic rhinitis*, common cold **Acts:** Antihistamine **Dose:** *Adults.* 4 mg PO q4–6h or 8–12 mg PO bid of SR *Peds.* 0.35 mg/kg/24 h PO ÷ q4–6h or 0.2 mg/kg/24 h SR **W/P:** [C, ?/–] BOO; NAG; hepatic Insuff **CI:** Allergy **Disp:** Tabs 4 mg; chew tabs 2 mg; SR tabs 8, 12 mg **SE:** Anticholinergic SE & sedation common, postural ↓ BP, QT changes, extrapyramidal Rxns, photosens **Notes:** Do not cut/crush/chew ER forms; deaths in pts < 2 y; associated w/ cough and cold meds [MMWR 2007;56(01):1–4]

Chlorpromazine (Thorazine) Uses: *Psychotic disorders, N/V*, apprehension, intractable hiccups **Acts:** Phenothiazine antipsychotic; antiemetic **Dose:** *Adults. Psychosis:* 30–800 mg/day in 1–4 ÷ doses, start low dose, ↑ PRN; typical 200–600 mg/day; 1–2 g/day may be needed in some cases. *Severe Sxs:* 25 mg IM/IV initial; may repeat in 1–4 h; then 25–50 mg PO or PR tid. *Hiccups:* 25–50 mg PO tid-qid. *Children > 6 mo: Psychosis & N/V:* 0.5–1 mg/kg/dose PO q4–6h or IM/IV q6–8h; **W/P:** [C, ?/–] Safety in children < 6 mo not established; Szs, avoid w/ hepatic impair, BM suppression **CI:** Sensitivity w/ phenothiazines; NAG **Disp:** Tabs 10, 25, 50, 100, 200 mg; soln 100 mg/mL; Inj 25 mg/mL **SE:** Extrapyramidal SE & sedation; α-adrenergic blocking properties; ↓ BP; ↑ QT interval **Notes:** Do not D/C abruptly; dilute PO conc in 2–4 oz of liq

Chlorpropamide (Diabinese) Uses: *Type 2 DM* **Acts:** Sulfonylurea; ↑ pancreatic insulin release; ↑ peripheral insulin sensitivity; ↓ hepatic glucose output **Dose:** 100–500 mg/d; w/ food, ↓ hepatic impair **W/P:** [C, ?/–] CrCl < 50 mL/min; ↓ in hepatic impair **CI:** Cross-sensitivity w/ sulfonamides **Disp:** Tabs 100, 250 mg **SE:** HA, dizziness, rash, photosens, hypoglycemia, SIADH **Notes:** Avoid EtOH (disulfiram-like Rxn)

Chlorthalidone (Hygroton, Others) Uses: *HTN* **Acts:** Thiazide diuretic **Dose:** *Adults.* 25–100 mg PO daily. *Peds.* (Not approved) 2 mg/kg/dose PO 3×/wk or

1–2 mg/kg/d PO; ↓ in renal impair; OK w/ food, milk **W/P:** [D, +] **CI:** Cross-sensitivity w/ thiazides or sulfonamides; anuria **Disp:** Tabs 15, 25, 50 mg **SE:** ↓ K+, dizziness, photosens, ↑ glucose, hyperuricemia, sexual dysfunction

Chlorzoxazone (Paraflex, Parafon Forte DSC, Others) Uses: *Adjunct to rest & physical therapy Rx to relieve discomfort associated w/ acute, painful musculoskeletal conditions* **Acts:** Centrally acting skeletal muscle relaxant **Dose:** *Adults.* 250–500 mg PO tid-qid. *Peds.* 20 mg/kg/d in 3–4 ÷ doses **W/P:** [C, ?] Avoid EtOH & CNS depressants **CI:** Severe liver Dz **Disp:** Tabs 250, 500 mg **SE:** Drowsiness, tachycardia, dizziness, hepatotox, angioedema

Cholecalciferol [Vitamin D₃] (Delta D) Uses: *Dietary supl to Rx vit D deficiency* **Acts:** ↑ intestinal Ca²⁺ absorption **Dose:** 400–1000 Int Units/d PO **W/P:** [A (D doses above the RDA), +] **CI:** ↑ Ca²⁺, hypervitaminosis, allergy **Disp:** Tabs 400, 1000 Int Units **SE:** Vit D tox (renal failure, HTN, psychosis) **Notes:** 1 mg cholecalciferol = 40,000 Int Units vit D activity

Cholestyramine (Questran, Questran Light, Prevalite) Uses: *Hypercholesterolemia; hyperlipidemia; pruritus associated w/ partial biliary obst; D associated w/ excess fecal bile acids* pseudomembranous colitis, dig tox, hyperoxaluria **Acts:** Binds intestinal bile acids, forms insoluble complexes **Dose:** *Adults.* Titrate: 4 g/d-bid ↑ to max 24 g/d ÷ 1–6 doses/d. *Peds.* 240 mg/kg/d in 3 ÷ doses **W/P:** [C, ?] Constipation, phenylketonuria, may interfere w/ other drug absorption; consider supl w/ fat-soluble vits **CI:** Complete biliary or bowel obst; w/ mycophenolate hyperlipoproteinemia types III, IV, V **Disp:** (*Questran*) 4 g cholestyramine resin/9 g powder; (*Prevalite*) 4 g resin w/ aspartame: 4 g resin/5.5 g powder; (*Questran Light*) 4 g resin/6.4 g powder **SE:** Constipation, Abd pain, bloating, HA, rash, vit K deficiency **Notes:** OD may cause GI obst; mix 4 g in 2–6 oz of noncarbonated beverage; take other meds 1–2 h before or 6 h after; ✔ lipids

Ciclesonide, Inhalation (Alvesco) Uses: *Asthma maint* **Acts:** Inhaled steroid **Dose:** *Adults & Peds > 12 y. On bronchodilators alone:* 80 mcg bid (320 mcg/d max). *Inhaled corticosteroids:* 80 mcg bid (640 mcg/d max). *On oral corticosteroids:* 320 mcg bid, 640 mcg/d max **W/P:** [C, ?] **CI:** Status asthmaticus or other acute episodes of asthma, hypersens **Disp:** Inh 80, 160 mcg/actuation **SE:** HA, nasopharyngitis, sinusitis, pharyngolaryngeal pain, URI, arthralgia, nasal congestion **Notes:** Oral *Candida* risk, rinse mouth and spit after, taper systemic steroids slowly when transferring to ciclesonide, monitor growth in pediatric pts, counsel on use of device, clean mouthpiece weekly

Ciclesonide, Nasal (Omnaris) Uses: *Allergic rhinitis* **Acts:** Nasal corticosteroid **Dose:** *Adults & Peds > 12 y.* 2 sprays each nostril 1×/d **W/P:** [C, ?/–] w/ Ketoconazole; monitor peds for growth reduction **CI:** Component allergy **Disp:** Intranasal spray susp, 50 mcg/spray, 120 doses **SE:** Adrenal suppression, delayed nasal wound healing, URI, HA, ear pain, epistaxis ↑ risk viral Dz (e.g., chickenpox), delayed growth in children

Ciclopirox (Loprox, Penlac) Uses: *Tinea pedis, tinea cruris, tinea corporis, cutaneous candidiasis, tinea versicolor, tinea rubrum* Acts: Antifungal antibiotic; cellular depletion of essential substrates &/or ions Dose: *Adults & Peds >10 y.* Massage into affected area bid. *Onychomycosis:* apply to nails daily, w/ removal q7d W/P: [B, ?] CI: Component sensitivity Disp: Cream 0.77%, gel 0.77%, topical susp 0.77%, shampoo 1%, nail lacquer 8% SE: Pruritus, local irritation, burning Notes: D/C w/ irritation; avoid dressings; gel best for athlete's foot

Cidofovir (Vistide) BOX: Renal impair is the major tox. Follow administration instructions; possible carcinogenic, teratogenic Uses: *CMV retinitis w/ HIV* Acts: Selective inhibition of viral DNA synth Dose: *Rx:* 5 mg/kg IV once/wk for 2 wk w/ probenecid. *Maint:* 5 mg/kg IV once/2 wk w/ probenecid (2 g PO 3 h prior to cidofovir, then 1 g PO at 2 h & 8 h after cidofovir); ↓ in renal impair W/P: [C, −] SCr > 1.5 mg/dL or CrCl < 55 mL/min or urine protein > 100 mg/dL; w/ other nephrotoxic drugs CI: Probenecid or sulfa allergy Disp: Inj 75 mg/mL SE: Renal tox, chills, fever, HA, N/V/D, thrombocytopenia, neutropenia Notes: Hydrate w/ NS prior to each Inf

Cilostazol (Pletal) Uses: *Reduce Sxs of intermittent claudication* Acts: Phosphodiesterase III inhib; ↑ s cAMP in plts & blood vessels, vasodilation & inhibit plt aggregation Dose: 100 mg PO bid, 1/2 h before or 2 h after breakfast & dinner W/P: [C, +/−] ↓ dose w/ drugs that inhibit CYP3A4 & CYP2C19 (Table 10, p 301) CI: CHF, hemostatic disorders, active pathologic bleeding Disp: Tabs 50, 100 mg SE: HA, palpitation, D

Cimetidine (Tagamet, Tagamet HB 200 [OTC]) Uses: *Duodenal ulcer; ulcer prophylaxis in hypersecretory states (e.g., trauma, burns); & GERD* Acts: H_2-receptor antagonist Dose: *Adults. Active ulcer:* 2400 mg/d IV cont Inf or 300 mg IV q6h; 400 mg PO bid or 800 mg hs. *Maint:* 400 mg PO hs. *GERD:* 300–600 mg PO q6h; maint 800 mg PO hs. *Peds Infants.* 10–20 mg/kg/24 h PO or IV ÷ q6–12h. *Children:* 20–40 mg/kg/24 h PO or IV ÷ q6h; ↓ w/ renal Insuff & in elderly W/P: [B, +] Many drug interactions (P-450 system); do not use w/ clopidogrel (↓ effect) CI: Component sensitivity Disp: Tabs 200 (OTC), 300, 400, 800 mg; liq 300 mg/5 mL; Inj 300 mg/2 mL SE: Dizziness, HA, agitation, ↓ plt, gynecomastia Notes: 1 h before or 2 h after antacids; avoid EtOH

Cinacalcet (Sensipar) Uses: *Secondary hyperparathyroidism in CRF; ↑ Ca^{2+} in parathyroid carcinoma* Acts: ↓ PTH by ↑ calcium-sensing receptor sensitivity Dose: *Secondary hyperparathyroidism:* 30 mg PO daily. *Parathyroid carcinoma:* 30 mg PO bid; titrate q2–4wk based on calcium & PTH levels; swallow whole; take w/ food W/P: [C, ?/−] w/ Szs, adjust w/ CYP3A4 inhib (Table 10, p 301) Disp: Tabs 30, 60, 90 mg SE: N/V/D, myalgia, dizziness, ↓ Ca^{2+} Notes: Monitor Ca^{2+}, PO_4^-, PTH

Ciprofloxacin (Cipro, Cipro XR, Proquin XR) BOX: ↑ risk of tendonitis and tendon rupture; ↑ risk w/ age > 60, transplant pts may worsen MG sxs Uses: *Rx lower resp tract, sinuses, skin & skin structure, bone/joints, complex intra abd Infxn (w/ metronidazole), typhoid, infectious D, uncomp GC, inhal anthrax UT Infxns, including prostatitis* **Acts:** Quinolone antibiotic; ↓ DNA gyrase. *Spectrum:* Broad gram(+) & (–) aerobics; little *Streptococcus*; good *Pseudomonas, E. coli, B. fragilis, P. mirabilis, K. pneumoniae, C. jejuni,* or *Shigella* **Dose:** *Adults.* 250–750 mg PO q12h; XR 500–1000 mg PO q24h; or 200–400 mg IV q12h; ↓ in renal impair **W/P:** [C, ?/–] Children < 18 y; avoid in MG **CI:** Component sensitivity; w/ tizanidine **Disp:** Tabs 100, 250, 500, 750 mg; Tabs XR 500, 1000 mg; susp 5 g/100 mL, 10 g/100 mL; Inj 200, 400 mg; premixed piggyback 200, 400 mg/100 mL **SE:** Restlessness, N/V/D, rash, ruptured tendons, ↑ LFTs **Notes:** Avoid antacids; reduce/restrict caffeine intake; interactions w/ theophylline, caffeine, sucralfate, warfarin, antacids, most tendon problems in Achilles, rare shoulder and hand

Ciprofloxacin, Ophthalmic (Ciloxan) **Uses:** *Rx & prevention of ocular Infxns (conjunctivitis, blepharitis, corneal abrasions)* **Acts:** Quinolone antibiotic; ↓ DNA gyrase **Dose:** 1–2 gtt in eye(s) q2h while awake for 2 d, then 1–2 gtt q4h while awake for 5 d, oint 1/2-inch ribbon in eye tid × 2 d, then bid × 5 d **W/P:** [C, ?/–] **CI:** Component sensitivity **Disp:** Soln 3.5 mg/mL; oint 0.3%, 35 g **SE:** Local irritation

Ciprofloxacin, Otic (Cetraxal) **Uses:** *Otitis externa* **Acts:** Quinolone antibiotic; ↓ DNA gyrase. *Spectrum: P. aeruginosa, S. aureus* **Dose:** *Adults & Peds > 1 yr.* 0.25 mL in ear(s) q 12 h × 7 d **W/P:** [C, ?/–] **CI:** Component sensitivity **Disp:** Sol 0.2% **SE:** hypersens rxn, ear pruritus/pain, HA, fungal superinfection

Ciprofloxacin & Dexamethasone, Otic (Ciprodex Otic) **Uses:** *Otitis externa, otitis media peds* **Acts:** Quinolone antibiotic; ↓ DNA gyrase; w/ steroid **Dose:** *Adults.* 4 gtt in ear(s) bid × 7 d. *Peds > 6 mo.* 4 gtt in ear(s) bid for 7 d **W/P:** [C, ?/–] **CI:** Viral ear infxns **Disp:** Susp ciprofloxacin 0.3% & dexamethasone 1% **SE:** Ear discomfort **Notes:** OK w/ tympanostomy tubes

Ciprofloxacin & Hydrocortisone, Otic (Cipro HC Otic) **Uses:** *Otitis externa* **Acts:** Quinolone antibiotic; ↓ DNA gyrase; w/ steroid **Dose:** *Adults & Peds > 1 mo.* 1–2 gtt in ear(s) bid × 7 d **W/P:** [C, ?/–] **CI:** Perforated tympanic membrane, viral Infxns of the external canal **Disp:** Susp ciprofloxacin 0.2% & hydrocortisone 1% **SE:** HA, pruritus

Cisplatin (Platinol, Platinol AQ) **BOX:** Anaphylactic-like Rxn, ototox, cumulative renal tox; doses > 100 mg/m^2 q3–4wk rarely used, do not confuse w/ carboplatin **Uses:** *Testicular, bladder, ovarian*, SCLC, NSCLC, breast, head & neck, & penile CAs; osteosarcoma; peds brain tumors **Acts:** DNA-binding; denatures double helix; intrastrand cross-linking **Dose:** 10–20 mg/m^2/d for 5 d q3wk; 50–120 mg/m^2 q3–4wk (per protocols); ↓ w/ renal impair **W/P:** [D, –] Cumulative renal tox may be severe; ↓ BM, hearing impair, preexisting renal Insuff **CI:** w/ Anthrax or live vaccines, platinum-containing compound allergy; w/ cidofovir **Disp:** Inj 1 mg/mL **SE:** Allergic Rxns, N/V, nephrotox (↑ w/ administration of other nephrotoxic drugs; minimize by NS Inf & mannitol diuresis), high-frequency hearing loss in 30%, peripheral "stocking glove"-type neuropathy, cardiotox (ST, T-wave changes),

↓ Mg^{2+}, mild ↓ BM, hepatotox; renal impair dose-related & cumulative **Notes:** Give taxanes before platinum derivatives; ✓ Mg^{2+}, lytes before & w/in 48 h after cisplatin

Citalopram (Celexa) BOX: Closely monitor for worsening depression or emergence of suicidality, particularly in pts < 24 y **Uses:** *Depression* **Acts:** SSRI **Dose:** Initial 20 mg/d, may ↑ to 40 mg/d max dose; ↓ 20 mg/day max > 60 yr, w/ cimetidine, or hepatic/renal Insuff **W/P:** [C, +/–] Hx of mania, Szs & pts at risk for suicide **CI:** MAOI or w/in 14 d of MAOI use **Disp:** Tabs 10, 20, 40 mg; soln 10 mg/5 mL **SE:** Somnolence, insomnia, anxiety, xerostomia, N, diaphoresis, sexual dysfunction; may ↑ Qt interval and cause arrhythmias; ↓ Na^+/SIADH

Cladribine (Leustatin) BOX: Dose-dependent reversible myelosuppression; neurotox, nephrotox, administer by physician with w/ experience in chemotherapy regimens **Uses:** *HCL, CLL, NHLs, progressive MS* **Acts:** Induces DNA strand breakage; interferes w/ DNA repair/synth; purine nucleoside analog **Dose:** 0.09–0.1 mg/kg/d cont IV Inf for 1–7 d (per protocols); ↓ w/ renal impair **W/P:** [D, ?/–] Causes neutropenia & Infxn **CI:** Component sensitivity **Disp:** Inj 1 mg/mL **SE:** ↓ BM, T lymphocyte ↓ may be prolonged (26–34 wk), fever in 46%, tumor lysis synd, Infxns (especially lung & IV sites), rash (50%), HA, fatigue, N/V **Notes:** Consider prophylactic allopurinol; monitor CBC

Clarithromycin (Biaxin, Biaxin XL) **Uses:** *Upper/lower resp tract, skin/ skin structure Infxns, H. pylori Infxns, & Infxns caused by non-tuberculosis (atypical) Mycobacterium; prevention of MAC Infxns in HIV Infxn* **Acts:** Macrolide antibiotic, ↓ protein synth. **Spectrum:** H. influenzae, M. catarrhalis, S. pneumoniae, M. pneumoniae, & H. pylori **Dose:** Adults. 250–500 mg PO bid or 1000 mg (2 × 500 mg XL tab)/d. Mycobacterium: 500 mg PO bid. Peds > 6 mo. 7.5 mg/kg/dose PO bid; ↓ w/ renal impair **W/P:** [C, ?] Antibiotic-associated colitis; rare QT prolongation & ventricular arrhythmias, including torsades de pointes **CI:** Macrolide allergy; w/ ranitidine in pts w/ Hx of porphyria or CrCl < 25 mL/min **Disp:** Tabs 250, 500 mg; susp 125, 250 mg/5 mL; tab 500 mg XL tab **SE:** ↑ QT interval, causes metallic taste, N/D, Abd pain, HA, rash **Notes:** Multiple drug interactions, ↑ theophylline & carbamazepine levels; do not refrigerate susp

Clemastine Fumarate (Tavist, Dayhist, Antihist-1) [OTC] **Uses:** *Allergic rhinitis & Sxs of urticaria* **Acts:** Antihistamine **Dose:** Adults & Peds > 12 y. 1.34 mg bid-2.68 mg tid; max 8.04 mg/d, 6–12 y: 0.67–1.34 mg bid (max 4.02 /d), < 6 y: 0.335–0.67 mg/d ÷ into 2–3 doses (max 1.34 mg/d), **W/P:** [B, M] BOO; Do not take w/ MAOI **CI:** NAG **Disp:** Tabs 1.34, 2.68 mg; syrup 0.67 mg/5 mL **SE:** Drowsiness, dyscoordination, epigastric distress, urinary retention **Notes:** Avoid EtOH

Clevidipine (Cleviprex) **Uses:** *HTN when PO not available/desirable* **Action:** Dihydropyridine CCB, potent arterial vasodilator **Dose:** 1-2 mg/h IV then maint 4–6 mg/h; 21 mg/h max **W/P:** [C, ?] ↓ BP, syncope, rebound HTN, reflex tachycardia, CHF **CI:** Hypersens: component or formulation (soy, egg products); impaired lipid metabolism; severe aortic stenosis **Disp:** Inj 0.5 mg/mL (50 mL, 100 mL) **SE:** AF, fever, insomnia, N/V, HA, renal impair

Clindamycin (Cleocin, Cleocin-T, Others) **BOX:** Pseudomembranous colitis may range from mild to life-threatening **Uses:** *Rx aerobic & anaerobic Infxns; topical for severe acne & vag Infxns* **Acts:** Bacteriostatic; interferes w/ protein synth. *Spectrum:* Streptococci (e.g., pneumococci), staphylococci, & gram(+) & (–) anaerobes; no activity against gram(–) aerobes **Dose:** *Adults. PO:* 150–450 mg PO q6–8h. *IV:* 300–600 mg IV q6h or 900 mg IV q8h. *Vaginal:* 1 applicator hs for 7 d. *Topical:* Apply 1% gel, lotion, or soln bid. *Peds Neonates.* (Avoid use; contains benzyl alcohol) 10–15 mg/kg/24 h ÷ q8–12h. *Children > 1 mo:* 10–30 mg/kg/24 h ÷ q6–8h, to a max of 1.8 g/d PO or 4.8 g/d IV. *Topical:* Apply 1%, gel, lotion, or soln bid; ↓ in severe hepatic impair **W/P:** [B, +] Can cause fatal colitis **CI:** Hx pseudomembranous colitis **Disp:** Caps 75, 150, 300 mg; susp 75 mg/5 mL; Inj 300 mg/2 mL; vag cream 2%, vag soln 1%, gel 1%, lotion 1%, vag supp 100 mg **SE:** D may be *C. difficile* pseudomembranous colitis, rash, ↑ LFTs **Notes:** D/C drug w/ D, evaluate for *C. difficile*

Clindamycin and Tretinoin (Veltin Gel) **Uses:** *Acne vulgaris* **Acts:** Lincosamide abx (↓ protein synthesis)w/ a retinoid; *Spectrum: P. acnes* **Dose:** *Adults (> 12 y).* Apply pea-size amount to area q/day **W/P:** [C, ?/–] do not use w/ erythromycin products **CI:** Hx regional enteritis/UC/abx assoc colitis **Disp:** Top Gel (clindamycin 1.2%/tretinoin 0.025%) **SE:** Dryness, irritation, erythema, pruritis, exfoliation, dermatitis, sunburn **Notes:** Avoid eyes, lips, mucous membranes

Clofarabine (Clolar) **Uses:** *Rx relapsed/refractory ALL after at least 2 regimens in children 1–21 y* **Acts:** Antimetabolite; ↓ ribonucleotide reductase w/ false nucleotide base-inhibiting DNA synth **Dose:** 52 mg/m^2 IV over 2 h daily × 5 d (repeat q2–6wk); per protocol **W/P:** [D, –] **Disp:** Inj 20 mg/20 mL **SE:** N/V/D, anemia, leukopenia, thrombocytopenia, neutropenia, Infxn, ↑ AST/ALT **Notes:** Monitor for tumor lysis synd & systemic inflammatory response synd (SIRS)/ capillary leak synd; hydrate well

Clomiphene (Clomid) **Uses:** *Tx ovulatory dysfunction in women desiring PRG* **Acts:** Nonsteroidal ovulatory stimulant; estrogen antagonist **Dose:** 50 mg × 5 d; if no ovulation ↑ to 100 mg × 5 d @ 30 d later; ovulation usually 5–10 d postcourse, time coitus w/ expected ovulation time **W/P:** [X, ?/–] r/o PRG & ovarian enlargement **CI:** Hypersens, uterine bleed, PRG, ovarian cysts, ovarian Dz, thyroid/ adrenal dysfunction **Disp:** Tabs 50 mg **SE:** Ovarian enlargement, vasomotor flushes

Clomipramine (Anafranil) **BOX:** Closely monitor for suicidal ideation or unusual behavior changes **Uses:** *OCD*, depression, chronic pain, panic attacks **Acts:** TCA; ↑ synaptic serotonin & norepinephrine **Dose:** *Adults.* Initial 25 mg/d PO in ÷ doses; ↑ over few wks 250 mg/d max QHS. *Peds > 10 y.* Initial 25 mg/d PO in ÷ doses; ↑ over few wks 200 mg/d or 3 mg/kg/d max given HS **W/P:** [C, +/–] **CI:** w/ MAOIs, TCA allergy, during acute MI recovery **Disp:** Caps 25, 50, 75 mg **SE:** Anticholinergic (xerostomia, urinary retention, constipation), somnolence

Clonazepam (Klonopin) [C-IV] **Uses:** *Lennox-Gastaut synd, akinetic & myoclonic Szs, absence Szs, panic attacks*, restless legs synd, neuralgia, parkinsonian dysarthria, bipolar disorder **Acts:** Benzodiazepine; anticonvulsant **Dose:** *Adults.* 1.5 mg/d PO in 3 ÷ doses; ↑ by 0.5–1 mg/d q3d PRN up to 20 mg/d. *Peds.* 0.01–0.03 mg/kg/24 h PO ÷ tid; ↑ to 0.1–0.2 mg/kg/24 h ÷ tid; avoid abrupt D/C **W/P:** [D, M] Elderly pts, resp Dz, CNS depression, severe hepatic impair, NAG **CI:** Severe liver Dz, acute NAG **Disp:** Tabs 0.5, 1, 2 mg, oral disintegrating tabs 0.125, 0.25, 0.5, 1, 2 mg **SE:** CNS (drowsiness, dizziness, ataxia, memory impair) **Notes:** Can cause retrograde amnesia; a CYP3A4 substrate

Clonidine, Oral (Catapres) Uses: *HTN*; opioid, EtOH, & tobacco withdrawal, ADHD **Acts:** Centrally acting α-adrenergic stimulant **Dose:** *Adults.* 0.1 mg PO bid, adjust daily by 0.1–0.2-mg increments (max 2.4 mg/d). *Peds.* 5–10 mcg/kg/d ÷ q8–12h (max 0.9 mg/d); ↓ in renal impair **W/P:** [C, +/–] Avoid w/ β-blocker, elderly, severe CV Dz, renal impair; use w/agents that affect sinus node may cause severe ↓ HR **CI:** Component sensitivity **Disp:** Tabs 0.1, 0.2, 0.3 mg **SE:** drowsiness, orthostatic ↓ BP, xerostomia, constipation, ↓ HR, dizziness **Notes:** More effective for HTN if combined w/ diuretics; withdraw slowly, rebound HTN w/ abrupt D/C of doses > 0.2 mg bid; ADHD use in peds needs CV assessment before starting epidural clonidine (Duraclon) used for chronic CA pain

Clonidine, Oral, Extended-Release (Kapvay, Jenloga) Uses: *ADHD alone or as adjunct (Kapvay)*, *hypertension, alone or combo (Jenloga)* **Acts:** Central α-adrenergic stimulant **Dose:** *Adults. Jenloga* 0.1 mg PO qhs, titrate, usual 0.2–0.6 mg/d; 0.6 mg/d max *Peds 6–17 y. Kapvay* 0.1 mg PO qhs, adjust weekly per table to response; am and hs doses may be ≠; max 0.4 mg/d; do not cut/crush/chew tabs; ↓ in renal impair. See *Kapvay* table below.

Kapvay Total Daily Dose	Morning Dose	Bedtime Dose
0.1 mg	N/A	0.1 mg
0.2 mg	0.1 mg	0.1 mg
0.3 mg	0.1 mg	0.2 mg
0.4 mg	0.2 mg	0.2 mg

W/P: [C, +/–] may cause severe ↓ HR and ↓BP; w/ BP meds **CI:** Component sensitivity **Disp:** Tabs ER *Kapvay* 0.1, 0.2 mg; *Jenloga* 0.1 mg **SE:** Somnolence, fatigue, URI, irritability, sore throat, insomnia, nightmares, emotional disorder, constipation, congestion, ↑ temperature, dry mouth, ear pain **Notes:** On D/C, ↓ no more than 0.1 mg q3–7d

Clonidine, Transdermal (Catapres TTS) Uses: *HTN* **Acts:** Centrally acting α-adrenergic stimulant **Dose:** 1 patch q7d to hairless area (upper arm/torso); titrate to effect; ↓ w/ severe renal impair; **W/P:** [C, +/–] Avoid w/ β-blocker, withdraw slowly, in elderly, severe CV Dz and w/ renal impair; use w/agents that affect sinus node may cause severe ↓ HR **CI:** Component sensitivity **Disp:** TTS-1, TTS-2, TTS-3 (delivers 0.1, 0.2, 0.3 mg, respectively, of clonidine/d for 1 wk) **SE:** Drowsiness, orthostatic ↓ BP, xerostomia, constipation, ↓ HR **Notes:** Do not D/C abruptly (rebound HTN); Doses > 2 TTS-3 usually not associated w/ ↑ efficacy; steady state in 2–3 d

Clopidogrel (Plavix) **Uses:** *Reduce atherosclerotic events*, administer ASAP in ECC setting w/ high-risk ST depression or T-wave inversion **Acts:** ↓ Plt aggregation **Dose:** 75 mg/d; *ECC 2010. ACS:* 300–600 mg PO loading dose, then 75 mg/d PO; full effects take several days **W/P:** [B, ?] Active bleeding; risk of bleeding from trauma & other; TTP; liver Dz; do not use w/ PPI, other CYP2C19 (e.g., fluconazole); OK with ranitidine, famotidine **CI:** Coagulation disorders, active/ intracranial bleeding; CABG planned w/in 5–7 d **Disp:** Tabs 75, 300 mg **SE:** ↑ bleeding time, GI intolerance, HA, dizziness, rash, thrombocytopenia, ↓ WBC **Notes:** Plt aggregation to baseline ~ 5 d after D/C, plt transfusion to reverse acutely; clinical response highly variable

Clorazepate (Tranxene) [C-IV] **Uses:** *Acute anxiety disorders, acute EtOH withdrawal Sxs, adjunctive therapy Rx in partial Szs* **Acts:** Benzodiazepine; antianxiety agent **Dose:** *Adults.* 15–60 mg/d in ÷ doses. *Elderly & debilitated pts:* Initial 7.5–15 mg/d in ÷ doses. *EtOH withdrawal:* Day 1: Initial 30 mg; then 30–60 mg ÷ doses; Day 2: 45–90 mg ÷ doses; Day 3: 22.5–45 mg ÷ doses; Day 4: 15–30 mg ÷ doses. *Peds.* 3.75–7.5 mg/dose bid to 60 mg/d max ÷ bid-tid **W/P:** [D, ?/–] Elderly; Hx depression **CI:** NAG; Not OK < 9 y of age **Disp:** Tabs 3.75, 7.5, 15 mg; Tabs-SD (daily) 11.25, 22.5 mg **SE:** CNS depressant effects (drowsiness, dizziness, ataxia, memory impair), ↓ BP **Notes:** Monitor pts w/ renal/ hepatic impair (drug may accumulate); avoid abrupt D/C; may cause dependence

Clotrimazole (Lotrimin, Mycelex, Others) [OTC] **Uses:** *Candidiasis & tinea Infxns* **Acts:** Antifungal; alters cell wall permeability. *Spectrum:* Oropharyngeal candidiasis, dermatophytes, superficial mycoses, cutaneous candidiasis, & vulvovaginal candidiasis **Dose:** *PO: Prophylaxis:* 1 troche dissolved in mouth tid *Rx:* 1 troche dissolved in mouth 5×/d for 14 d. *Vaginal 1% Cream:* 1 applicator-full hs for 7 d. *2% Cream:* 1 applicator-full hs for 3 d *Tabs:* 100 mg vaginally hs for 7 d or 200 mg (2 tabs) vaginally hs for 3 d or 500-mg tabs vaginally hs once. *Topical:* Apply bid 10–14 d **W/P:** [B (C if PO), ?] Not for systemic fungal Infxn; safety in children < 3 y not established **CI:** Component allergy **Disp:** 1% cream; soln; lotion; troche 10 mg; vag tabs 100, 200, 500 mg; vag cream 1%, 2% **SE:** *Topical:* Local irritation; *PO:* N/V, ↑ LFTs **Notes:** PO prophylaxis immunosuppressed pts

Clotrimazole & Betamethasone (Lotrisone) **Uses:** *Fungal skin Infxns* **Acts:** Imidazole antifungal & anti-inflammatory. *Spectrum:* Tinea pedis, cruris, & corporis **Dose:** ≥*17 y.* Apply & massage into area bid for 2–4 wk **W/P:** [C, ?] Varicella Infxn **CI:** Children < 12 y **Disp:** Cream 1/0.05% 15, 45 g; lotion

1/0.05% 30 mL **SE:** Local irritation, rash **Notes:** Not for diaper dermatitis or under occlusive dressings

Clozapine (Clozaril & FazaClo) BOX: Myocarditis, agranulocytosis, Szs, & orthostatic ↓ BP associated w/ clozapine; ↑ mortality in elderly w/ dementia-related psychosis **Uses:** *Refractory severe schizophrenia*; childhood psychosis; obsessive-compulsive disorder (OCD); bipolar disorder **Acts:** "Atypical" TCA **Dose:** 25 mg daily-bid initial; ↑ to 300–450 mg/d over 2 wk; maintain lowest dose possible; do not D/C abruptly **W/P:** [B, +/–] Monitor for psychosis & cholinergic rebound **CI:** Uncontrolled epilepsy; comatose state; WBC < 3500 cells/mm³ and ANC < 2000 cells/mm³ before Rx or < 3000 cells/mm³ during Rx **Disp:** Orally disintegrating tabs (ODTs) 12.5, 25, 100 mg; tabs 25, 100 mg **SE:** Sialorrhea, tachycardia, drowsiness, ↑ wgt, constipation, incontinence, rash, Szs, CNS stimulation, hyperglycemia **Notes:** Avoid activities where sudden loss of consciousness could cause harm; benign temperature ↑ may occur during the 1st 3 wk of Rx, weekly CBC mandatory 1st 6 mo, then q other wk

Cocaine [C-II] **Uses:** *Topical anesthetic for mucous membranes* **Acts:** Narcotic analgesic, local vasoconstrictor **Dose:** Lowest topical amount that provides relief; 1 mg/kg max **W/P:** [C, ?] **CI:** PRG, ocular anesthesia **Disp:** Topical soln & viscous preparations 4–10%; powder **SE:** CNS stimulation, nervousness, loss of taste/smell, chronic rhinitis, CV tox, abuse potential **Notes:** Use only on PO, laryngeal, & nasal mucosa; do not use on extensive areas of broken skin

Codeine [C-II] **Uses:** *Mild–mod pain; symptomatic relief of cough* **Acts:** Narcotic analgesic; ↓ cough reflex **Dose:** *Adults. Analgesic:* 15–20 mg PO or IM qid PRN. *Antitussive:* 10–20 mg PO q4h PRN; max 120 mg/d. *Peds. Analgesic:* 0.5–1 mg/kg/dose PO q4–6h PRN. *Antitussive:* 1–1.5 mg/kg/24 h PO ÷ q4h; max 30 mg/24 h; ↓ in renal/hepatic impair **W/P:** [C (D if prolonged use or high dose at term), +] CNS depression, Hx drug abuse, severe hepatic impair **CI:** Component sensitivity **Disp:** Tabs 15, 30, 60 mg; soln 15 mg/5 mL; Inj 15, 30 mg/mL **SE:** Drowsiness, constipation, ↓ BP **Notes:** Usually combined w/ APAP for pain or w/ agents (e.g., terpin hydrate) as an antitussive; 120 mg IM = 10 mg IM morphine

Colchicine (Colcrys) **Uses:** *Acute gouty arthritis & prevention of recurrences; familial Mediterranean fever*; primary biliary cirrhosis **Acts:** ↓ migration of leukocytes; ↓ leukocyte lactic acid production **Dose:** *Initial:* 0.6–1.2 mg PO, then 0.6 mg q1–2h until relief or GI SE develop (max 8 mg/d); do not repeat for 3 d. *Prophylaxis:* PO: 0.6 mg/d or 3–4 d/wk; ↓ renal impair **W/P:** [D, +] w/ P-glycoprotein or CYP3A4 inhib in pt w/renal or hepatic impair, ↓ dose or avoid in elderly or w/indinavir **CI:** Serious renal, GI, hepatic, or cardiac disorders; blood dyscrasias **Disp:** Tabs 0.6 mg **SE:** N/V/D, Abd pain, BM suppression, hepatotox; local Rxn w/ SQ/IM **Notes:** IV no longer available

Colesevelam (Welchol) **Uses:** *↓ LDL & total cholesterol alone or in combo w/ an HMG-CoA reductase inhib, improve glycemic control in type 2 DM*

Acts: Bile acid sequestrant **Dose:** 3 tabs PO bid or 6 tabs daily w/ meals **W/P:** [B, ?] Severe GI motility disorders; in pts w/ triglycerides > 300 mg/dL (may ↑ levels); use not established in peds **CI:** Bowel obst, serum triglycerides > 500; Hx hyper-triglyceridemia-pancreatitis **Disp:** Tabs 625 mg; oral susp 1.875, 3.75 gm **SE:** Constipation, dyspepsia, myalgia, weakness **Notes:** May ↓ absorption of fat-soluble vits

Colestipol (Colestid) **Uses:** *Adjunct to ↓ serum cholesterol in primary hypercholesterolemia, relieve pruritus associated w/ ↑ bile acids* **Acts:** Binds intestinal bile acids to form insoluble complex **Dose:** *Granules:* 5–30 g/d ÷ 2–4 doses; tabs: 2–16 g/d ÷ daily-bid **W/P:** [C, ?] Avoid w/ high triglycerides, GI dysfunction **CI:** Bowel obst **Disp:** Tabs 1 g; granules 5 g/pack or scoop **SE:** Constipation, Abd pain, bloating, HA, GI irritation & bleeding **Notes:** Do not use dry powder; mix w/ beverages, cereals, etc; may ↓ absorption of other meds and fat-soluble vits

Conivaptan HCL (Vaprisol) **Uses:** Euvolemic & hypervolemic hyponatremia **Acts:** Dual arginine vasopressin V_{1A}/V_2 receptor antagonist **Dose:** 20 mg IV × 1 over 30 min, then 20 mg cont IV Inf over 24 h; 20 mg/d cont IV Inf for 1–3 more d; may ↑ to 40 mg/d if Na⁺ not responding; 4 max use; use large vein, change site q24h **W/P:** [C, ?/–] Rapid ↑ Na⁺ (> 12 mEq/L/24 h) may cause osmotic demyelination synd; impaired renal/hepatic Fxn; may ↑ digoxin levels; CYP3A4 inhib (Table 10, p 301) **CI:** Hypovolemic hyponatremia; w/ CYP3A4 inhib; anuria **Disp:** Amp 20 mg/4 mL **SE:** Inf site Rxns, HA, N/V/D, constipation, ↓ K⁺, orthostatic ↓ BP, thirst, dry mouth, pyrexia, pollakiuria, polyuria, Infxn **Notes:** Monitor Na⁺, vol and neurologic status; D/C w/ very rapid ↑ Na⁺; mix only w/ 5% dextrose

Copper IUD Contraceptive (ParaGard T 380A) **Uses:** *Contraception, long-term (up to 10 y)* **Acts:** ?, interfere w/ sperm survival/transport **Dose:** Insert any time during menstrual cycle; replace at 10 y max **W/P:** [C, ?] Remove w/ intrauterine PRG, increased risk of comps w/ PRG and device in place **CI:** Acute PID or in high-risk behavior, postpartum endometritis, cervicitis **Disp:** 52 mg IUD **SE:** PRG, ectopic PRG, pelvic Infxn w/ or w/o immunocompromised, embedment, perforation, expulsion, Wilson Dz, fainting w/ insert, vag bleeding, expulsion **Notes:** Counsel pt does not protect against STD/HIV; see PI for detailed instructions; 99% effective

Cortisone, Systemic and Topical See Steroids, p 244, and Tables 2 & 3, pp 283 & 284

Cromolyn Sodium (Intal, NasalCrom, Opticrom, Others) **Uses:** *Adjunct to the Rx of asthma; prevent exercise-induced asthma; allergic rhinitis; ophthal allergic manifestations*; food allergy, systemic mastocytosis, IBD **Acts:** Antiasthmatic; mast cell stabilizer **Dose:** *Adults & Children > 12 y. Inh:* 20 mg (as powder in caps) inhaled qid or metered-dose inhaler 2 puffs qid. *PO:* 200 mg qid 15–20 min ac, up to 400 mg qid. *Nasal instillation:* Spray once in each nostril 2–6×/d. *Ophthal:* 1–2 gtt in each eye 4–6 × d. *Peds. Inh:* 2 puffs qid of metered-dose inhaler. *PO: Infants < 2 y:* (not OK) 20 mg/kg/d in 4 ÷ doses. *2–12 y:* 100 mg qid ac **W/P:** [B, ?] w/ Renal/hepatic impair **CI:** Acute asthmatic attacks **Disp:** PO conc 100 mg/5 mL; soln for nebulizer 20 mg/2 mL; metered-dose inhaler (contains ozone-depleting CFCs; will be gradually removed from US market); nasal soln 40 mg/mL; ophthal soln 4% **SE:** Unpleasant taste, hoarseness, coughing **Notes:** No benefit in acute Rx; 2–4 wk for maximal effect in perennial allergic disorders

Cyanocobalamin [Vitamin B₁₂] (Nascobal)   **Uses:** *Pernicious anemia & other vit B₁₂ deficiency states; ↑ requirements d/t PRG; thyrotoxicosis; liver or kidney Dz* **Acts:** Dietary vit B₁₂ supl **Dose:** *Adults.* 30 mcg/d × 5–10 d intranasal: 500 mcg once/wk for pts in remission, 100 mcg IM or SQ daily for 5–10 d, then 100 mcg IM 2×/wk for 1 mo, then 100 mcg IM monthly. *Peds.* Use 0.2 mcg/kg × 2 d test dose; if OK 30–50 mcg/d for 2 or more wk (total 1000 mcg) then maint: 100 mg/mo. **W/P:** [A (C if dose exceeds RDA), +] **CI:** Allergy to cobalt; hereditary optic nerve atrophy; Leber Dz **Disp:** Tabs 50, 100, 250, 500, 1000, 2500, 5000 mcg; Inj 100, 1000 mcg/mL; intranasal (Nascobal) gel 500 mcg/ 0.1 mL **SE:** Itching, D, HA, anxiety **Notes:** PO absorption erratic and not; OK for use w/ hyperalimentation

Cyclobenzaprine (Flexeril)   **Uses:** *Relief of muscle spasm* **Acts:** Centrally acting skeletal muscle relaxant; reduces tonic somatic motor activity **Dose:** 5–10 mg PO bid-qid (2–3 wk max) **W/P:** [B, ?] Shares the toxic potential of the TCAs; urinary hesitancy, NAG **CI:** Do not use concomitantly or w/in 14 d of MAOIs; hyperthyroidism; heart failure; arrhythmias **Disp:** Tabs 5, 10 mg **SE:** Sedation & anticholinergic effects **Notes:** May inhibit mental alertness or physical coordination

Cyclobenzaprine, Extended-Release (Amrix)   **Uses:** *Muscle spasm* **Acts:** ? Centrally acting long-term muscle relaxant **Dose:** 15–30 mg PO daily 2–3 wk; 30 mg/d max **W/P:** [B, ?/–] w/ Urinary retention, NAG, w/ EtOH/CNS depressant **CI:** MAOI w/in 14 d, elderly, arrhythmias, heart block, CHF, MI recovery phase, ↑ thyroid **Disp:** Caps 15, 30 ER **SE:** Dry mouth, drowsiness, dizziness, HA, N, blurred vision, dysgeusia **Notes:** Avoid abrupt D/C w/ long-term use

Cyclopentolate, Ophthalmic (Cyclogyl, Cylate)   **Uses:** *Cycloplegia, mydriasis* **Acts:** Cycloplegic mydriatic, anticholinergic inhibits iris sphincter and ciliary body **Dose:** *Adults.* 1 gtt in eye 40–50 min preprocedure, may repeat × 1 in 5–10 min *Peds.* As adult, children 0.5%; infants use 0.5% **W/P:** [C (may cause late-term fetal anoxia/↓ HR), +/–], w/premature infants, HTN, Down synd, elderly, **CI:** NAG **Disp:** Ophthal soln 0.5, 1, 2% **SE:** Tearing, HA, irritation, eye pain, photophobia, arrhythmia, tremor, ↑ IOP, confusion **Notes:** Compress lacrimal sac for several min after dose; heavily pigmented irises may require ↑ strength; peak 25–75 min, cycloplegia 6–24 h, mydriasis up to 24 h; 2% soln may result in psychotic Rxns and behavioral disturbances in peds

Cyclopentolate With Phenylephrine (Cyclomydril)   **Uses:** *Mydriasis greater than cyclopentolate alone* **Acts:** Cycloplegic mydriatic, α-adrenergic agonist w/ anticholinergic to inhibit iris sphincter **Dose:** 1 gtt in eye q 5–10 min (max 3 doses) 40–50 min preprocedure **W/P:** [C (may cause late-term fetal anoxia/↓ HR), +/−] HTN, w/ elderly w/ CAD **CI:** NAG **Disp:** Ophthal soln cyclopentolate 0.2%/phenylephrine 1% (2, 5 mL) **SE:** Tearing, HA, irritation, eye pain, photophobia, arrhythmia, tremor **Notes:** Compress lacrimal sac for several min after dose; heavily pigmented irises may require ↑ strength; peak 25–75 min, cycloplegia 6–24 h, mydriasis up to 24 h

Cyclophosphamide (Cytoxan, Neosar) Uses: *Hodgkin Dz & NHLs;
multiple myeloma; small cell lung, breast, & ovarian CAs; mycosis fungoides; neuroblastoma; retinoblastoma; acute leukemias; allogeneic & ABMT in high doses; severe rheumatologic disorders (SLE, JRA, Wegner granulomatosis)* **Acts:** Alkylating agent **Dose:** *Adults.* (per protocol) 500–1500 mg/m^2; single dose at 2- to 4-wk intervals; 1.8 g/m^2 to 160 mg/kg (or at 12 g/m^2 in 75-kg individual) in the BMT setting (per protocols). *Peds. SLE:* 500–750 mg/m^2 q mo. *JRA:* 10 mg/kg q 2 wk; ↓ w/ renal impair **W/P:** [D, ?] w/ BM suppression, hepatic Insuff **CI:** Component sensitivity **Disp:** Tabs 25, 50 mg; Inj 500 mg, 1 g, 2 g **SE:** ↓ BM; hemorrhagic cystitis, SIADH, alopecia, anorexia; N/V; hepatotox; rare interstitial pneumonitis; irreversible testicular atrophy possible; cardiotox rare; 2nd malignancies (bladder, ALL), risk 3.5% at 8 y, 10.7% at 12 y **Notes:** Hemorrhagic cystitis prophylaxis: cont bladder irrigation & MESNA uroprotection; encourage hydration, long-term bladder Ca screening

Cyclosporine (Sandimmune, Neoral, Gengraf) BOX: ↑ risk neoplasm, ↑ risk skin malignancies, ↑ risk HTN and nephrotox Uses: *Organ rejection
in kidney, liver, heart, & BMT w/ steroids; RA; psoriasis* **Acts:** Immunosuppressant; reversible inhibition of immunocompetent lymphocytes **Dose:** *Adults & Peds. PO:* 15 mg/kg/d12h pretransplant; after 2 wk, taper by 5 mg/wk to 5–10 mg/kg/d. *IV:* If NPO, give 1/3 PO dose IV; ↓ in renal/hepatic impair **W/P:** [C, ?] Dose-related risk of nephrotox/hepatotox/serious fatal infections; live, attenuated vaccines may be less effective; may induce fatal malignancy; many drug interactions; ↑ risk of infections after D/C **CI:** Renal impair; uncontrolled HTN **Disp:** Caps 25, 100 mg; PO soln 100 mg/mL; Inj 50 mg/mL **SE:** May ↑ BUN & Cr & mimic transplant rejection; HTN; HA; hirsutism **Notes:** Administer in glass container; *Neoral & Sandimmune* not interchangeable; monitor BP, Cr, CBC, LFTs, interaction w/ St. John's wort; Levels: *Trough:* Just before next dose: *Therapeutic:* Variable 150–300 ng/mL RIA

Cyclosporine, Ophthalmic (Restasis) Uses: *↑ Tear production sup-
pressed d/t ocular inflammation* **Acts:** Immune modulator, anti-inflammatory **Dose:** 1 gtt bid each eye 12 h apart; OK w/ artificial tears, allow 15 min between **W/P:** [C, −] **CI:** Ocular Infxn, component allergy **Disp:** Single-use vial 0.05% **SE:** Ocular burning/hyperemia **Notes:** Mix vial well

Cyproheptadine (Periactin) Uses: *Allergic Rxns; itching* Acts: Phenothi-
azine antihistamine; serotonin antagonist **Dose:** *Adults.* 4–20 mg PO + q8h; max 0.5 mg/kg/d. *Peds 2–6 y.* 2 mg bid-tid (max 12 mg/24 h). *7–14 y:* 4 mg bid-tid; ↓ in hepatic impair **W/P:** [B, ?] Elderly, CV Dz, Asthma, thyroid Dz, BPH **CI:** Neonates

or < 2 y; NAG; BOO; acute asthma; GI obst; w/ MAOI **Disp:** Tabs 4 mg; syrup 2 mg/5 mL **SE:** Anticholinergic, drowsiness **Notes:** May stimulate appetite

Cytarabine [ARA-C] (Cytosar-U) **BOX:** Administration by experienced physician in properly equipped facility; potent myelosuppressive agent **Uses:** *Acute leukemias, CML, NHL; IT for leukemic meningitis or prophylaxis* **Acts:** Antimetabolite; interferes w/ DNA synth **Dose:** 100–150 mg/m²/d for 5–10 d (low dose); 3 g/m² q12h for 6–12 doses (high dose); 1 mg/kg 1–2/wk (SQ maint); 5–70 mg/m² up to 3/wk IT (per protocols); ↓ in renal/hepatic impair **W/P:** [D, ?] in elderly, w/ marked BM suppression, ↓ dosage by ↓ the number of days of administration **CI:** Component sensitivity **Disp:** Inj 100, 500 mg, 1, 2 g, also 20, 100 mg/mL **SE:** ↓ BM, N/V/D, stomatitis, flu-like synd, rash on palms/soles, hepatic/cerebellar dysfunction w/ high doses, noncardiogenic pulm edema, neuropathy, fever **Notes:** Little use in solid tumors; high-dose tox limited by corticosteroid ophthal soln

Cytarabine Liposome (DepoCyt) **BOX:** Can cause chemical arachnoiditis (N/V/HA, fever) ↓ severity w/ dexamethasone. Administer by experienced physician in properly equipped facility **Uses:** *Lymphomatous meningitis* **Acts:** Antimetabolite; interferes w/ DNA synth **Dose:** 50 mg IT q14d for 5 doses, then 50 mg IT q28d × 4 doses; use dexamethasone prophylaxis **W/P:** [D, ?] May cause neurotox; blockage to CSF flow may ↑ the risk of neurotox; use in peds not established **CI:** Active meningeal Infxn **Disp:** IT Inj 50 mg/5 mL **SE:** Neck pain/rigidity, HA, confusion, somnolence, fever, back pain, N/V, edema, neutropenia, ↓ plt, anemia **Notes:** Cytarabine liposomes are similar in microscopic appearance to WBCs; caution in interpreting CSF studies

Cytomegalovirus Immune Globulin [CMV-IG IV] (CytoGam) **Uses:** *Prophylaxis/attenuation CMV Dz w/ transplantation* **Acts:** IgG antibodies to CMV **Dose:** 150 mg/kg/dose w/in 72 hrs of transplant and, wks 2, 4, 6, 8, and 100 mg/kg/dose wks 12, 16 post-transplant; see PI **W/P:** [C, ?] Anaphylactic Rxns; renal dysfunction **CI:** Allergy to immunoglobulins; IgA deficiency **Disp:** Inj 50 mg/mL **SE:** Flushing, N/V, muscle cramps, wheezing, HA, fever, non-cardiogenic pulm edema, renal insuff, aseptic meningitis **Notes:** IV only in separate line; do not shake

Dabigatran (Pradaxa) **Uses:** *↓ risk stroke/systemic embolism w/nonvalvular afib* **Acts:** Thrombin inhibitor **Dose:** *Adults.* CrCl > 30 mL/min: 150 mg PO bid; CrCl 15–30 mL/min: 75 mg PO bid **W/P:** [C, ?/–] avoid w/ P-gp inducers (i.e., rifampin) **CI:** Active bleeding **Disp:** Caps 75, 150 mg **SE:** Bleeding, gastritis, dyspepsia **Notes:** Do not chew/break/open caps; see label to convert between other anticoagulants

Dacarbazine (DTIC) **BOX:** Causes hematopoietic depression, hepatic necrosis, may be carcinogenic, teratogenic **Uses:** *Melanoma, Hodgkin Dz, sarcoma* **Acts:** Alkylating agent; antimetabolite as a purine precursor; ↓ protein synth, RNA, & especially DNA **Dose:** 2–4.5 mg/kg/d for 10 consecutive d or 250 mg/m²/d for 5 d (per protocols); ↓ in renal impair **W/P:** [C, ?] in BM suppression; renal/hepatic impair **CI:** Component sensitivity **Disp:** Inj 100, 200 mg **SE:** ↓ BM, N/V, hepatotox, flu-like synd, ↓ BP, photosens, alopecia, facial flushing, facial paresthesias, urti-caria, phlebitis at Inj site **Notes:** Avoid extrav, ✓ CBC, plt

Daclizumab (Zenapax) **BOX:** Administer under skilled supervision in properly equipped facility **Uses:** *Prevent acute organ rejection* **Acts:** IL-2 recep-tor antagonist **Dose:** 1 mg/kg/dose IV; 1st dose pretransplant, then 1 mg/kg q14d × 4 doses **W/P:** [C, ?] **CI:** Component sensitivity **Disp:** Inj 5 mg/mL **SE:** Hypergly-cemia, edema, HTN, ↓ BP, constipation, HA, dizziness, anxiety, nephrotox, pulm edema, pain, anaphylaxis/hypersens **Notes:** Administer w/in 4 h of prep

Dactinomycin (Cosmegen) **BOX:** Administer under skilled supervision in properly equipped facility; powder and soln toxic, corrosive, mutagenic, carcino-genic, and teratogenic; avoid exposure and use precautions **Uses:** *Choriocarci-noma, Wilms tumor, Kaposi and Ewing sarcomas, rhabdomyosarcoma, uterine and testicular CA* **Acts:** DNA-intercalating agent **Dose:** *Adults.* 0.5 mg/d for 5 d; 2 mg/wk for 3 consecutive wk; 15 mcg/kg or 0.45 mg/m²/d (max 0.5 mg) for 5 d q3–8wk *Peds.* Sarcoma (per protocols); ↓ in renal impair **W/P:** [C, ?] **CI:** Concur-rent/recent chickenpox or herpes zoster; infants < 6 mo **Disp:** Inj 0.5 mg **SE:** Myelo-/immunosuppression, severe N/V/D, alopecia, acne, hyperpigmentation, radiation recall phenomenon, tissue damage w/ extrav, hepatotox **Notes:** Classified as antibiotic but not used as antimicrobial

Dalfampridine (Ampyra) **Uses:** *Improve walking w/ MS* **Acts:** K⁺ chan-nel blocker **Dose:** 10 mg PO q12h **W/P:** [C, ?/–] not w/ other 4-aminopyridines **CI:** Hx seizure; w/ CrCl ≤ 50 mL/min **Disp:** Tab ER 10 mg **SE:** HA, N, constipa-tion, dyspepsia, dizziness, insomnia, UTI, nasopharyngitis, back pain, pharyngola-ryngeal pain, asthenia, balance disorder, MS relapse, paresthesia, seizure **Notes:** Do not cut/chew/crush/dissolve tab

Dalteparin (Fragmin) **BOX:** ↑ Risk of spinal/epidural hematoma w/LP **Uses:** *Unstable angina, non–Q-wave MI, prevent & Rx DVT following surgery (hip, Abd), pt w/ restricted mobility, extended therapy Rx for PE DVT in CA pt* **Acts:** LMW heparin **Dose:** *Angina/MI:* 120 units/kg (max 10,000 units) SQ q12h w/ ASA. *DVT prophylaxis:* 2500–5000 units SQ 1–2 h pre-op, then daily for 5–10 d. *Systemic anticoagulation:* 200 units/kg/d SQ or 100 units/kg bid SQ. *CA:* 200 Int Units/kg (max 18,000 Int Units) SQ q24h × 30 d, mo 2–6 150 Int Units/kg SQ q24h (max 18,000 Int Units) SQ q24h **W/P:** [B, ?] In renal/hepatic impair, active hemor-rhage, cerebrovascular Dz, cerebral aneurysm, severe HTN **CI:** HIT; pork product allergy; w/ mifepristone **Disp:** Inj 2500 (16 mg/0.2 mL), 5000 (32 mg/0.2 mL), 7500 (48 mg/0.3 mL), 10,000 units (64 mg/mL), 25,000 units (3.8 mL); prefilled vials 10,000 units/mL (9.5 mL) **SE:** Bleeding, pain at site, ↓ plt **Notes:** Predictable effects eliminates lab monitoring; not for IM/IV use

Dantrolene (Dantrium) **BOX:** Hepatotox reported; D/C after 45 d if no benefit observed **Uses:** *Rx spasticity d/t upper motor neuron disorders (e.g., spinal cord injuries, stroke, CP, MS); malignant hyperthermia* **Acts:** Skeletal muscle relaxant **Dose:** *Adults. Spasticity:* 25 mg PO daily; ↑ 25 mg to effect to 100 mg max PO qid PRN. *Peds.* 0.5 mg/kg/dose bid; ↑ by 0.5 mg/kg to effect, to 3 mg/kg/dose max qid PRN. *Adults & Peds. Malignant hyperthermia: Rx:* Cont rapid IV, start 1 mg/kg until Sxs subside or 10 mg/kg is reached. *Post-crisis follow-up:* 4–8 mg/kg/d in 3–4 ÷ doses for 1–3 d to prevent recurrence **W/P:** [C, ?] Impaired cardiac/pulm/hepatic Fxn **CI:** Active hepatic Dz; where spasticity needed to maintain posture or balance **Disp:** Caps 25, 50, 100 mg; powder for Inj 20 mg/vial **SE:** Hepatotox, ↑ LFTs, drowsiness, dizziness, rash, muscle weakness, D/N/V, pleural effusion w/ pericarditis, D, blurred vision, hep, photosens **Notes:** Monitor LFTs; avoid sunlight/EtOH/CNS depressants

Dapsone, Oral **Uses:** *Rx & prevent PCP; toxoplasmosis prophylaxis; leprosy* **Acts:** Unknown; bactericidal **Dose:** *Adults. PCP* prophylaxis 50–100 mg/d PO; Rx PCP 100 mg/d PO w/ TMP 15–20 mg/kg/d for 21 d. *Peds. PCP prophylaxis alternated dose:* (> 1 mo) 4 mg/kg/dose once/wk (max 200 mg); prophylaxis of PCP 1–2 mg/kg/24 h PO daily; max 100 mg/d **W/P:** [C, +] G6PD deficiency; severe anemia **CI:** Component sensitivity **Disp:** Tabs 25, 100 mg **SE:** Hemolysis, methemoglobinemia, agranulocytosis, rash, cholestatic jaundice **Notes:** Absorption ↑ by an acidic environment; for leprosy, combine w/ rifampin & other agents

Dapsone, Topical (Aczone) **Uses:** *Topical for acne vulgaris* **Acts:** Unknown; bactericidal **Dose:** Apply pea-size amount and rub into areas bid; wash hands after **W/P:** [C, +] G6PD deficiency; severe anemia **CI:** Component sensitivity **Disp:** 5% gel **SE:** Skin oiliness/peeling, dryness erythema **Notes:** Not for oral, ophthal, or intravag use; check G6PD levels before use; follow CBC if G6PD deficient

Daptomycin (Cubicin) **Uses:** *Complicated skin/skin structure Infxns d/t gram(+) organisms* *S. aureus,* bacteremia, MRSA endocarditis **Acts:** Cyclic lipopeptide; rapid membrane depolarization & bacterial death. *Spectrum: S. aureus* (including MRSA), *S. pyogenes, S. agalactiae, S. dysgalactiae* subsp *Equisimilis,* & *E. faecalis* (vancomycin-susceptible strains only) **Dose:** *Skin:* 4 mg/kg IV daily × 7–14 d (over 2 min); *Bacteremia & Endocarditis:* 6 mg/kg q48h; ↓ w/ CrCl < 30 mL/min or dialysis: q48h **W/P:** [B, ?] w/ HMG-CoA inhib **Disp:** Inj 250, 500 mg/10 mL **SE:** Anemia, constipation, N/V/D, HA, rash, site Rxn, muscle pain/weakness, edema, cellulitis, hypo-/hyperglycemia, ↑ alkaline phosphatase, cough, back pain, Abd pain, ↓ K^+, anxiety, chest pain, sore throat, cardiac failure, confusion, *Candida* Infxns **Notes:** ✓ CPK baseline & weekly; consider D/C HMG-CoA reductase inhib to ↓ myopathy risk; not for Rx PNA

Darbepoetin Alfa (Aranesp) **BOX:** Associated w/ ↑ CV, thromboembolic events and/or mortality; D/C if Hgb > 12 g/dL; may increase tumor progression and death in CA pts **Uses:** *Anemia associated w/ CRF*, anemia in nonmyeloid malignancy w/ concurrent chemotherapy **Acts:** ↑ Erythropoiesis, recombinant erythropoietin variant **Dose:** 0.45 mcg/kg single IV or SQ q wk; titrate, do not exceed target Hgb of 12 g/dL; use lowest doses possible, see PI to convert from *Epogen* **W/P:** [C, ?] May ↑ risk of CV &/or neurologic SE in renal failure; HTN; w/ Hx Szs **CI:**

Uncontrolled HTN, component allergy **Disp:** 25, 40, 60, 100, 150, 200, 300 mcg/mL, 150 mcg/0.075 mL in polysorbate or albumin excipient **SE:** May ↑ cardiac risk, CP, hypo-/hypertension, N/V/D, myalgia, arthralgia, dizziness, edema, fatigue, fever, ↑ risk Infxn **Notes:** Longer 1/2-life than *Epogen*; weekly CBC until stable

Darifenacin (Enablex) **Uses:** *OAB* **Urinary antispasmodic Acts:** Muscarinic receptor antagonist **Dose:** 7.5 mg/d PO; 15 mg/d max (7.5 mg/d w/ mod hepatic impair or w/ CYP3A4 inhib); w/ drugs metabolized by CYP2D (Table 10, p 301); swallow whole **W/P:** [C, ?/–] w/ Hepatic impair **CI:** Urinary/gastric retention, uncontrolled NAG, paralytic ileus **Disp:** Tabs ER 7.5, 15 mg **SE:** Xerostomia/eyes, constipation, dyspepsia, Abd pain, retention, abnormal vision, dizziness, asthenia

Darunavir (Prezista) **Uses:** *Rx HIV w/ resistance to multiple protease inhib* **Acts:** HIV-1 protease inhib **Dose:** *Adults.* Rx-naïve and w/o darunavir resistance substitutions: 800 mg w/ ritonavir 100 mg QD. Rx experienced w/ one darunavir resistance: 600 mg w/ ritonavir 100 mg BID w/ food. *Peds 6–18 y and > 20 kg.* Dose based on body weight (see label); do not exceed the Rx experienced adult dose. Do not use QD dosing in peds; w/ food **W/P:** [B, ?/–] Hx Sulfa allergy, CYP3A4 substrate, changes levels of many meds (↑ amiodarone, ↑ dihydropyridine, ↑ HMG-CoA reductase inhib [statins], ↓ SSRIs, ↓ rifampin, ↓ methadone); do not use w/salmeterol, colchicine (w/ renal impair; do not use w/ severe hepatic impair); adjust dose w/ bosentan, tadalafil for PAH **CI:** w/ Astemizole, rifampin, St. John's Wort, terfenadine, dihydroergotamine, ergonovine, ergotamine, methylergonovine, pimozide, midazolam, triazolam, alpha 1-adrenoreceptor antagonist (alfuzosin), PDE5 inhibitors (e.g., sildenafil) **Supplied:** Tabs 75, 150, 400, 600 mg **SE:** ↑ glucose, cholesterol, triglycerides, central redistribution of fat (metabolic synd), N, ↓ neutrophils & ↑ amylase

Dasatinib (Sprycel) **Uses:** CML, Ph + ALL **Acts:** Multi-TKI **Dose:** 100–140 mg PO day; adjust w/ CYP3A4 inhib/inducers (Table 10, p 301) **W/P:** [D, ?/–] **CI:** None **Disp:** Tabs 20, 50, 70, 100 mg **SE:** ↓ BM, edema, fluid retention, pleural effusions, N/V/D, Abd pain, bleeding, fever, ↑ QT **Notes:** Replace K⁺, Mg⁺² before Rx

Daunorubicin (Daunomycin, Cerubidine) **BOX:** Cardiac Fxn should be monitored d/t potential risk for cardiac tox & CHF, renal/hepatic dysfunction **Uses:** *Acute leukemias* **Acts:** DNA-intercalating agent; ↓ topoisomerase II; generates oxygen free radicals **Dose:** 45–60 mg/m²/d for 3 consecutive d; 25 mg/m²/wk (per protocols); ↓ w/renal/hepatic impair **W/P:** [D, ?] **CI:** Component sens **Disp:** Inj 20, 50 mg **SE:** ↓ BM, mucositis, N/V, orange urine, alopecia, radiation recall phenomenon, hepatotx (↑ bili), tissue necrosis w/ extrav, cardiotox (1–2% CHF w/ 550 mg/m² cumulative dose) **Notes:** Prevent cardiotox w/ dexrazoxane (w/ > 300 mg/m² daunorubicin cum dose);IV use only; allopurinol prior to ↓ hyperuricemia

Decitabine (Dacogen) **Uses:** *MDS* **Acts:** Inhibits DNA methyltransferase **Dose:** 15 mg/m² cont Inf over 3 h; repeat q8h × 3 d; repeat cycle q6wk, min 4 cycles; delay Tx and ↓ dose if inadequate hematologic recovery at 6 wk (see PI);

delay Tx w/ Cr > 2 mg/dL or bili > 2× ULN **W/P:** [D, ?/–]; avoid PRG; males should not father a child during or 2 mo after; renal/hepatic impair **Disp:** Powder 50 mg/vial **SE:** ↓ WBC, ↓ HgB,↓ plt, febrile neutropenia, edema, petechiae, N/V/D, constipation, stomatitis, dyspepsia, cough, fever, fatigue, ↑ LFTs/bili, hyperglycemia, Infxn, HA **Notes:** ✓ CBC & plt before cycle and prn; premedicate w/ antiemetic

Deferasirox (Exjade) Uses: *Chronic iron overload d/t transfusion in pts > 2 y* **Acts:** Oral iron chelator **Dose:** 20 mg/kg PO/d; adjust by 5–10 mg/kg q3–6mo based on monthly ferritin; 30 mg/kg/d max; on empty stomach 30 min ac; hold dose w/ferritin < 500 mcg/L; dissolve in water, orange/apple juice (< 1 g/3.5 oz; > 1 g in 7 oz) drink immediately; resuspend residue and swallow; do not chew, swallow whole tabs or take w/ Al-containing antacids **W/P:** [B, ?/–] elderly, renal impair, hepatic impair, heme disorders; ↑ MDS in pt 60 yrs **Disp:** Tabs for oral susp 125, 250, 500 mg **SE:** N/V/D, Abd pain, skin rash, HA, fever, cough, ↑ Cr & LFTs, Infxn, hearing loss, dizziness, cataracts, retinal disorders, ↑ IOP **Notes:** ARF, cytopenias possible; ✓ Cr weekly 1st mo then q mo, ✓ CBC, urine protein, LFTs; do not use w/ other iron-chelator therapies; dose to nearest whole tab; instead auditory/ophthal testing and q12mo

Degarelix (Firmagon) Uses:* Advanced PCa* **Action:** Reversible LHRH antagonist, ↓ LH and testosterone w/o flare seen w/ LHRH agonists (transient ↑ in testosterone **Dose:** Initial 240 mg SQ in two 120 mg doses (40 mg/mL); maint 80 mg SQ (20 mg/mL) q28d **W/P:** [not for women] **CI:** Women **Supplied:** Inj vial 120 mg (initial); 80 mg (maint) **SE:** inj site Rxns, hot flashes, ↑ wgt, ↑ serum GGT **Notes:** Requires 2 inj initial (volume); 44% testosterone castrate (<50 ng/dL) at day 1, 96% day 3

Delavirdine (Rescriptor) Uses: *HIV Infxn* **Acts:** Nonnucleoside RT inhib **Dose:** 400 mg PO tid **W/P:** [C, ?] CDC rec: HIV-infected others not breastfeed (transmission risk); w/ renal/hepatic impair **CI:** w/ Drugs dependent on CYP3A (Table 10, p 301) **Disp:** Tabs 100, 200 mg **SE:** Fat redistribution, immune reconstitution synd, HA, fatigue, rash, ↑ transaminases, N/V/D **Notes:** Avoid antacids; ↓ cytochrome P-450 enzymes; numerous drug interactions; monitor LFTs

Demeclocycline (Declomycin) Uses: *SIADH* **Acts:** Antibiotic, antagonizes ADH action on renal tubules **Dose:** 300–600 mg PO q12h on empty stomach; ↓ in renal failure; avoid antacids **W/P:** [D, +] Avoid in hepatic/renal impair & children **CI:** Tetracycline allergy **Disp:** Tabs 150, 300 mg **SE:** D, Abd cramps, photosens, DI **Notes:** Avoid sunlight, numerous drug interactions; not for peds < 8 y

Denosumab (Prolia, Xgeva) Uses: *Tx osteoporosis postmenopausal women ↑ BMD in men on ADT (Prolia); prevent skeletal events w/ bone mets from solid tumors (Xgeva)* **Acts:** RANK ligand (RANKL) inhibitor (human IgG2 MoAb); inhibits osteoclasts **Dose:** Prolia: 60 mg SQ q6mo; Xgeva: 120 mg SQ q4wk; in upper arm, thigh, abd **W/P:** [C, ?/–] **CI:** Hypocalcemia **Disp:** Inj **SE:** ↓ Ca^{+2}, hypophosphatemia, serious Infxns, dermatitis, rashes, eczema, jaw osteonecrosis, pancreatitis, pain (musculoskeletal, back), fatigue, asthenia, dyspnea, N, abd pain, flatulence, hypercholesterolemia, anemia, cystitis **Notes:** Give w/ calcium 1000 mg & vit D 400 IU/d

Desipramine (Norpramin)   **BOX:** Closely monitor for worsening depression or emergence of suicidality ↑ **Uses:** *Endogenous depression*, chronic pain, peripheral neuropathy **Acts:** TCA; ↑ synaptic serotonin or norepinephrine in CNS **Dose:** *Adults.* 100–200 mg/d single or ÷ dose; usually single hs dose (max 300 mg/d) *Peds 6–12 y.* 1–3 mg/kg/d ÷ dose, 5 mg/kg/d max; ↓ dose in elderly **W/P:** [C, ?/–] CV Dz, Sz disorder, hypothyroidism, elderly, liver impair **CI:** MAOIs w/in 14 d; during AMI recovery phase **Disp:** Tabs 10, 25, 50, 75, 100, 150 mg; caps 25, 50 mg **SE:** Anticholinergic (blurred vision, urinary retention, xerostomia); orthostatic ↓ BP; ↑ QT, arrhythmias **Notes:** Numerous drug interactions; blue-green urine; avoid sunlight

Desirudin (Iprivask)   **BOX:** Recent/planned epidural/spinal anesthesia, ↑ epidural/spinal hematoma risk w/ paralysis; consider risk vs benefit before neuraxial intervention **Uses:** *DVT Px in hip replacement* **Acts:** Thrombin inhibitor **Dose:** *Adults.* 15 mg SQ q12h, initial 5–15 min prior to surgery; CrCl 31–60 mL/min: 5 mg SQ q12h; CrCl < 31 mL/min: 1.7 mg SQ q12h; ✓ aPTT & SCr daily for dosage mod **W/P:** [C, ?/–] **CI:** Active bleeding, irreversible coags, hypersens to hirudins **Disp:** Inj **SE:** Hemorrhage, N/V, Inj site mass, wound secretion, anemia, thrombophlebitis, ↓ BP, dizziness, anaphylactic Rxn, fever

Desloratadine (Clarinex)   **Uses:** *Seasonal & perennial allergic rhinitis; chronic idiopathic urticaria* **Acts:** Active metabolite of Claritin, H₁-antihistamine, blocks inflammatory mediators **Dose:** *Adults & Peds > 12 y.* 5 mg PO daily; 5 mg PO q other day w/ hepatic/renal impair **W/P:** [C, ?/–] RediTabs contain phenylalanine **Disp:** Tabs & RediTabs (rapid dissolving) 5 mg, syrup 0.5 mg/mL **SE:** Allergy, anaphylaxis, somnolence, HA, dizziness, fatigue, pharyngitis, xerostomia, N, dyspepsia, myalgia

Desmopressin (DDAVP, Stimate)   **BOX:** Not for hemophilia B or w/ factor VIII antibody; not for hemophilia A w/ factor VIII levels < 5% **Uses:** *DI (intranasal & parenteral); bleeding d/t uremia, hemophilia A, & type I von Willebrand Dz (parenteral), nocturnal enuresis* **Acts:** Synthetic analog of vasopressin (human ADH); ↑ factor VIII **Dose:** *DI: Intranasal: Adults.* 0.1–0.4 mL (10–40 mcg/d in 1–3 ÷ doses). *Peds 3 mo–12 y.* 0.05–0.3 mL/d in 1 or 2 doses. *Parenteral: Adults.* 0.5–1 mL (2–4 mcg/d in 2 ÷ doses); converting from nasal to parenteral, use 1/10 nasal dose. *PO: Adults.* 0.05 mg bid; ↑ to max of 1.2 mg. *Hemophilia A & von Willebrand Dz (type I): Adults & Peds > 10 kg.* 0.3 mcg/kg in 50 mL NS, Inf over 15–30 min. *Peds < 10 kg.* As above w/ dilution to 10 mL w/ NS. *Nocturnal enuresis: Peds > 6 y.* 20 mcg intranasally hs **W/P:** [B, M] Avoid overhydration **CI:** Hemophilia B; CrCl < 50 mL/min, severe classic von Willebrand Dz; pts w/ factor VIII antibodies; hyponatremia **Disp:** Tabs 0.1, 0.2 mg; Inj 4, 15 mcg/mL; nasal spray 0.1 mL (10 mcg)/spray **SE:** Facial flushing, HA, dizziness, vulval pain, nasal congestion, pain at Inj site, ↓ Na⁺, H₂O intoxication **Notes:** In very young & old pts, ↓ fluid intake to avoid H₂O intoxication & ↓ Na⁺; ↓ urine output, ↑ urine osm; ↓ plasma osm

Desvenlafaxine (Pristiq) **BOX:** Monitor for worsening or emergence of suicidality, particularly in peds, adolescent, and young adult pts **Uses:** *Major depressive disorder* **Acts:** Selective serotonin and norepinephrine reuptake inhib **Dose:** 50 mg PO daily, ↓ w/ renal impair **W/P:** [C, ±/M] **CI:** Hypersens, MAOI w/ or w/in 14 d of stopping MAOI **Disp:** Tabs 50, 100 mg **SE:** N, dizziness, insomnia, hyperhidrosis, constipation, somnolence, decreased appetite, anxiety, and specific male sexual Fxn disorders **Notes:** Tabs should be taken whole, allow 7 d after stopping before starting an MAOI

Dexmedetomidine (Precedex) **Uses:** *Sedation in intubated & nonintubated pts* **Acts:** Sedative; selective α₂-agonist **Dose:** *Adults. ICU Sedation:* 1 mcg/kg IV over 10 min then 0.2–0.7 mcg/kg/h; *Procedural sedation:* 0.5–1 mcg/kg IV over 10 min then 0.2–1 mcg/kg/h; ↓ in elderly, liver Dz **W/P:** [C, ?/–] **CI:** none **Disp:** Inj 200 mcg/2 mL **SE:** Hypotension, bradycardia **Notes:** Tachyphylaxis & tolerance assoc w/ exposure > 24 h

Dexamethasone, Nasal (Dexacort Phosphate Turbinaire) **Uses:** *Chronic nasal inflammation or allergic rhinitis* **Acts:** Anti-inflammatory corticosteroid **Dose:** *Adults & Peds > 12 y.* 2 sprays/nostril bid–tid, max 12 sprays/d. *Peds 6–12 y.* 1–2 sprays/nostril bid, max 8 sprays/d **W/P:** [C, ?] **CI:** Untreated Infxn **Disp:** Aerosol, 84 mcg/activation **SE:** Local irritation

Dexamethasone, Ophthalmic (AK-Dex Ophthalmic, Decadron Ophthalmic) **Uses:** *Inflammatory or allergic conjunctivitis* **Acts:** Anti-inflammatory corticosteroid **Dose:** Instill 1–2 gtt tid–qid **W/P:** [C, ?/–] **CI:** Active untreated bacterial, viral, & fungal eye infxns **Disp:** Susp & soln 0.1%; oint 0.05% **SE:** Long-term use associated w/ cataracts

Dexamethasone, Systemic, Topical (Decadron) See Steroids, Systemic. *Peds. ECC 2010.* Croup: 0.6 mg/kg IV/IM/PO once; max dose 16 mg; *Asthma:* 0.6 mg/kg IV/IM/PO q24h; max dose 16 mg

Dexmethylphenidate (Focalin, Focalin XR)[C-II] **BOX:** Caution w/ Hx drug dependence/alcoholism. Chronic abuse may lead to tolerance, psychological dependence & abnormal behavior; monitor closely during withdrawal **Uses:** *ADHD* **Acts:** CNS stimulant, blocks reuptake of norepinephrine & DA **Dose:** *Adults. Focalin:* 2.5 mg PO twice daily, ↑ by 2.5–5 mg weekly; max 20 mg/d *Focalin XR:* 10 mg PO daily, ↑ 10 mg weekly; max 40 mg/d *Peds ≥ 6 y. Focalin:* 2.5 mg PO bid, ↑ 2.5–5 mg weekly; max 20 mg/d *Focalin XR:* 5 mg PO daily, ↑ 5 mg weekly; max 30 mg/d; if already on methylphenidate, start w/ half of current total daily dose **W/P:** [C, ?/–] avoid w/ known cardiac abnorm; may ↓ metabolism of warfarin/anticonvulsants/antidepressants **CI:** Agitation, anxiety, tension, glaucoma, Hx motor tic, fam Hx/dx Tourette's w/ or w/in 14 d of MAOI; hypersens to methylphenidate **Disp:** Tabs 2.5, 5, 10 mg; Caps ER 5, 10, 15, 20, 30, 40 mg **SE:** HA, anxiety, dyspepsia, ↓ appetite, weight loss, dry mouth, visual disturbances, ↑ HR, HTN, MI, stroke, sudden death, seizures, growth suppression, aggression, mania, psychosis **Notes:** ✓CBC w/prolonged use; swallow ER caps whole or sprinkle contents on applesauce (do not crush/chew)

Dexlansoprazole (Dexilant, Kapidex) **Uses:** *Heal and maint of erosive esophagitis (EE), GERD* PUD **Acts:** PPI, delayed release **Dose:** EE: 60 mg QD up to 8 wks; maint healed EE: 30 mg QD up to 6 mos; GERD 30 mg/QD × 4 wks; ↓ w/ hepatic impair **W/P:** [B, +/–] do not use w/ clopidogrel/atazanavir or drugs w/pH based absorption (e.g., ampicillin, iron salts, ketoconazole); may alter warfarin and tacrolimus levels **CI:** Component hypersensitivity **Disp:** Caps 30,60 mg **SE:** N/V/D, flatulence, abd pain, URI **Notes:** w or w/o food; take whole or sprinkle on tsp applesauce; clinical response does not r/o gastric malignancy; see also lansoprazole; 2 ↑ risk of fractures w/ all PPI; risk of hypomagnesemia w/ long-term use, monitor

Dexpanthenol (Ilopan-Choline [Oral], Ilopan) **Uses:** *Minimize paralytic ileus, Rx post-op distention* **Acts:** Cholinergic agent **Dose:** *Adults.* Relief of gas: 2–3 tabs PO tid. *Prevent post-op ileus:* 250–500 mg IM stat, repeat in 2 h, then q6h PRN. *Ileus:* 500 mg IM stat, repeat in 2 h, then q6h, PRN **W/P:** [C, ?] **CI:** Hemophilia, mechanical bowel obst **Disp:** Inj 250 mg/mL; tabs 50 mg; cream 2% (Panthoderm Cream [OTC]) **SE:** GI cramps

Dexrazoxane (Zinecard, Totect) **Uses:** *Prevent anthracycline-induced (e.g., doxorubicin) cardiomyopathy (Zinecard), extrav of anthracycline chemotherapy (Totect)* **Acts:** Chelates heavy metals; binds intracellular iron & prevents anthracycline-induced free radicals **Dose:** *Systemic (cardiomyopathy, Zinecard):* 10:1 ratio dexrazoxane:doxorubicin 30 min before each dose, 5:1 ratio w/ CrCl < 40 mL/min. *Extrav (Totect):* IV Inf over 1–2 h q day × 3 d, w/in 6 h of extrav. *Day 1:* 1000 mg/m² (max 2000 mg); *Day 2:* 1000 mg/m² (max 2000 mg); *Day 3:* 500 mg/m² (max: 1000 mg); w/ CrCl < 40 mL/min, ↓ dose by 50% **W/P:** [D, –] **CI:** Component sensitivity **Disp:** Inj powder 250, 500 mg (10 mg/mL) **SE:** ↓ BM, fever, Infxn, stomatitis, alopecia, N/V/D; ↑ LFTs, Inj site pain

Dextran 40 (Gentran 40, Rheomacrodex) **Uses:** *Shock, prophylaxis of DVT & thromboembolism, adjunct in peripheral vascular surgery* **Acts:** Expands plasma vol; ↓ blood viscosity **Dose:** *Shock:* 10 mL/kg Inf rapidly; 20 mL/kg max 1st 24 h; beyond 24 h 10 mL/kg max; D/C after 5 d. *Prophylaxis of DVT & thromboembolism:* 10 mL/kg IV day of surgery, then 500 mL/d IV for 2–3 d, then 500 mL IV q2–3d based on risk for up to 2 wk **W/P:** [C, ?] Inf Rxns; w/ corticosteroids **CI:** Major hemostatic defects; cardiac decompensation; renal Dz w/ severe oliguria/anuria **Disp:** 10% dextran 40 in 0.9% NaCl or 5% dextrose **SE:** Allergy/anaphylactoid Rxn (observe during 1st min of Inf), arthralgia, cutaneous Rxns, ↓ BP, fever **Notes:** Monitor Cr & lytes; stay well hydrated

Dextroamphetamine (Dexedrine) [C-II] **BOX:** Amphetamines have a high potential for abuse. Long-term use may lead to dependence. **Uses:** *ADHD, Narcolepsy* **Acts:** CNS stimulant; ↑ DA & norepinephrine release **Dose:** *ADHD ≥ 6 y:* 5 mg daily-bid, ↑ by 5 mg/d weekly PRN, max 60 mg/d ÷ bid-tid; *Peds 3–5 y.*

2.5 mg PO daily, ↑ 2.5 mg/d weekly PRN to response; *Peds < 3 y.* Not recommended; *Narcolepsy 6–12 y: 5 mg daily,* ↑ by 5 mg/d weekly PRN max 60 mg/d ÷ bid–tid; ≥ *12 y:* 10-60 mg/d ÷ bid–tid; ER caps once daily **W/P:** [C, +/–] Hx drug abuse; separate 14 days from MAOIs **CI:** Advanced arteriosclerosis, CVD, mod-severe HTN, hyperthyroidism, glaucoma **Disp:** Tabs 5, 10 mg; ER capsules 5, 10, 15 mg **SE:** HTN, ↓ appetite, insomnia **Notes:** May open ER capsules, do not crush beads

Dextromethorphan (Benylin DM, Delsym, Mediquell, PediaCare 1, Others) [OTC] Uses: *Control nonproductive cough* **Acts:** Suppresses medullary cough center **Dose:** *Adults.* 10–30 mg PO q4h PRN (max 120 mg/24 h). *Peds 2–6 y.* 2.5–7.5 mg q4–8h (max 30 mg/24 h). *7–12 y:* 5–10 mg q4–8h (max 60 mg/24 h) **W/P:** [C, ?/–] Not for persistent or chronic cough **CI:** < 2 y **Disp:** Caps 30 mg; lozenges 2.5, 5, 7.5, 15 mg; syrup 15 mg/15 mL, 10 mg/5 mL; liq 10 mg/15 mL, 3.5, 7.5, 15 mg/5 mL; sustained-action liq 30 mg/5 mL **SE:** GI disturbances **Notes:** Found in combo OTC products w/ guaifenesin; deaths reported in pts < 2 y; abuse potential; efficacy in children debated; do not use w/in 14 d of D/C MAOI

Dextrose 50%/25% Uses: Hypoglycemia, insulin OD **Acts:** Sugar source in the form of d-glucose **Dose:** *Adults.* 1 50 mL amp of 50% soln IV *Peds. ECC 2010.* Hypoglycemia: 0.5–1 g/kg (25% max IV/IO conc); 50% Dextrose (0.5 g/mL): 1–2 mL/kg; 25% Dextrose (0.25 g/mL): 2–5 mL/kg; 10% Dextrose (0.1 g/mL): 5–10 mL/kg; 5% Dextrose (0.95 g/mL): 10–20 mL/kg if volume tolerated **W/P:** [C, M] w/ suspected intracranial bleeding can ↑ ICP **CI:** None if used w/ documented hypoglycemia **Disp:** Inj forms **SE:** Burning at IV site, local tissue necrosis w/ extravasation; neurologic Sxs (Wernicke encephalopathy) if pt thiamine deficient **Notes:** If pt well enough to protect airway, use oral glucose first; do not routinely use in altered mental status w/o low glucose, can worsen outcome in stroke; lower concentrations dextrose used in IV fluids

Diazepam (Valium, Diastat) [C-IV] Uses: *Anxiety, EtOH withdrawal, muscle spasm, status epilepticus, panic disorders, amnesia, pre-op sedation* **Acts:** Benzodiazepine **Dose:** *Adults. Status epilepticus:* 5–10 mg q10–20min to 30 mg max in 8-h period. *Anxiety, muscle spasm:* 2–10 mg PO bid-qid or IM/IV q3–4h PRN. *Pre-op:* 5–10 mg PO or IM 20–30 min or IV just prior to procedure. *EtOH withdrawal:* Initial 2–5 mg IV, then 5–10 mg q5–10min, 100 mg in 1 h max. May require up to 1000 mg/24 h for severe withdrawal; titrate to agitation; avoid excessive sedation; may lead to aspiration or resp arrest. *Peds. Status epilepticus: < 5 y:* 0.05–0.3 mg/kg/dose IV q15–30min up to a max of 5 mg. *> 5 y:* to max of 10 mg. *Sedation, muscle relaxation:* 0.04–0.3 mg/kg/dose q2–4h IM or IV to max of 0.6 mg/kg in 8 h, or 0.12–0.8 mg/kg/24 h PO ÷ tid-qid; ↓ w/ hepatic impair **W/P:** [D, ?/–] **CI:** Coma, CNS depression, resp depression, NAG, severe uncontrolled pain, PRG **Disp:** Tabs 2, 5, 10 mg; soln 1, 5 mg/mL; inj 5 mg/mL; rectal gel 2.5, 5, 10, 20 mg/mL **SE:** Sedation, amnesia, ↓ HR, ↓ BP, rash, ↓ resp rate **Notes:** 5 mg/min IV max in adults or 1–2 mg/min in peds (resp arrest possible); IM absorption erratic; avoid abrupt D/C

Diazoxide (Proglycem) Uses: *Hypoglycemia d/t hyperinsulinism (Proglycem); hypertensive crisis (Hyperstat)* Acts: ↓ Pancreatic insulin release; antihypertensive Dose: Repeat in 5–15 min until BP controlled; repeat q4–24h; monitor BP closely. *Hypoglycemia: Adults & Peds.* 3–8 mg/kg/24 h PO ÷ q8–12h. *Neonates.* 8–15 mg/kg/24 h ÷ in 3 equal doses; maint 8–10 mg/kg/24 h PO in 2–3 equal doses W/P: [C, ?] ↓ Effect w/ phenytoin; ↑ effect w/ diuretics, warfarin CI: Allergy to thiazides or other sulfonamide-containing products; HTN associated w/ aortic coarctation, AV shunt, or pheochromocytoma Disp: Caps 50 mg; PO susp 50 mg/mL; IV 15 mg/mL SE: Hyperglycemia, ↓ BP, dizziness, Na⁺ & H₂O retention, N/V, weakness Notes: Can give false(−) insulin response to glucagons; Rx extrav w/ warm compress

Dibucaine (Nupercainal) Uses: *Hemorrhoids & minor skin conditions* Acts: Topical anesthetic Dose: Insert PR w/ applicator bid & after each bowel movement; apply sparingly to skin W/P: [C, ?] topical use only CI: Component sensitivity Disp: 1% oint w/ rectal applicator; 0.5% cream SE: Local irritation, rash

Diclofenac and Misoprostol (Arthrotec) BOX: May induce abortion, birth defects; do not take if PRG; may ↑ risk of CV events & GI bleeding; CI in post-op CABG Uses: *OA and RA w/ ↑ risk GI bleed* Acts: NSAID w/ GI protective PGE₁ Dose: OA: 50–75 mg PO bid-tid; RA 50 mg bid-qid or 75 mg bid; w/ food or milk W/P: [X, ?] CHF, HTN, renal/hepatic dysfunction, & Hx PUD, asthma; avoid w/ porphyria CI: PRG; GI bleed; renal/hepatic failure; severe CHF; NSAID/ aspirin ASA allergy; following CABG Disp: Tabs *Arthrotec* 50: 50 mg diclofenac w/ 200 mcg misoprostol; *Arthrotec*: 75 mg diclofenac w/ 200 mcg misoprostol SE: *Oral:* Abd cramps, heartburn, GI ulcers, rash, interstitial nephritis Notes: Do not crush tabs; watch for GI bleed; ✓CBC, LFTs; PRG test females before use

Diclofenac, Oral (Cataflam, Voltaren, Voltaren-XR) BOX: May ↑ risk of CV events & GI bleeding; CI in post-op CABG Uses: *Arthritis & pain, oral and topical, actinic keratosis* Acts: NSAID Dose: 50–75 mg PO bid; w/ food or milk W/P: [C (avoid after 30 wks), ?] CHF, HTN, renal/hepatic dysfunction, & Hx PUD, asthma CI: NSAID/aspirin ASA allergy; porphyria; following CABG Disp: Tabs 50 mg; tabs DR 25, 50, 75, 100 mg; XR tabs 100 mg SE: *Oral:* Abd cramps, heartburn, GI ulceration, rash, interstitial nephritis Notes: Do not crush tabs; watch for GI bleed; ✓CBC, LFTs periodically

Diclofenac, Topical (Flector Patch, Pennsaid, Solaraze, Voltaren Gel) BOX: May ↑ risk CV events & GI bleeding; CI in post-op CABG Uses: *Arthritis of the knee (Pennsaid); arthritis of knee/hands (Voltaren Gel); pain due to strain, sprain, and contusions (Flector Patch); actinic keratosis (Solaraze)* Acts: NSAID Dose: *Flector Patch:* 1 patch to painful area. *Pennsaid:* 10 drops spread around knee; repeat until 40 drops applied. Usual *dose:* 40 drops/knee qid; wash hands; wait until dry before dressing. *Solaraze:* 0.5 g to each 5 × 5 cm lesion 60–90 days; *Voltaren Gel:* upper extremity 2 g qid (max 8 g/d); lower extremity 4 g qid (max 16 g/d) **W/P:** [C (avoid after 30 wk), ?] avoid nonintact skin; CV events possible w/ CHF, ↑ BP, renal/hepatic dysfunct, w/ Hx PUD, asthma; avoid w/ PO NSAID **CI:** NSAID/ASA allergy; following CABG; component allergy **Disp:** *Flector Patch:* 180 mg (10 × 14 cm); *Voltaren Gel 1%; Solaraze 3%* **SE:** Pruritus, dermatitis, burning, dry skin, N, HA **Notes:** Do not apply patch/gel to damaged skin or while bathing; w/ CDC, LFTs periodically; no box warning on *Solaraze*

Diclofenac, Ophthalmic (Voltaren Ophthalmic) **Uses:** *Inflammation postcataract or pain/photophobia post corneal refractive surgery * **Acts:** NSAID **Dose:** *Post-op cataract:* 1 gtt qid, start 24 h post-op × 2 wk. *Post-op refractive:* 1–2 gtt w/in 1 h pre-op and w/in 15 min post-op then qid up to 3 d **W/P:** [C, ?] May ↑ bleed risk in ocular tissues **CI:** NSAID/ASA allergy **Disp:** ophthal soln 0.1% 2.5-, 5-mL bottle **SE:** Burning/stinging/itching, keratitis, ↑ IOP, lacrimation, abnormal vision, conjunctivitis, lid swelling, discharge, iritis

Dicloxacillin (Dynapen, Dycill) **Uses:** *Rx of pneumonia, skin, & soft-tissue infxns, & osteomyelitis caused by penicillinase-producing staphylococci* **Acts:** Bactericidal; ↓ cell wall synth. *Spectrum:* S. aureus & Streptococcus **Dose:** *Adults.* 150–500 mg qid (2 g/d max) *Peds < 40 kg.* 12.5–100 mg/kg/d ÷ qid; take on empty stomach **W/P:** [B, ?] **CI:** Component or PCN sensitivity **Disp:** Caps 125, 250, 500 mg; soln 62.5 mg/5 mL **SE:** N/D, Abd pain **Notes:** Monitor PTT if pt on warfarin

Dicyclomine (Bentyl) **Uses:** *Functional IBS* **Acts:** Smooth-muscle relaxant **Dose:** *Adults.* 20 mg PO qid; ↑ to 160 mg/d max or 20 mg IM q6h, 80 mg/d ÷ qid then ↑ to 160 mg/d, max 2 wk *Peds Infants > 6 mo.* 5 mg/dose tid-qid. *Children:* 10 mg/dose tid-qid **W/P:** [B, −] **CI:** Infants < 6 mo, NAG, MyG, severe UC, BOO, GI obst, reflux esophagitis **Disp:** Caps 10, 20 mg; tabs 20 mg; syrup 10 mg/5 mL; Inj 10 mg/mL **SE:** Anticholinergic SEs may limit dose **Notes:** Take 30–60 min ac; avoid EtOH, do not administer IV

Didanosine (ddI) (Videx) **BOX:** Allergy manifested as fever, rash, fatigue, GI/resp Sxs reported; stop drug immediately & do not rechallenge; lactic acidosis & hepatomegaly/steatosis reported **Uses:** *HIV Infxn in zidovudine-intolerant pts* **Acts:** NRTI **Dose:** *Adults.* > 60 kg: 400 mg/d PO or 200 mg PO bid. < 60 kg: 250 mg/d PO or 125 mg PO bid; adults should take 2 tabs/administration *Peds 2 wk–8 mo.* 100 mg/m². *> 8 mo:* 120 mg/m² PO bid; on empty stomach; ↓ w/ renal impair **W/P:** [B, −] CDC rec: HIV-infected mothers not breast-feed **CI:** Component sensitivity **Disp:** Chew tabs 25, 50, 100, 150, 200 mg; powder packets 100, 167, 250, 375 mg; powder for soln 2, 4 g **SE:** Pancreatitis, peripheral neuropathy, D, HA **Notes:** Do not take w/ meals; thoroughly chew tabs, do not mix w/ fruit juice or acidic beverages; reconstitute powder w/ H₂O, watch for drug interactions

Diflunisal (Dolobid) **BOX:** May ↑ risk of CV events & GI bleeding; CI in post-op CABG **Uses:** *Mild–mod pain; OA* **Acts:** NSAID **Dose:** *Pain:* 500 mg PO bid. *OA:* 500–1500 mg PO in 2–3 ÷ doses; ↓ in renal impair, take w/ food/milk **W/P:** [C (D 3rd tri or near delivery), ?] CHF, HTN, renal/hepatic dysfunction, &

Hx PUD **CI:** Allergy to NSAIDs or ASA, active GI bleed, post-CABG **Disp:** Tabs 250, 500 mg **SE:** May ↑ bleeding time; HA, Abd cramps, heartburn, GI ulceration, rash, interstitial nephritis, fluid retention

Digoxin (Lanoxin, Lanoxicaps, Digitek) Uses: *CHF, AF & A flutter, & PAT* **Acts:** Positive inotrope; ↑ AV node refractory period **Dose: Adults.** *PO digitalization:* 0.5–0.75 mg PO, then 0.25 mg PO q6–8h to total 1–1.5 mg. *IV or IM digitalization:* 0.25–0.5 mg IM or IV, then 0.25 mg q4–6h to total 0.25–0.5 mg PO, IM, or IV (average daily dose 0.125–0.25 mg). **Peds. Preterm infants.** Digitalization: 30 mcg/kg PO or 25 mcg/kg IV; give 1/2 of initial dose, then 1/4 of dose at 8–12-h intervals for 2 doses. *Maint:* 5–7.5 mcg/kg/24 h PO or 4–6 mcg/kg/24 h IV ÷ q12h. *Term infants: Digitalization:* 25–35 mcg/kg PO or 20–30 mcg/kg IV; give 1/2 the initial dose, then 1/3 of dose at 8–12 h. *Maint:* 6–10 mcg/kg/24 h PO or 5–8 mcg/kg/24 h ÷ q12h. *1 mo–2 y:* Digitalization: 35–60 mcg/kg PO or 30–50 mcg/kg IV; give 1/2 the initial dose, then 1/3 dose at 8–12-h intervals for 2 doses. *Maint:* 10–15 mcg/kg/24 h PO or 7.5–15 mcg/kg/24 h IV ÷ q12h. *2–10 y:* Digitalization: 30–40 mcg/kg PO or 25 mcg/kg IV; give 1/2 initial dose, then 1/3 of the dose at 8–12-h intervals for 2 doses. *Maint:* 8–10 mcg/kg/24 h PO or 6–8 mcg/kg/24 h IV ÷ q12h. *7–10 y:* Same as for adults; ↓ in renal impair **W/P:** [C, +] w/ ↓ K⁺, Mg²⁺, renal failure **CI:** AV block; idiopathic hypertrophic subaortic stenosis; constrictive pericarditis **Disp:** Caps 0.05, 0.1, 0.2 mg; tabs 0.125, 0.25, 0.5 mg; elixir 0.05 mg/mL; Inj 0.1, 0.25 mg/mL **SE:** Can cause heart block; ↓ K⁺ potentiates tox; N/V, HA, fatigue, visual disturbances (yellow-green halos around lights), cardiac arrhythmias **Notes:** Multiple drug interactions; IM Inj painful, has erratic absorption & should not be used. *Levels:* Trough: Just before next dose: *Therapeutic:* 0.8–2 ng/mL; *Toxic:* > 2 ng/mL; *1/2-life:* 36 h

Digoxin Immune Fab (Digibind, DigiFab) Uses: *Life-threatening digoxin intoxication* **Acts:** Antigen-binding fragments bind & inactivate digoxin **Dose:** *Adults & Peds.* Based on serum level & pt's wgt; see charts provided w/ drug **W/P:** [C, ?] **CI:** Sheep product allergy **Disp:** Inj 38 mg/vial **SE:** Worsening of cardiac output or CHF, ↓ K⁺, facial swelling, & redness **Notes:** Each vial binds ~ 0.6 mg of digoxin; renal failure may require redosing in several days

Diltiazem (Cardizem, Cardizem CD, Cardizem LA, Cardizem SR, Cartia XT, Dilacor XR, Diltia XT, Taztia XT, Tiamate, Tiazac) Uses: *Angina, prevention of reinfarction, HTN, AF or A flutter, & PAT* **Acts:** **Dose:** *Stable angina PO:* Initial, 30 mg PO qid; ↑ to 180–360 mg/d in 3–4 ÷ doses PRN; XR 120 mg/d (540 mg/d max), *LA:* 180–360 mg/d. *HTN:* SR: 60–120 mg PO bid; ↑ to 360 mg/d max. *CD or XR:* 120–360 mg/d (max 540 mg/d) or LA 180–360 mg/d. *IV:* 0.25 mg/kg IV bolus over 2 min; may repeat in 15 min at 0.35 mg/kg; begin INF of 5–15 mg/h. *ECC 2010.* Acute rate control: 0.25 mg/kg (15–20 mg) over 2 min, followed in 15 min by 0.35 mg/kg (20–25 mg) over 2 min; maint inf 5–15 mg/h **W/P:** [C, +] ↑ effect w/ amiodarone, cimetidine, fentanyl, Li, cyclosporine, digoxin, β-blockers, theophylline **CI:** SSS, AV block, ↓ BP, AMI, pulm congestion **Disp:**

Cardizem CD: Caps 120, 180, 240, 300, 360 mg; *Cardizem LA:* Tabs 120, 180, 240, 300, 360, 420 mg; *Cardizem SR:* caps 60, 90, 120 mg; *Cardizem:* Tabs 30, 60, 90, 120 mg; *Cartia XT:* Caps 120, 180, 240, 300 mg; *Dilacor XR:* Caps 180, 240 mg; *Diltia XT:* Caps 120, 180, 240 mg; *Tiazac:* Caps 120, 180, 240, 300, 360, 420 mg; *Tiamate (XR):* Tabs 120, 180, 240 mg; Inj 5 mg/mL; *Taztia XT:* 120, 180, 240, 300, 360 mg **SE:** Gingival hyperplasia, ↓ HR, AV block, ECG abnormalities, peripheral edema, dizziness, HA **Notes:** *Cardizem CD, Dilacor XR, & Tiazac* **not** interchangeable

Dimenhydrinate (Dramamine, Others)   Uses: *Prevention & Rx of N/V, dizziness, or vertigo of motion sickness* **Acts:** Antiemetic, action unknown **Dose:** *Adults.* 50–100 mg PO q4–6h, max 400 mg/d; 50 mg IM/IV PRN. *Peds 2–6 y.* 12.5–25 mg q6–8h max 75 mg/d. *6–12 y:* 25–50 mg q6–8h max 150 mg/d **W/P:** [B, ?] **CI:** Component sensitivity **Disp:** Tabs 50 mg; chew tabs 50 mg; liq 12.5 mg/4 mL, 12.5 mg/5 mL, 15.62 mg/5 mL **SE:** Anticholinergic SE **Notes:** Take 30 min before travel for motion sickness

Dimethyl Sulfoxide [DMSO] (Rimso-50)   Uses: *Interstitial cystitis* **Acts:** Unknown **Dose:** Intravesical, 50 mL, retain for 15 min; repeat q2wk until relief **W/P:** [C, ?] **CI:** Component sensitivity **Disp:** 50% & 100% soln **SE:** Cystitis, eosinophilia, GI, & taste disturbance

Dinoprostone (Cervidil Vaginal Insert, Prepidil Vaginal Gel, Prostin E2)   BOX: Should only be used by trained personnel in an appropriate hospital setting Uses: *Induce labor; terminate PRG (12–20 wk); evacuate uterus in missed abortion or fetal death* **Acts:** Prostaglandin, changes consistency, dilatation, & effacement of the cervix; induces uterine contraction **Dose:** *Gel:* 0.5 mg; if no cervical/uterine response, repeat 0.5 mg q6h (max 24-h dose 1.5 mg). *Vaginal insert:* 1 insert (10 mg = 0.3 mg dinoprostone/h over 12 h); remove w/ onset of labor or 12 h after insertion. *Vaginal supp:* 20 mg repeated q3–5h; adjust PRN supp: 1 high in vagina, repeat at 3–5-h intervals until abortion (240 mg max) **W/P:** [X, ?] **CI:** Ruptured membranes, allergy to prostaglandins, placenta previa or AUB, when oxytocic drugs CI or if prolonged uterine contractions are inappropriate (Hx C-section, cephalopelvic disproportion, etc) **Disp:** *Endocervical gel:* 0.5 mg in 3-g syringes (w/ 10- & 20-mm shielded catheter). *Vaginal gel:* 0.5 mg/3 g *Vaginal supp:* 20 mg. *Vaginal insert, CR:* 10 mg **SE:** N/V/D, dizziness, flushing, HA, fever, abnormal uterine contractions

Diphenhydramine (Benadryl) [OTC]   Uses: *Rx & prevent allergic Rxns, motion sickness, potentiate narcotics, sedation, cough suppression, & Rx of extrapyramidal Rxns* **Acts:** Antihistamine, antiemetic **Dose:** *Adults.* 25–50 mg PO, IV, or IM bid–tid. *Peds > 2 y.* 5 mg/kg/24 h PO or IM ÷ q6h (max 300 mg/d); ↑ dosing interval w/ mod–severe renal Insuff **W/P:** [B, –] elderly, NAG, BPH, w/ MAOI **CI:** acute asthma **Disp:** Tabs & caps 25, 50 mg; chew tabs 12.5 mg; elixir 12.5 mg/ 5 mL; syrup 12.5 mg/5 mL; liq 6.25 mg/5 mL, 12.5 mg/5 mL; Inj 50 mg/mL, cream 2% **SE:** Anticholinergic (xerostomia, urinary retention, sedation)

Diphenoxylate + Atropine (Lomotil, Lonox) [C-V] Uses: *D* Acts: Constipating meperidine congener, ↓ GI motility Dose: **Adults.** Initial, 5 mg PO tid-qid until controlled, then 2.5–5 mg PO bid; 20 mg/d max **Peds > 2 y.** 0.3–0.4 mg/kg/24 h (of diphenoxylate) bid-qid, 10 mg/d max W/P: [C, +] elderly, w/ renal impair CI: Obstructive jaundice, D d/t bacterial Infxn; children < 2 y Disp: Tabs 2.5 mg diphenoxylate/0.025 mg atropine; liq 2.5 mg diphenoxylate/0.025 mg atropine/5 mL SE: Drowsiness, dizziness, xerostomia, blurred vision, urinary retention, constipation

Diphtheria & Tetanus Toxoids (Td) (Decavac—for > 7 y) Uses: primary immunization, booster (peds 7–9 y; peds 11–12 y if 5 y since last shot then q 10 y); tetanus protection after wound. Acts: Active immunization Dose: 0.5 mL IM × 1; W/P: [C, ?/–] CI: Component sensitivity Disp: Single-dose syringes 0.5 mL SE: Inj site pain, redness, swelling; fever, fatigue, HA, malaise, neuro disorders rare Notes: If IM, use only preservative-free Inj; Use DTaP (*Adacel*) rather than TT or Td all adults 19–64 y who have **not** previously received one dose of DTaP (protection adult pertussis) and Tdap for ages 10–18 y (*Boostrix*); do not confuse Td (for adults) w/ DT (for children < 7 y)

Diphtheria & Tetanus Toxoids (DT) (Generic Only for < 7 y) Uses: primary immunization ages < 7 y (DTaP is recommended vaccine) Acts: Active immunization Dose: 0.5 mL IM ×1 W/P: [C, N/A] CI: Component sensitivity Disp: Single-dose syringes 0.5 mL SE: Inj site pain, redness, swelling; fever, fatigue, myalgias/arthralgias, N/V, seizures, other neurological disorders rare Notes: If IM, use only preservative-free Inj. Do not confuse DT (for children < 7 y) w Td (for adults); DTaP is recommended for primary immunization

Diphtheria, Tetanus Toxoids, & Acellular Pertussis Adsorbed (Tdap) (Ages > 10–11 y) (Boosters: Adacel, Boostrix) Acts: active immunization, ages > 10–11 y Uses: "Catch-up" vaccination if 1 or more of the 5 childhood doses of DTP or DTaP missed; all adults 19–64 y who have **not** received one dose previously (adult pertussis protection) or if around infants < 12 mo; booster q10y; tetanus protection after fresh wound. Actions: Active immunization Dose: 0.5 mL IM ×1; W/P: [C, ?/–] w/ latex allergy CI: Component sensitivity; if previous pertussis vaccine caused progressive neurologic disorder/encephalopathy w/in 7 d of shot Disp: Single-dose vials 0.5 mL SE: Inj site pain, redness, swelling; abd pain, arthralgias/myalgias, fatigue, fever, headache, N/V/D, rash, tiredness Notes: If IM, use only preservative-free Inj; ACIP rec: Tdap for ages 10–18 y (*Boostrix*) or 11–64 y (*Adacel*); Td should be used in children 7–9 y; CDC recommends pts > age 65 who have close contact with infants get a dose of Tdap (protection against pertussis).

Diphtheria, Tetanus Toxoids, & Acellular Pertussis, Adsorbed (DTaP) (Ages < 7 y) (Daptacel, Infanrix, Tripedia) Uses: primary vaccination; 5 Inj at 2, 4, 6, 15–18 mo and 4–6 y Acts: Active immunization Dose: 0.5 mL IM ×1 as in above; W/P: [C, N/A] CI: Component sensitivity; if previous pertussis vaccine caused progressive neurologic disorder/

encephalopathy w/in 7 d of shot **Disp:** Single-dose vials 0.5 mL **SE:** Inj site nodule/pain/swelling/redness; drowsiness, fatigue, fever, fussiness, irritability, lethargy, V, prolonged crying; rare ITP and neurologic disorders **Notes:** If IM, use only preservative-free Inj; DTaP recommended for primary immunization age < 7 y, if age 7–9 y use Td, ages > 10–11 y use Tdap; if encephalopathy or other neurologic disorder w/in 7 d of previous dose **DO NOT USE** DTaP use DT or Td depending on age

Diphtheria, Tetanus Toxoids, Acellular Pertussis Adsorbed, Inactivated Poliovirus Vaccine [IPV], & Haemophilus b Conjugate Vaccine Combined (Pentacel) **Uses:** * immunization against diphtheria, tetanus, pertussis, poliomyelitis and invasive disease due to *Haemophilus influenzae* type b* **Acts:** Active immunization **Dose:** *Infants:* 0.5-mL IM at 2, 4, 6 and 15–18 months of age. **W/P:** [C, N/A] W/ fever > 40.5°C (105°F), hypotonic-hyporesponsive episode (HHE) or persistent, inconsolable crying >3h w/in 48 h after a previous pertussis-containing vaccine; Sz w/in 3 d after a previous pertussis-containing vaccine; Guillain-Barré w/in 6 wks of previous tetanus toxoid vaccine; w/ Hx Sz antipyretic may be administered w/ vaccine × 24 h w/ bleeding disorders **CI:** allergy to any components; encephalopathy w/in 7 d of previous pertussis vaccine; w/progressive neurologic disorders **Disp:** Single-dose vials 0.5 mL **SE:** fussiness/irritability and inconsolable crying; fever >38.0°C inj site Rxn

Diphtheria, Tetanus Toxoids, & Acellular Pertussis Adsorbed, Hep B (Recombinant), & Inactivated Poliovirus Vaccine [IPV], Combined (Pediarix) **Uses:** *Vaccine against diphtheria, tetanus, pertussis, HBV, polio (types 1, 2, 3) as a 3-dose primary series in infants & children < 7 y, born to HBsAg(–) mothers* **Acts:** Active immunization **Dose:** *Infants:* Three 0.5-mL doses IM, at 6–8-wk intervals, start at 2 mo; child given 1 dose of hep B vaccine, same; previously vaccinated w/ 1 or more doses inactivated poliovirus vaccine, use to complete series **W/P:** [C, N/A] w/ bleeding disorders **CI:** HBsAg(+) mother, adults, children > 7 y, immunosuppressed, component sensitivity or allergy to yeast/neomycin/polymyxin B; encephalopathy, or progressive neurologic disorders **Disp:** Single-dose vials 0.5 mL **SE:** Drowsiness, restlessness, fever, fussiness, ↓ appetite, Inj site pain/swelling/nodule/redness **Notes:** If IM, use only preservative-free Inj

Dipivefrin (Propine) **Uses:** *Open-angle glaucoma* **Acts:** α-Adrenergic agonist **Dose:** 1 gtt in eye q12h **W/P:** [B, ?] **CI:** NAG **Disp:** 0.1% soln **SE:** HA, local irritation, blurred vision, photophobia, HTN

Dipyridamole (Persantine) **Uses:** *Prevent post-op thromboembolic disorders, often in combo w/ ASA or warfarin (e.g., CABG, vascular graft); w/ warfarin after artificial heart valve; chronic angina; w/ ASA to prevent coronary artery thrombosis; dipyridamole IV used in place of exercise stress test for CAD* **Acts:** Anti-plt activity; coronary vasodilator **Dose:** *Adults.* 75–100 mg PO tid-qid; stress test 0.14 mg/kg/min (max 60 mg over 4 min). *Peds > 12 y.* 3–6 mg/kg/d ÷ tid (safety/efficacy not established) **W/P:** [B, ?/–] w/ Other drugs that affect coagulation **CI:** Component sensitivity **Disp:** Tabs 25, 50, 75 mg; Inj 5 mg/mL **SE:** HA, ↓ BP, N, Abd distress, flushing rash, dizziness, dyspnea **Notes:** IV use can worsen angina

Dipyridamole & Aspirin (Aggrenox) Uses: =↓ Reinfarction after MI; prevent occlusion after CABG; ↓ risk of stroke* **Acts:** ↓ Plt aggregation (both agents) **Dose:** 1 cap PO bid **W/P:** [C, ?] **CI:** Ulcers, bleeding diathesis **Disp:** Dipyridamole (XR) 200 mg/ASA 25 mg **SE:** ASA component: allergic Rxns, skin Rxns, ulcers/GI bleed, bronchospasm; dipyridamole component: dizziness, HA, rash **Notes:** Swallow caps whole

Disopyramide (Norpace, Norpace CR, NAPAmide, Rythmodan)
BOX: Excessive mortality or nonfatal cardiac arrest rate w/ use in asymptomatic non–life-threatening ventricular arrhythmias w/ MI 6 d to 2 y prior. Restrict use to life-threatening arrhythmias only Uses: *Suppression & prevention of VT* **Acts:** Class IA antiarrhythmic; stabilizes membranes, ↓ action potential **Dose:** *Adults.* Immediate < 50 kg 200 mg, > 50 kg 300 mg, maint 400–800 mg/d ÷ q6h or q12h for CR, max 1600 mg/d. *Peds < 1 y.* 10–30 mg/kg/24 h PO (÷ qid). *1–4 y:* 10–20 mg/kg/24 h PO (÷ qid). *4–12 y:* 10–15 mg/kg/24 h PO (÷ qid). *12–18 y:* 6–15 mg/kg/24 h PO (÷ qid); ↓ in renal/hepatic impair **W/P:** [C, +] Elderly, w/ abnormal ECG, lytes, liver/renal impair, NAG **CI:** AV block, cardiogenic shock, ↓ BP, CHF **Disp:** Caps 100, 150 mg; CR caps 100, 150 mg **SE:** Anticholinergic SEs; negative inotrope, may induce CHF **Notes:** Levels: *Trough:* just before next dose; *Therapeutic:* 2–5 mcg/mL; *Toxic* > 5 mcg/mL; half-life: 4–10 h

Dobutamine (Dobutrex) Uses: *Short-term in cardiac decompensation secondary to ↓ contractility* **Acts:** Positive inotrope **Dose:** *Adults. ECC 2010.* 2–20 mcg/kg/min; titrate to HR not > 10% of baseline. *Peds. ECC 2010. Shock w/ high SVR:* 2–20 mcg/kg/min; titrate **W/P:** [C, ?] w/ Arrhythmia, MI, severe CAD, ↑ vol **CI:** Sensitivity to sulfites, IHSS **Disp:** Inj 250 mg/20 mL, 12.5/mL **SE:** Chest pain, HTN, dyspnea **Notes:** Monitor PWP & cardiac output if possible; ✓ ECG for ↑ HR, ectopic activity; follow BP

Docetaxel (Taxotere) **BOX:** Do not administer if neutrophil count < 1500 cell/mm³; severe Rxns possible in hepatic dysfunction Uses: *Breast (anthracycline-resistant), ovarian, lung, & prostate CA* **Acts:** Antimitotic agent; promotes microtubular aggregation; semisynthetic taxoid **Dose:** 100 mg/m² over 1 h IV q3wk (per protocols); dexamethasone 8 mg bid prior & continue for 3–4 d; ↓ dose w/ ↑ bili levels **W/P:** [D, –] **CI:** Sensitivity to meds w/ polysorbate 80, component sensitivity **Disp:** Inj 20 mg/0.5 mL, 80 mg/2 mL **SE:** ↓ BM, neuropathy, N/V, alopecia, fluid retention synd; cumulative doses of 300–400 mg/m² w/o steroid prep & 600–800 mg/m² w/ steroid prep; allergy possible (rare w/ steroid prep) **Notes:** ✓ Bili/SGOT/SGPT prior to each cycle; frequent CBC during Rx

Docusate Calcium (Surfak)/Docusate Potassium (Dialose)/ Docusate Sodium (DOSS, Colace) Uses: *Constipation; adjunct w/o painful anorectal conditions (hemorrhoids)* **Acts:** Stool softener **Dose:** *Adults.* 50–500 mg PO ÷ daily–qid. *Peds Infants–3 y.* 10–40 mg/24 h ÷ daily–qid. *3–6 y:* 20–60 mg/24 h ÷ daily–qid. *6–12 y:* 40–120 mg/24 h ÷ daily–qid **W/P:** [C, ?] CI: Use w/ mineral oil; intestinal obst, acute Abd pain, N/V **Disp:** *Ca:* Caps 50, 240 mg. *K:* Caps 100, 240 mg. *Na:* Caps 50, 100 mg; syrup 50, 60 mg/15 mL; liq 150 mg/15 mL; soln 50 mg/mL **SE:** Rare Abd cramping, D **Notes:** Take w/ full glass of H$_2$O; no laxative action; do not use > 1 wk

Dofetilide (Tikosyn)   BOX: To minimize the risk of induced arrhythmia, hospitalize for minimum of 3 d to provide calculations of CrCl, cont ECG monitoring, & cardiac resuscitation **Uses:** *Maintain nl sinus rhythm in AF/A flutter after conversion* **Acts:** Class III antiarrhythmic, prolongs action potential **Dose:** Based on CrCl & QTc; CrCl > 60 mL/min 500 mcg PO q12h, ✓ QTc 2–3 h after, if QTc > 15% over baseline or > 500 msec, ↓ to 250 mcg q 12h, ✓ after each dose; if CrCl < 60 mL/min, see PI; D/C if QTc > 500 msec after dosing adjustments **W/P:** [C, −] w/ AV block, renal Dz, electrolyte imbalance **CI:** Baseline QTc > 440 msec, CrCl < 20 mL/min; w/ verapamil, cimetidine, trimethoprim, ketoconazole, quinolones, ACE inhib/HCTZ combo **Disp:** Caps 125, 250, 500 mcg **SE:** Ventricular arrhythmias, QT ↑, torsades de pointes, rash, HA, CP, dizziness **Notes:** Avoid w/ other drugs that ↑ QT interval; hold class I/III antiarrhythmics for 3 1/2-lives prior to dosing; amiodarone level should be < 0.3 mg/L before use, do not initiate if HR < 60 BPM; restricted to participating prescribers; correct K$^+$ and Mg^{2+} before use

Dolasetron (Anzemet)   **Uses:** *Prevent chemotherapy and post-op–associated N/V* **Acts:** 5-HT$_3$ receptor antagonist **Dose:** *Adults. PO:* 100 mg PO as a single dose 1 h prior to chemotherapy. *Post-op:* 12.5 mg IV, or 100 mg PO 2 h pre-op *Peds 2–16 y.* 1.8 mg/kg PO (max 100 mg) as single dose. *Post-op:* 0.35 mg/kg IV or 1.2 mg/kg PO **W/P:** [B, ?] w/ Cardiac conduction problems **CI:** IV use w/ chemo Component sensitivity **Disp:** Tabs 50, 100 mg; Inj 20 mg/mL **SE:** ↑ QT interval, D, HTN, HA, Abd pain, urinary retention, transient ↑ LFTs **Notes:** IV form no longer approved for chemo-induced N&V due to heart rhythm abnormalities.

Donepezil (Aricept)   **Uses:** *Severe Alzheimer dementia* ADHD; behavioral synds in dementia; dementia w/ Parkinson Dz; Lewy-body dementia **Acts:** ACH inhib **Dose:** *Adults.* 5 mg qhs, ↑ to 10 mg PO qhs after 4–6 wk *Peds. ADHD:* 5 mg/d **W/P:** [C, ?] risk for ↓ HR w/ preexisting conduction abnormalities, may exaggerate succinylcholine-type muscle relaxation w/ anesthesia, ↑ gastric acid secretion **CI:** Hypersens **Disp:** Tabs 5, 10, 23 mg; ODT tab 5, 10 mg **SE:** N/V/D, insomnia, Infxn, muscle cramp, fatigue, anorexia **Notes:** N/V/D dose-related & resolves in 1–3 wk

Dopamine (Intropin)   BOX: Tissue vesicant, give phentolamine w/ extrav **Uses:** *Short-term use in cardiac decompensation secondary to ↓ contractility; ↑ organ perfusion (at low dose)* **Acts:** Positive inotropic agent w/ dose response: 1–10 mcg/kg/min β effects (↑ CO); 10–20 mcg/kg/min β-effects (peripheral vasoconstriction, pressor); > 20 mcg/kg/min peripheral & renal vaso-constriction **Dose:** *Adults.* 5 mcg/kg/min by cont Inf, ↑ by 5 mcg/kg/min to 50 mcg/kg/min max to effect; *ECC 2010.* 2–20 mcg/kg/min. *Peds. ECC 2010. Shock w/ adequate intravascular volume and stable rhythm:* 2–20 mcg/kg/min; titrate, if > 20 mcg/kg/min needed, consider alternative adrenergic **W/P:** [C, ?] ↓ Dose w/ MAOI UI **Contra:** Pheochromocytoma, VF, sulfite sensitivity **Disp:** Inj 40, 80, 160 mg/mL, premixed 0.8, 1.6, 3.2 mg/mL **SE:** Tachycardia, vasoconstriction, ↓ BP, HA, N/V, dyspnea **Notes:** > 10 mcg/kg/min ↓ renal perfusion; monitor urinary output & ECG if possible for ↑ HR, BP, ectopy; monitor PCWP & cardiac output if possible, phen-tolamine used for extrav 10 to 15 mL NS w/ 5 to 10 mg of phentolamine

Doripenem (Doribax) Uses: *Complicated intra-Abd infection and UTI including pyelo* **Acts:** Carbapenem, ↓ cell wall synth, a β-lactam *Spectrum:* Excellent gram(+) (except MRSA and *Enterococcus* sp.), excellent gram(−) cover-age including β-lactamase producers, good anaerobic **Dose:** 500 mg IV q8h, ↓ w/ renal impair **W/P:** [B, ?] **CI:** carbapenem β-lactams hypersens **Disp:** 500 mg single-use vial **SE:** HA, N/D, rash, phlebitis **Notes:** May ↓ valproic acid levels; over-use may ↑ bacterial resistance; monitor for *C. difficile*-associated D

Dornase Alfa (Pulmozyme, DNase) Uses: *↓ Frequency of resp infxns in CF* **Acts:** Enzyme cleaves extracellular DNA, ↓ mucous viscosity **Dose:** *Adults.* Inh 2.5 mg/bid dosing w/ FVC > 85% w/ recommended nebulizer *Peds* > 5 y. Inh 2.5 mg/daily-bid if forced vital capacity > 85% **W/P:** [B, ?] **CI:** Chinese ham-ster product allergy **Disp:** Soln for Inh 1 mg/mL **SE:** Pharyngitis, voice alteration, CP, rash

Dorzolamide (Trusopt) Uses: *Open-angle glaucoma, ocular hypertension* **Acts:** Carbonic anhydrase inhib **Dose:** 1 gtt in eye(s) tid **W/P:** [C, ?] w/ NAG, CrCl < 30 mL/min **CI:** Component sensitivity **Disp:** 2% soln **SE:** irritation, bitter taste, punctate keratitis, ocular allergic Rxn

Dorzolamide & Timolol (Cosopt) Uses: *Open-angle glaucoma, ocular hypertension* **Acts:** Carbonic anhydrase inhib w/ β-adrenergic blocker **Dose:** 1 gtt in eye(s) bid **W/P:** [C, ?] CrCl < 30 mL/min **CI:** Component sensitivity, asthma, severe COPD, sinus bradycardia, AV block **Disp:** Soln dorzolamide 2% & timolol 0.5% **SE:** Irritation, bitter taste, superficial keratitis, ocular allergic Rxn

Doxazosin (Cardura, Cardura XL) Uses: *HTN & symptomatic BPH* **Acts:** α₁-Adrenergic blocker; relaxes bladder neck smooth muscle **Dose:** *HTN:* Initial 1 mg/d PO; may be ↑ to 16 mg/d PO. *BPH:* Initial 1 mg/d PO, may ↑ to 8 mg/d; XL 2–8 mg q A.M. **W/P:** [B, ?] w/ Liver impair **CI:** Component sensitivity; use w/ PDE5 inhib (e.g., sildenafil) can cause ↓ BP **Disp:** Tabs 1, 2, 4, 8 mg; XL 4, 8 mg **SE:** Dizziness, HA, drowsiness, fatigue, malaise, sexual dysfunction, doses > 4 mg ↑ postural ↓ BP risk; intraoperative floppy iris synd **Notes:** 1st dose hs; syn-cope may occur w/in 90 min of initial dose

Doxepin (Adapin) **BOX:** Closely monitor for worsening depression or emergence of suicidality Uses: *Depression, anxiety, chronic pain* **Acts:** TCA; ↑ synaptic

CNS serotonin or norepinephrine **Dose:** 25–150 mg/d PO, usually hs but can ÷ doses; up to 300 mg/d for depression; ↓ in hepatic impair **W/P:** [C, ?/–] w/ EtOH abuse, elderly, w/ MAOI **CI:** NAG, urinary retention, MAOI use w/in 14 d, in recovery phase of MI **Disp:** Caps 10, 25, 50, 75, 100, 150 mg; PO conc 10 mg/mL **SE:** Anticholinergic SEs, ↓ BP, tachycardia, drowsiness, photosens

Doxepin (Silenor) **Uses:** *Insomnia* **Acts:** TCA **Dose:** Take w/in 30 min HS 6 mg qd; 3 mg in elderly; 6 mg/d max; not w/in 3 h of a meal **W/P:** [C, ?/–] w/ EtOH abuse/elderly/sleep apnea/CNS depressants; may cause abnormal thinking and hallucinations; may worsen depression **CI:** NAG, urinary retention, MAOI w/ in 14 d **Disp:** Tabs 3, 6 mg **SE:** somnolence/sedation, N, URI

Doxepin, Topical (Zonalon, Prudoxin) **Uses:** *Short-term Rx pruritus (atopic dermatitis or lichen simplex chronicus)* **Acts:** Antipruritic; H_1- & H_2-receptor antagonism **Dose:** Apply thin coating qid, 8 d max **W/P:** [C, ?/–] **CI:** Component sensitivity **Disp:** 5% cream **SE:** ↓ BP, tachycardia, drowsiness, photosens **Notes:** Limit application area to avoid systemic tox

Doxorubicin (Adriamycin, Rubex) **Uses:** *Acute leukemias; Hodgkin Dz & NHLs; soft tissue, osteo- & Ewing sarcoma; Wilms tumor; neuroblastoma; bladder, breast, ovarian, gastric, thyroid, & lung CAs* **Acts:** Intercalates DNA; ↓ DNA topoisomerase I & II **Dose:** 60–75 mg/m² q3wk; ↓ w/ hepatic impair; IV use only ↓ cardiotox w/ weekly (20 mg/m²/wk) or cont Inf (60–90 mg/m² over 96 h); (per protocols) **W/P:** [D, ?] **CI:** Severe CHF, cardiomyopathy, preexisting ↓ BM, previous Rx w/ total cumulative doses of doxorubicin, idarubicin, daunorubicin **Disp:** Inj 10, 20, 50, 75, 150, 200 mg **SE:** ↓ BM, venous streaking & phlebitis, N/V/D, mucositis, radiation recall phenomenon, cardiomyopathy rare (dose-related) **Notes:** Limit of 550 mg/m² cumulative dose (400 mg/m² w/ prior mediastinal irradiation); dexrazoxane may limit cardiac tox; tissue damage w/ extrav; red/orange urine; tissue vesicant w/ extrav, Rx w/ dexrazoxane

Doxycycline (Adoxa, Periostat, Oracea, Vibramycin, Vibra-Tabs) **Uses:** *Broad-spectrum antibiotic* acne vulgaris, uncomplicated GC, chlamydia, PID, Lyme Dz, skin Infxns, anthrax, malaria prophylaxis **Acts:** Tetracycline; bacteriostatic; ↓ protein synth. *Spectrum:* Limited gram(+) and (–), *Rickettsia* sp, *Chlamydia, M. pneumoniae, B. anthracis* **Dose:** *Adults.* 100 mg PO q12h on 1st d, then 100 mg PO daily–bid or 100 mg IV q12h; acne q day, chlamydia × 7 d, Lyme × 21 d, PID × 14 d *Peds > 8 y.* 5 mg/kg/24 h PO, 200 mg/d max + daily-bid **W/P:** [D, +] hepatic impair **CI:** Children < 8 y, severe hepatic dysfunction **Disp:** Tabs 20, 50, 75, 100, 150 mg; caps 50, 100 mg; Oracea 40 mg caps (30 mg timed release, 10 mg DR); syrup 50 mg/5 mL; susp 25 mg/5 mL; Inj 100, 200 mg/vial **SE:** D, GI disturbance, photosens **Notes:** ↓ effect w/ antacids; tetracycline of choice w/in renal impair; for inhalational anthrax use w/ 1–2 additional antibiotics, not for CNS anthrax

Dronabinol (Marinol) [C-II] **Uses:** *N/V associated w/ CA chemotherapy; appetite stimulation* **Acts:** Antiemetic; ↓ V center in the medulla **Dose:** *Adults & Peds.* Antiemetic: 5–15 mg/m²/dose q4–6h PRN. *Adults. Appetite stimulant:*

2.5 mg PO before lunch & dinner; max 20 mg/d **W/P:** [C, ?] elderly, Hx psychological disorder, Sz disorder, substance abuse **CI:** Hx schizophrenia, sesame oil hypersens **Disp:** Caps 2.5, 5, 10 mg **SE:** Drowsiness, dizziness, anxiety, mood change, hallucinations, depersonalization, orthostatic ↓ BP, tachycardia **Notes:** Principal psychoactive substance present in marijuana

Droperidol (Inapsine) BOX: Cases of QT interval prolongation and torsades de pointes (some fatal) reported **Uses:** *N/V; anesthetic premedication* **Acts:** Tranquilizer, sedation, antiemetic **Dose:** *Adults. N:* initial max 2.5 mg IV/IM, may repeat 1.25 mg based on response; *Premed:* 2.5–10 mg IV, 30–60 min pre-op. *Peds. Premed:* 0.1–0.15 mg/kg/dose **W/P:** [C, ?] w/ Hepatic/renal impair **CI:** Component sensitivity **Disp:** Inj 2.5 mg/mL **SE:** Drowsiness, ↓ BP, occasional tachycardia & extrapyramidal Rxns, ↑ QT interval, arrhythmias **Notes:** Give IV push slowly over 2–5 min

Dronedarone (Multaq) BOX: CI w/ NYHA Class IV HF or NYHA Class II-III HF w/ decompensation **Uses:** *A Fib/A Flutter* **Acts:** Antiarrhythmic **Dose:** 400 mg PO bid w/ A.M. and P.M. meal **W/P:** [X, −] w/ other drugs (see PI); increased risk of death and serious CV events **CI:** See Box; 2nd- /3rd-degree AV block or SSS (unless w/ pacemaker), HR < 50 BPM, w/ strong CYP3A inhib, w/ drugs/ herbals ↑ QT interval, QTc interval ≥500 ms, severe hepatic impair, PRG **Disp:** Tabs 400 mg **SE:** N/V/D, Abd pain, asthenia, heart failure, ↑ K+, ↑ Mg2+, ↑ QTc, ↓ HR,↑ SCr, rash **Notes:** Avoid grapefruit juice

Drotrecogin Alfa (Xigris) **Uses:** *↑↓ Mortality in adults w/ severe sepsis (w/ acute organ dysfunction) at high risk of death (e.g., determined by APACHE II score [www.ncemi.org])* **Acts:** Recombinant human-activated protein C; antithrombotic and anti-inflammatory, unclear mechanism **Dose:** 24 mcg/kg/h, total of 96 h **W/P:** [C, ?] w/ Anticoagulation, INR > 3, plt 30,000 cells/mm³, GI bleed w/ in 6 wk **CI:** Active bleeding, recent CNS surgery, head trauma/CNS lesion w/ herniation risk, trauma w/ bleeding risk, epidural catheter, mifepristone **Disp:** 5-, 20-mg vials **SE:** Bleeding **Notes:** Single-organ dysfunction & recent surgery may not be at high risk of death irrespective of APACHE II score & therefore not indicated. *Percutaneous procedures:* Stop Inf 2 h before & resume 1 h after; major surgery: stop Inf 2 h before & resume 12 h after in absence of bleeding

Duloxetine (Cymbalta) BOX: Antidepressants may ↑ risk of suicidality; consider risks/benefits of use. Closely monitor for clinical worsening, suicidality, or behavior changes **Uses:** *Depression, DM peripheral neuropathic pain, generalized anxiety disorder (GAD), fibromyalgia, chronic OA & back pain* **Acts:** Selective serotonin & norepinephrine reuptake inhib (SSNRI) **Dose:** *Depression:* 40–60 mg/d PO ÷ bid. *DM neuropathy:* 60 mg/d PO; *GAD:* 60 mg, max 120 mg/d; *Fibromyalgia, OA/back pain:* 30–60 mg/d, 60 mg/d max **W/P:** [C, ?/−]; use in 3rd tri; avoid if CrCl < 30 mL/min, NAG, w/ fluvoxamine, inhib of CYP2D6 (Table 10, p 301), TCAs, phenothiazines, type class 1C antiarrhythmics (Table 9, p 300) **CI:** MAOI use w/in 14 d, w/ thioridazine, NAG, hepatic Insuff **Disp:** Caps delayed-release 20, 30, 60 mg **SE:** N, dry mouth, somnolence, fatigue, constipation, ↓ appetite, hyperhydrosis **Notes:** Swallow whole; monitor BP; avoid abrupt D/C

Dutasteride (Avodart) **Uses:** *Symptomatic BPH to improve Sxs, ↓ risk of retention and BPH surgery alone or in combo w/ tamsulosin* **Acts:** 5α-Reductase inhib; ↓ intracellular dihydrotestosterone (DHT) **Dose:** *Monotherapy:* 0.5 mg PO/d. *Combo:* 0.5 mg PO q day w/ tamsulosin 0.4 mg q day **W/P:** [X, −] Hepatic impair; pregnant women should not handle pills; R/O cancer before starting **CI:** Women, peds **Disp:** Caps 0.5 mg **SE:** ↑ testosterone, ↑ TSH, impotence, ↓ libido, gynecomastia, ejaculatory disturbance, may ↑ risk of high-grade prostate Ca **Notes:** No blood donation until 6 mo after D/C; ↓ PSA, ✓ new baseline PSA at 6 mo (corrected PSA × 2); any PSA rise on dutasteride suspicious for cancer; now available in fixed dose combination w/tamsulosin (see *Jalyn*)

Dutasteride and Tamsulosin (Jalyn) **Uses:** *Symptomatic BPH to improve Sxs* **Acts:** 5α-Reductase inhib (↓ intracellular DHT) w/ alpha blocker **Dose:** 1 capsule daily after same meal **W/P:** [X, −] w/ CYP3A4 and CYP2D6 inhib may ↑ SEs; pregnant women should not handle pills; R/O cancer before starting; IFIS (tamsulosin) discuss w/ophthalmologist before cataract surgery; rare priapism; w/ warfarin; may ↑ risk of high grade prostate cancer **CI:** Women, peds, component sens **Disp:** Caps 0.5 mg dutasteride w/0.4 mg tamsulosin **SE:** impotence, decreased libido, ejaculation disorders, and breast disorders **Notes:** No blood donation until 6 mo after D/C; ↓ PSA, ✓ new baseline PSA at 6 mo (corrected PSA × 2); any PSA rise on dutasteride suspicious for cancer (see also dutasteride and tamsulosin)

Ecallantide (Kalbitor) **BOX:** Anaphylaxis reported, administer in a setting able to manage anaphylaxis and HAE, monitor closely **Uses:** *Acute attacks of hereditary angioedema (HAE)* **Acts:** Plasma kallikrein inhibitor **Dose:** *Adult & > 16 y.* 30 mg SC in three 10-mg injections; if attack persists may repeat 30-mg dose w/in 24 h **W/P:** [C, ?/−] Hypersens Rxns **CI:** Hypersens to ecallantide **Disp:** Inj 10 mg/mL **SE:** HA, N/V/D, pyrexia, Inj site Rxn, nasopharyngitis, fatigue, and pain

Echothiophate Iodine (Phospholine Ophthalmic) **Uses:** *Glaucoma* **Acts:** Cholinesterase inhib **Dose:** 1 gtt eye(s) bid w/ 1 dose hs **W/P:** [C, ?] **CI:** Active uveal inflammation, inflammatory Dz of iris/ciliary body, glaucoma iridocyclitis **Disp:** Powder, reconstitute 1.5 mg/0.03%; 3 mg/0.06%; 6.25 mg/0.125%; 12.5 mg/0.25% **SE:** Local irritation, myopia, blurred vision, ↓ BP, ↓ HR

Econazole (Spectazole) **Uses:** *Tinea, cutaneous Candida, & tinea versicolor Infxns* **Acts:** Topical antifungal **Dose:** Apply to areas bid (daily for tinea versicolor) for 2–4 wk **W/P:** [C, ?] **CI:** Component sensitivity **Disp:** Topical cream 1% **SE:** Local irritation, pruritus, erythema **Notes:** Early Sx/clinical improvement; complete course to avoid recurrence

Eculizumab (Soliris) **BOX:** ↑ Risk of meningococcal infections (give meningococcal vaccine 2 wk prior to 1st dose and revaccinate per guidelines) **Uses:** *Rx paroxysmal nocturnal hemoglobinuria* **Acts:** Complement inhib **Dose:** 600 mg IV q 7 d × 4 wk, then 900 mg IV 5th dose 7 d later, then 900 mg IV q14d **W/P:** [C, ?]

CI: Active *N. meningitidis* Infxn; if not vaccinated against *N. meningitidis* **Disp:** 300-mg vial **SE:** Meningococcal Infxn, HA, nasopharyngitis, N, back pain, infxns, fatigue, severe hemolysis on D/C **Notes:** IV over 35 min (2-h max Inf time); monitor for 1 h for S/Sx of Inf Rxn

Edrophonium (Tensilon, Reversol) **Uses:** *Diagnosis of MyG; acute MyG crisis; curare antagonist, reverse of nondepolarizing neuromuscular blockers* **Acts:** Anticholinesterase **Dose:** *Adults. Test for MyG:* 2 mg IV in 1 min; if tolerated, give 8 mg IV; (+) test is brief ↑ in strength. *Peds. Test for MyG:* Total dose 0.2 mg/kg; 0.04 mg/kg test dose; if no Rxn, give remainder in 1-mg increments to 10 mg max; ↓ in renal impair **W/P:** [C, ?] **CI:** GI or GU obst; allergy to sulfite **Disp:** Inj 10 mg/mL **SE:** N/V/D, excessive salivation, stomach cramps, ↑ aminotransferases **Notes:** Can cause severe cholinergic effects; keep atropine available

Efalizumab (Raptiva) Withdrawn from US market in 2009 due to progressive multifocal leukoencephalopathy (PML)

Efavirenz (Sustiva) **Uses:** *HIV Infxns* **Acts:** Antiretroviral; nonnucleoside RT inhib **Dose:** *Adults.* 600 mg/d PO q hs. *Peds ≥3 y 10–< 15 kg.* 200 mg PO q day; *15–< 20 kg:* 250 mg PO q day; *20–< 25 kg:* 300 mg PO q day; *25–< 32.5 kg:* 350 mg PO q day; *32.5–< 40 kg:* 400 mg PO q day ≥*40 kg:* 600 mg PO q day; on empty stomach **W/P:** [D, ?] CDC rec: HIV-infected mothers not breast-feed **CI:** w/ Astemizole, bepridil, cisapride, midazolam, pimozide, triazolam, ergot derivatives, voriconazole **Disp:** Caps 50, 100, 200; 600 mg tab **SE:** Somnolence, vivid dreams, depression, CNS Sxs, dizziness, rash, N/V/D **Notes:** ✓ LFTs (especially w/underlying liver Dz), cholesterol; not for monotherapy

Efavirenz, Emtricitabine, Tenofovir (Atripla) **BOX:** Lactic acidosis and severe hepatomegaly w/ steatosis, including fatal cases, reported w/ nucleoside analogs alone or combo w/ other antiretrovirals **Uses:** *HIV Infxns* **Acts:** Triple fixed-dose combo nonnucleoside RT inhib/nucleoside analog **Dose:** *Adults.* 1 tab q day on empty stomach; HS dose may ↓ CNS SE **W/P:** [D, ?] CDC rec: HIV-infected mothers not breast-feed, w/ obesity **CI:** < 18 y, w/ astemizole, midazolam, triazolam, or ergot derivatives (CYP3A4 competition by efavirenz could cause serious/life-threatening SE) **Disp:** Tab (efavirenz 600 mg/emtricitabine 200 mg/tenofovir 300 mg) **SE:** Somnolence, vivid dreams, HA, dizziness, rash, N/V/D, ↓ BMD **Notes:** Monitor LFTs, cholesterol; see individual agents for additional info, not for HIV/hep B coinfection

Eletriptan (Relpax) **Uses:** *Acute Rx of migraine* **Acts:** Selective serotonin receptor (5-HT$_{1B/1D}$) agonist **Dose:** 20–40 mg PO, may repeat in 2 h; 80 mg/24 h max **W/P:** [C, +] **CI:** Hx ischemic heart Dz, coronary artery spasm, stroke or TIA, peripheral vascular Dz, IBD, uncontrolled HTN, hemiplegic or basilar migraine, severe hepatic impair, w/in 24 h of another 5-HT₁ agonist or ergot, w/in 72 h of CYP3A4 inhib **Disp:** Tabs 20, 40 mg **SE:** Dizziness, somnolence, N, asthenia, xerostomia, paresthesias; pain, pressure, or tightness in chest, jaw, or neck; serious cardiac events

Eltrombopag (Promacta) **BOX:** May cause hepatotoxicity. ✓ baseline ALT/AST/bili, q 2 wks w/dosage adjustment, then monthly. D/C if ALT is > 3× ULN w/ ↑ bili, or Sx of liver injury **Uses:** *Tx ↑ plt in idiopathic thrombocytopenia refractory to steroids, immune globulins, splenectomy* **Acts:** Thrombopoietin receptor agonist **Dose:** 50 mg PO daily, adjust to keep plt ≥50,000 cells/mm³; 75 mg/d max; start 25 mg/d if East-Asian or w/ hepatic impair; on an empty stomach; not w/in 4 hrs of product w/ polyvalent cations **W/P:** [C, ?/–] ↑ risk for BM reticulin fiber deposition, heme malignancies, rebound ↓ plt on D/C, thromboembolism **CI:** None **Disp:** Tabs 25, 50 mg **SE:** rash, bruising, menorrhagia, N/V, dyspepsia, ↓ plt, ↑ ALT/AST, limb pain, myalgia, paresthesia, cataract, conjunctival hemorrhage **Notes:** D/C if no ↑ plt count after 4 wks; restricted distribution *Promacta Cares (1-877-9-PROMACTA)*

Emedastine (Emadine) **Uses:** *Allergic conjunctivitis* **Acts:** Antihistamine; selective H₁-antagonist **Dose:** 1 gtt in eye(s) up to qid **W/P:** [B, ?] **CI:** Allergy to ingredients (preservatives benzalkonium, tromethamine) **Disp:** 0.05% soln **SE:** HA, blurred vision, burning/stinging, corneal infiltrates/staining, dry eyes, foreign body sensation, hyperemia, keratitis, tearing, pruritus, rhinitis, sinusitis, asthenia, bad taste, dermatitis, discomfort **Notes:** Do not use contact lenses if eyes are red

Emtricitabine (Emtriva) **BOX:** Lactic acidosis, & severe hepatomegaly w/ steatosis reported; not for HBV Infxn **Uses:** HIV-1 Infxn **Acts:** NRTI **Dose:** 200 mg caps or 240 mL soln PO daily; ↓ w/ renal impair **W/P:** [B, –] risk of liver Dz **CI:** Component sensitivity **Disp:** Soln 10 mg/mL, caps 200 mg **SE:** HA, N/D, rash, rare hyperpigmentation of feet & hands, posttreatment exacerbation of hep **Notes:** 1st one-daily NRTI; caps/soln not equivalent; not ok as monotherapy; screen for hep B, do not use w/ HIV and HBV coinfection

Enalapril (Vasotec) **BOX:** ACE inhib used during PRG can cause fetal injury & death **Uses:** *HTN, CHF, LVD*, DN* **Acts:** ACE inhib **Dose:** *Adults.* 2.5–40 mg/d PO; 1.25 mg IV q6h. *Peds.* 0.05–0.08 mg/kg/d PO q12–24h; ↓ w/ renal impair **W/P:** [C (1st tri); D 2nd & 3rd tri), +] D/C immediately w/PRG, w/ NSAIDs, K⁺ supplements **CI:** Bilateral RAS, angioedema **Disp:** Tabs 2.5, 5, 10, 20 mg; IV 1.25 mg/mL (1, 2 mL) **SE:** ↓ BP w/ initial dose (especially w/ diuretics), ↑ K⁺, ↑ Cr nonproductive cough, angioedema **Notes:** Monitor Cr; D/C diuretic for 2–3 d prior to start

Enfuvirtide (Fuzeon) **BOX:** Rarely causes allergy; never rechallenge **Uses:** *w/ Antiretroviral agents for HIV-1 in Tx-experienced pts w/ viral replication despite ongoing Rx** **Acts:** Viral fusion inhib **Dose:** *Adults.* 90 mg (1 mL) SQ bid in upper arm, anterior thigh, or abd; rotate site *Peds.* See PI **W/P:** [B, –] **CI:** Previous allergy to drug **Disp:** 90 mg/mL recons; pt kit w/ supplies × 1 mo **SE:** Inj site Rxns; pneumonia, D, N, fatigue, insomnia, peripheral neuropathy **Notes:** Available via restricted distribution system; use immediately on recons or refrigerate (24 h max)

Enoxaparin (Lovenox) **BOX:** Recent or anticipated epidural/spinal anesthesia, ↑ risk of spinal/epidural hematoma w/ subsequent paralysis **Uses:** *Prevention &*

Rx of DVT; Rx PE; unstable angina & non–Q-wave MI* **Acts:** LMW heparin; inhibit thrombin by complexing w/ antithrombin III **Dose: Adults. Prevention:** 30 mg SQ bid or 40 mg SQ q24h. *DVT/PE Rx:* 1 mg/kg SQ q12h or 1.5 mg/kg SQ q24h. *Angina:* 1 mg/kg SQ q12h; *Ancillary to AMI fibrinolysis:* 30 mg IV bolus, then 1 mg/kg SQ bid *(ECC 2005);* CrCl < 30 mL/min ↓ to 1 mg/kg SQ q day *Peds. Prevention:* 0.5 mg/kg SQ q12h. *DVT/PE Rx:* 1 mg/kg SQ q12h; ↓ dose w/ CrCl < 30 mL/min **W/P:** [B, ?] Not for prophylaxis in prosthetic heart valves **CI:** Active bleeding, HIT Ab **Disp:** Inj 10 mg/0.1 mL (30-, 40-, 60-, 80-, 100-, 120-, 150-mg syringes); 300-mg/mL multidose vial **SE:** Bleeding, hemorrhage, bruising, thrombocytopenia, fever, pain/hematoma at site, ↑ AST/ALT **Notes:** No effect on bleeding time, plt Fxn, PT, or aPTT; monitor plt for HIT, clinical bleeding; may monitor antifactor Xa; not for IM

Entacapone (Comtan) **Uses:** *Parkinson Dz* **Acts:** Selective & reversible carboxymethyl transferase inhib **Dose:** 200 mg w/ each levodopa/carbidopa dose; max 1600 mg/d; ↓ levodopa/carbidopa dose 25% w/ levodopa dose > 800 mg **W/P:** [C, ?] Hepatic impair **CI:** Use w/ MAOI **Disp:** Tabs 200 mg **SE:** Dyskinesia, hyperkinesia, N, D, dizziness, hallucinations, orthostatic ↓ BP, brown-orange urine **Notes:** ✓ LFTs; do not D/C abruptly

Ephedrine **Uses:** *Acute bronchospasm, bronchial asthma, nasal congestion*, ↓ BP, narcolepsy, enuresis, & MyG **Acts:** Sympathomimetic; stimulates α- & β-receptors; bronchodilator **Dose: Adults. Congestion:** 25–50 mg PO q6h PRN; ↓ *BP:* 25–50 mg IV q5–10min, 150 mg/d max. *Peds.* 0.2–0.3 mg/kg/dose IV q4–6h PRN **W/P:** [C, ?/–] **CI:** Arrhythmias; NAG **Disp:** Nasal soln 0.48%, 0.5%; caps 25 mg; Inj 50 mg/mL; nasal spray 0.25% **SE:** CNS stimulation (nervousness, anxiety, trembling), tachycardia, arrhythmia, HTN, xerostomia, dysuria **Notes:** Protect from light; monitor BP, HR, urinary output; can cause false (+) amphetamine EMIT; take last dose 4–6 h before hs; abuse potential, OTC sales mostly banned/ restricted

Epinephrine (Adrenalin, Sus-Phrine, EpiPen, EpiPen Jr., Others) **Uses:** *Cardiac arrest, anaphylaxis Rxn, bronchospasm, open-angle glaucoma* **Acts:** β-Adrenergic agonist, some α-effects **Dose: Adults. ECC 2010.** 1-mg (10 mL of 1:1000 soln) IV/IO push, repeat q3–5min (0.2 mg/kg max) if 1-mg dose fails. Inf: 0.1–0.5 mcg/kg/min, titrate. ET 2–2.5 mg in 20 mL NS. *Profound bradycardia/ hypotension:* 2–10 mcg/min (1 mg in 250 mL D5W). *Allergic Rxn:* 0.3–0.5 mg (0.3–0.5 mL of 1:1000 soln) SQ. *Anaphylaxis:* 0.3–0.5 (3–5 mL of 1:1000 soln) IV. *Asthma:* 0.1–0.5 mL of 1:1000 dilution, repeat q20min to 4 h, or 1 Inh (metered-dose) repeat in 1–2 min, or susp 0.1–0.3 mL SQ for extended effect. *Peds. ECC 2010.* Pulseless arrest: 0.01 mg/kg (0.1 mL/kg 1:1000) IV/IO q3–5min; max dose 1 mg; OK via ET tube 0.1 mg/kg (0.1 mL/kg 1:1000) until IV/IO access. *Symptomatic bradycardia:* 0.01 mg/kg (0.1 mL/kg 1:1000) cont inf: typical 0.1–1 mcg/kg/min, titrate. *Anaphylaxis/status asthmaticus:* 0.01 mg/kg (0.01 ml/kg 1:1000) IM, repeat PRN; max single dose 0.3 mg **W/P:** [C, ?] ↓ bronchodilation w/ β-blockers **CI:** Cardiac arrhythmias, NAG **Disp:** Inj 1:1000, 1:2000, 1:10,000, 1:100,000; susp for Inj

1:200; aerosol 220 mcg/spray; 1% Inh soln; EpiPen Autoinjector 1 dose = 0.30 mg; EpiPen Jr. 1 dose = 0.15 mg **SE:** CV (tachycardia, HTN, vasoconstriction), CNS stimulation (nervousness, anxiety, trembling), ↓ renal blood flow **Notes:** Can give via ET tube if no central line (use 2–2.5 × IV dose); EpiPen for pt self-use (www.EpiPen.com)

Epinastine (Elestat)   **Uses:** Itching w/ allergic conjunctivitis **Acts:** Antihistamine **Dose:** 1 gtt bid **W/P:** [C, ?/–] **Disp:** Soln 0.05% **SE:** Burning, folliculosis, hyperemia, pruritus, URI, HA, rhinitis, sinusitis, cough, pharyngitis **Notes:** Remove contacts before, reinsert in 10 min

Epirubicin (Ellence)   **BOX:** Do not give IM or SQ. Extrav causes tissue necrosis; potential cardiotox; severe myelosuppression; ↓ dose w/ hepatic impair **Uses:** *Adjuvant Rx for (+) axillary nodes after resection of primary breast CA* **Actions:** Anthracycline cytotoxic agent **Dose:** Per protocols; ↓ dose w/ hepatic impair **W/P:** [D, –] **CI:** Baseline neutrophil count < 1500 cells/mm³, severe cardiac Insuff, recent MI, severe arrhythmias, severe hepatic dysfunction, previous anthracyclines Rx to max cumulative dose **Disp:** Inj 50 mg/25 mL, 200 mg/100 mL **SE:** Mucositis, N/V/D, alopecia, ↓ BM, cardiotox, secondary AML, tissue necrosis w/ extrav (see Adriamycin for Rx), lethargy **Notes:** ✓ CBC, bili, AST, Cr, cardiac Fxn before/during each cycle

Eplerenone (Inspra)   **Uses:** *HTN, ↑ survival after MI with LVEF < 40% and CHF* **Acts:** Selective aldosterone antagonist **Dose:** *Adults.* 50 mg PO daily-bid, doses > 100 mg/d no benefit w/ ↑ K⁺; ↓ to 25 mg PO daily if giving w/ CYP3A4 inhib **W/P:** [B, +/–] w/ CYP3A4 inhib (Table 10, p 301); monitor K⁺ w/ ACE inhib, ARBs, NSAIDs, K⁺-sparing diuretics; grapefruit juice, St. John's wort **CI:** K⁺ > 5.5 mEq/L; non–insulin-dependent diabetes mellitus (NIDDM) w/ microalbuminuria; SCr > 2 mg/dL (males), > 1.8 mg/dL (females); CrCl < 30 mL/min; w/ K⁺ supls/K⁺-sparing diuretics, ketoconazole **Disp:** Tabs 25, 50 mg **SE:** ↑ cholesterol/triglycerides, ↑ K⁺, HA, dizziness, gynecomastia, D, orthostatic ↓ BP **Notes:** May take 4 wk for full effect

Epoetin Alfa [Erythropoietin, EPO] (Epogen, Procrit)   **BOX:** ↑ Mortality, serious CV/thromboembolic events, and tumor progression. Renal failure pts experienced ↑ greater risks (death/CV events) on erythropoiesis-stimulating agents (ESAs) to target higher Hgb levels. Maintain Hgb 10–12g/dL. In cancer pt, ESAs ↓ survival/time to progression in some cancers when dosed Hgb ≥12 g/dL. Use lowest dose needed. Use only for myelosuppressive chemo-therapy. D/C following chemotherapy. Pre-op ESA ↑ DVT. Consider DVT prophylaxis **Uses:** *CRF-associated anemia, zidovudine Rx in HIV-infected pts, CA chemotherapy; ↓ transfusions associated w/ surgery* **Acts:** Induces erythropoiesis **Dose:** *Adults & Peds.* 50–150 units/kg IV/SQ 3×/wk; adjust dose q4–6wk PRN. *Surgery:* 300 units/kg/d × 10 d before to 4 d after; ↓ dose if Hct ~36% or Hgb, ↑ > ≅ 12 g/dL or Hgb ↑ > 1 g/dL in 2-wk period; hold dose if Hgb > 12 g/dL **W/P:** [C, +] **CI:** Uncontrolled HTN **Disp:** Inj 2000, 3000, 4000, 10,000, 20,000, 40,000 units/mL **SE:**

HTN, HA, fatigue, fever, tachycardia, N/V **Notes:** Refrigerate; monitor baseline & posttreatment Hct/Hgb, BP, ferritin

Epoprostenol (Flolan) **Uses:** *Pulm HTN* **Acts:** Dilates pulm/systemic arterial vascular beds; ↓ plt aggregation **Dose:** Initial 2 ng/kg/min; ↑ by 2 ng/kg/min q15min until dose-limiting SE (CP, dizziness, N/V, HA, ↓ BP, flushing); IV cont Inf 4 ng/kg/min < max tolerated rate; adjust based on response; per protocol **W/P:** [B, ?] ↑ tox w/ diuretics, vasodilators, acetate in dialysis fluids, anticoagulants **CI:** Chronic use in CHF 2nd degree, if pt develops pulm edema w/ dose initiation, severe LVSD **Disp:** Inj 0.5, 1.5 mg **SE:** Flushing, tachycardia, CHF, fever, chills, nervousness, HA, N/V/D, jaw pain, flu-like Sxs **Notes:** Abrupt D/C can cause rebound pulm HTN; monitor bleeding w/ other antiplatelet/anticoagulants; watch ↓ BP w/ other vasodilators/diuretics

Eprosartan (Teveten) **Uses:** *HTN*, DN, CHF **Acts:** ARB **Dose:** 400–800 mg/d single dose or bid **W/P:** [C (1st tri); D (2nd & 3rd tri), D/C immediately when PRG detected] w/ Li, ↑ K⁺ w/ K⁺-sparing diuretics/supls/high-dose trimethoprim **CI:** Bilateral RAS, 1st-degree aldosteronism **Disp:** Tabs 400, 600 mg **SE:** Fatigue, depression, URI, UTI, Abd pain, rhinitis/pharyngitis/cough, hypertriglyceridemia

Eptifibatide (Integrilin) **Uses:** *ACS, PCI* **Acts:** Glycoprotein IIb/IIIa inhib **Dose:** 180 mcg/kg IV bolus, then 2 mcg/kg/min cont Inf; ↓ in renal impair (SCr > 2 mg/dL, < 4 mg/dL: 135 mcg/kg bolus & 0.5 mcg/kg/min Inf); *PCI:* 135 mcg/kg IV bolus then 0.5 mcg/kg/min; bolus again in 10 min; *ECC 2010. ACS:* 180 mcg/kg/min IV bolus over 1–2 min, then 2 mcg/kg/min, then repeat bolus in 10 min; continue infusion 18–24 h post PCI **W/P:** [B, ?] Monitor bleeding w/ other anticoagulants **CI:** Other glycoprotein IIb/IIIa inhib, Hx abnormal bleeding, hemorrhagic stroke (w/in 30 d), severe HTN, major surgery (w/in 6 wk), plt count < 100,000 cells/mm³, renal dialysis **Disp:** Inj 0.75, 2 mg/mL **SE:** Bleeding, ↓ BP, Inj site Rxn, thrombocytopenia **Notes:** Monitor bleeding, coagulants, plts, SCr, activated coagulation time (ACT) w/ prothrombin consumption index (keep ACT 200–300 s)

Eribulin (Halaven) **Uses:** *Met breast Ca after 2 chemo regimens (including anthracycline & taxane)* **Acts:** Microtubule inhibitor **Dose:** *Adults.* 1.4 mg/m² IV (over 2–5 min) days 1 & 8 of 21-d cycle; ↓ dose w/ hepatic & mod renal impair; delay/↓ for toxicity (see label) **W/P:** [D, –] **CI:** None **Disp:** Inj **SE:** ↓ WBC/Hct/plt, fatigue/asthenia, neuropathy, N/V/D, constipation, pyrexia, alopecia,↑ QT, arthralgia/myalgia, back/pain, cough, dyspnea, UTI **Notes:** ✓ CBC & monitor for neuropathy prior to dosing

Erlotinib (Tarceva) **Uses:** *NSCLC after failing 1 chemotherapy; maint NSCLC who have not progressed after 4 cycles cisplatin based therapy, CA pancreas* **Acts:** HER2/EGFR TKI **Dose:** CA pancreas 100 mg, others 150 mg/d PO 1 h ac or 2 h pc; ↓ (in 50-mg decrements) w/ severe Rxn or w/ CYP3A4 inhib (Table 10, p 301) **W/P:** [D, ?/–] avoid pregnancy; w/ CYP3A4 inhib (Table 10, p 301) **Disp:** Tabs 25, 100, 150 mg **SE:** Rash, N/V/D, anorexia, Abd pain, fatigue, cough, dyspnea, edema, stomatitis, conjunctivitis, pruritus, skin/nail changes, infxn, ↑ LFTs, interstitial lung Dz Notes: May ↑ INR w/ warfarin, monitor INR

Ertapenem (Invanz) Uses: *Complicated intra-Abd, acute pelvic, & skin infxns, pyelonephritis, CAP* Acts: α-carbapenem; β-lactam antibiotic, ↓ cell wall synth. Spectrum: Good gram(+/–) & anaerobic coverage, not Pseudomonas, PCN-resistant pneumococci, MRSA, Enterococcus, β-lactamase (+) H. influenzae, Mycoplasma, Chlamydia Dose: Adults. 1 g IM/IV daily; 500 mg/d in CrCl < 30 mL/min. Peds 3 mo–12 y. 15 mg/kg bid IM/IV, max 1 g/d W/P: [B, ?/–] Sz Hx, CNS disorders, β-lactam & multiple allergies, probenecid ↓ renal clearance CI: component hypersens or amide anesthetics Disp: Inj 1 g/vial SE: HA, N/V/D, Inj site Rxns, thrombocytosis, ↑ LFTs Notes: Can give IM × 7 d, IV × 14 d; 137 mg Na⁺ (6 mEq)/g ertapenem

Erythromycin (E-Mycin, E.E.S., Ery-Tab, EryPed, Ilotycin) Uses: *Bacterial Infxns; bowel prep*; ↑ GI motility (prokinetic); *acne vulgaris* Acts: Bacteriostatic; interferes w/ protein synth. Spectrum: Group A streptococci (S. pyogenes), S. pneumoniae, N. meningitidis, N. gonorrhoeae (if PCN-allergic), Legionella, M. pneumoniae Dose: Adults. Base 250–500 mg PO q6–12h or ethylsuccinate 400–800 mg q6–12h; 500 mg–1 g IV q6h. Prokinetic: 250 mg PO tid 30 min ac. Peds. 30–50 mg/kg/d PO ÷ q6–8h or 20–40 mg/kg/d IV ÷ q6h, max 2 g/d W/P: [B, +] ↑ tox of carbamazepine, cyclosporine, digoxin, methylprednisolone, theophylline, felodipine, warfarin, simvastatin/lovastatin; ↓ sildenafil dose w/ use CI: Hepatic impair, preexisting liver Dz (estolate), use w/ pimozide Disp: Lactobionate (Ilotycin): Powder for Inj 500 mg, 1 g. Base: Tabs 250, 333, 500 mg; caps 250 mg. Estolate (Ilosone): Susp 125, 250 mg/5 mL. Stearate (Erythrocin): Tabs 250, 500 mg. Ethylsuccinate (EES, EryPed): Chew tabs 200 mg; tabs 400 mg; susp 200, 400 mg/5 mL SE: HA, Abd pain, N/V/D; [QT prolongation, torsades de pointes, ventricular arrhythmias/tachycardias (rarely)]; cholestatic jaundice (estolate) Notes: 400 mg ethylsuccinate = 250 mg base/estolate; w/ food minimizes GI upset; lactobionate contains benzyl alcohol (caution in neonates)

Erythromycin & Benzoyl Peroxide (Benzamycin) Uses: *Topical for acne vulgaris* Acts: Macrolide antibiotic w/ keratolytic Dose: Apply bid (A.M. & P.M.) W/P: [C, ?] CI: Component sensitivity Disp: Gel erythromycin 30 mg/benzoyl peroxide 50 mg/g SE: Local irritation, dryness

Erythromycin & Sulfisoxazole (Eryzole, Pediazole) Uses: *Upper & lower resp tract; bacterial infxns; H. influenzae otitis media in children*; Infxns in PCN-allergic pts Acts: Macrolide antibiotic w/ sulfonamide Dose: Adults. Based on erythromycin content; 400 mg erythromycin/1200 mg sulfisoxazole PO q6h. Peds > 2 mo. 40–50 mg/kg/d erythromycin & 150 mg/kg/d sulfisoxazole PO ÷ q6h; max 2 g/d erythromycin or 6 g/d sulfisoxazole × 10 d; ↓ in renal impair W/P: [C (D if near term), +] w/ PO anticoagulants, hypoglycemics, phenytoin, cyclosporine CI: Infants < 2 mo Disp: Susp erythromycin ethylsuccinate 200 mg/sulfisoxazole 600 mg/5 mL (100, 150, 200 mL) SE: GI upset

Erythromycin, Ophthalmic (Ilotycin Ophthalmic)   Uses: *Conjunctival/corneal Infxns* Acts: Macrolide antibiotic Dose: 1/2 inch 2–6×/d W/P: [B, +] CI: Erythromycin hypersens Disp: 0.5% oint SE: Local irritation

Erythromycin, Topical (A/T/S, Eryderm, Erycette, T-Stat)   Uses: *Acne vulgaris* Acts: Macrolide antibiotic Dose: Wash & dry area, apply 2% product over area bid W/P: [B, +] CI: Component sensitivity Disp: Soln 1.5%, 2%; gel 2%; pads & swabs 2% SE: Local irritation

Escitalopram (Lexapro)   BOX: Closely monitor for worsening depression or emergence of suicidality, particularly in ped pts Uses: Depression, anxiety Acts: SSRI Dose: Adults. 10–20 mg PO daily; 10 mg/d in elderly & hepatic impair W/P: [C, +/–] Serotonin synd (Table 11, p 303); use of escitalopram, w/ NSAID, ASA, or other drugs affecting coagulation associated w/ ↑ bleeding risk CI: w/ or w/in 14 d of MAOI Disp: Tabs 5, 10, 20 mg; soln 1 mg/mL SE: N/V/D, sweating, insomnia, dizziness, xerostomia, sexual dysfunction Notes: Full effects may take 3 wk

Esmolol (Brevibloc)   Uses: *SVT & noncompensatory sinus tachycardia, AF/A flutter* Acts: β_1-Adrenergic blocker; class II antiarrhythmic Dose: Adults & Peds. ECC 2010. 0.5 mg/kg (500 mcg/kg) over 1 min, then 0.05 mg/kg/min (50 mcg/kg/min) inf; if inadequate response after 5 min, repeat 0.5 mg/kg bolus, then titrate inf up to 0.2 mg/kg/min (200 mcg/kg/min); max 0.3 mg/kg/min (300 mcg/kg/min) W/P: [C (1st tri; D 2nd or 3rd tri), ?] CI: Sinus bradycardia, heart block, uncompensated CHF, cardiogenic shock, ↓ BP Disp: Inj 10, 20, 250 mg/mL; premix Inf 10 mg/mL SE: ↓ BP; ↓ HR, diaphoresis, dizziness, pain on Inj Notes: Hemodynamic effects back to baseline w/in 30 min after D/C Inf

Esomeprazole (Nexium)   Uses: *Short-term (4–8 wk) for erosive esophagitis/GERD; H. pylori Infxn in combo w/ antibiotics* Acts: Proton pump inhib, ↓ gastric acid Dose: Adults. GERD/erosive gastritis: 20–40 mg/d PO × 4–8 wk; 20–40 mg IV 10–30 min Inf or > 3 min IV push, 10 d max; Maint: 20 mg/d PO. H. pylori Infxn: 40 mg/d PO, plus clarithromycin 500 mg PO bid & amoxicillin 1000 mg/bid for 10 d; W/P: [B, ?/–] CI: Component sensitivity; do not use w/ clopidogrel (↓ effect) Disp: Caps 20, 40 mg; IV 20, 40 mg SE: HA, D, Abd pain Notes: Do not chew; may open caps & sprinkle on applesauce; ? ↑ risk of fractures w/ all PPI; risk of hypomagnesemia w/ long-term use, monitor

Estazolam (ProSom) [C-IV]   Uses: *Short-term management of insomnia* Acts: Benzodiazepine Dose: 1–2 mg PO qhs PRN; ↓ in hepatic impair/elderly/debilitated W/P: [X, –] Effects w/ CNS depressants; cross-sensitivity w/ other benzodiazepines CI: PRG, component hypersens, w/ itraconazole or ketoconazole Disp: Tabs 1, 2 mg SE: Somnolence, weakness, palpitations, anaphylaxis, angioedema, amnesia Notes: May cause psychological/physical dependence; avoid abrupt D/C after prolonged use

Esterified Estrogens (Estratab, Menest)   BOX: ↑ Risk endometrial CA. Do not use in the prevention of CV Dz or dementia; ↑ risk of MI, stroke, breast CA, PE, DVT, in postmenopausal Uses: *Vasomotor Sxs or vulvar/vag atrophy w/ menopause*; female hypogonadism, PCa, prevent osteoporosis **Acts:** Estrogen supl **Dose:** *Menopausal vasomotor Sx:* 0.3–1.25 mg/d, cyclically 3 wk on, 1 wk off; add progestin 10–14 d w/ 28-d cycle w/ uterus intact; *Vulvovaginal atrophy:* same regimen except use 0.3–1.25 mg; *Hypogonadism:* 2.5–7.5 mg/d PO × 20 d, off × 10 d; add progestin 10–14 d w/ 28-d cycle w/uterus intact **W/P:** [X, –] **CI:** Undiagnosed genital bleeding, breast CA, estrogen-dependent tumors, thromboembolic disorders, thrombophlebitis, recent MI, PRG, severe hepatic Dz **Disp:** Tabs 0.3, 0.625, 1.25, 2.5 mg **SE:** N, HA, bloating, breast enlargement/tenderness, edema, venous thromboembolism, hypertriglyceridemia, gallbladder Dz **Notes:** Use lowest dose for shortest time (see WHI data [www.whi.org])

Esterified Estrogens + Methyltestosterone (Estratest, Estratest HS, Syntest DS, HS)   **BOX:** ↑ Risk endometrial CA. Avoid in PRG. Do not use in the prevention of CV Dz or dementia; ↑ risk of MI, stroke, breast CA, PE, DVT in postmenopause women **Uses:** *Vasomotor Sxs*; postpartum breast engorgement **Acts:** Estrogen & androgen supl **Dose:** 1 tab/d × 3 wk, 1 wk off **W/P:** [X, –] **CI:** Genital bleeding of unknown cause, breast CA, estrogen-dependent tumors, thromboembolic disorders, thrombophlebitis, recent MI, PRG **Disp:** Tabs (estrogen/methyltestosterone) 0.625 mg/1.25 mg, 1.25 mg/2.5 mg **SE:** N, HA, bloating, breast enlargement/tenderness, edema, ↑ triglycerides, venous thromboembolism, gallbladder Dz **Notes:** Use lowest dose for shortest time; (see WHI data [www.whi.org])

Estradiol, Gel (Divigel)   **BOX:** ↑ Risk of endometrial CA. Do not use in the prevention of CV Dz or dementia; ↑ risk MI, stroke, breast CA, PE, and DVT in postmenopausal women (50–79 y). ↑ Dementia risk in postmenopausal women (≥65 y) **Uses:** *Vasomotor Sx in menopause* **Acts:** Estrogen **Dose:** 0.25 g q day on right or left upper thigh **W/P:** [X, +/–] may ↑ PT/PTT/plt aggregation w/ thyroid Dz **CI:** Undiagnosed genital bleeding, breast CA, estrogen-dependent tumors, thromboembolic disorders, thrombophlebitis, recent MI, PRG, severe hepatic Dz **Disp:** 0.1% gel 0.25/0.5/1 g single-dose foil packets w/ 0.25, 0.5, 1-mg estradiol, respectively **SE:** N, HA, bloating, breast enlargement/tenderness, edema, venous thromboembolism, ↑ hypertriglyceridemia, gallbladder Dz **Notes:** if person other than pt applies, glove should be used, keep dry immediately after, rotate site; contains alcohol, caution around flames until dry, not for vag use

Estradiol, Gel (Elestrin)   **BOX:** Do not use in the prevention of CV Dz or dementia; ↑ risk MI, stroke, breast CA, PE, and DVT in postmenopausal women **Uses:** *Postmenopausal vasomotor Sxs* **Acts:** Estrogen **Dose:** Apply 0.87–1.7 g to skin q day; add progestin × 10–14 d/28-d cycle w/ intact uterus; use lowest effective estrogen dose **W/P:** [X, ?] **CI:** AUB, breast CA, estrogen-dependent tumors, thromboembolic disorders, recent MI, PRG, severe hepatic Dz **Disp:** Gel 0.06% **SE:** Thromboembolic events, MI, stroke, ↑ BP, breast/ovarian/endometrial CA, site Rxns, vag spotting, breast changes, Abd bloating, cramps, HA, fluid retention

Notes: Apply to upper arm, wait > 25 min before sunscreen; avoid concomitant use for > 7 d; BP, breast exams

Estradiol, Oral (Estrace, Delestrogen, Femtrace) **BOX:** ↑ Risk of endometrial CA; avoid in PRG **Uses:** *Atrophic vaginitis, menopausal vasomotor Sxs,↑ low estrogen levels, palliation breast and PCa* **Acts:** Estrogen **Dose:** *PO:* 1–2 mg/d, adjust PRN to control Sxs. *Vaginal cream:* 2–4 g/d ×2 wk, then 1 g 1–3×/wk. *Vasomotor Sx/vag Atrophy:* 10–20 mg IM q4wk, D/C or taper at 3–6-mo intervals. *Hypoestrogenism:* 10–20 mg IM q4wk. *PCa:* 30 mg IM q12wk **W/P:** [X, –] **CI:** Genital bleeding of unknown cause, breast CA, porphyria, estrogen-dependent tumors, thromboembolic disorders, thrombophlebitis; recent MI; hepatic impair **Disp** Ring 0.05, 0.1, 2 mg; gel 0.061%; tabs 0.5, 1, 2 mg; vag cream 0.1 mg/g, depot Inj (Delestrogen) 10, 20, 40 mg/mL **SE:** N, HA, bloating, breast enlargement/tenderness, edema, ↑ triglycerides, venous thromboembolism, gallbladder Dz

Estradiol, Spray (Evamist) **BOX:** ↑ Risk of endometrial CA. Do not use in the prevention of CV Dz or dementia; ↑ risk MI, stroke, breast CA, PE, and DVT in postmenopausal women (50–79 y). ↑ Dementia risk in postmenopausal women (≥65 y) **Uses:** *Vasomotor Sx in menopause* **Acts:** Estrogen supl **Dose:** 1 spray on inner surface of forearm **W/P:** [X, +/–] May ↑ PT/PTT/plt aggregation w/ thyroid Dz **CI:** Undiagnosed genital bleeding, breast CA, estrogen-dependent tumors, thromboembolic disorders, thrombophlebitis, recent MI, PRG, severe hepatic Dz **Disp:** 1.53 mg/spray (56-spray container) **SE:** N, HA, bloating, breast enlargement/tenderness, edema, venous thromboembolism, ↑ BP, hypertriglyceridemia, gallbladder Dz **Notes:** Contains alcohol, caution around flames until dry; not for vag use

Estradiol, Transdermal (Estraderm, Climara, Vivelle, Vivelle Dot) **BOX:** ↑ Risk of endometrial CA. Do not use in the prevention of CV Dz or dementia; ↑ risk MI, stroke, breast CA, PE, and DVT in postmenopausal women (50–79 y). ↑ Dementia risk in postmenopausal women (≥65 y) **Uses:** *Severe menopausal vasomotor Sxs; female hypogonadism* **Acts:** Estrogen supl **Dose:** Start 0.0375–0.05 mg/d patch 2×/wk based on product; adjust PRN to control Sxs; w/ intact uterus cycle 3 wk on 1 wk off or use cyclic progestin 10–14 d **W/P:** [X, –] See Estradiol **CI:** PRG, AUB, porphyria, breast CA, estrogen-dependent tumors, Hx thrombophlebitis, thrombosis **Disp:** Transdermal patches (mg/24 h) 0.025, 0.0375, 0.05, 0.06, 0.075, 0.1 **SE:** N, bloating, breast enlargement/tenderness, edema, HA, hypertriglyceridemia, gallbladder Dz **Notes:** Do not apply to breasts, place on trunk, rotate sites

Estradiol, Vaginal (Estring, Femring, Vagifem) **BOX:** ↑ Risk of endometrial CA. Do not use in the prevention of CV Dz or dementia; ↑ risk MI, stroke, breast CA, PE, and DVT in postmenopausal women (50–79 y) **Uses:** *Postmenopausal vag atrophy (Estring)* *vasomotor Sxs and vulvar/vag atrophy associated w/ menopause (Femring)* *atrophic vaginitis (Vagifem)* **Acts:** Estrogen supl **Dose:** *Estring:* Insert ring into upper third of vag vault; remove and replace after 90 d; reassess 3–6 mo; *Femring:* use lowest effective dose, insert vaginally, replace q3mo; *Vagifem:* 1 tab vaginally q day × 2 wk, then maint 1 tab 2×/wk, D/C or taper at 3–6 mo **W/P:** [X, –] May ↑ PT/PTT/plt aggregation w/ thyroid Dz, toxic shock reported **CI:** Undiagnosed genital bleeding, breast CA, estrogen-dependent tumors, thromboembolic disorders, thrombophlebitis, recent MI, PRG, severe hepatic Dz **Disp:** *Estring ring:* 0.0075 mg/24 h; *Femring ring:* 0.05 and 0.1 mg/d *Vagifem tab (vag):* 25 mcg **SE:** HA, leukorrhea, back pain, candidiasis, vaginitis, vag discomfort/hemorrhage, arthralgia, insomnia, Abd pain

Estradiol/Levonorgestrel, Transdermal (Climara Pro) **BOX:** ↑ Risk of endometrial CA. Do not use in the prevention of CV Dz or dementia; ↑ risk MI, stroke, breast CA, PE, and DVT in postmenopausal women (50–79 y). ↑ Dementia risk in postmenopausal women (≥65 y) **Uses:** *Menopausal vasomotor Sx; prevent postmenopausal osteoporosis* **Acts:** Estrogen & progesterone **Dose:** 1 Patch 1×/wk **W/P:** [X, –] w/ ↓ Thyroid Dz AUB, estrogen-sensitive tumors, Hx thromboembolism, liver impair, PRG, hysterectomy **Disp:** Estradiol 0.045 mg/levonorgestrel 0.015/mg day patch **SE:** Site Rxn, vag bleed/spotting, breast changes, Abd bloating/cramps, HA, retention fluid, edema, ↑ BP **Notes:** Apply lower Abd; for osteoporosis give Ca^{2+}/vit D supl; follow breast exams

Estradiol/Medroxyprogesterone (Lunelle) **BOX:** Cigarette smoking ↑ risk of serious CV SEs from contraceptives w/ estrogen. This risk ↑ w/ age & w/ heavy smoking (> 15 cigarettes/d) & is marked in women > 35 y. Women who use Lunelle should not smoke **Uses:** *Contraceptive* **Acts:** Estrogen & progestin **Dose:** 0.5 mL IM (deltoid, anterior thigh, buttock) monthly, do not exceed 33 d **W/P:** [X, M] HTN, gallbladder Dz, ↑ lipids, migraines, sudden HA, valvular heart Dz w/ comps **CI:** PRG, heavy smokers > 35 y, DVT, PE, cerebro-/CV Dz, estrogen-dependent neoplasm, undiagnosed AUB, porphyria, hepatic tumors, cholestatic jaundice **Disp:** Estradiol cypionate (5 mg), medroxyprogesterone acetate (25 mg) single-dose vial or syringe (0.5 mL) **SE:** Arterial thromboembolism, HTN, cerebral hemorrhage, MI, amenorrhea, acne, breast tenderness **Notes:** Start w/in 5 d of menstruation

Estradiol/Norethindrone (FemHRT, Activella) **BOX:** ↑ Risk of endometrial CA. Do not use in the prevention of CV Dz or dementia; ↑ risk MI, stroke, breast CA, PE, and DVT in postmenopausal women (50–79 y). ↑ Dementia risk in postmenopausal women (≥65 y) **Uses:** *Menopause vasomotor Sxs; prevent osteoporosis* **Acts:** Estrogen/progestin; plant derived **Dose:** 1 tab/d start w/ lowest dose combo **W/P:** [X, –] w/ ↓ Ca^{2+}/thyroid **CI:** PRG; Hx breast CA; estrogen-dependent tumor; abnormal genital bleeding; Hx DVT, PE, or related disorders; recent (w/in past year) arterial thromboembolic Dz (CVA, MI) **Disp:** *Femhrt:* Tabs 2.5/0.5, 5 mcg/1 mg; *Activella:* tabs 1/0.5, 0.5 mg/0.1 mg **SE:** Thrombosis, dizziness, HA, libido changes, insomnia, emotional instability, breast pain **Notes:** Use in women w/ intact uterus; caution in heavy smokers

Estramustine Phosphate (Emcyt) **Uses:** *Advanced PCa* **Acts:** estradiol w/ nitrogen mustard; exact mechanism unknown **Dose:** 14 mg/kg/d in 3–4 ÷ doses;

on empty stomach, no dairy products **W/P:** [NA, not used in females] **CI:** Active thrombophlebitis or thromboembolic disorders **Disp:** Caps 140 mg **SE:** N/V, exacerbation of preexisting CHF, edema, hepatic disturbances, thrombophlebitis, MI, PE, gynecomastia in 20–100% **NOTE:** low-dose breast irradiation before may ↓ gynecomastia

Estrogen, Conjugated (Premarin) **BOX:** ↑ Risk of endometrial CA. Do not use in the prevention of CV Dz or dementia; ↑ risk MI, stroke, breast CA, PE, and DVT in postmenopausal women (50–79 y). ↑ Dementia risk in postmenopausal women (≥65 y) **Uses:** *Mod–severe menopausal vasomotor Sxs; atrophic vaginitis, dyspareunia*; palliative advanced CAP; prevention & Tx of estrogen deficiency osteoporosis **Acts:** Estrogen replacement **Dose:** 0.3–1.25 mg/d PO; intravaginal cream 0.5–2g × 21 d, then off × 7 d or 0.5 mg twice weekly **W/P:** [X, –] **CI:** Severe hepatic impair, genital bleeding of unknown cause, breast CA, estrogen-dependent tumors, thromboembolic disorders, thrombosis, thrombophlebitis, recent MI **Disp:** Tabs 0.3, 0.45, 0.625, 0.9, 1.25, 2.5 mg; vag cream 0.625 mg/g **SE:** ↑ Risk of endometrial CA, gallbladder Dz, thromboembolism, HA, & possibly breast CA **Notes:** generic products not equivalent

Estrogen, Conjugated Synthetic (Cenestin, Enjuvia) **BOX:** ↑ Risk of endometrial CA. Do not use in the prevention of CV Dz or dementia; ↑ risk MI, stroke, breast CA, PE, and DVT in postmenopausal women (50–79 y). ↑ Dementia risk in postmenopausal women (≥65 y) **Uses:** *Vasomotor menopausal Sxs, vulvovaginal atrophy, prevent postmenopausal osteoporosis* **Acts:** Multiple estrogen replacement **Dose:** For all w/ intact uterus progestin × 10–14 d/28-d cycle; *Vasomotor:* 0.3–1.25 mg (Enjuvia) 0.625–1.25 mg (Cenestin) PO daily; *Vag atrophy:* 0.3 mg/d; *Osteoporosis:* (Cenestin) 0.625 mg/d **W/P:** [X, –] **CI:** See Estrogen, conjugated **Disp:** Tabs, Cenestin 0.3, 0.45, 0.625, 0.9 mg; Enjuvia ER 0.3, 0.45, 0.625, 1.25 mg **SE:** ↑ Risk endometrial/breast CA, gallbladder Dz, thromboembolism

Estrogen, Conjugated + Medroxyprogesterone (Prempro, Premphase) **BOX:** Should not be used for the prevention of CV Dz or dementia; ↑ risk of MI, stroke, breast CA, PE, & DVT; ↑ risk of dementia in postmenopausal women **Uses:** *Mod–severe menopausal vasomotor Sxs; atrophic vaginitis; prevent postmenopausal osteoporosis* **Acts:** Hormonal replacement **Dose:** *Prempro* 1 tab PO daily; *Premphase* 1 tab PO daily **W/P:** [X, –] **CI:** Severe hepatic impair, genital bleeding of unknown cause, breast CA, estrogen-dependent tumors, thromboembolic disorders, thrombosis, thrombophlebitis **Disp:** (As estrogen/medroxyprogesterone) *Prempro:* Tabs 0.3/1.5, 0.45/1.5, 0.625/2.5, 0.625/5 mg; *Premphase:* Tabs 0.625/0 (d 1–14) & 0.625/5 mg (d 15–28) **SE:** Gallbladder Dz, thromboembolism, HA, breast tenderness **Notes:** See WHI (www.whi.org); use lowest dose/shortest time possible

Estrogen, Conjugated + Methyl Progesterone (Premarin + Methyl Progesterone) **BOX:** Do not use in the prevention of CV Dz or dementia; ↑ risk of endometrial CA **Uses:** *Menopausal vasomotor Sxs; osteoporosis* **Acts:**

Estrogen & androgen combo **Dose:** 1 tab/d **W/P:** [X, –] **CI:** Severe hepatic impair, AUB, breast CA, estrogen-dependent tumors, thromboembolic disorders, thrombosis, thrombophlebitis **Disp:** Tabs 0.625 mg estrogen, conjugated, & 2.5 or 5 mg of methyl progesterone **SE:** N, bloating, breast enlargement/tenderness, edema, HA, hypertriglyceridemia, gallbladder Dz

Estrogen,   Conjugated   +   Methyltestosterone   (Premarin   +   Methyltestosterone)   **BOX:** Do not use in the prevention of CV Dz or dementia; ↑ risk of endometrial CA **Uses:** *Mod–severe menopausal vasomotor Sxs*; postpartum breast engorgement **Acts:** Estrogen & androgen combo **Dose:** 1 tab/d × 3 wk, then 1 wk off **W/P:** [X, –] **CI:** Severe hepatic impair, genital bleeding of unknown cause, breast CA, estrogen-dependent tumors, thromboembolic disorders, thrombophlebitis **Disp:** Tabs (estrogen/methyltestosterone) 0.625 mg/5 mg, 1.25 mg/10 mg **SE:** N, bloating, breast enlargement/tenderness, edema, HA, hypertriglyceridemia, gallbladder Dz

Eszopiclone (Lunesta) [C-IV]   **Uses:** *Insomnia* **Acts:** Nonbenzodiazepine hypnotic **Dose:** 2–3 mg/d hs *Elderly:* 1–2 mg/d hs; w/ hepatic impair use w/ CYP3A4 inhib (Table 10, p 301): 1 mg/d hs **W/P:** [C, ?/–] **Disp:** Tabs 1, 2, 3 mg **SE:** HA, xerostomia, dizziness, somnolence, hallucinations, rash, Infxn, unpleasant taste, anaphylaxis, angioedema **Notes:** High-fat meals ↓ absorption

Etanercept (Enbrel)   **BOX:** Serious infxns (bacterial sepsis, TB, reported); D/C w/ severe Infxn. Evaluate for TB risk; test for TB before use; lymphoma/other CA possible in children/adolescents possible **Uses:** *↓ Sxs of RA in pts who fail other DMARD*, Crohn Dz **Acts:** TNF receptor blocker **Dose:** *Adults.* RA 50 mg SQ weekly or 25 mg SQ 2×/wk (separated by at least 72–96 h). *Peds 4–17 y.* 0.8 mg/kg/wk (max 50 mg/wk) or 0.4 mg/kg (max 25 mg/dose) 2×/wk 72–96 h apart **W/P:** [B, ?] w/ Predisposition to Infxn (i.e., DM); may ↑ risk of malignancy in peds and young adults **CI:** Active Infxn **Disp:** Inj 25 mg/vial, 50 mg/mL syringe **SE:** HA, rhinitis, Inj site Rxn, URI, new onset psoriasis **Notes:** Rotate Inj sites

Ethambutol (Myambutol)   **Uses:** *Pulm TB* & other mycobacterial Infxns, MAC **Acts:** ↓ RNA synth **Dose:** *Adults & Peds > 12 y.* 15–25 mg/kg/d PO single dose; ↓ in renal impair, take w/ food, avoid antacids **W/P:** [C, +] **CI:** unconscious pts, optic neuritis **Disp:** Tabs 100, 400 mg **SE:** HA, hyperuricemia, acute gout, Abd pain, ↑ LFTs, optic neuritis, GI upset

Ethinyl Estradiol (Estinyl, Feminone)   **BOX:** ↑ Risk endometrial CA. Avoid in PRG. Do not use in the prevention of CV Dz or dementia; ↑ risk of MI, stroke, breast CA, PE, DVT, in postmenopausal women **Uses:** *Menopausal vasomotor Sxs; female hypogonadism* **Acts:** Estrogen supl **Dose:** 0.02–1.5 mg/d ÷ daily–tid **W/P:** [X, –] **CI:** Severe hepatic impair; genital bleeding of unknown cause, breast CA, estrogen-dependent tumors, thromboembolic disorders, thrombophlebitis **Disp:** Tabs 0.02, 0.05, 0.5 mg **SE:** N, bloating, breast enlargement/tenderness, edema, HA, hypertriglyceridemia, gallbladder Dz

Ethinyl Estradiol & Norelgestromin (Ortho Evra)   **Uses:** *Contraceptive patch* **Acts:** Estrogen & progestin **Dose:** Apply patch to abd, buttocks, upper torso (not breasts), or upper outer arm at the beginning of the menstrual cycle; new patch is applied weekly for 3 wk; wk 4 is patch-free **W/P:** [X, M] **CI:** PRG, Hx or current DVT/PE, stroke, MI, CV Dz, CAD; SBP ≥ 160 systolic mm Hg or DBP ≥ 100 diastolic mm Hg severe HTN; severe HA w/ focal neurologic Sx; breast/endometrial CA; estrogen-dependent neoplasms; hepatic dysfunction; jaundice; major surgery w/ prolonged immobilization; heavy smoking if > 35 y **Disp:** 20 cm^2 patch (6 mg norelgestromin [active metabolite norgestimate] & 0.75 mg of ethinyl estradiol) **SE:** Breast discomfort, HA, site Rxns, N, menstrual cramps; thrombosis risks similar to OCP **Notes:** Less effective in women > 90 kg; instruct pt does not protect against STD/HIV; discourage smoking

Ethosuximide (Zarontin)   Uses: *Absence (petit mal) Szs* **Acts:** Anticonvulsant; ↑ Sz threshold **Dose:** *Adults & peds > 6 y.* Initial, 500 mg PO ÷ bid; ↑ by 250 mg/d q4–7d PRN (max 1500 mg/d) usual maint 20–30 mg/kg. *Peds 3–6 y.* *Initial:* 15 mg/kg/d PO ÷ bid. *Maint:* 15–40 mg/kg/d ÷ bid, max 1500 mg/d **W/P:** [D, +] In renal/hepatic impair; antiepileptics may ↑ risk of suicidal behavior or ideation **CI:** Component sensitivity **Disp:** Caps 250 mg; syrup 250 mg/5 mL **SE:** Blood dyscrasias, GI upset, drowsiness, dizziness, irritability **Notes:** Levels: *Trough:* just before next dose; *Therapeutic: Peak:* 40–100 mcg/mL; *Toxic Trough:* > 100 mcg/mL; *Half-life:* 25–60 h

Etidronate Disodium (Didronel)   Uses: *↑ Ca^{2+} of malignancy, Paget Dz, & heterotopic ossification* **Acts:** ↓ nl & abnormal bone resorption **Dose:** *Paget Dz:* 5–10 mg/kg/d PO ÷ doses (for 3–6 mo). ↑ *Ca^{2+}:* 7.5 mg/kg/d IV Inf over 2 h × 3 d, then 20 mg/kg/d PO on last day of Inf × 1–3 mo **W/P:** [B PO (C parenteral), ?] Bisphosphonates may cause severe musculoskeletal pain **CI:** Overt osteomalacia, SCr > 5 mg/dL **Disp:** Tabs 200, 400 mg; Inj 50 mg/mL **SE:** GI intolerance (↓ by ÷ daily doses); hyperphosphatemia, hypomagnesemia, bone pain, abnormal taste, fever, convulsions, nephrotox **Notes:** Take PO on empty stomach 2 h before or 2 h po

Etodolac   BOX: May ↑ risk of CV events & GI bleeding; may worsen ↑ BP **Uses:** *OA & pain*, RA **Acts:** NSAID **Dose:** 200–400 mg PO bid-qid (max 1200 mg/d) **W/P:** [C (D 3rd tri), ?] ↑ Bleeding risk w/ ASA, warfarin; ↑ nephrotox w/ cyclosporine; Hx CHF, HTN, renal/hepatic impair, PUD **CI:** Active GI ulcer **Disp:** Tabs 400, 500 mg; ER tabs 400, 500, 600 mg; caps 200, 300 mg **SE:** N/V/D, gastritis, Abd cramps, dizziness, HA, depression, edema, renal impair **Notes:** Do not crush tabs

Etomidate (Amidate)   Uses: *Induce general or short-procedure anesthesia* **Acts:** Short-acting hypnotic **Dose:** *Adults & Peds > 10 y.* Induce anesthesia 0.2–0.6 mg/kg IV over 30–60 s; *Peds < 10 y.* Not recommended *Peds. ECC 2010. Rapid sedation:* 0.2–0.4 mg/kg IV/IO over 30–60 s; max dose 20 mg **W/P:** [C, ?] **CI:** Hypersens **Disp:** Inj 2 mg/mL **SE:** Inj site pain, myoclonus

Etonogestrel/Ethinyl Estradiol Vaginal Insert (NuvaRing)   Uses: *Contraceptive* **Acts:** Estrogen & progestin combo **Dose:** Rule out PRG first; insert ring vaginally for 3 wk, remove for 1 wk; insert new ring 7 d after last removed (even if bleeding) at same time of day ring removed. 1st day of menses is day 1, insert before day 5 even if bleeding. Use other contraception for 1st 7 d of starting Rx. See PI if converting from other contraceptive; after delivery or 2nd tri abortion, insert 4 wk postpartum (if not breast-feeding) **W/P:** [X, ?/–] HTN, gall-bladder Dz, ↑ lipids, migraines, sudden HA **CI:** PRG, heavy smokers > 35 y, DVT, PE, cerebro-/CV Dz, estrogen-dependent neoplasm, undiagnosed abnormal genital bleeding, hepatic tumors, cholestatic jaundice **Disp:** Intravag ring: ethinyl estradiol 0.015 mg/d & etonogestrel 0.12 mg/d **Notes:** If ring removed, rinse w/ cool/luke-warm H_2O (not hot) & reinsert ASAP; if not reinserted w/in 3 h, effectiveness ↓; do not use w/ diaphragm

Etonogestrel Implant (Implanon) Uses: *Contraception* **Acts:** Trans-forms endometrium from proliferative to secretory **Dose:** 1 Implant subdermally q3y **W/P:** [X, +] Exclude PRG before implant **CI:** PRG, hormonally responsive tumors, breast CA, AUB, hepatic tumor, active liver Dz, Hx thromboembolic Dz **Disp:** 68-mg implant **SE:** Spotting, irregular periods, amenorrhea, dysmenorrhea, HA, tender breasts, N, wgt gain, acne, ectopic PRG, PE, ovarian cysts, stroke, ↑ BP **Notes:** 99% Effective; remove implant and replace; restricted distribution; phy-sician must register and train; does not protect against STDs

Etoposide [VP-16] (VePesid, Toposar) Uses: *Testicular, NSCLC, Hodgkin Dz, & NHLs, peds ALL, & allogeneic/autologous BMT in high doses* **Acts:** Topoisomerase II inhib **Dose:** 50 mg/m^2/d IV for 3–5 d; 50 mg/m^2/d PO for 21 d (PO availability = 50% of IV); 2–6 g/m^2 or 25–70 mg/kg in BMT (per proto-cols); ↓ in renal/hepatic impair **W/P:** [D, –] **CI:** IT administration **Disp:** Caps 50 mg; Inj 20 mg/mL **SE:** N/V (emesis in 10–30%), ↓ BM, alopecia, ↓ BP w/ rapid IV, anorexia, anemia, leukopenia, ↑ risk secondary leukemias

Etravirine (Intelence) Uses: *HIV* **Acts:** Non-NRTI **Dose:** 200 mg PO bid following a meal **W/P:** [B, ±] Many interactions: substrate/inducer (CYP3A4), substrate/inhib (CYP2C9, CYP2C19); do not use w/ tipranavir/ritonavir, fosampre-navir/ritonavir, atazanavir/ritonavir, protease inhib w/o ritonavir, and non-NRTIs **CI:** None **Disp:** Tabs 100 mg **SE:** N/V/D, rash, severe/potentially life-threatening skin Rxns, fat redistribution

Everolimus (Afinitor) Uses: *Advanced RCC w/ sunitinib or sorafenib fail-ure, subependymal giant cell astrocytoma in nonsurgical candidates w/ tuberous sclerosis* **Action:** mTOR inhib (mammalian rapamycin target) **Dose:** 10 mg PO daily, ↓ to 5 mg SE or hepatic impair; avoid w/high fat meal **W/P:** [D, ?] Avoid w/ or if received live vaccines; w/ CYP3A4 inhib **CI:** compound/ rapamycin deriv-ative hypersens **Disp:** Tabs 5, 10 mg **SE:** Non-infectious pneumonitis, ↑ Infxn risk, oral ulcers, asthenia, cough, fatigue, diarrhea, ↑ glucose/SCr/lipids; ↓ hemoglobin/WBC/plt **Notes:** Follow CBC, LFT, glucose, lipids; see also everolimus (Zortress)

Everolimus (Zortress) Uses: * Prevent renal transplant rejection; combo w/ basiliximab w/ ↓ dose of steroids and cyclosporine * **Action:** mTOR inhib (mam-malian rapamycin target) **Dose:** 7.5 mg PO bid, adjust to trough levels 3–8 ng/mL

W/P: [D, ?] **CI:** compound/ rapamycin derivative hypersens **Disp:** Tabs 0.25, 0.5,0.75 mg **SE:** peripheral edema, constipation, ↑ BP, N, ↓ Hct, UTI, ↑ lipids **Notes:** Follow CBC, LFT, glucose, lipids; see also everolimus (Afinitor); trough level 3–8 ng/mL w/ cyclosporina

Exemestane (Aromasin) **Uses:** *Advanced breast CA in postmenopausal women w/ progression after tamoxifen* **Acts:** Irreversible, steroidal aromatase inhib; ↓ estrogens **Dose:** 25 mg PO daily after a meal **W/P:** [D, ?/–] **CI:** PRG, component sensitivity **Disp:** Tabs 25 mg **SE:** Hot flashes, N, fatigue,↑ alkaline phosphate

Exenatide (Byetta) **Uses:** Type 2 DM combined w/ metformin &/or sulfony-lurea **Acts:** Incretin mimetic: ↑ insulin release, ↓ glucagon secretion, ↓ gastric emptying, promotes satiety **Dose:** 5 mcg SQ bid w/in 60 min before A.M. & P.M. meals; ↑ to 10 mcg SQ bid after 1 mo PRN; do not give pc **W/P:** [C, ?/–] may ↓ absorption of other drugs (take antibiotics/contraceptives 1 h before) **CI:** CrCl < 30 mL/min **Disp:** Soln 5, 10 mcg/dose in prefilled pen **SE:** Hypoglycemia, N/V/D, dizziness, HA, dyspepsia, ↓ appetite, jittery; acute pancreatitis **Notes:** Consider ↓ sulfonylurea to ↓ risk of hypoglycemia; discard pen 30 d after 1st use; monitor Tcr

Ezetimibe (Zetia) **Uses:** *Hypercholesterolemia alone or w/ a HMG-CoA reductase inhib* **Acts:** ↓ cholesterol & phytosterols absorption **Dose:** *Adults & Peds >10 y.* 10 mg/d PO **W/P:** [C, +/–] Bile acid sequestrants ↓ bioavailability **CI:** Hepatic impair **Disp:** Tabs 10 mg **SE:** HA, D, Abd pain, ↑ transaminases w/ HMG-CoA reductase inhib, erythema multiforme **Notes:** See ezetimibe/simvastatin

Ezetimibe/Simvastatin (Vytorin) **Uses:** *Hypercholesterolemia* **Acts:** ↓ Absorption of cholesterol & phytosterols w/ HMG-CoA-reductase inhib **Dose:** 10/10–10/80 mg/d PO; w/ cyclosporine/ or danazol: 10/10 mg/d max; w/ amio-darone/ or verapamil: 10/20 mg/d max; ↓ w/ severe renal Insuff; give 2 h before or 4 h after bile acid sequestrants **W/P:** [X, –] w/ CYP3A4 inhib (Table 10, p 301), gemfibrozil, niacin > 1 g/d, danazol, amiodarone, verapamil; avoid high dose w/ diltiazem; w/Chinese pt on lipid modifying meds **CI:** PRG/lactation; liver Dz, ↑ LFTs **Disp:** Tabs (mg ezetimibe/mg simvastatin) 10/10, 10/20, 10/40, 10/80 **SE:** HA, GI upset, myalgia, myopathy (muscle pain, weakness, or tenderness w/ cre-atine kinase 10 × ULN, rhabdomyolysis), hep, Infxn **Notes:** Monitor LFTs, lipids; ezetimibe/simvastatin combo lowered LDL more than simvastatin alone in ENHANCE study, but was no difference in carotid-intima media thickness; pts to report muscle pain

Famciclovir (Famvir) **Uses:** *Acute herpes zoster (shingles) & genital her-pes* **Acts:** ↓ Viral DNA synth **Dose:** *Zoster:* 500 mg PO q8h × 7 d. *Simplex:* 125–250 mg PO bid; ↓ w/ renal impair **W/P:** [B, –] **CI:** Component sensitivity **Disp:** Tabs 125, 250, 500 mg **SE:** Fatigue, dizziness, HA, pruritus, N/D **Notes:** Best w/in 72 h of initial lesion

Famotidine (Pepcid, Pepcid AC) [OTC] **Uses:** *Short-term Tx of duodenal ulcer & benign gastric ulcer; maint for duodenal ulcer, hypersecretory conditions,

GERD, & heartburn* **Acts:** H$_2$-antagonist; ↓ gastric acid **Dose: *Adults. Ulcer:*** 20 mg IV q12h or 20–40 mg PO qhs × 4–8 wk. *Hypersecretion:* 20–160 mg PO q6h. *GERD:* 20 mg PO bid × 6 wk; maint: 20 mg PO hs. *Heartburn:* 10 mg PO PRN q12h. ***Peds.*** 0.5–1 mg/kg/d; ↓ in severe renal Insuff **W/P:** [B, M] **CI:** Component sensitivity **Disp:** Tabs 10, 20, 40 mg; chew tabs 10 mg; susp 40 mg/5 mL; gelatin caps 10 mg, Inj 10 mg/2 mL **SE:** Dizziness, HA, constipation, N/V/D, ↓ plt, hepatitis **Notes:** Chew tabs contain phenylalanine

Febuxostat (Uloric) **Uses:** *Hyperuricemia and gout* **Action:** Xanthine oxidase inhib (enzyme that converts hypoxanthine to xanthine to uric acid) **Dose:** 40 mg PO 1× daily, ↑ 80 mg if uric acid not < 6 mg/dL after 2 wks **W/P:** [C, ?/–] **CI:** use w/azathioprine, mercaptopurine, theophylline **Supplied:** Tabs 40, 80 mg **SE:** ↑ LFTs, rash, myalgia **Notes:** OK to continue w/ gouty flare or use w/ NSAIDs

Felodipine (Plendil) **Uses:** *HTN & CHF* **Acts:** CCB **Dose:** 2.5–10 mg PO daily; swallow whole; ↓ in hepatic impair **W/P:** [C, ?] ↑ effect w/ azole antifungals, erythromycin, grapefruit juice **CI:** Component sensitivity **Disp:** ER tabs 2.5, 5, 10 mg **SE:** Peripheral edema, flushing, tachycardia, HA, gingival hyperplasia **Notes:** Follow BP in elderly & w/ hepatic impair

Fenofibrate (TriCor, Antara, Lofibra, Lipofen, Triglide) **Uses:** *Hypertriglyceridemia, hypercholesteremia* **Acts:** ↓ Triglyceride synth **Dose:** 43–160 mg/d; ↓ w/ renal impair; take w/ meals **W/P:** [C, ?] **CI:** Hepatic/severe renal Insuff, primary biliary cirrhosis, unexplained ↑ LFTs, gallbladder Dz **Disp:** Caps 50, 100, 150 mg; caps (micronized): (*Lofibra*) 67, 134, 200 mg, tabs 54, 160 mg (*Antara*) 43, 130 mg; **SE:** GI disturbances, cholecystitis, arthralgia, myalgia, dizziness, ↑ LFTs **Notes:** Monitor LFTs

Fenofibric Acid (Trilipix) **Uses:** * Adjunct to diet for ↑ triglycerides, to ↓ LDL-C, cholesterol, triglycerides, and apo B, to ↑ HDL-C in hypercholesterolemia/ mixed dyslipidemia; adjunct to diet w/ a statin to ↓ triglycerides and ↑ HDL-C w/ CHD or w/ CHD risk* **Action:** Agonist of peroxisome proliferator-activated receptor-alpha (PPAR-α),causes ↑ VLDL catabolism, fatty acid oxidation, and clearing of triglyceride-rich particles w/ ↓ VLDL, triglycerides; ↑ HDL in some **Dose:** Mixed dyslipidemia w/ a statin 135 mg PO × 1 daily; *Hypertriglyceridemia:* 45–135 mg 1× daily; Maint based on response; *Primary hypercholesterolemia/ mixed dyslipidemia:* 135 mg PO 1 × daily; 135 mg/d max **W/P:** [C, /–], Multiple interactions, ↑ embolic phenomenon **CI:** Severe renal impair, pt on dialysis, active liver/gall bladder Dz, nursing **Disp:** DR Caps 45, 135 mg **SE:** HA, back pain, nasopharyngitis, URI, N/D, myalgia, gall stones, ↓ CBC (usually stabilizes), rare myositis/rhabdomyolysis **Notes:** ✓CBC, lipid panel, LFTs; D/C if LFT > 3× ULN

Fenoldopam (Corlopam) **Uses:** *Hypertensive emergency* **Acts:** Rapid vasodilator **Dose:** Initial 0.03–0.1 mcg/kg/min IV Inf, titrate q15min by 1.6 mcg/kg/min, to max 0.05–0.1 mcg/kg/min **W/P:** [B, ?] ↓ BP w/ β-blockers **CI:** Allergy to sulfites **Disp:** Inj 10 mg/mL **SE:** ↓ BP, edema, facial flushing, N/V/D, atrial flutter/fibrillation, ↑ IOP **Notes:** Avoid concurrent β-blockers

Fenoprofen (Nalfon) BOX: May ↑ risk of CV events and GI bleeding Uses: *Arthritis & pain* Acts: NSAID Dose: 200–600 mg q4–8h, to 3200 mg/d max; w/ food W/P: [B (D 3rd tri), +/–] CHF, HTN, renal/hepatic impair, Hx PUD CI: NSAID sensitivity Disp: Caps 200, 300, 600 mg SE: GI disturbance, dizziness, HA, rash, edema, renal impair, hep Notes: Swallow whole

Fentanyl (Sublimaze) [C-II] Uses: *Short-acting analgesic* in anesthesia & PCA Acts: Narcotic analgesic Dose: *Adults.* 25–100 mcg/kg/dose IV/IM titrated; *Anesthesia:* 5–15 mcg/kg; *Pain:* 200 mcg over 15 min, titrate to effect *Peds.* 1–2 mcg/kg IV/IM q1–4h titrate; ↓ in renal impair W/P: [B, +] CI: Paralytic ileus ↑ ICP, resp depression, severe renal/hepatic impair Disp: Inj 0.05 mg/mL SE: Sedation, ↓ BP, ↓ HR, constipation, N, resp depression, miosis Notes: 0.1 mg fentanyl = 10 mg morphine IM

Fentanyl Iontophoretic Transdermal System (Ionsys) BOX: Use only w/ hospitalized pts, D/C on discharge; fentanyl may result in potentially life-threatening resp depression and death Uses: *Short-term in-hospital analgesia* Acts: Opioid narcotic, iontophoretic transdermal Dose: 40 mcg/activation by pt; dose given over 10 min; max over 24 h 3.2 mg (80 doses) W/P: [C, –] CI: See fentanyl Disp: Battery-operated self-contained transdermal system, 40 mcg/activation, 80 doses SE: See fentanyl, site Rxn Notes: Choose nl skin site chest or upper outer arm; titrate; to comfort, pts must have access to supplemental analgesia; instruct in device use; dispose properly at discharge

Fentanyl, Transdermal (Duragesic) [C-II] BOX: Potential for abuse and fatal OD Uses: *Persistent mod–severe chronic pain in pts already tolerant to opioids* Acts: Narcotic Dose: Apply Patch to upper torso q72h; dose based on narcotic requirements in previous 24 h; start 25 mcg/h patch q72h; ↓ in renal impair W/P: [B, +] w/ CYP3A4 inhib (Table 10, p 301) may ↑ fentanyl effect, w/ Hx substance abuse CI: Not opioid tolerant, short-term pain management, post-op outpatient pain in outpatient surgery, mild pain, PRN use, ↑ ICP, resp depression, severe renal/hepatic impair, peds < 2 y Disp: Patches 12.5, 25, 50, 75, 100 mcg/h SE: Resp depression (fatal), sedation, ↓ BP, ↓ HR, constipation, N, miosis Notes: 0.1 mg fentanyl = 10 mg morphine IM; do not cut patch; peak level in PRG 24–72 h

Fentanyl, Transmucosal (Abstral, Actiq, Fentora, Onsolis) [C-II] BOX: Potential for abuse and fatal OD; use only in pts w/ chronic pain who are opioid tolerant; CI in acute/post-op pain; do not substitute for other fentanyl products; fentanyl can be fatal to children, keep away; use w/ strong CYP3A4 inhib may ↑ fentanyl levels. *Abstral, Onsolis* restricted distribution Uses: *Breakthrough CA pain w/ tolerance to opioids* Acts: Narcotic analgesic, transmucosal absorption Dose: Titrate to effect

- *Abstral:* Start 100 mcg SL, 2 doses max per pain breakthrough episode; wait 2 h for next breakthrough dose; limit to < 4 breakthrough doses w/ successful baseline dosing
- *Actiq:* Start 200 mcg PO × 1, may repeat × 1 after 30 min

- *Fentora*: Start 100 mcg buccal tab × 1, may repeat in 30 min, 4 tabs/dose max
- *Onsolis*: Start 200 mcg film, ↑ 200 mcg increments to max 4 200-mcg films or single 1200-mcg film

W/P: [B, +] resp/CNS depression possible; CNS depressants/CYP3A4 inhib may ↑ effect; may impair tasks (driving, machinery); w/ severe renal/hepatic impair **CI:** Opioid intolerant patient, acute/post-op pain **Disp:**

- *Abstral*: SL tab 100, 200, 300, 400, 600, 800 mcg
- *Actiq*: Lozenges on stick 200, 400, 600, 800, 1200, 1600 mcg
- *Fentora*: Buccal tabs 100, 200, 300, 400, 600, 800 mcg
- *Onsolis*: Buccal soluble film 200, 400, 600, 800, 1200 mcg

SE: Sedation, ↓ BP, ↓ HR, constipation, N/V, ↓ resp, dyspnea, HA, miosis, anxiety, confusion, depression, rash dizziness **Notes:** 0.1 mg fentanyl = 10 mg IM morphine

Ferrous Gluconate (Fergon [OTC], Others)   **BOX:** Accidental OD of iron-containing products is a leading cause of fatal poisoning in children < 6 y. Keep out of reach of children **Uses:** *Iron-deficiency anemia* & Fe supl **Acts:** Dietary supl **Dose:** *Adults.* 100–200 mg of elemental Fe/d ÷ doses. *Peds.* 4–6 mg/kg/d ÷ doses; on empty stomach (OK w/ meals if GI upset occurs); avoid antacids **W/P:** [A, ?] **CI:** Hemochromatosis, hemolytic anemia **Disp:** Tabs Fergon 240 (27 mg Fe), 246 (28 mg Fe), 300 (34 mg Fe), 325 (36 mg Fe) **SE:** GI upset, constipation, dark stools, discoloration of urine, may stain teeth **Notes:** 12% Elemental Fe; false(+) stool guaiac; keep away from children; severe tox in OD

Ferrous Gluconate Complex (Ferrlecit)   **Uses:** *Iron deficiency anemia or supl to erythropoietin Rx therapy* **Acts:** Fe supl **Dose:** *Test dose:* 2 mL (25 mg Fe) IV over 1 h, if OK, 125 mg (10 mL) IV over 1 h. *Usual cumulative dose:* 1 g Fe over 8 sessions (until favorable Hct) **W/P:** [B, ?] **CI:** non–Fe-deficiency anemia; CHF; Fe overload **Disp:** Inj 12.5 mg/mL Fe **SE:** ↓ BP, serious allergic Rxns, GI disturbance, Inj site Rxn **Notes:** Dose expressed as mg Fe; may infuse during dialysis

Ferrous Sulfate (OTC)   **Uses:** *Fe-deficiency anemia & Fe supl* **Acts:** Dietary supl **Dose:** *Adults.* 100–200 mg elemental Fe/d in ÷ doses. *Peds.* 1–6 mg/kg/d ÷ daily–tid; on empty stomach (OK w/ meals if GI upset occurs); avoid antacids **W/P:** [A, ?] ↑ Absorption w/ vit C; ↓ absorption w/ tetracycline, fluoroquinolones, antacids, H_2 blockers, proton pump inhib **CI:** Hemochromatosis, hemolytic anemia **Disp:** Tabs 187 (60 mg Fe), 200 (65 mg Fe), 324 (65 mg Fe), 325 (65 mg Fe); SR caplets & tabs 160 (50 mg Fe), 200 mg (65 mg Fe); gtt 75 mg/0.6 mL (15 mg Fe/0.6 mL); elixir 220 mg/5 mL (44 mg Fe/5 mL); syrup 90 mg/5 mL (18 mg Fe/5 mL) **SE:** GI upset, constipation, dark stools, discolored urine

Ferumoxytol (Feraheme)   **Uses:** *Iron deficiency anemia in chronic kidney disease* **Acts:** Fe replacement **Dose:** *Adults.* 510 mg IV × 1, then 510 mg IV × 1 3–8 days later; give 1 mL/s **W/P:** [C, ?/–] Monitor for hypersens & ↓ BP for 30 mins after dose, may alter MRI studies **CI:** Iron overload; hypersens to ferumoxytol **Disp:** IV sol 30 mg/mL (510 mg elemental Fe/17 mL) **SE:** N/D, constipation, dizziness, hypotension, peripheral edema, hypersens Rxn **Notes:** ✓ hematologic response 1 month after 2nd dose

Fesoterodine Fumarate (Toviaz) Uses: * OAB w/ urge urinary incontinence, urgency, frequency * **Action:** Competitive muscarinic receptor antagonist, ↓ bladder muscle contractions **Dose:** 4 mg PO q day, ↑ to 8 mg PO daily PRN **W/P:** [C, /?] Avoid > 4 mg w/ severe renal insuff or w/ CYP3A4 inhib (e.g., ketoconazole, clarithromycin); w/ BOO, ↓ GI motility/constipation, NAG, MyG **CI:** urinary/gastric retention, or uncontrolled NAG, hypersens to class **Disp:** Tabs 5, 10 mg **SE:** Dry mouth, constipation, ↓ sweating can cause heat prostration

Fexofenadine (Allegra, Allegra-D) Uses: *Allergic rhinitis; chronic idiopathic urticaria* **Acts:** Selective antihistamine, antagonizes H_1-receptors; Allegra D contains w/ pseudoephedrine **Dose:** *Adults & Peds > 12 y.* 60 mg PO bid or 180 mg/d; 12-h ER form bid, 24-h ER form q day. *Peds 6–11 y.* 30 mg PO bid; ↓ in renal impair **W/P:** [C, ?] w/ Nevirapine **CI:** Component sensitivity **Disp:** Tabs 30, 60, 180 mg; susp 6 mg/mL; *Allegra-D* 12-h ER tab (60 mg fexofenadine/120 mg pseudoephedrine), *Allegra-D 24-h ER* (180 mg fexofenadine/240 mg pseudoephedrine) **SE:** Drowsiness (rare), HA, ischemic colitis

Fibrinogen Concentrate, Human (Riastap) Uses: *Rx acute bleeding associated w/ congenital fibrinogen deficiency * **Action:** Fibrinogen replacement **Dose:** *Adults & Peds.* 70 mg/kg IV, when baseline fibrinogen is known: Dose (mg/kg) = (Target fibrinogen level − actual fibrinogen level) ÷ 1.7. **W/P:** [C, ?] **Disp:** Inj 900–1300 mg (✓ vial label) **SE:** Fever, HA, hypersens rxn, thromboembolism **Notes:** Target fibrinogen level of 100 mg/dL

Fidaxomicin (Dificid) Uses: * *Clostridium difficile*-associated diarrhea* **Acts:** Macrolide antibiotic **Dose:** 200 mg PO bid × 10 d **W/P:** [B, +/–] Not for systemic Infxn or < 18 y; to ↓ resistance, use only when diagnosis suspected/proven **Disp:** Tabs 200 mg **SE:** N/V, abd pain, GI bleed, anemia, neutropenia

Filgrastim [G-CSF] (Neupogen) Uses: *↓ Incidence of Infxn in febrile neutropenic pts; Rx chronic neutropenia* **Acts:** Recombinant G-CSF **Dose:** *Adults & Peds.* 5 mcg/kg/d SQ or IV single daily dose; D/C when ANC > 10,000 cells/mm^3 **W/P:** [C, ?] w/ Drugs that potentiate release of neutrophils (e.g., Li) **CI:** Allergy to E. coli–derived proteins or G-CSF **Disp:** Inj 300, 600 mcg/mL **SE:** Fever, alopecia, N/V/D, splenomegaly, bone pain, HA, rash **Notes:** ✓ CBC & plt; monitor for cardiac events; no benefit w/ ANC > 10,000 cells/mm^3

Finasteride (Proscar [Generic], Propecia) Uses: *BPH & androgenetic alopecia* **Acts:** ↓ 5α-Reductase **Dose:** *BPH:* 5 mg/d PO. *Alopecia:* 1 mg/d PO; food ↓ absorption **W/P:** [X, −] Hepatic impair **CI:** Pregnant women should avoid handling pills, teratogen to male fetus **Disp:** Tabs 1 mg (Propecia), 5 mg (Proscar) **SE:** ↓ Libido, vol ejaculate, ED, gynecomastia; may slightly ↑ risk of high grade prostate Ca **Notes:** ↓ PSA by ~50%; reestablish PSA baseline 6 mo (double PSA for "true" reading); 3–6 mo for effect on urinary Sxs; continue to maintain new hair, not for use in women

Fingolimod (Gilenya) Uses: *Relapsing MS* Acts: Sphingosine 1-phosphate receptor modulator; ↓ lymphocyte migration into CNS Dose: Adults. 0.5 mg PO once/d; monitor for 6 h after 1st dose for bradycardia; monitor W/P: [C, −] monitor w/ severe hepatic impair and if on Class 1a or III antiarrhythmics/β-blockers/CCBs (rhythm disturbances); avoid live vaccines during & 2 mo after D/C; ketoconazole ↑ level Disp: Caps 0.5 mg SE: HA, D, back pain, dizziness, bradycardia, AV block, HTN, Infxns, macular edema, ↑ LFTs, cough, dyspnea Notes: Obtain baseline ECG, CBC, LFTs & eye exam; women of childbearing potential should use contraception during & 2 months after D/C

Flavoxate (Urispas) Uses: *Relief of Sx of dysuria, urgency, nocturia, suprapubic pain, urinary frequency, incontinence* Acts: Antispasmodic Dose: 100–200 mg PO tid-qid W/P: [B, ?] CI: GI obst, GI hemorrhage, ileus, achalasia, BPH Disp: Tabs 100 mg SE: Drowsiness, blurred vision, xerostomia

Flecainide (Tambocor) BOX: ↑ Mortality in pts w/ ventricular arrhythmias and recent MI; pulm effects reported; ventricular proarrhythmic effects in AF/A flutter, not ok for chronic AF Uses: Prevent AF/A flutter & PSVT, *prevent/suppress life-threatening ventricular arrhythmias* Acts: Class 1C antiarrhythmic Dose: Adults. 100 mg PO q12h; ↑ by 50 mg q12h q4d, to max 4400 mg/d max Peds. 3–6 mg/kg/d in 3 ÷ doses; ↓ w/ renal impair, W/P: [C, +] Monitor w/ hepatic impair, ↑ conc w/ amiodarone, digoxin, quinidine, ritonavir/amprenavir, β-blockers, verapamil; may worsen arrhythmias CI: 2nd-/3rd-degree AV block, right BBB w/ bifascicular or trifascicular block, cardiogenic shock, CAD, ritonavir/amprenavir, alkalinizing agents Disp: Tabs 50, 100, 150 mg SE: Dizziness, visual disturbances, dyspnea, palpitations, edema, chest pain, tachycardia, CHF, HA, fatigue, rash, N Notes: Initiate Rx in hospital; dose q8h if pt is intolerant/uncontrolled at q12h; Levels: Trough: Just before next dose; Therapeutic: 0.2–1 mcg/mL; Toxic: > 1 mcg/mL; 1/2-life: 11–14 h

Floxuridine (FUDR) BOX: Administration by experienced physician only; pts should be hospitalized for 1st course d/t risk for severe Rxn Uses: *GI adenoma, liver, renal CAs*; colon & pancreatic CAs Acts: Converted to 5-FU; inhibits thymidylate synthase; ↓ DNA synthase (S-phase specific) Dose: 0.1–0.6 mg/kg/d for 1–6 wk (per protocols) usually intraarterial for liver mets W/P: [D, −] Interaction w/ vaccines CI: BM suppression, poor nutritional status, serious Infxn, PRG, component sensitivity Disp: Inj 500 mg SE: ↓ BM, anorexia, Abd cramps, N/V/D, mucositis, alopecia, skin rash, & hyperpigmentation; rare neurotox (blurred vision, depression, nystagmus, vertigo, & lethargy); intraarterial catheter-related problems (ischemia, thrombosis, bleeding, & Infxn) Notes: Need effective birth control; palliative Rx for inoperable/incurable pts

Fluconazole (Diflucan) Uses: *Candidiasis (esophageal, oropharyngeal, urinary tract, vag, prophylaxis); cryptococcal meningitis, prophylaxis w/ BMT* Acts: Antifungal; ↓ cytochrome P-450 sterol demethylation. Spectrum: All Candida sp except C. krusei Dose: Adults. 100–400 mg/d PO or IV. Vaginitis: 150 mg PO daily. Crypto: doses up to 800 mg/d reported; 400 mg d 1, then 200 mg × 10–12 wk after CSF (−). **Peds.** 3–6 mg/kg/d PO or IV; 12 mg/kg/d/systemic Infxn; ↓ in renal impair **W/P:** [C, vag candidiasis (D high or prolonged dose) −] do not use w/ clopidogrel (↓ effect) **CI:** None **Disp:** Tabs 50, 100, 150, 200 mg; susp 10, 40 mg/mL; Inj 2 mg/mL **SE:** HA, rash, GI upset, ↓ K⁺, ↑ LFTs **Notes:** PO (preferred) = IV levels; cong anomalies w/ high dose 1st tri

Fludarabine Phosphate (Flamp, Fludara) **BOX:** Administer only under supervision of qualified physician experienced in chemotherapy. Can ↓ BM and cause severe CNS effects (blindness, coma, and death). Severe/fatal autoimmune hemolytic anemia reported; monitor for hemolysis. Use w/ pentostatin not ok (fatal pulm tox) **Uses:** *Autoimmune hemolytic anemia, CLL, cold agglutinin hemolysis*, low-grade lymphoma, mycosis fungoides **Acts:** ↓ Ribonucleotide reductase; blocks DNA polymerase-induced DNA repair **Dose:** 18–30 mg/m²/d for 5 d, as a 30-min Inf (per protocols); ↓ w/ renal impair **W/P:** [D, −] Give cytarabine before fludarabine (↓ its metabolism) **CI:** w/ Pentostatin, severe Infxns, CrCl < 30 mL/min, hemolytic anemia **Disp:** Inj 50 mL **SE:** ↓ BM, N/V/D, ↑ LFTs, edema, CHF, fever, chills, fatigue, dyspnea, nonproductive cough, pneumonitis, severe CNS tox rare in leukemia, autoimmune hemolytic anemia

Fludrocortisone Acetate (Florinef) **Uses:** *Adrenocortical Insuff, Addison Dz, salt-wasting synd* **Acts:** Mineralocorticoid **Dose:** **Adults.** 0.1–0.2 mg/d PO. **Peds.** 0.05–0.1 mg/d PO **W/P:** [C, ?] **CI:** Systemic fungal infxns; known allergy **Disp:** Tabs 0.1 mg **SE:** HTN, edema, CHF, HA, dizziness, convulsions, acne, rash, bruising, hyperglycemia, hypothalamic–pituitary–adrenal suppression, cataracts **Notes:** For adrenal Insuff, use w/ glucocorticoid; dose changes based on plasma renin activity

Flumazenil (Romazicon) **Uses:** *Reverse sedative effects of benzodiazepines & general anesthesia* **Acts:** Benzodiazepine receptor antagonist **Dose:** **Adults.** 0.2 mg IV over 15 s; repeat PRN, to 1 mg max (5 mg max in benzodiazepine OD). **Peds.** 0.01 mg/kg (0.2 mg/dose max) IV over 15 s; repeat 0.005 mg/kg at 1-min intervals to max 1 mg total; ↓ in hepatic impair **W/P:** [C, ?] **CI:** TCA OD; if pts given benzodiazepines to control life-threatening conditions (ICP/status epilepticus) **Disp:** Inj 0.1 mg/mL **SE:** N/V, palpitations, HA, anxiety, nervousness, hot flashes, tremor, blurred vision, dyspnea, hyperventilation, withdrawal synd **Notes:** Does not reverse narcotic Sx or amnesia, use associated w/ Szs

Flunisolide (AeroBid, Aerospan, Nasarel) **Uses:** *Asthma in pts requiring chronic steroid Rx; relieve seasonal/perennial allergic rhinitis* **Acts:** Topical steroid **Dose:** **Adults.** Metered-dose Inh: 2 Inh bid (max 8/d). Nasal: 2 sprays/nostril bid (max 8/d). **Peds > 6 y.** Metered-dose Inh: 2 Inh bid (max 4/d). Nasal: 1–2 sprays/nostril bid (max 4/d) **W/P:** [C, ?] w/ Adrenal Insuff **Disp:** AeroBid 0.25 mg/Inh; Nasarel 29 mcg/spray; Aerospan 80 mcg/Inh (CFC-free) **SE:** Tachycardia, bitter taste, local effects, oral candidiasis **Notes:** Not for acute asthma

Fluorouracil [5-FU] (Adrucil) **BOX:** Administration by experienced chemotherapy physician only; pts should be hospitalized for 1st course d/t risk for severe

Rxn Uses: *Colorectal, gastric, pancreatic, breast, basal cell*, head, neck, bladder, CAs **Acts:** Inhibits thymidylate synthetase (↓ DNA synth, S-phase specific) **Dose:** 370–1000 mg/m²/d × 1–5 d IV push to 24-h cont Inf; protracted venous Inf of 200–300 mg/m²/d (per protocol); 800 mg/d max **W/P:** [D, ?] ↑ tox w/ allopurinol; do not give live vaccine before 5-FU **CI:** Poor nutritional status, depressed BM Fxn, thrombocytopenia, major surgery w/in past mo, G6PD enzyme deficiency, PRG, serious Infxn, bili > 5 mg/dL **Disp:** Inj 50 mg/mL **SE:** Stomatitis, esophago- pharyngitis, N/V/D, anorexia, ↓ BM, rash/dry skin/photosens, tingling in hands/feet w/ pain (palmar–plantar erythrodysesthesia), phlebitis/discoloration at Inj sites **Notes:** ↑ Thiamine intake; contraception OK

Fluorouracil, Topical [5-FU] (Efudex) **Uses:** *Basal cell carcinoma; actinic/solar keratosis* **Acts:** Inhibits thymidylate synthetase (↓ DNA synth, S-phase specific) **Dose:** 5% cream bid × 2–6 wk **W/P:** [D, ?] Irritant chemotherapy **CI:** Component sensitivity **Disp:** Cream 0.5, 1, 5%; soln 1, 2, 5% **SE:** Rash, dry skin, photosens **Notes:** Healing may not be evident for 1–2 mo; wash hands thoroughly; avoid occlusive dressings; do not overuse

Fluoxetine (Prozac, Sarafem) **BOX:** Closely monitor for worsening depression or emergence of suicidality, particularly in ped pt **Uses:** *Depression, OCD, panic disorder, bulimia (Prozac)* *PMDD (Sarafem)* **Acts:** SSRI **Dose:** 20 mg/d PO (max 80 mg/d ÷ dose); weekly 90 mg/wk after 1–2 wk of standard dose. *Bulimia:* 60 mg q A.M. *Panic disorder:* 20 mg/d. *OCD:* 20–80 mg/d. *PMDD:* 20 mg/d or 20 mg intermittently, start 14 d prior to menses, repeat w/ each cycle; ↓ in hepatic failure **W/P:** [C, ?/–] Serotonin syndr w/ MAOI, SSRI, serotonin agonists, linezolid; QT prolongation w/ phenothiazines; do not use w/ clopidogrel (↓ effect) **CI:** w/ MAOI/thioridazine (wait 5 wk after D/C before MAOI) **Disp:** *Prozac:* Caps 10, 20, 40 mg; scored tabs 10, 20 mg; SR caps 90 mg; soln 20 mg/5 mL. *Sarafem:* Caps 10, 20 mg **SE:** N, nervousness, wgt loss, HA, insomnia

Fluoxymesterone (Halotestin, Androxy) [C-III] **Uses:** Androgen-responsive metastatic *breast CA, hypogonadism* **Acts:** ↓ Secretion of LH & FSH (feedback inhibition) **Dose:** *Breast CA:* 10–40 mg/d ÷ × 1–3 mo. *Hypogonadism:* 5–20 mg/d **W/P:** [X, ?/–] ↑ Effect w/ anticoagulants, cyclosporine, insulin, Li, narcotics **CI:** Serious cardiac, liver, or kidney Dz; PRG **Disp:** Tabs 10 mg **SE:** Priapism, edema, virilization, amenorrhea & menstrual irregularities, hirsutism, alopecia, acne, N, cholestasis; suppression of factors II, V, VII, & X, & polycythemia; ↑ libido, HA, anxiety **Notes:** Radiographic exam of hand/wrist q6mo in prepubertal children; ↓ total T₄ levels

Flurazepam (Dalmane) [C-IV] **Uses:** *Insomnia* **Acts:** Benzodiazepine **Dose:** *Adults & Peds > 15 y.* 15–30 mg PO qhs PRN; ↓ in elderly **W/P:** [X, ?/–] Elderly, low albumin, hepatic impair **CI:** NAG; PRG **Disp:** Caps 15, 30 mg **SE:** "Hangover" d/t accumulation of metabolites, apnea, anaphylaxis, angioedema, amnesia **Notes:** May cause dependency

Flurbiprofen (Ansaid, Ocufen) BOX: May ↑ risk of CV events and GI bleeding Uses: *Arthritis, ocular surgery* Acts: NSAID Dose: 50–300 mg/d ÷ bid-qid, max 300 mg/d w/ food, ocular 1 gtt q 30 min × 4, beginning 2 h pre-op W/P: [B (D in 3rd tri), +] CI: PRG (3rd tri); ASA allergy Disp: Tabs 50, 100 mg SE: Dizziness, GI upset, peptic ulcer Dz, ocular irritation

Flutamide (Eulexin) BOX: Liver failure & death reported. Measure LFTs before, monthly, & periodically after; D/C immediately if ALT 2 × ULN or jaundice develops Uses: Advanced *PCa* (w/ LHRH agonists, e.g., leuprolide or goserelin); w/ radiation & GnRH for localized CAP Acts: Nonsteroidal antiandrogen Dose: 250 mg PO tid (750 mg total) W/P: [D, ?] CI: Severe hepatic impair Disp: Caps 125 mg SE: Hot flashes, loss of libido, impotence, N/V/D, gynecomastia, hepatic failure Notes: ✓ LFTs, avoid EtOH

Fluticasone Furoate, Nasal (Veramyst) Uses: *Seasonal allergic rhinitis* Acts: Topical steroid Dose: *Adults & Peds > 12 y.* 2 sprays/nostril/d, then 1 spray /d maint. *Peds 2–11 y.* 1–2 sprays/nostril/d W/P: [C, M] Avoid w/ ritonavir, other steroids, recent nasal surgery/trauma CI: None Disp: Nasal spray 27.5 mcg/actuation SE: HA, epistaxis, nasopharyngitis, pyrexia, pharyngolaryngeal pain, cough, nasal ulcers, back pain, anaphylaxis

Fluticasone Propionate, Nasal (Flonase) Uses: *Seasonal allergic rhinitis* Acts: Topical steroid Dose: *Adults & Peds > 12 y.* 2 sprays/nostril/d *Peds 4–11 y.* 1–2 sprays/nostril/d W/P: [C, M] CI: Primary Rx of status asthmaticus Disp: Nasal spray 50 mcg/actuation SE: HA, dysphonia, oral candidiasis

Fluticasone Propionate, Inhalation (Flovent HFA, Flovent Diskus) Uses: *Chronic asthma* Acts: Topical steroid Dose: *Adults & Peds > 12 y.* 2–4 puffs bid. *Peds 4–11 y.* 44 or 50 mcg bid W/P: [C, M] CI: Status asthmaticus Disp: *Diskus dry powder:* 50, 100, 250 mcg/action; HFA; MDI 44/110/220 mcg/ Inh SE: HA, dysphonia, oral candidiasis Notes: Risk of thrush, rinse mouth after; counsel on use of devices

Fluticasone Propionate & Salmeterol Xinafoate (Advair Diskus, Advair HFA) BOX: Increased risk of worsening wheezing or asthma-related death w/ long-acting β_2-adrenergic agonists; use only if asthma not controlled on agent such as inhaled steroid Uses: *Maint Rx for asthma* Acts: Corticosteroid w/ LA bronchodilator β_2 agonist Dose: *Adults & Peds > 12 y.* 1 Inh bid q12h; titrate to lowest effective dose (4 Inh or 920/84 mcg/d max) W/P: [C, M] CI: Acute asthma attack; conversion from PO steroids; w/ phenothiazines Disp: Diskus = metered-dose Inh powder (fluticasone/salmeterol in mcg) 100/50, 250/50, 500/50; HFA = aerosol 45/21, 115/21, 230/21 mg SE: Upper resp Infxn, pharyngitis, HA Notes: Combo of Flovent & Serevent; do not wash mouthpiece, do not exhale into device; Advair HFA for pts not controlled on other meds (e.g., low-medium dose Inh steroids) or whose Dz severity warrants 2 maint therapies

Fluvastatin (Lescol) Uses: *Atherosclerosis, primary hypercholesterolemia, heterozygous familial hypercholesterolemia hypertriglyceridemia* Acts: HMG-CoA reductase inhib **Dose:** 20–40 mg bid PO or XL 80 mg/d ↓ w/ hepatic impair **W/P:** [X, −] **CI:** Active liver Dz, ↑ LFTs, PRG, breast-feeding **Disp:** Caps 20, 40 mg; XL 80 mg **SE:** HA, dyspepsia, N/D, Abd pain **Notes:** Dose no longer limited to HS; ✓ LFTs; OK w/ grapefruit

Fluvoxamine (Luvox, Luvox CR)   **BOX:** Closely monitor for worsening depression or emergence of suicidality, particularly in ped pts **Uses:** *OCD, SAD* **Acts:** SSRI **Dose:** Initial 50-mg single qhs dose, ↑ to 300 mg/d in ÷ doses; *CR:* 100–300 mg PO qhs, may ↑ by 50 mg/d q wk, max 300 mg/d ↓ in elderly/hepatic impair, titrate slowly; ÷ doses > 100 mg **W/P:** [C, ?/−] multiple interactions (see PI: MAOIs, phenothiazines, SSRIs, serotonin agonists, others); do not use w/ clopidogrel **CI:** MAOI w/in 14 d, w/ alosetron, tizanidine, thioridazine, pimozide **Disp:** Tabs 25, 50, 100 mg; Caps ER 100, 150 mg **SE:** HA, N/D, somnolence, insomnia, ↓ Na⁺, **Notes:** gradual taper to D/C

Folic Acid   **Uses:** *Megaloblastic anemia; folate deficiency* **Acts:** Dietary supl **Dose:** *Adults.* *Supl:* 0.4 mg/d PO. *PRG:* 0.8 mg/d PO. *Folate deficiency:* 1 mg PO daily–tid. *Peds.* *Supl:* 0.04–0.4 mg/24 h PO, IM, IV, or SQ. *Folate deficiency:* 0.5–1 mg/24 h PO, IM, IV, or SQ **W/P:** [A, +] **CI:** Pernicious, aplastic, normocytic anemias **Disp:** Tabs 0.4, 0.8, 1 mg; Inj 5 mg/mL **SE:** Well tolerated **Notes:** OK for all women of childbearing age; ↓ fetal neural tube defects by 50%; no effect on normocytic anemias

Fondaparinux (Arixtra)   **BOX:** When epidural/spinal anesthesia or spinal puncture is used, pts anticoagulated or scheduled to be anticoagulated w/ LMW heparins, heparinoids, or fondaparinux are at risk for epidural or spinal hematoma, which can result in long-term or permanent paralysis **Uses:** *DVT prophylaxis* w/ hip fracture, hip or knee replacement, Abd surgery; w/ DVT or PE in combo w/ warfarin **Acts:** Synth inhib of activated factor X; a pentasaccharide **Dose:** *Prophylaxis* 2.5 mg SQ daily, up to 5–9 d; start > 6 h post-op; *Tx:* 7.5 mg SQ daily (< 50 kg: 5 mg SQ daily; > 100 kg: 10mg SQ daily); ↓ w/ renal impair **W/P:** [B, ?] ↑ Bleeding risk w/ anticoagulants, anti-plts, drotrecogin alfa, NSAIDs **CI:** Wgt < 50 kg, CrCl < 30 mL/min, active bleeding, SBE ↓ plt w/ anti-plt Ab **Disp:** Prefilled syringes w/ 27-gauge needle: 2.5/0.5, 5/0.4, 7.5 /0.6, 10/0.8, mg/mL **SE:** Thrombocytopenia, anemia, fever, N **Notes:** D/C if plts < 100,000 cells/mcL; only give SQ; may monitor antifactor Xa levels

Formoterol Fumarate (Foradil, Perforomist)   **BOX:** May ↑ risk of asthma-related death **Uses:** *Long-term Rx of bronchoconstriction in COPD, EIB (only Foradil)* **Acts:** LA β₂-agonist **Dose:** *Adults. Perforomist:* 20-mcg Inh q12h; *Foradil:* 12-mcg Inh q12h, 24 mcg/d max; *EIB:* 12 mcg 15 min before exercise *Peds* > 5y. (Foradil) See Adults **W/P:** [C, M] Not for acute Sx, w/ CV Dz, w/ adrenergic meds, xanthine derivatives meds that ↑ QT; β-blockers may ↓ effect, D/C w/ ECG change **CI:** None **Disp:** Foradil caps 12 mcg for Aerolizer Inhaler (12 & 60 doses) **SE:** N/D, nasopharyngitis, dry mouth, angina, HTN, ↓ BP, tachycardia, arrhythmias, nervousness, HA, tremor, muscle cramps, palpitations, dizziness **Notes:** excess use may ↑ ↑ CV risks; not for oral use

Fosamprenavir (Lexiva) **BOX:** Do not use w/ severe liver dysfunction, reduce dose w/ mild–mod liver impair (fosamprenavir 700 mg bid w/o ritonavir) **Uses:** HIV Infxn **Acts:** Protease inhib **Dose:** 1400 mg bid w/o ritonavir; w/ritonavir, fosamprenavir 1400 mg + ritonavir 200 mg daily or fosamprenavir 700 mg + ritonavir 100 mg bid; w/ efavirenz & ritonavir: fosamprenavir 1400 mg + ritonavir 300 mg daily **W/P:** [C, ?/–] do not use w/salmeterol, colchicine (w/ renal/hepatic failure); adjust dose w/ bosentan, tadalafil for PAH **CI:** w/ CYPA4 drugs (Table 10, p 301) such as w/ rifampin, lovastatin, simvastatin, delavirdine, ergot alkaloids, midazolam, triazolam, or pimozide; sulfa allergy; w/ alpha 1-adrenoceptor antagonist (alfuzosin); w/ PDE5 inhibitor sildenafil **Disp:** Tabs 700 mg **SE:** N/V/D, HA, fatigue, rash **Notes:** Numerous drug interactions because of hepatic metabolism; replaced amprenavir

Fosaprepitant (Emend, Injection) **Uses:** *Prevent chemotherapy-associated N/V* **Acts:** Substance P/neurokinin 1 receptor antagonist **Dose:** *Chemotherapy:* 115 mg IV 30 min before chemotherapy on d 1 (followed by aprepitant [Emend, Oral] 80 mg PO days 2 and 3) in combo w/ other antiemetics **W/P:** [B, ?/–] Potential for drug interactions, substrate and mod CYP3A4 inhib (dose-dependent); ↓ effect of OCP and warfarin **CI:** w/ Pimozide, terfenadine, astemizole, or cisapride **Disp:** Inj 115 mg **SE:** N/D, weakness, hiccups, dizziness, HA, dehydration, hot flushing, dyspepsia, Abd pain, neutropenia, ↑ LFTs, Inj site discomfort **Notes:** See also Aprepitant (Emend, Oral)

Foscarnet (Foscavir) **Uses:** *CMV retinitis*; acyclovir-resistant *herpes infxns* **Acts:** ↓ Viral DNA polymerase & RT **Dose:** *CMV retinitis: Induction:* 60 mg/kg IV q8h or 100 mg/kg q12h × 14–21 d. *Maint:* 90–120 mg/kg/d IV (Mon–Fri). *Acyclovir-resistant HSV: Induction:* 40 mg/kg IV q8–12h × 14–21 d; use central line; ↓ w/ renal impair **W/P:** [C, –] ↑ Sz potential w/ fluoroquinolones; avoid nephrotoxic Rx (cyclosporine, aminoglycosides, amphotericin B, protease inhib) **CI:** CrCl < 0.4 mL/min/kg **Disp:** Inj 24 mg/mL **SE:** Nephrotox, electrolyte abnormalities **Notes:** Sodium loading (500 mL 0.9% NaCl) before & after helps minimize nephrotox; monitor-ionized Ca^{2+}

Fosfomycin (Monurol) **Uses:** *Uncomplicated UTI* **Acts:** ↓ cell wall synth *Spectrum:* gram(+) *Enterococcus,* staphylococci, pneumococci; gram(–) (*E. coli, Salmonella, Shigella, H. influenzae, Neisseria,* indole(–) *Proteus, Providencia*); *B. fragilis* & anaerobic gram(–) cocci are resistant **Dose:** 3 g PO in 90–120 mL of H_2O single dose; ↓ in renal impair **W/P:** [B, ?] ↓ Absorption w/ antacids/Ca salts **CI:** Component sensitivity **Disp:** Granule packets 3 g **SE:** HA, GI upset **Notes:** May take 2–3 d for Sxs to improve

Fosinopril (Monopril) **Uses:** *HTN, CHF*, DN **Acts:** ACE inhib **Dose:** 10 mg/d PO initial; max 40 mg/d PO; ↓ in elderly; ↓ in renal impair **W/P:** [D, +] ↑ K^+ w/ K^+ supls, ARBs, K^+-sparing diuretics; ↑ renal after effects w/ NSAIDs, diuretics, hypovolemia **CI:** Hereditary/idiopathic angioedema or angioedema w/ ACE inhib, bilateral RAS **Disp:** Tabs 10, 20, 40 mg **SE:** Cough, dizziness, angioedema, ↑ K^+

Fosphenytoin (Cerebyx) Uses: *Status epilepticus* Acts: ↓ Sz spread in motor cortex Dose: As phenytoin equivalents (PE). *Load:* 15–20 mg PE/kg. *Maint:* 4–6 mg PE/kg/d; ↓ dosage, monitor levels in hepatic impair W/P: [D, +] May ↑ phenobarbital CI: Sinus bradycardia, SA block, 2nd-/3rd-degree AV block, Adams–Stokes synd, rash during Rx Disp: Inj 75 mg/mL SE: ↓ BP, dizziness, ataxia, pruritus, nystagmus Notes: 15 min to convert fosphenytoin to phenytoin; administer < 150 mg PE/min to prevent ↓ BP; administer w/ BP monitoring

Frovatriptan (Frova) Uses: *Rx acute migraine* Acts: Vascular serotonin receptor agonist Dose: 2.5 mg PO repeat in 2 h PRN; max 7.5 mg/d W/P: [C, ?/–] CI: Angina, ischemic heart Dz, coronary artery vasospasm, hemiplegic or basilar migraine, uncontrolled HTN, ergot use, MAOI use w/in 14 d Supplied: Tabs 2.5 mg SE: N, V, dizziness, hot flashes, paresthesias, dyspepsia, dry mouth, hot/cold sensation, chest pain, skeletal pain, flushing, weakness, numbness, coronary vasospasm, HTN

Fulvestrant (Faslodex) Uses: *HR(+) metastatic breast CA in postmenopausal women w/ progression following antiestrogen Rx therapy* Acts: Estrogen receptor antagonist Dose: 250 mg IM monthly, as single 5-mL Inj or 2 concurrent 2.5-mL IM Inj in buttocks W/P: [X, ?/–] ↑ Effects w/ CYP3A4 inhib (Table 10, p 301); w/ hepatic impair CI: PRG Disp: Prefilled syringes 50 mg/mL (single 5 mL, dual 2.5 mL) SE: N/V/D, constipation, Abd pain, HA, back pain, hot flushes, pharyngitis, Inj site Rxns Notes: Only use IM

Furosemide (Lasix) Uses: *CHF, HTN, edema*, ascites Acts: Loop diuretic; ↓ Na & Cl reabsorption in ascending loop of Henle & distal tubule Dose: *Adults* 20–80 mg PO or IV bid. *Peds.* 1 mg/kg/dose IV q6–12h; 2 mg/kg/dose PO q12–24h (max 6 mg/kg/dose); ↑ doses w/ renal impair W/P: [C, +] ↓ K⁺, ↑ risk digoxin tox & ototox w/ aminoglycosides, cisplatin (especially in renal dysfunction) CI: Sulfonylurea allergy; anuria; hepatic coma; electrolyte depletion Disp: Tabs 20, 40, 80 mg; soln 10 mg/mL, 40 mg/5 mL; Inj 10 mg/mL SE: ↓ BP, hyperglycemia, ↓ K⁺ Notes: ✓ Lytes, renal Fxn; high doses IV may cause ototox

Gabapentin (Neurontin) Uses: Adjunct in *partial Szs*; postherpetic neuralgia (PHN)*; chronic pain synds Acts: Anticonvulsant; GABA analog Dose: *Adults & Peds > 12 y. Anticonvulsant:* 300 mg PO tid, ↑ max 3600 mg/d. *PHN:* 300 mg day 1, 300 mg bid day 2, 300 mg tid day 3, titrate (1800–3600 mg/d); *Peds 3–12 y.* Start 0–15 mg/kg/d ÷ tid, ↑ over 3 d: *3–4 y:* 40 mg/kg/d given tid ≥5 y: 25–35 mg/kg/d ÷ tid, 50 mg/kg max; ↓ w/ renal impair W/P: [C, ?] Use in peds 3–12 y w/ epilepsy may ↑ CNS-related adverse events CI: Component sensitivity Disp: Caps 100, 300, 400 mg; soln 250 mg/5 mL; scored tab 600, 800 mg SE: Somnolence, dizziness, ataxia, fatigue Notes: Not necessary to monitor levels; taper ↑ or ↓ over 1 wk

Galantamine (Razadyne, Razadyne ER) Uses: *Mild–mod Alzheimer Dz* Acts: ? acetylcholinesterase inhib Dose: *Razadyne* 4 mg PO bid, ↑ to 8 mg bid after 4 wk; may ↑ to 16 mg bid in 4 wk; target 16–24 mg/d ÷ bid. *Razadyne ER*

Start 8 mg/d, ↑ to 16 mg/d after 4 wk, then to 24 mg/d after 4 more wk; give q A.M. w/ food **W/P:** [B, ?] w/ heart block, ↑ effect w/ succinylcholine, bethanechol, amiodarone, diltiazem, verapamil, NSAIDs, digoxin; ↓ effect w/ anticholinergics; ↑ risk of death w/ mild impair **CI:** Severe renal/hepatic impair **Disp:** *Razadyne* Tabs 4, 8, 12 mg; soln 4 mg/mL. *Razadyne ER* Caps 8, 16, 24 mg **SE:** GI disturbances, ↓ wgt, sleep disturbances, dizziness, HA **Notes:** Caution w/ urinary outflow obst, Parkinson Dz, ↑ w/ severe asthma/COPD, severe heart Dz or ↓ BP

Gallium Nitrate (Ganite)   BOX: ↑ Risk of severe renal Insuff w/ concurrent use of nephrotoxic drugs (e.g., aminoglycosides, amphotericin B). D/C if use of potentially nephrotoxic drug is indicated; hydrate several days after administration. D/C w/ SCr > 2.5 mg/dL **Uses:** *↑ Ca^{2+} of malignancy*; bladder CA **Acts:** ↓ Bone resorption of Ca^{2+} **Dose:** ↑ Ca^{2+}: 100–200 mg/m²/d × 5 d. *CA:* 350 mg/m² cont Inf × 5 d to 700 mg/m² rapid IV Inf q2wk in antineoplastic settings (per protocols) **W/P:** [C, ?] Do not give w/ live or rotavirus vaccine **CI:** SCr > 2.5 mg/dL **Disp:** Inj 25 mg/mL **SE:** Renal Insuff, ↓ Ca^{2+}, hypophosphatemia, ↓ bicarb, < 1% acute optic neuritis **Notes:** Bladder CA, use in combo w/ vinblastine & ifosfamide

Ganciclovir (Cytovene, Vitrasert)   Uses: *Rx & prevent CMV retinitis, prevent CMV Dz* in transplant recipients **Acts:** ↓ viral DNA synth **Dose:** *Adults & Peds*. *IV:* 5 mg/kg IV q12h for 14–21 d, then maint 5 mg/kg/d IV × 7 d/wk or 6 mg/kg/d IV × 5 d/wk. *Ocular implant:* One implant q5–8mo. **Adults.** *PO:* Following induction, 1000 mg PO tid. *Prevention:* 1000 mg PO tid; w/ food; ↓ in renal impair **W/P:** [C, –] ↑ Effect w/ immunosuppressives, imipenem/cilastatin, zidovudine, didanosine, other nephrotoxic Rx **CI:** ANC < 500 cells/mm³, plt < 25,000 cells/mm³, intravitreal implant **Disp:** Caps 250, 500 mg; Inj 500 mg, ocular implant 4.5 mg **SE:** Granulocytopenia & thrombocytopenia, fever, rash, GI upset **Notes:** Not a cure for CMV; handle Inj w/ cytotoxic cautions; no systemic benefit w/ implant

Ganciclovir, Ophthalmic Gel (Zirgan)   Uses: *Acute herpetic keratitis (dendritic ulcers* **Acts:** ↓ viral DNA synth **Dose:** *Adult & Peds ≥2 y.* 1 gtt affected eye/s 5 × daily (q3h while awake) until ulcer heals, then 1 gtt tid × 7 d **W/P:** [C, ?/–] Remove contacts during therapy **CI:** None **Disp:** Gel, 5-g tube **SE:** Blurred vision, eye irritation, punctate keratitis, conjunctival hyperemia **Notes:** Correct ↓ Ca^{2+} before use; ✓ Ca^{2+}

Gefitinib (Iressa)   Uses: *Rx locally advanced or metastatic NSCLC after platinum-based & docetaxel chemotherapy fails* **Acts:** selective TKI of EGFR **Dose:** 250 mg/d PO **W/P:** [D, –] **Disp:** Tabs 250 mg **SE:** D, rash, acne, dry skin, N/V, interstitial lung Dz, ↑ transaminases **Notes:** ✓ LFTs, only give to pts who have already received drug; no new pts because it has not been shown to increase survival

Gemcitabine (Gemzar)   Uses: *Pancreatic CA (single agent), breast CA w/ paclitaxel, NSCLC w/cisplatin, ovarian CA w/carboplatin*, gastric CA **Acts:** Antimetabolite; nucleoside metabolic inhibitor; ↓ ribonucleotide reductase; produces false nucleotide base-inhibiting DNA synth **Dose:** 1000–1250 mg/m^2 over 30 min–1 h IV Inf/wk × 3–4 wk or 6–8 wk; modify dose based on hematologic Fxn (per protocol) **W/P:** [D, ?/–] **CI:** PRG **Disp:** Inj 200 mg, 1 g **SE:** ↓ BM, N/V/D, drug fever, skin rash **Notes:** Reconstituted soln 38 mg/mL; monitor hepatic/renal Fxn

Gemfibrozil (Lopid)   **Uses:** *Hypertriglyceridemia, coronary heart Dz* **Acts:** Fibric acid **Dose:** 1200 mg/d PO ÷ bid 30 min ac A.M. & P.M. **W/P:** [C, ?] ↑ Warfarin effect, sulfonylureas; ↑ risk of myopathy w/ HMG-CoA reductase inhib; ↓ effects w/ cyclosporine **CI:** Renal/hepatic impair (SCr > 2.0 mg/dL), gallbladder Dz, primary biliary cirrhosis, use w/ repaglinide (↓ glucose) **Disp:** Tabs 600 mg **SE:** Cholelithiasis, GI upset **Notes:** Avoid w/HMG-CoA reductase inhib; ✓ LFTs & serum lipids

Gemifloxacin (Factive)   **Uses:** *CAP, acute exacerbation of chronic bronchitis* **Acts:** ↓ DNA gyrase & topoisomerase IV; *Spectrum:* S. pneumoniae (including multidrug-resistant strains), H. influenzae, H. parainfluenzae, M. catarrhalis, M. pneumoniae, C. pneumoniae, K. pneumoniae **Dose:** 320 mg PO daily × 5–7 d; CrCl < 40 mL/min: 160 mg PO/d **W/P:** [C, ?/–]; Peds < 18 y; Hx of ↑ QTc interval, electrolyte disorders, w/ class IA/III antiarrhythmics, erythromycin, TCAs, antipsychotics, ↑ INR and bleeding risk w/ warfarin **CI:** Fluoroquinolone allergy **Disp:** Tab 320 mg **SE:** Rash, N/V/D, *C. difficile* enterocolitis, ↑ risk of Achilles tendon rupture, tendonitis, Abd pain, dizziness, xerostomia, arthralgia, allergy/anaphylactic Rxns, peripheral neuropathy, tendon rupture **Notes:** Take 3 h before or 2 h after Al/Mg antacids, Fe 2^{2+}, Zn^{2+} or other metal cations; ↑ rash risk w/ ↑ duration of Rx

Gemtuzumab Ozogamicin (Mylotarg) [Withdrawn From Market 2010]   Fatal induction phase toxicity and lack of efficacy issues. Patients under treatment can complete course.

Gentamicin (Garamycin, G-mycitin, Others)   **Uses:** *Septicemia, serious bacterial Infxn of CNS, urinary tract, resp tract, GI tract, including peritonitis, skin, bone, soft tissue, including burns; severe Infxn P. aeruginosa w/ carbenicillin; group D streptococci endocarditis w/ PCN-type drug; serious staphylococcal Infxns, but not the antibiotic of 1st choice; mixed Infxn w/ staphylococci and gram(–)* **Acts:** Aminoglycoside, bactericidal; ↓ protein synth *Spectrum:* gram(–) (not *Neisseria, Legionella, Acinetobacter*); weaker gram(+) but synergy w/ PCNs **Dose:** *Adults. Standard:* 1–2 mg/kg IV q8–12h or daily dosing 4–7 mg/kg q24h IV. *Gram(+) Synergy:* 1 mg/kg q8h **Peds.** *Infants < 7 d < 1200 g.* 2.5 mg/kg/dose q18–24h. *Infants > 1200 g:* 2.5 mg/kg/dose q12–18h. *Infants > 7 d:* 2.5 mg/kg/dose IV q8–12h. *Children:* 2.5 mg/kg/d IV q8h; ↓ w/ renal Insuff; if obese, dose based on IBW **W/P:** [C, +/–] Avoid other nephrotoxics **CI:** Aminoglycoside sensitivity **Disp:** Premixed Inf 40, 60, 70, 80, 90, 100, 120 mg; ADD-Vantage Inj vials 10 mg/mL; Inj 40 mg/mL; IT preservative-free 2 mg/mL **SE:** Nephro-/oto-/neurotox **Notes:** Follow CrCl, SCr & serum conc for dose adjustments; use IBW to dose (use adjusted if obese > 30% IBW); OK to use intraperitoneal for peritoneal dialysis-related Infxns *Levels: Peak:* 30 min after Inf; *Trough:* < 0.5 h before next dose; *Therapeutic: Peak:* 5–8 mcg/mL, *Trough:* < 2 mcg/mL, if > 2 mcg/mL associated w/ renal tox

Gentamicin, Ophthalmic (Garamycin, Genoptic, Gentacidin, Gentak, Others) Uses: *Conjunctival infxns* Acts: Bactericidal; ↓ protein synth Dose: *Oint:* Apply 1/2 inch bid-tid. *Soln:* 1–2 gtt q2–4h, up to 2 gtt/h for severe Infxn W/P: [C, ?] CI: Aminoglycoside sensitivity Disp: Soln & oint 0.1% and 0.3% SE: Local irritation Notes: Do not use other eye drops w/in 5–10 min; do not touch dropper to eye

Gentamicin, Topical (Garamycin, G-mycitin) Uses: *Skin Infxns* caused by susceptible organisms Acts: Bactericidal; ↓ protein synth Dose: *Adults & Peds > 1 y:* Apply tid-qid W/P: [C, ?] CI: Aminoglycoside sensitivity Disp: Cream & oint 0.1% SE: Irritation

Gentamicin & Prednisolone, Ophthalmic (Pred-G Ophthalmic) Uses: *Steroid-responsive ocular & conjunctival Infxns* sensitive to gentamicin Acts: Bactericidal; ↓ protein synth w/ anti-inflammatory. *Spectrum: Staphylococcus, E. coli, H. influenzae, Klebsiella, Neisseria, Pseudomonas, Proteus, & Serratia* sp Dose: *Oint:* 1/2 inch in conjunctival sac daily-tid. *Susp:* 1 gtt bid-qid, up to 1 gtt/h for severe Infxn CI: Aminoglycoside sensitivity W/P: [C, ?] Disp: *Oint, ophthal:* Prednisolone acetate 0.6% & gentamicin sulfate 0.3% (3.5 g). *Susp, ophthal:* Prednisolone acetate 1% & gentamicin sulfate 0.3% (2, 5, 10 mL) SE: Local irritation

Glimepiride (Amaryl) Uses: *Type 2 DM* Acts: Sulfonylurea; ↑ pancreatic insulin release; ↑ peripheral insulin sensitivity; ↓ hepatic glucose output/production Dose: 1–4 mg/d, max 8 mg W/P: [C, –] CI: DKA Disp: Tabs 1, 2, 4 mg SE: HA, hypoglycemia Notes: Give w/ 1st meal of day

Glimepiride/Pioglitazone (Duetact) Uses: *Adjunct to exercise type 2 DM not controlled by single agent* Acts: Sulfonylurea (↓ glucose) w/ agent that ↑ insulin sensitivity & ↓ gluconeogenesis Dose: initial 30 mg/2 mg PO q A.M; 45 mg pioglitazone/8 mg glimepiride/d max; w/food W/P: [C, ?/–] w/ Liver impair, elderly. w/ Hx bladder CA; do not use w/ active bladder CA CI: Component hypersens, DKA Disp: Tabs 30/2, 30 mg/4 mg SE: Hct, ↑ ALT, ↓ glucose, URI, ↑ wgt, edema, HA, N/D, may ↑ CV mortality Notes: Monitor CBC, ALT, Cr, wgt

Glipizide (Glucotrol, Glucotrol XL) Uses: *Type 2 DM* Acts: Sulfonylurea; ↑ pancreatic insulin release; ↑ peripheral insulin sensitivity; ↓ hepatic glucose output/production; ↓ intestinal glucose absorption Dose: 5 mg initial, ↑ by 2.5–5 mg/d, max 40 mg/d; XL max 20 mg; 30 min ac; hold if NPO W/P: [C, ?/–] Severe liver Dz CI: DKA, type 1 DM, sulfonamide sensitivity Disp: Tabs 5, 10 mg; XL tabs 2.5, 5, 10 mg SE: HA, anorexia, N/V/D, constipation, fullness, rash, urticaria, photosens Notes: Counsel about DM management; wait several days before adjusting dose; monitor glucose

Glucagon Uses: Severe *hypoglycemic* Rxns in DM w/ sufficient liver glycogen stores; β-blocker/CCB OD **Acts:** Accelerates liver gluconeogenesis **Dose:** *Adults.* 0.5–1 mg SQ, IM, or IV; repeat in 20 min PRN. *ECC 2010.* β-*Blocker or CCB overdose:* 3–10 mg slow IV over 3–5 min; follow w/ inf of 3–5 mg/h; Hypoglycemia: 1 mg IV, IM, or SQ. *Peds. Neonates:* 0.3 mg/kg/dose SQ, IM, or IV q4h PRN. *Children:* 0.025–0.1 mg/kg/dose SQ, IM, or IV; repeat in 20 min PRN **W/P:** [B, M] **CI:** Pheochromocytoma **Disp:** Inj 1 mg SE: N/V, ↓ BP **Notes:** Administration of dextrose IV necessary; ineffective in starvation, adrenal Insuff, or chronic hypoglycemia

Glyburide (DiaBeta, Micronase, Glynase) Uses: *Type 2 DM* **Acts:** Sulfonylurea; ↑ pancreatic insulin release; ↑ peripheral insulin sensitivity; ↓ hepatic glucose output/production; ↓ intestinal glucose absorption **Dose:** 1.25–10 mg daily-bid, max 20 mg/d. *Micronized:* 0.75–6 mg daily-bid, max 12 mg/d **W/P:** [C, ?] Renal impair, sulfonamide allergy **CI:** DKA, type 1 DM **Disp:** Tabs 1.25, 2.5, 5 mg; micronized tabs 1.5, 3, 6 mg **SE:** HA, hypoglycemia, cholestatic jaundice, and hepatitis may cause liver failure **Notes:** Not OK for CrCl < 50 mL/min; hold dose if NPO; hypoglycemia may be difficult to recognize; many medications can enhance hypoglycemic effects

Glyburide/Metformin (Glucovance) Uses: *Type 2 DM* **Acts:** *Sulfonylurea:* ↑ Pancreatic insulin release. *Metformin:* Peripheral insulin sensitivity; ↓ hepatic glucose output/production; ↓ intestinal glucose absorption **Dose:** 1st line (naïve pts), 1.25/250 mg PO daily-bid; 2nd line, 2.5/500 mg or 5/500 mg bid (max 20/2000 mg); take w/ meals, slowly ↑ dose; hold before & 48 h after ionic contrast media **W/P:** [C, –] **CI:** SCr > 1.4 mg/dL in females or > 1.5 mg/dL in males; hypoxemic conditions (sepsis, recent MI); alcoholism; metabolic acidosis; liver Dz; **Disp:** Tabs 1.25/250 mg, 2.5/500 mg, 5/500 mg **SE:** HA, hypoglycemia, lactic acidosis, anorexia, N/V, rash **Notes:** Avoid EtOH; hold dose if NPO; monitor folate levels (megaloblastic anemia)

Glycerin Suppository Uses: *Constipation* **Acts:** Hyperosmolar laxative **Dose:** *Adults.* 1 Adult supp PR PRN. *Peds.* 1 Infant supp PR daily-bid PRN **W/P:** [C, ?] **Disp:** Supp (adult, infant); liq 4 mL/applicator-full **SE:** D

Golimumab (Simponi) **BOX:** Serious Infxns (bacterial, fungal, TB, opportunistic) possible. D/C w/ severe Infxn/sepsis, test and monitor for TB w/treatment; lymphoma/other CA possible in children/adolescents Uses: *Mod/severe RA w/ methotrexate, psoriatic arthritis w/ or w/o methotrexate, ankylosing spondylitis* **Acts:** TNF blocker **Dose:** 50 mg SQ 1 × mo **W/P:** [B, ?/–] do use w/active infxn; w/ malignancies, CHF, demyelinating dz; do use w/ abatacept, anakinra, live vaccines **CI:** None **Disp:** Prefilled syringe & SmartJect auto-injector 50 mg/0.5 mL **SE:** URI, nasopharyngitis, Inj site Rxn, ↑ LFTs, Infxn, hep B reactivation, new onset psoriasis

Gonadorelin (Factrel) Uses: *Primary hypothalamic amenorrhea* **Acts:** ↑ Pituitary release of LH & FSH **Dose:** 5 mcg IV over 1 min q 90 min × 21 d using pump kit **W/P:** [B, M] ↑ Levels w/ androgens, estrogens, progestins, glucocorticoids, spironolactone, levodopa; ↓ levels w/ OCP, digoxin, dopamine antagonists **CI:** Condition exacerbated by PRG or reproductive hormones, ovarian cysts, causes of anovulation other than hypothalamic, hormonally dependent tumor **Disp:** Inj 100 mcg **SE:** Multiple PRG risk; Inj site pain **Notes:** Monitor LH, FSH

Goserelin (Zoladex) **Uses:** Advanced *CA Prostate* & w/ radiation for localized high-risk Dz, *endometriosis,* breast CA* **Acts:** LHRH agonist, transient ↑ then ↓ in LH, w/ ↓ testosterone **Dose:** 3.6 mg SQ (implant) q28d or 10.8 mg SQ q3mo; usually upper Abd wall **W/P:** [X, −] **CI:** PRG, breast-feeding, 10.8-mg implant not for women **Disp:** SQ implant 3.6 (1 mo), 10.8 mg (3 mo) **SE:** Hot flashes, ↓ libido, gynecomastia, & transient exacerbation of CA-related bone pain ("flare Rxn") 7–10 d after 1st dose) **Notes:** Inject SQ into fat in Abd wall; do not aspirate; females must use contraception

Granisetron (Kytril) **Uses:** *Rx and Prevention of N/V (chemo/radiation/postoperation)* **Acts:** Serotonin (5-HT$_3$) receptor antagonist **Dose:** *Adults & Peds. Chemotherapy:* 10 mcg/kg/dose IV 30 min prior to chemotherapy *Adults. Chemotherapy:* 2 mg PO q day 1 h before chemotherapy, then 12 h later. *Post-op N/V:* 1 mg IV over 30 s before end of case **W/P:** [B, +/−] St. John's wort ↓ levels **CI:** Liver Dz, children < 2 y **Disp:** Tabs 1 mg; Inj 1 mg/mL; soln 2 mg/10 mL **SE:** HA, asthenia, somnolence, D, constipation, Abd pain, dizziness, insomnia, ↑ LFTs

Guaifenesin (Robitussin, Others) **Uses:** *Relief of dry, nonproductive cough* **Acts:** Expectorant **Dose:** *Adults.* 200–400 mg (10–20 mL) PO q4h SR 600–1200 mg PO bid (max 2.4 g/d). *Peds 2–5 y.* 50–100 mg (2.5–5 mL) PO q4h (max 600 mg/d). *6–11 y:* 100–200 mg (5–10 mL) PO q4h (max 1.2 g/d) **W/P:** [C, ?] **Disp:** Tabs 100, 200 mg; SR tabs 600, 1200 mg; caps 200 mg; SR caps 300 mg; liq 100 mg/5 mL **SE:** GI upset **Notes** Give w/ large amount of H$_2$O; some dosage forms contain EtOH

Guaifenesin & Codeine (Robitussin AC, Brontex, Others) [C-V] **Uses:** *Relief of dry cough* **Acts:** Antitussive w/ expectorant **Dose:** *Adults.* 5–10 mL or 1 tab PO q4–6h (max 60 mL/24 h). *Peds 2–6 y.* 1–1.5 mg/kg codeine/d ÷ dose q4–6h (max 30 mg/24 h). *6–12 y:* 5 mL q4h (max 30 mL/24 h) **W/P:** [C, +] **Disp:** Brontex tab 10 mg codeine/300 mg guaifenesin; liq 2.5 mg codeine/75 mg guaifenesin/5 mL; others 10 mg codeine/100 mg guaifenesin/5 mL **SE:** Somnolence, constipation

Guaifenesin & Dextromethorphan (Many OTC Brands) **Uses:** *Cough d/t upper resp tract irritation* **Acts:** Antitussive w/ expectorant **Dose:** *Adults & Peds > 12 y.* 10 mL PO q6–8h (max 40 mL/24 h). *Peds 2–6 y.* Dextromethorphan 1–2 mg/kg/24 h ÷ 3–4 × d (max 10 mL/d). *6–12 y:* 5 mL q6–8h (max 20 mL/d) **W/P:** [C, +] **CI:** Administration w/ MAOI **Disp:** Many OTC formulations **SE:** Somnolence **Notes:** Give w/ plenty of fluids; some forms contain EtOH

Guanfacine (Intuniv, Tenex) **Uses:** *ADHD (peds > 6 y)*; *HTN (adults)* **Acts:** central α$_{2a}$-adrenergic agonist; **Dose:** *Adults.* 1–3 mg/d IR PO h (*Tenex*),

↑ by 1 mg q3–4wk PRN 3 mg/d max; *Peds.* 1–4 mg/d XR PO (*Intuniv*), ↑ by 1 mg q1wk PRN 4 mg/d max **W/P:** [B, +/−] **Disp:** Tabs IR 1, 2 mg; tabs XR 1, 2, 3, 4 mg **SE:** somnolence, dizziness, HA, fatigue, constipation, abd pain, xerostomia, hypotension, bradycardia, syncope **Notes:** rebound ↑ BP, anxiety, nervousness w/ abrupt D/C; metabolized by CYP3A4

Haemophilus B Conjugate Vaccine (ActHIB, HibTITER, Hiberix, PedvaxHIB, Prohibit, TriHIBit, Others) Uses: *Immunize children against *H. influenzae* type B Dzs* **Acts:** Active immunization **Dose:** *Peds.* 0.5 mL (25 mg) IM (deltoid or vastus lateralis muscle) 2 doses 2 and 4 mos; booster 12–15 mos or 2, 4, and 6 mos booster at 12–15 mos depending on formulation; **W/P:** [C, +] **CI:** Component sensitivity; febrile illness, immunosuppression, thimerosal allergy **Disp:** Inj 7.5, 10, 15, 25 mcg/0.5 mL **SE:** Fever, restlessness, fussiness, anorexia, pain/redness inj site; observe for anaphylaxis; edema, ↑ risk of *Haemophilus* B Infxn the wk after vaccination **Notes:** *Prohibit* and *TriHIBit* cannot be used in children < 12 mo. *Hiberix* approved ages 15 mo–4 y, single dose; booster beyond 5 y old not required; report SAE to Vaccine Adverse Events Reporting System (VAERS: 1-800-822-7967); dosing varies, check with each product

Haloperidol (Haldol) BOX: ↑ Mortality in elderly w/ dementia-related psychosis. Risk for torsade de pointes and QT prolongation, death w/ IV administration at higher doses Uses: *Psychotic disorders, agitation, Tourette disorders, hyperactivity in children* **Acts:** Butyrophenone; antipsychotic, neuroleptic **Dose:** *Adults.* Mod *Sxs:* 0.5–2 mg PO bid–tid. *Severe Sxs/agitation:* 3–5 mg PO bid–tid or 1–5 mg IM q4h PRN (max 100 mg/d). *ICU psychosis:* 2–10 mg IV q 30 min to effect, the 25% max dose q6h *Peds 3–6 y.* 0.01–0.03 mg/kg/24 h PO daily. *6–12 y:* Initial, 0.5–1.5 mg/24 h PO; ↑ by 0.5 mg/24 h to maint of 2–4 mg/24 h (0.05–0.1 mg/kg/24 h) or 1–3 mg/dose IM q4–8h to 0.1 mg/kg/24 h max; Tourette Dz may require up to 15 mg/24 h PO; ↓ in elderly **W/P:** [C, ?] ↑ Effects w/ SSRIs, CNS depressants, TCA, indomethacin, metoclopramide; avoid levodopa (↓ antiparkinsonian effects) **CI:** NAG, severe CNS depression, coma, Parkinson Dz, ↓ BM suppression, severe cardiac/hepatic Dz **Disp:** Tabs 0.5, 1, 2, 5, 10, 20 mg; conc liq 2 mg/mL; Inj 5 mg/mL; decanoate Inj 50, 100 mg/mL **SE:** Extrapyramidal Sxs (EPS), tardive dyskinesia, neuroleptic malignant synd, ↓ BP, anxiety, dystonias, risk for torsades de pointes and QT prolongation; leukopenia, neutropenia and agranulocytosis **Notes:** Do not give decanoate IV; dilute PO conc liq w/ H₂O/juice; monitor for EPS; ECG monitoring w/ off-label IV use; follow CBC if WBC counts decreased

Heparin (Generic) Uses: *Rx & prevention of DVT & PE*, unstable angina, AF w/ emboli, & acute arterial occlusion **Acts:** Acts w/ antithrombin III to inactivate thrombin & ↓ thromboplastin formation **Dose:** *Adults.* Prophylaxis. 3000–5000 units SQ q8–12h. *DVT/PE Rx:* Load 50–80 units/kg IV (max 10,000 units), then 10–20 units/kg IV qh (adjust based on PTT); *ECC 2010. STEMI:* Bolus 60 units/kg (max 4000 units); then 12 units/kg/h (max 1000 units/h) round to nearest 50 units; keep aPTT 1.5–2 × control 48 h or until angiography. *Peds Infants.*

Load 50 units/kg IV bolus, then 20 units/kg/h IV by cont Inf. ***Children:*** Load 50 units/kg IV, then 15–25 units/kg cont Inf or 100 units/kg/dose q4h IV intermittent bolus (adjust based on PTT) **W/P:** [B, +] ↑ Risk of hemorrhage w/ anticoagulants, ASA, anti-plt, cephalosporins w/ MTT side chain **CI:** Uncontrolled bleeding, severe thrombocytopenia, suspected ICH **Disp:** Unfractionated Inj 10, 100, 1000, 2000, 2500, 5000, 7500, 10,000, 20,000, 40,000 units/mL **SE:** Bruising, bleeding, thrombocytopenia **Notes:** Follow PTT, thrombin time, or activated clotting time; little PT effect; therapeutic PTT 1.5–2 control for most conditions; monitor for HIT w/ plt counts; New "USP" formulation heparin is approximately 10% less effective than older formulations

Hepatitis A Vaccine (HAVRIX, VAQTA) Uses: *Prevent hep A* in high-risk individuals (e.g., travelers, certain professions, day-care workers if 1 or more children or workers are infected, high-risk behaviors, children at ↑ risk); in chronic liver Dz **Acts:** Active immunity **Dose:** *Adults.* *HAVRIX* 1.0-mL IM w/ 1.0-mL booster 6–12 mo later; *VAQTA:* 1.0 mL IM w/ 1.0 ml IM booster 6–18 mo later *Peds > 12 mo.* HAVRIX 0.5-mL IM, w/ 0.5-mL booster 6–18 mo later; VAQTA 0.5 mL IM w/ booster 0.5 mL 6–18 mo later **W/P:** [C, +/–] **CI:** Component sensitivity; syringes contain latex **Disp:** *HAVRIX:* Inj 720 EL.U./0.5 mL, 1440 EL.U./1 mL; *VAQTA* 50 units/mL **SE:** Fever, fatigue, HA, Inj site pain **Notes:** Give primary at least 2 wks before anticipated exposure; do not give HAVRIX in gluteal region; report SAE to VAERS (1-800-822-7967)

Hepatitis A (Inactivated) & Hepatitis B (Recombinant) Vaccine (Twinrix) Uses: *Active immunization against hep A/B in pts > 18 y* **Acts:** Active immunity **Dose:** 1 mL IM at 0, 1, & 6 mo; accelerated regimen 1 mL IM day 0, 7 and 21–20 then booster at 12 mo; 720 ELISA EL.U. units hep A antigen, 20 mcg/mL hep B surface antigen **W/P:** [C, +/–] **CI:** Component sensitivity **Disp:** Single-dose vials, syringes **SE:** Fever, fatigue, HA, pain/redness at site **Notes:** Booster OK 6–12 mo after vaccination; report SAE to Vaccine Adverse Events Reporting System (VAERS: 1-800-822-7967)

Hepatitis B Immune Globulin (HyperHep, HepaGam B, Nabi-HB, H-BIG) Uses: *Exposure to HBsAg(+) material (e.g., blood, accidental needlestick, mucous membrane contact, PO or sexual contact), prevent hep B in HBsAg(+) liver Tx pt* **Acts:** Passive immunization **Dose:** *Adults & Peds.* 0.06 mL/kg IM 5 mL max; w/in 24 h of exposure; w/in 14 d of sexual contact; repeat 1 mo if nonresponder or refused initial tx; liver Tx per protocols **W/P:** [C, ?] **CI:** Allergies to γ-globulin, anti-immunoglobulin Ab, or thimerosal; IgA deficiency **Disp:** Inj **SE:** Inj site pain, dizziness, HA, myalgias, arthralgias, anaphylaxis **Notes:** IM in gluteal or deltoid; w/ continued exposure, give hep B vaccine; not for active hep B; ineffective for chronic hep B

Hepatitis B Vaccine (Engerix-B, Recombivax HB) Uses: *Prevent hep B*: men who have sex w/ men, people who inject street drugs; chronic renal/liver Dz, healthcare workers exposed to blood, body fluids; sexually active not in monogamous relationship, people seeking evaluation for or w/ STDs, household

contacts and partners of hep B infected persons, travelers to countries w/ ↑ hep B prevalence, clients/staff working w/ people w/ developmental disabilities **Acts:** Active immunization; recombinant DNA **Dose:** *Adults.* 3 IM doses 1 mL each; 1st 2 doses 1 mo apart; the 3rd 6 mo after the 1st. *Peds.* 0.5 mL IM adult schedule **W/P:** [C, +] ↓ Effect w/ immunosuppressives **CI:** Yeast allergy, component sensitivity **Disp:** *Engerix-B:* Inj 20 mcg/mL; peds Inj 10 mcg/0.5 mL. *Recombivax HB:* Inj 10 & 40 mcg/mL; peds Inj 5 mcg/0.5 mL **SE:** Fever, HA, Inj site pain **Notes:** Deltoid IM Inj adults/older peds; younger peds, use anterolateral thigh

Hetastarch (Hespan) **Uses:** *Plasma vol expansion* adjunct in shock & leukapheresis **Acts:** Synthetic colloid; acts similar to albumin **Dose:** *Vol expansion:* 500–1000 mL (1500 mL/d max) IV (20 mL/kg/h max rate). *Leukapheresis:* 250–700 mL; ↓ in renal failure **W/P:** [C, +] **CI:** Severe bleeding disorders, CHF, oliguric/anuric renal failure **Disp:** Inj 6 g/100 mL **SE:** Bleeding (↑ PT, PTT, bleeding time) **Notes:** Not blood or plasma substitute

Human Papillomavirus Recombinant Vaccine (Cervarix [Types 16, 18], Gardasil, [Types 6, 11, 16, 18]) **Uses:** *Prevent cervical CA, precancerous genital lesions (Cervarix and Gardasil), genital warts, anal cancer and oral cancer (Gardasil) d/t to human papillomavirus (HPV) types 16, 18 (Cervarix) and types 6, 11, 16, 18 (Gardasil) in females 9–26 y*; prevent genital warts, anal cancer, and anal intraepithelial neoplasia in males 9–26 y (Gardasil)* **Acts:** Recombinant vaccine, passive immunity **Dose:** 0.5 mL IM, then 1 and 6 mo (Cervarix), or 2 and 6 mo (Gardasil) (upper thigh or deltoid) **W/P:** [B, ?/–] **Disp:** Single-dose vial & prefilled syringe: 0.5 mL **SE:** Erythema, pain at inj site, fever, syncope, venous thromboembolism **Notes:** First cancer prevention vaccine, 90% effective in preventing CIN 2 or more severe dx in HPV naive populations; report adverse events to Vaccine Adverse Events Reporting System (VAERS: 1-800-822-7967); continue cervical CA screening. Hx of genital warts, abn Pap smear, or + HPV DNA test is **not** CI to vaccination

Hydralazine (Apresoline, Others) **Uses:** *Mod–severe HTN; CHF* (w/ Isordil) **Acts:** Peripheral vasodilator **Dose:** *Adults.* Initial 10 mg PO 3–4×/d, ↑ to 25 mg 3–4×/d, 300 mg/d max. *Peds.* 0.75–3 mg/kg/24 h PO ÷ q6–12h; ↓ in renal impair; ✓ CBC & ANA before **W/P:** [C, +] ↓ Hepatic Fxn & CAD; ↑ tox w/ MAOI, indomethacin, β-blockers **CI:** Dissecting aortic aneurysm, mitral valve/ rheumatic heart Dz **Disp:** Tabs 10, 25, 50, 100 mg; Inj 20 mg/mL **SE:** SLE-like synd w/ chronic high doses; SVT following IM route;, peripheral neuropathy **Notes:** Compensatory sinus tachycardia eliminated w/ β-blocker

Hydrochlorothiazide (HydroDIURIL, Esidrix, Others) **Uses:** *Edema, HTN* prevent stones in hypercalcuria **Acts:** Thiazide diuretic; ↓ distal tubule Na+ reabsorption **Dose:** *Adults.* 25–100 mg/d PO single or ÷ doses; 200 mg/d max. *Peds < 6 mo.* 2–3 mg/kg/d in 2 ÷ doses. *> 6 mo:* 2 mg/kg/d in 2 ÷ doses **W/P:** [D, +] **CI:** Anuria, sulfonamide allergy, renal Insuff **Disp:** Tabs 25, 50, mg; caps 12.5 mg; PO soln 50 mg/5 mL **SE:** ↓ K+, hyperglycemia, hyperuricemia, ↓ Na+; sun sensitivity **Notes:** Follow K+, may need supplementation

Hydrochlorothiazide & Amiloride (Moduretic) Uses: *HTN* Acts: Combined thiazide & K⁺-sparing diuretic Dose: 1–2 tabs/d PO W/P: [D, ?] CI: Renal failure, sulfonamide allergy Disp: Tabs (amiloride/HCTZ) 5 mg/50 mg each SE: ↓ BP, photosens, ↑ K⁺/↓ K⁺, hyperglycemia, ↓ Na⁺, hyperlipidemia, hyperuricemia

Hydrochlorothiazide & Spironolactone (Aldactazide) Uses: *Edema, HTN* Acts: Thiazide & K⁺-sparing diuretic Dose: 25–200 mg each component/d, ÷ doses W/P: [D, +] CI: Sulfonamide allergy Disp: Tabs (HCTZ/ spironolactone) 25 mg/25 mg, 50 mg/50 mg SE: Photosens, ↓ BP, ↑ or ↓ K⁺, ↓ Na⁺, hyperglycemia, hyperlipidemia, hyperuricemia

Hydrochlorothiazide & Triamterene (Dyazide, Maxzide) Uses: *Edema & HTN* Acts: Combo thiazide & K⁺-sparing diuretic Dose: *Dyazide:* 1–2 caps PO daily-bid. *Maxzide:* 1 tab/d PO W/P: [D, +/–] CI: Sulfonamide allergy Disp: (Triamterene/HCTZ) 37.5 mg/25 mg, 75 mg/50 mg SE: Photosens, ↓ BP, ↑ or ↓ K⁺, ↓ Na⁺, hyperglycemia, hyperlipidemia, hyperuricemia Notes: HCTZ component in Maxzide more bioavailable than in Dyazide

Hydrocodone & Acetaminophen (Lorcet, Vicodin, Hycet, Others) [C-III] Uses: *Mod–severe pain*; Acts: Narcotic analgesic w/ nonnarcotic analgesic Dose: *Adults.* 1–2 caps or tabs PO q4–6h PRN; soln 15 mL q4–6h *Peds.* Soln (Hycet) 0.27 mL/kg q4–6h W/P: [C, M] CI: CNS depression, severe resp depression Disp: Many formulations; specify hydrocodone/APAP dose: caps 5/500 mg; tabs 2.5/500, 5/325, 5/400, 5/500, 7.5/325, 7.5/400, 7.5/500, 7.5/650, 7.5/750, 10/325, 10/400, 10/500, 10/650, 10/660, 10/750 mg; soln Hycet (fruit punch) 7.5 mg hydrocodone/325 mg acetaminophen/15 mL SE: GI upset, sedation, fatigue Notes: Do not exceed > 4 g APAP/d; see Acetaminophen note p 34

Hydrocodone & Aspirin (Lortab ASA, Others) [C-III] Uses: *Mod–severe pain* Acts: Narcotic analgesic w/ NSAID Dose: 1–2 PO q4–6h PRN, w/ food/milk W/P: [C, M] ↓ Renal Fxn, gastritis/PUD, CI: Component sensitivity; children w/chickenpox (Reye synd) Disp: 5 mg hydrocodone/500 mg ASA/tab SE: GI upset, sedation, fatigue Notes: Monitor for GI bleed

Hydrocodone & Guaifenesin (Hycotuss Expectorant, Others) [C-III] Uses: *Nonproductive cough* associated w/ resp Infxn Acts: Expectorant w/ cough suppressant Dose: *Adults & Peds > 12 y.* 5 mL q4h pc & hs. *Peds < 2 y.* 0.3 mg/kg/d ÷ qid. *2–12 y:* 2.5 mL q4h pc & hs W/P: [C, M] CI: Component sensitivity Disp: Hydrocodone 5 mg/guaifenesin 100 mg/5 mL SE: GI upset, sedation, fatigue

Hydrocodone & Homatropine (Hycodan, Hydromet, Others) [C-III] Uses: *Relief of cough* Acts: Combo antitussive Dose: (Based on hydrocodone) *Adults.* 5–10 mg q4–6h. *Peds.* 0.6 mg/kg/d ÷ tid-qid W/P: [C, M] CI: NAG, ↑ ICP, depressed ventilation Disp: Syrup 5 mg hydrocodone/5 mL; tabs 5 mg hydrocodone/5 mL SE: Sedation, fatigue, GI upset Notes: Do not give < q4h; see individual drugs

Hydrocodone & Ibuprofen (Vicoprofen) [C-III] Uses: *Mod–severe pain (< 10 d)* Acts: Narcotic w/ NSAID Dose: 1–2 tabs q4–6h PRN W/P: [C, M]

Renal Insuff; ↓ effect w/ ACE inhib & diuretics; ↑ effect w/ CNS depressants, EtOH, MAOI, ASA, TCA, anticoagulants **CI:** Component sensitivity **Disp:** Tabs 7.5 mg hydrocodone/200 mg ibuprofen **SE:** Sedation, fatigue, GI upset

Hydrocodone & Pseudoephedrine (Detussin, Histussin-D, Others) [C-III]

Uses: *Cough & nasal congestion* **Acts:** Narcotic cough suppressant w/ decongestant **Dose:** 5 mL qid, PRN **W/P:** [C, M] **CI:** MAOIs **Disp:** hydrocodone/pseudoephedrine 5 mg/60 mg, 3 mg/15 mg 5 mL; tab 5 mg/60 mg **SE:** ↑ BP, GI upset, sedation, fatigue

Hydrocodone, Chlorpheniramine, Phenylephrine, Acetaminophen, & Caffeine (Hycomine Compound) [C-III]

Uses: *Cough & Sxs of URI* **Acts:** Narcotic cough suppressant w/ decongestants & analgesic **Dose:** 1 tab PO q4h PRN **W/P:** [C, M] **CI:** NAG **Disp:** Hydrocodone 5 mg/chlorpheniramine 2 mg/phenylephrine 10 mg/APAP 250 mg/caffeine 30 mg/tab **SE:** ↑ BP, GI upset, sedation, fatigue

Hydrocortisone, Rectal (Anusol-HC Suppository, Cortifoam Rectal, Proctocort, Others)

Uses: *Painful anorectal conditions*, radiation proctitis, ulcerative colitis **Acts:** Anti-inflammatory steroid **Dose:** *Adults.* Ulcerative colitis: 10–100 mg PR daily-bid for 2–3 wk **W/P:** [B, ?/–] **CI:** Component sensitivity **Disp:** *Hydrocortisone acetate:* Rectal aerosol 90 mg/applicator; supp 25 mg. *Hydrocortisone base:* Rectal 0.5%, 1%, 2.5%; rectal susp 100 mg/60 mL **SE:** Minimal systemic effect

Hydrocortisone, Topical & Systemic (Cortef, Solu-Cortef)

See Steroids p 244, 246 and Tables 2, p 283 & 3, p 284 *Peds. ECC 2010.* Adrenal insufficiency: 2 mg/kg IV/IO bolus; max dose 100 mg **W/P:** [B, –] **CI:** Viral, fungal, or tubercular skin lesions; serious Infxns (except septic shock or TB meningitis) **SE:** *Systemic:* ↑ Appetite, insomnia, hyperglycemia, bruising **Notes:** May cause hypothalamic–pituitary–adrenal axis suppression

Hydromorphone (Dilaudid, Dilaudid HP) [C-II]

BOX: A potent Schedule II opioid agonist; highest potential for abuse and risk of resp depression. HP formula is highly concentrated; do not confuse w/ standard formulations, OD and death could result. Alcohol, other opioids, CNS depressants ↑ resp depressant effects **Uses:** *Mod/severe pain* **Acts:** Narcotic analgesic **Dose:** 1–4 mg PO, IM, IV, or PR q4–6h PRN; 3 mg PR q6–8h PRN; ↓ w/ hepatic failure **W/P:** [B (D if prolonged use or high doses near term), ?] ↑ Resp depression and CNS effects, CNS depressants, phenothiazines, TCA **CI:** CNS lesion w/ ↑ ICP, COPD, cor pulmonale, emphysema, kyphoscoliosis, status asthmaticus; HP-Inj form in OB analgesia **Disp:** Tabs 2, 4 mg, 8 mg scored; liq 5 mg/5 mL or 1 mg/mL; Inj 1, 2, 4 mg, *Dilaudid HP* is 10 mg/mL; supp 3 mg **SE:** Sedation, dizziness, GI upset **Notes:** Morphine 1mg IM = hydromorphone 1.5 mg IM

Hydromorphone, Extended-Release (Exalgo) [C-II]

BOX: Use in opioid tolerant only; high potential for abuse, criminal diversion and resp depression. Not for post-op pain or PRN use. OD and death especially in children. Do not break/crush/chew tabs, may result in OD **Uses:** *Mod/severe chronic pain requiring*

around-the-clock opioid analgesic *Acts:* Narcotic analgesic **Dose:** 8–64 mg PO/d titrate to effect; ↓ w/ hepatic/renal impair and elderly **W/P:** [C, –] Abuse potential; ↑ Resp depression and CNS effects, w/ CNS depressants, patients susceptible to intracranial effects of CO_2 retention **CI:** Opioid-intolerant patients, ↓ pulmonary function, ileus, GI tract narrowing/obstr, component hypersens; w/in 14 d of MAOI; anticholinergics may ↑ SE **Disp:** Tabs 8, 12, 16 mg **SE:** constipation, N/V, somnolence, HA, dizziness **Notes:** See label for opioid conversion

Hydroxocobalamin (Cyanokit) Uses: *Cyanide poisoning* **Acts:** Binds cyanide to form nontoxic cyanocobalamin excreted in urine **Dose:** 5 g IV over 15 min, repeat PRN 5 g IV over 15 min–2 h, total dose 10 g **W/P:** [C, ?] **CI:** None known **Disp:** Kit 2 to 2.5 g vials w/ Inf set **SE:** ↑ BP (can be severe) anaphylaxis, chest tightness, edema, urticaria, rash, chromaturia, N, HA, Inj site Rxns

Hydroxyurea (Hydrea, Droxia) Uses: *CML, head & neck, ovarian & colon CA, melanoma, ALL, sickle cell anemia, polycythemia vera, HIV* **Acts:** ↓ Ribonucleotide reductase **Dose:** (per protocol) 50–75 mg/kg for WBC > 100,000 cells/mL; 20–30 mg/kg in refractory CML. *HIV:* 1000–1500 mg/d in single or ÷ doses; ↓ in renal Insuff **W/P:** [D, –] ↑ Effects w/ zidovudine, zalcitabine, didanosine, stavudine, fluorouracil **CI:** Severe anemia, BM suppression, WBC < 2500 cells/mL or plt < 100,000 cells/mm³, PRG **Disp:** Caps 200, 300, 400, 500 mg, tabs 1000 mg **SE:** ↓ BM (mostly leukopenia), N/V, rashes, facial erythema, radiation recall Rxns, renal impair **Notes:** Empty caps into H_2O

Hydroxyzine (Atarax, Vistaril) Uses: *Anxiety, sedation, itching* **Acts:** Antihistamine, antianxiety **Dose:** *Adults. Anxiety/sedation:* 50–100 mg PO or IM qid or PRN (max 600 mg/d). *Itching:* 25–50 mg PO or IM tid-qid. *Peds.* 0.5–1.0 mg/kg/24 h PO or IM q6h; ↓ w/hepatic impair **W/P:** [C, +/–] ↑ Effects w/ CNS depressants, anticholinergics, EtOH **CI:** Component sensitivity **Disp:** Tabs 10, 25, 50 mg; caps 25, 50 mg; syrup 10 mg/5 mL; susp 25 mg/5 mL; Inj 25, 50 mg/mL **SE:** Drowsiness, anticholinergic effects **Notes:** Used to potentiate narcotic effects; not for IV/SQ (thrombosis & digital gangrene possible)

Hyoscyamine (Anaspaz, Cystospaz, Levsin, Others) Uses: *Spasm w/ GI & bladder disorders* **Acts:** Anticholinergic **Dose:** *Adults.* 0.125–0.25 mg (1–2 tabs) SL/PO tid-qid, ac & hs; 1 SR caps q12h **W/P:** [C, +] ↑ Effects w/ amantadine, antihistamines, antimuscarinics, haloperidol, phenothiazines, TCA, MAOI **CI:** BOO, GI obst, NAG, MyG, paralytic ileus, ulcerative colitis, MI **Disp:** (Cystospaz-M, Levsinex) time-release caps 0.375 mg; elixir (EtOH); soln 0.125 mg/5 mL; Inj 0.5 mg/mL; tab 0.125 mg; tab (Cystospaz) 0.15 mg; XR tab (Levbid) 0.375 mg; SL (Levsin SL) 0.125 mg **SE:** Dry skin, xerostomia, constipation, anticholinergic SE, heat prostration w/ hot weather **Notes:** Administer tabs ac

Hyoscyamine, Atropine, Scopolamine, & Phenobarbital (Donnatal, Others) Uses: *Irritable bowel, spastic colitis, peptic ulcer, spastic bladder* **Acts:** Anticholinergic, antispasmodic **Dose:** 0.125–0.25 mg (1–2 tabs) tid-qid, 1 caps q12h (SR), 5–10 mL elixir tid-qid or q8h **W/P:** [D, M] **CI:** NAG **Disp:**

Many combos/manufacturers. *Caps (Donnatal, others):* Hyoscyamine 0.1037 mg/atropine 0.0194 mg/scopolamine 0.0065 mg/phenobarbital 16.2 mg. *Tabs (Donnatal, others):* Hyoscyamine 0.1037 mg/atropine 0.0194 mg/scopolamine 0.0065 mg/phenobarbital 16.2 mg. *LA (Donnatal):* Hyoscyamine 0.311 mg/atropine 0.0582 mg/scopolamine 0.0195 mg/phenobarbital 48.6 mg. *Elixirs (Donnatal, others):* Hyoscyamine 0.1037 mg/atropine 0.0194 mg/scopolamine 0.0065 mg/phenobarbital 16.2 mg/5 mL **SE:** Sedation, xerostomia, constipation

Ibandronate (Boniva) Uses: *Rx & prevent osteoporosis in postmenopausal women* Acts: Bisphosphonate, ↓ osteoclast-mediated bone resorption Dose: 2.5 mg PO daily or 150 mg once/month on same day (do not lie down for 60 min after); 3 mg IV over 15–30 s q3mo W/P: [C, ?/–] Avoid w/ CrCl < 30 mL/min CI: Uncorrected ↓ Ca²⁺; inability to stand/sit upright for 60 min (PO) Disp: Tabs 2.5, 150 mg, Inj IV 3 mg/3 mL SE: Jaw osteonecrosis (avoid extensive dental procedures) N/D, HA, dizziness, asthenia, HTN, Infxn, dysphagia, esophagitis, esophageal/gastric ulcer, musculoskeletal pain Notes: Take 1st thing in AM. w/ H_2O (6–8 oz) > 60 min before 1st food/beverage & any meds w/ multivalent cations; give adequate Ca²⁺ & vit D supls; possible association between bisphosphonates & severe muscle/bone/joint pain; may ↑ atypical subtrochanteric femur fractures

Ibuprofen, Oral (Motrin, Motrin IB, Rufen, Advil, Others) [OTC] BOX: May ↑ risk of CV events & GI bleeding Uses: *Arthritis, pain, fever* Acts: NSAID Dose: *Adults.* 200–800 mg PO bid-qid (max 2.4 g/d). *Peds.* 30–40 mg/kg/d in 3–4 ÷ doses (max 40 mg/kg/d); w/ food W/P: [B, +] May interfere w/ ASAs anti-plt effect if given < 8 h before ASA CI: 3rd tri PRG, severe hepatic impair, allergy, use w/ other NSAIDs, upper GI bleeding, ulcers Disp: Tabs 100, 200, 400, 600, 800 mg; chew tabs 50, 100 mg; caps 200 mg; susp 50 mg/1.25 mL, 100 mg/2.5 mL, 100 mg/5 mL, 40 mg/mL (Motrin IB & Advil OTC 200 mg are the OTC forms) SE: Dizziness, peptic ulcer, plt inhibition, worsening of renal insuff

Ibuprofen, Parenteral (Caldolor) BOX: May ↑ risk of CV events & GI bleeding Uses: *Mild/moderate pain, as adjunct to opioids, ↓ fever* Acts: NSAID Dose: *Pain:* 400–800 mg IV over 30 min q6h PRN; *Fever:* 400 mg IV over 30 min, the 400 mg q4–6h or 100–200 mg q4–6h PRN W/P: [C < 30 wks, D after 30 wks, ?/–] may ↓ ACE effects; avoid w/ ASA, and < 17 yrs CI: Hypersens NSAIDs; asthma, urticaria, or allergic Rxns w/ NSAIDs, peri-op CABG Disp: Vials 400 mg/4 mL, 800 mg/8 mL SE: N/V, HA, flatulence, hemorrhage, dizziness Notes: Make sure pt well hydrated; use lowest dose/shortest duration possible

Ibutilide (Corvert) Uses: *Rapid conversion of AF/A flutter* Acts: Class III antiarrhythmic Dose: *Adults > 60 kg.* 1 mg IV over 10 min; may repeat × 1; < 60 kg use 0.01 mg/kg IV *ECC 2010.* SVT (AFib about AFlutter): *Adults > 60 kg.* 1 mg (10 mL) over 10 min; a second dose may be used; < 60 kg 0.01 mg/kg over 10 min. Consider DC cardioversion W/P: [C, –] CI: w/ Class I/III antiarrhythmics (Table 9, p 300); QTc > 440 msec Disp: Inj 0.1 mg/mL SE: Arrhythmias, HA Notes: Give w/ ECG monitoring; ✓ K⁺, Mg²⁺

Idarubicin (Idamycin) **BOX:** Administer only under supervision of an MD experienced in leukemia and in an institution w/ resources to maintain a pt compromised by drug tox **Uses:** *Acute leukemias* (AML, ALL), *CML in blast crisis, breast CA* **Acts:** DNA-intercalating agent; ↓ DNA topoisomerase I & II **Dose:** (Per protocol) 10–12 mg/m²/d for 3–4 d; ↓ in renal/hepatic impair **W/P:** [D, –] **CI:** Bilirubin > 5 mg/dL, PRG **Disp:** Inj 1 mg/mL (5-, 10-, 20-mg vials) **SE:** ↓ BM, cardiotox, N/V, mucositis, alopecia, & IV site Rxns, rarely ↓ renal/hepatic Fxn **Notes:** Avoid extrav, potent vesicant; IV only

Ifosfamide (Ifex, Holoxan) **BOX:** Administer only under supervision by an MD experienced in chemotherapy; hemorrhagic cystitis, myelosupp; confusion, coma possible **Uses:** *Testis*, lung, breast, pancreatic & gastric CA, Hodgkin lymphoma/NHL, soft-tissue sarcoma **Acts:** Alkylating agent **Dose:** (Per protocol) 1.2 g/m²/d for 5 d bolus or cont Inf; 2.4 g/m²/d for 3 d; w/ MESNA uroprotection; ↓ in renal/hepatic impair **W/P:** [D, M] ↑ Effect w/ phenobarbital, carbamazepine, phenytoin; St. John's wort may ↓ levels **CI:** ↓ BM Fxn, PRG **Disp:** Inj 1, 3 g **SE:** Hemorrhagic cystitis, nephrotox, N/V, mild–mod leukopenia, lethargy & confusion, alopecia, ↑ LFT **Notes:** Administer w/ MESNA to prevent hemorrhagic cystitis; WBC nadir 10–14 d; recovery 21–28 d

Iloperidone (Fanapt) **BOX:** Risk for torsades de pointes and ↑ QT. Elderly pts at ↑ risk of death, CVA **Uses:** *Acute schizophrenia* **Action:** Atypical antipsychotic **Dose:** *Initial:* 1 mg PO, ↑ daily to goal 12–24 mg/d ÷ bid **W/P:** [?/–] **CI:** component hypersens **Disp:** Tabs:1, 2, 4, 6, 8, 10, 12 mg **SE:** Orthostatic ↓ BP, dizziness, dry mouth, ↑ wgt **Notes:** Titrate to ↓ BP risk. Monitor QT interval

Iloprost (Ventavis) **BOX:** Associated w/ syncope; may require dosage adjustment **Uses:** *NYHA class III/IV pulm arterial HTN* **Acts:** Prostaglandin analog **Dose:** Initial 2.5 mcg; if tolerated, ↑ to 5 mcg Inh 6–9×/d at least 2 h apart while awake **W/P:** [C, ?/–] All-pit effects, ↑ bleeding risk w/ anticoagulants; additive hypotensive effects **CI:** SBP < 85 mm Hg **Disp:** Inh soln 10 mcg/mL **SE:** Syncope, ↓ BP, vasodilation, cough, HA, trismus, D, dysgeusia, rash, oral irritation **Notes:** Requires *Pro-Dose AAD* or *I-neb ADD* system nebulizer; counsel on syncope risk; do not mix w/ other drugs; monitor vitals during initial Rx

Imatinib (Gleevec) **Uses:** *Rx CML Ph (+), CML blast crisis, ALL Ph(+), myelodysplastic/myeloproliferative Dz, aggressive systemic mastocytosis, chronic eosinophilic leukemia, GIST, dermatofibrosarcoma protuberans* **Acts:** ↓ BCL-ABL; TKI **Dose:** *Adults. Typical dose* 400–600 mg PO daily; w/ meal *Peds.* CML Ph(+) newly diagnosed 340 mg/m²/d, 600 mg/d max; recurrent 260 mg/m²/d PO ÷ daily-bid, to 340 mg/m²/d max **W/P:** [D, ?/–] w/ CYP3A4 meds (Table 10, p 301), warfarin **CI:** Component sensitivity **Disp:** Tab 100, 400 mg **SE:** GI upset, fluid retention, muscle cramps, musculoskeletal pain, arthralgia, rash, HA, neutropenia, thrombocytopenia **Notes:** Follow CBCs & LFTs baseline & monthly; w/ large glass of H_2O & food to ↓ GI irritation

Imipenem–Cilastatin (Primaxin) Uses: *Serious infxns* d/t susceptible bacteria Acts: Bactericidal; ↓ cell wall synth. *Spectrum:* Gram(+) (*S. aureus*, group A & B streptococci), gram(–) (not *Legionella*), anaerobes Dose: *Adults.* 250–1000 mg (imipenem) IV q6–8h, 500–750 mg IM. Peds. 60–100 mg/kg/24 h IV ÷ q6h; ↓ if CrCl is < 70 mL/min W/P: [C, +/–] Probenecid ↑ tox CI: Peds pts w/ CNS Infxn (↑ Sz risk) & < 30 kg w/ renal impair Disp: Inj (imipenem/cilastatin) 250/250, 500/500 mg SE: Szs if drug accumulates, GI upset, thrombocytopenia

Imipramine (Tofranil) BOX: Close observation for suicidal thinking or unusual changes in behavior Uses: *Depression, enuresis*, panic attack, chronic pain Acts: TCA; ↑ CNS synaptic serotonin or norepinephrine Dose: *Adults. Hospitalized:* Initial 100 mg/24 h PO in ÷ doses; ↑ over several wk 300 mg/d max. *Outpatient:* Maint 50–150 mg PO hs, 300 mg/24 h max. *Peds. Antidepressant:* 1.5–5 mg/kg/24 h ÷ daily-qid. *Enuresis:* > *6 y:* 10–25 mg PO qhs; ↑ by 10–25 mg at 1–2-wk intervals (max 50 mg for 6–12 y, 75 mg for > 12 y); Rx for 2–3 mo, then taper W/P: [D, ?/–] CI: Use w/ MAOIs, NAG, acute recovery from MI, PRG, CHF, angina, CV Dz, arrhythmias Disp: Tabs 10, 25, 50 mg; caps 75, 100, 125, 150 mg SE: CV Sxs, dizziness, xerostomia, discolored urine Notes: Less sedation than amitriptyline

Imiquimod Cream, 5% (Aldara) Uses: *Anogenital warts, HPV, condylomata acuminata* Acts: Unknown; ? cytokine induction Dose: Apply 3×/wk, leave on 6–10 h & wash off w/ soap & water, continue 16 wk max W/P: [B, ?] CI: Component sensitivity Disp: Single-dose packets (5% 250-mg cream) SE: Local skin Rxns Notes: Not a cure; may weaken condoms/vag diaphragms, wash hands before & after use

Immune Globulin, IV (Gamimune N, Gammaplex, Gammar IV, Sandoglobulin, Others) Uses: *IgG deficiency Dz states, B-cell CLL, CIDP, HIV, hep A prophylaxis, ITP*, Kawasaki dx, travel to ? prevalence area and Hep A vaccination within 2 weeks of travel Acts: IgG supl Dose: *Adults & Peds. Immunodeficiency:* 200-(300 *Gammaplex*)-800 mg/kg/mo IV at 0.01–0.04 (0.08 *Gammaplex*) mL/kg/min; initial dose 0.01 mL/kg/min. *B-cell CLL:* 400 mg/kg/dose IV q 3 wks, *CIDP:* 2,000 over 2–4 days then 1,000 mg/kg/day every 3 wks, *ITP:* 400 mg/kg/dose IV daily × 5 d. *BMT:* 500 mg/kg/wk; ↓ in renal Insuff W/P: [C, ?] Separate live vaccines by 3 mo CI: IgA deficiency w/ Abs to IgA, severe ↓ plt, coag disorders Disp: Inj SE: Associated mostly w/ Inf rate; GI upset, thrombotic events, hemolysis, renal failure/dysfun, TRALI Notes: Monitor vitals during infusion; do not give if volume depleted; Hep A prophylaxis with immunoglobulin is no better than with vaccination; advantages to using vaccination, cost similar

Immune Globulin, Subcutaneous (Hizentra) Uses: *Primary immunodeficiency* Acts: IgG supl Dose: See label for dosage calculation/adjustment; for SQ inf only W/P: [C, ?] CI: Hx anaphylaxis to immune globulin; some IgA deficiency Disp: Sol for SQ Inj 0.2 g/mL (20%) SE: Inj site Rxns, HA, GI complaint, fatigue, fever, N, D, rash, sore throat Notes: May instruct in home administration; keep refrigerated; discard unused drug; use up to 4 Inj sites, max flow rate not > 50 mL/h for all sites combined

Inamrinone [Amrinone] (Inocor) Uses: *Acute CHF, ischemic cardiomyopathy* Acts: Inotrope w/ vasodilator Dose: *Adults.* IV bolus 0.75 mg/kg over 2–3 min; maint 5–10 mcg/kg/min, 10 mg/kg/d max; ↓ if CrCl < 10 mL/min *Peds. ECC 2010. CHF in postop CV surg pts, shock w/* ↑ SVR: 0.75–1 mg/kg IV/IO load over 5 min; repeat X 2 PRN; max 3 mg/kg; cont inf 5–10 mcg/kg/min W/P: [C, ?] CI: Bisulfate allergy Disp: Inj 5 mg/mL SE: Monitor fluid, electrolyte, & renal changes Notes: Incompatible w/ dextrose solns, ✓ LFTs, observe for arrhythmias

Indacaterol (Arcapta Neohaler) BOX: may ↑ risk of asthma related death; may ↑ relative to salmeterol; not for acute asthma Uses: *Long-term maint of COPD (chronic bronchitis/emphysema)* Acts: Long-acting β₂-agonist (LABA)bronchodilator Dose: 75 mcg inhal QD using NEOHALER device W/P: [C, ?/-]not for acute Sx; paradoxical bronchospasm possible; w/ CV Sz disorders, thyrotoxicosis; w/MAOI, TCA, xanthine derivatives, steroids, diuretics may ↑ hypokalemia or ECG changes; β-blocker may ↓ effect CI: asthma w/o long-term asthma med Disp: 75 mcg inhal capsule blister pack SE: cough, oropharyngeal pain, nasopharyngitis, H/A, N

Indapamide (Lozol) Uses: *HTN, edema, CHF* Acts: Thiazide diuretic; ↑ Na, Cl, & H₂O excretion in distal tubule Dose: 1.25–5 mg/d PO W/P: [D, ?] ↑ Effect w/ loop diuretics, ACE inhib, cyclosporine, digoxin, Li CI: Anuria, thiazide/ sulfonamide allergy, renal Insuff, PRG Disp: Tabs 1.25, 2.5 mg SE: ↓ BP, dizziness, photosens Notes: No additional effects w/ doses > 5 mg; take early to avoid nocturia; use sunscreen; OK w/ food/milk

Indinavir (Crixivan) Uses: *HIV Infxn* Acts: Protease inhib; ↓ maturation of noninfectious virions to mature infectious virus Dose: Typical 800 mg PO q8h in combo w/ other antiretrovirals (dose varies); on empty stomach; ↓ w/ hepatic impair W/P: [C, ?] Numerous drug interactions, especially CYP3A4 inhib (Table 10, p 301) CI: w/ Triazolam, midazolam, pimozide, ergot alkaloids, simvastatin, lovastatin, sildenafil, St. John's wort, amiodarone, salmeterol, PDE5 inhib, alpha 1-adrenoreceptor antagonist (alfuzosin); colchicine Disp: Caps 100, 200, 333, 400 mg SE: Nephrolithiasis, dyslipidemia, lipodystrophy, N/V, ↑ bili Notes: Drink six 8-oz glasses of H₂O/d

Indomethacin (Indocin) BOX: May ↑ risk of CV events & GI bleeding Uses: *Arthritis; close ductus arteriosus; ankylosing spondylitis* Acts: ↓ Prostaglandins Dose: *Adults.* 25–50 mg PO bid-tid, max 200 mg/d **Infants:** 0.2–0.25 mg/kg/dose IV; may repeat in 12–24 h up to 3 doses; w/ food W/P: [B, +] CI: ASA/NSAID sensitivity, peptic ulcer/active GI bleed, precipitation of asthma/ urticaria/rhinitis by NSAIDs/ASA, premature neonates w/ NEC, ↓ renal Fxn, active bleeding, thrombocytopenia, 3rd tri PRG Disp: Inj 1 mg/vial; caps 25, 50 mg; SR caps 75 mg; susp 25 mg/5 mL SE: GI bleeding or upset, dizziness, edema Notes: Monitor renal Fxn

Infliximab (Remicade) BOX: TB, invasive fungal Infxns, & other opportunistic Infxns reported, some fatal; perform TB skin testing prior to use; possible association w/ rare lymphoma Uses: *Mod–severe Crohn Dz; fistulizing Crohn Dz;*

ulcerative colitis; RA (w/ MTX) psoriasis, ankylosing spondilitis* **Acts:** IgG1K neutralizes TNF-α **Dose: *Adults. Crohn Dz: Induction:*** 5 mg/kg IV Inf, w/ doses 2 & 6 wk after. ***Maint:*** 5 mg/kg IV Inf q8wk. ***RA:*** 3 mg/kg IV Inf at 0, 2, 6 wk, then q8wk. ***Peds > 6 y.*** 5 mg/kg IV q8wk **W/P:** [B. ?/–] Active Infxn, hepatic impair, Hx or risk of TB, hep B **CI:** Murine allergy, mod–severe CHF, w/ live vaccines (e.g. smallpox) **Disp:** 100 mg Inj **SE:** Allergic Rxns; HA, fatigue, GI upset, Inf Rxns; hepatotox; reactivation hep B, pneumonia, BM suppression, systemic vasculitis, pericardial effusion, new psoriasis **Notes:** Monitor LFTs, PPD at baseline, monitor hep B carrier, skin exam for malignancy w/ psoriasis; can premedicate w/ antihistamines, APAP, and/or steroids to ↓ Inf Rxns

Influenza Vaccine, Inactivated (Afluria, Fluarix, FluLaval, Fluvirin, Fluzone, Fluzone High Dose, Fluzone Intradermal) **Uses:** *Prevent influenza (not H1N1/swine flu)* adults > 50 y, children 6–59 mo, pregnant women (2nd/3rd tri during flu season), nursing home residents, chronic dzs (asthma, CAD, DM, chronic liver or renal dx, hematologic Dzs, immunosuppression), health care workers, household contacts and caregivers of high-risk pts (children < 5 yrs and adults > 50 yrs) **Acts:** Active immunization **Dose: *Adults and Peds > 9 y.*** 0.5 mL/dose IM annually except Fluzone Intradermal for adults 18–64 y, intradermal. ***Peds 6 mo–3 y.*** 0.25 mL IM annually; 0.25 mL IM × 2 doses > 4 wk apart 1st vaccination; give 2 doses in 2nd vaccination year if only 1 dose given in 1st year. ***3–8 y:*** 0.5 mL IM annually, start 0.5 mL IM × 2 doses > 4 wk apart 1st vaccination **W/P:** [C, +] **CI:** Egg hypersensitivity; neomycin, polymyxin (*Afluria*), kanamycin, neomycin (*Agriflu*), gentamicin (*Fluarix*), polymyxin, neomycin (*Fluvirin*)/thimerosal allergy (*FluLaval, Fluvirin,* and *multi-dose Fluzone*); infection at site, acute resp or febrile illness, Hx Guillain-Barré, immunocompromised **Disp:** Based on manufacturer, 0.25-, 0.5-mL prefilled syringes **SE:** Inj site soreness, fever, chills, headache, insomnia, myalgia, malaise, rash, urticaria, anaphylactoid rxns, Guillain-Barré synd **Notes:** Not for swine flu H1N1; can be administered at same time. *Fluarix* and *Fluzone Intradermal* not for peds; US Oct-Nov best, protection 1–2 wk after, lasts up to 6 mo; given yearly, vaccines based on predictions of flu season (Nov-April in US, though sporadic cases all year); whole or split virus for adults; peds < 13 y split virus or purified surface antigen to ↑ febrile Rxns; see www.cdc.gov/flu; 2011–2012 US trivalent vaccines will protect against 3 different flu viruses: A/California/7/09 (H1N1)-like virus [pandemic (H1N1) 2009 influenza virus]; A/Perth/16/2009 (H3N2)-like virus; B/Brisbane/60/2008-like virus

Influenza Monovalent Vaccine (H1N1), Inactivated (CSL, ID Biomedical, Novartis, Sanofi Pasteur) The 2011-12 flu vaccines in the US/Canada will be the trivalent influenza vaccine that includes pandemic H1N1 influenza A. The monovalent vaccine against H1N1 influenza A will no longer be administered.

Influenza Virus Vaccine, Live, Intranasal [LAIV] (FluMist) **Uses:** *Prevent influenza* **Acts:** Live-attenuated vaccine **Dose: *Adults 18–49 y.*** 0.1 mL

each nostril ×1 annually *Peds 2–8 y.* 0.1 mL each nostril ×1 annually; initial 0.1 mL each nostril ×2 doses > 6 wk apart in 1st vaccination year > *9 y:* See adults **W/P:** [C, ?/–] **CI:** Age < 2 years, egg, gentamicin, gelatin, or arginine allergy, peds 2–17 y on ASA, PRG, Hx Guillain-Barré, known/suspected immune deficiency, asthma or reactive airway Dz, acute febrile illness, **Disp:** Prefilled, single-use, intranasal sprayer; shipped frozen, store 35–46°F **SE:** Runny nose, nasal congestion, HA, cough **Notes:** Do not give w/ other vaccines; avoid contact w/ immunocompromised individuals for 21 d; live influenza vaccine more effective in children than inactivated influenza vaccine; 2011-12 US trivalent vaccine will protect against 3 different flu viruses: H3N2, influenza B, H1N1

Insulin, Injectable (See Table 4, p 287)

Uses: *Type 1 or type 2 DM refractory to diet or PO hypoglycemic agents; acute life-threatening ↑ K^+* **Acts:** Insulin supl **Dose:** Based on serum glucose; usually SQ (upper arms, abd wall [most rapid absorption site], upper legs, buttocks); can give IV (only regular)/IM; type 1 typical start dose 0.5–1 units/kg/d; type 2 0.3–0.4 units/kg/d; renal failure ↓ insulin needs **W/P:** [B, +] **CI:** Hypoglycemia **Disp:** Table 4, p 287. Some can dispensed w/preloaded insulin cartridge pens w/ 29-, 30-, or 31-gauge needles and dosing adjustments. **SE:** Hypoglycemia. Highly purified insulins ↑ free insulin; monitor for several wks when changing doses/agents **Notes:** Specific agent/regimen based on patient and physician choices that maintain glycemic control. Typical type 1 regimens use a basal daily insulin w/ premeal Inj of rapidly acting insulins. Insulin pumps may achieve basal insulin levels. ↑ malignancy risk w/ glargine controversial.

Interferon Alfa-2b (Intron-A)

BOX: Can cause or aggravate fatal or life-threatening neuropsychological, autoimmune, ischemic, and infectious disorders. Monitor closely **Uses:** *Hairy cell leukemia, Kaposi sarcoma, melanoma, CML, chronic hep B & C, follicular NHL, condylomata acuminata* **Acts:** Antiproliferative; modulates host immune response; ↓ viral replication in infected cells **Dose:** Per protocols. *Adults.* Per protocols. *Hairy cell leukemia:* 2 mill units/m² IM/SQ 3×/wk for 2–6 mo. *Chronic hep B:* 3 mill units/m² SQ 3×/wk × 1 wk, then 6 mill units/m² 3×/wk (max 10 mill units 3×/wk, total duration 16–24 wk). *Follicular NHL:* 5 mill units SQ 3×/wk for 18 mo. *Melanoma:* 20 mill units/m² IV × 5 d/wk × 4 wk, then 10 mill units/m² SQ 3×/wk × 48 wk. *Kaposi sarcoma:* 30 mill units/m² IM/SQ 3×/wk, then 36 mill units IM/SQ 3×/wk. *Chronic hep C* (Intron-A): 3 mill units 3×/wk × 16 wk (continue 18–24 mo if response). *Condyloma:* 1 mill units/lesion (max 5 lesions) 3×/wk for 3 wk. *Peds. CML:* Chronic hep B: 3 mill units/m² SQ 3×/wk × 1 wk, then 6 mill units/m² 3×/wk × 16–24 wk. **CI:** Benzyl alcohol sensitivity, decompensated liver Dz, autoimmune Dz, immunosuppressed, neonates, infants **Disp:** Inj forms (see also polyethylene glycol [PEG]-interferon) **SE:** Flu-like Sxs, fatigue, anorexia, neurotox at high doses; up to 40% neutralizing Ab w/ Rx

Interferon Alfa-2b & Ribavirin Combo (Rebetron) BOX: Can cause/ or aggravate fatal or life-threatening neuropsychological, autoimmune, ischemic, & infectious disorders. Monitor pts closely. CI in pregnant females & their male partners **Uses:** *Chronic hep C w/ compensated liver Dz who relapse after α-interferon Rx therapy* **Acts:** Combo antiviral agents (see individual agents) **Dose:** 3 mill units Intron A SQ 3× wk w/ 1000–1200 mg of Rebetron PO ÷ bid dose for 24 wk. *Pts < 75 kg:* 1000 mg of Rebetron/d **W/P:** [X, ?] **CI:** PRG, males w/ PRG female partner, autoimmune hep, CrCl < 50 mL/min. *Pts > 75 kg:* Combo packs: 6 vials Intron A (3 mill units/0.5 mL) w/ 6 syringes & EtOH swabs, 70 Rebetol caps; one 18-mill units multidose vial of Intron A Inj (22.8 mill units/3.8 mL; 3 mill units/0.5 mL) & 6 syringes & swabs, 70 Rebetol caps; one 18-mill units Intron A Inj multidose pen (22.5 mill units/1.5 mL; 3 mill units/0.2 mL) w/ 6 needles & swabs, 70 Rebetol caps. *Pts > 75 kg:* Identical except 84 Rebetol caps/pack **SE:** See Box, flu-like synd, HA, anemia **Notes:** Monthly PRG test; instruct in self-administration of SQ Intron A

Interferon Alfacon-1 (Infergen) BOX: Can cause or aggravate fatal or life-threatening neuropsychological, autoimmune, ischemic, & infectious disorders. Monitor closely **Uses:** *Chronic hep C* **Acts:** Biologic response modifier **Dose:** 9 mcg SQ 3×/wk × 24 wk **W/P:** [C, M] **CI:** E. coli product allergy **Disp:** Inj 9, 15 mcg **SE:** Flu-like synd, depression, blood dyscrasias, colitis, pancreatitis, hepatic decompensation, ↑ SCr, eye disorders, ↓ thyroid **Notes:** Allow > 48 h between Inj; monitor CBC, plt, SCr, TFT

Interferon Beta-1a (Rebif) BOX: Can cause or aggravate fatal or life-threatening neuropsychological, autoimmune, ischemic, & infectious disorders. Monitor closely **Uses:** *MS, relapsing* **Acts:** Biologic response modifier **Dose:** 44 mcg SQ 3×/wk; start 8.8 mcg SQ 3×/wk × 2 wk, then 22 mcg SQ 3×/wk × 2 wk **W/P:** [C, ?] w/ Hepatic impair, depression, Sz disorder, thyroid Dz **CI:** Human albumin allergy **Disp:** 0.5- mL prefilled syringes w/ 29-gauge needle *Titrate Pak* 8.8 and 22 mcg; 22 or 44 mcg **SE:** Inj site Rxn, HA, flu-like Sx, malaise, fatigue, rigors, myalgia, depression w/ suicidal ideation, hepatotox, ↓ BM **Notes:** Dose > 48 h apart; ✓ CBC 1, 3, 6 mo; ✓ TFTs q6mo w/ Hx thyroid Dz

Interferon Beta-1b (Betaseron, Extavia) Uses: *MS, relapsing/remitting/ secondary progressive* **Acts:** Biologic response modifier **Dose:** 0.0625 mg (2 mill units) (0.25 mL) q other day SQ, ↑ by 0.0625 mg q2wk to target dose 0.25 mg (1 mL) q other day **W/P:** [C, ?/–] **CI:** Human albumin sensitivity **Disp:** Powder for Inj 0.3 mg (32 mill units interferon [IFN]) **SE:** Flu-like synd, depression, suicide, blood dyscrasias, ↑ AST/ALT/GGT, inj site necrosis, anaphylaxis **Notes:** Teach pt self-injection, rotate sites; ✓ LFTs, CBC 1, 3, 6 mo; TFT q6mo; consider stopping w/depression

Interferon Gamma-1b (Actimmune) Uses: *↓ Incidence of serious infxns in chronic granulomatous Dz (CGD), osteoporosis* **Acts:** Biologic response modifier **Dose:** *Adults. CGD:* 50 mcg/m² SQ (1.5 mill units/m²) BSA > 0.5 m²; if BSA < 0.5 m², give 1.5 mcg/kg/dose; given 3×/wk **W/P:** [C, ?] **CI:** Allergy to E. coli-derived products **Disp:** Inj 100 mcg (2 mill units) **SE:** Flu-like synd, depression, blood dyscrasias, dizziness, altered mental status, gait disturbance, hepatic tox **Notes:** may ↑ deaths in interstitial pulm fibrosis

Ipecac Syrup [OTC] **Uses:** *Drug OD, certain cases of poisoning* **Editorial Note: Usage is falling out of favor & is no longer recommended by some groups** **Acts:** Irritation of the GI mucosa; stimulation of the chemoreceptor trigger zone **Dose:** *Adults.* 15–30 mL PO, followed by 200–300 mL of H_2O; if no emesis in 20 min, repeat once. *Peds 6–12 mo.* 5–10 mL PO, followed by 10–20 mL/kg of H_2O; if no emesis in 20 min, repeat once. *1–12 y:* 15 mL PO followed by 10–20 mL/kg of H_2O; if no emesis in 20 min, repeat once **W/P:** [C, ?] **CI:** Ingestion of petroleum distillates, strong acid, base, or other caustic agents; comatose/unconscious **Disp:** Syrup 15, 30 mL (OTC) **SE:** Lethargy, D, cardiotox, protracted V **Notes:** Caution in CNS depressant OD; activated charcoal considered more effective (www.clintox.org/PosStatements/Ipecac.html)

Ipilimumab (Yervoy) **BOX:** Severe fatal immune Rxns possible; D/C and Tx w/ high-dose steroids w/ severe Rxn; assess for enterocolitis, dermatitis, neuropathy, endocrinopathy before each dose **Uses:** *Unresectable/metastatic melanoma* **Acts:** Human cytotoxic T-lymphocyte antigen 4 (CTLA-4)-blocking Ab; ↑ T cell proliferation/activation **Dose:** 3 mg/kg IV q3wk × 4 doses; inf over 90 min **W/P:** [X, –] can cause immune-mediated adverse Rxns; endocrinopathies may require Rx; hepatitis **CI:** None **Disp:** IV 50 mg/10 mL, 200 mg/40 mL **SE:** fatigue, D, pruritus, rash, colitis **Notes:** ✓ LFTs, TFT, chemistries baseline/pre-inf

Ipratropium (Atrovent HFA, Atrovent Nasal) **Uses:** *Bronchospasm w/ COPD, rhinitis, rhinorrhea* **Acts:** Synthetic anticholinergic similar to atropine; antagonizes acetylcholine receptors, inhibits mucous gland secretions **Dose:** *Adults & Peds > 12 y.* 2–4 puffs qid, max 12 Inh/d *Nasal:* 2 sprays/nostril bid-tid; *Nebulization:* 500 mcg 3–4 ×/d; *ECC 2010. Asthma:* 250–500 mcg by neb/MDI q20min × 3 **W/P:** [B, +/–] w/ Inhaled insulin **CI:** Allergy to soya lecithin-related foods **Disp:** *HFA* Metered-dose inhaler 18 mcg/dose; Inh soln 0.02%; nasal spray 0.03, 0.06% **SE:** Nervousness, dizziness, HA, cough, bitter taste, nasal dryness, URI, epistaxis **Notes:** Not for acute bronchospasm

Irbesartan (Avapro) **BOX:** D/C immediately if PRG detected **Uses:** *HTN, DN*, CHF* **Acts:** Angiotensin II receptor antagonist **Dose:** 150 mg/d PO, may ↑ to 300 mg/d **W/P:** [C (1st tri; D 2nd/3rd), ?/–] **CI:** PRG, component sensitivity **Disp:** Tabs 75, 150, 300 mg **SE:** Fatigue, ↓ BP ↑ K

Irinotecan (Camptosar) **BOX:** D & myelosuppression **Uses:** *Colorectal* & lung CA **Acts:** Topoisomerase I inhib; ↓ DNA synth **Dose:** Per protocol; 125–350 mg/m² q wk–q3wk (↓ hepatic dysfunction, as tolerated per tox) **W/P:** [D, –] **CI:** Allergy to component **Disp:** Inj 20 mg/mL **SE:** ↓ BM, N/V/D, Abd cramping, alopecia; D is dose limiting; Rx acute D w/ atropine; Rx subacute D w/ loperamide **Notes:** D correlated to levels of metabolite SN-38

Iron Dextran (Dexferrum, INFeD) **BOX:** Anaphylactic Rxn w/ death reported; proper personnel and equipment should be available. Use test dose on only if PO iron not possible. **Uses:** *Iron deficiency anemia where PO administration not possible* **Dose:** See also label for tables/formula to calculate dose. Estimate Fe deficiency; total dose (mL) = $(0.0442 \times (\text{desired Hgb} - \text{observed Hgb}) \times \text{lean body wgt}) + (0.26 \times \text{lean body wgt})$; Fe replacement, blood loss: total dose (mg) = blood loss (mL) × Hct (as decimal fraction) max 100 mg/d. **IV use:** *Test dose:* 0.5 mL IV over 30 s, if OK, 2 mL or less daily IV over 1 mL/min to calculated total dose IM u**se:** *Test dose* 0.5 mL deep IM in buttock. Administer calculated total dose not to exceed daily doses as follows: Infants < 5 kg: 1.0 mL; children < 10 kg; all others 2.0 mL (100 mg of iron). **W/P:** [C, M] w/Hx allergy/asthma. Keep Epi available (1:1000) for acute rxn **CI:** Component hypersens, non–Fe-deficiency anemia **Disp:** Inj 50 mg Fe/mL in 2 mL vials (*INFeD*) and 1 & 2 mL vials (*Dexferrum*) **Notes:** Not rec in infants < 4 mo. ✓ Hgb/Hct. Also Fe, TIBC and % saturation transferrin may be used to monitor. Reticulocyte count best early indicator of response (several days). IM use "Z-track" technique

Iron Sucrose (Venofer) **Uses:** *Iron deficiency anemia in CKD, w/wo dialysis, w/wo erythropoietin* **Acts:** Fe supl **Dose:** 100 mg on dialysis; 200 mg slow IV over 25 min ×5 doses over 14-day period. Total cum dose 1000 mg **W/P:** [B, ?] hypersens, ↓ BP, Fe overload, may interfere w/ MRI **CI:** non–Fe-deficiency anemia; Fe overload; component sens **Disp:** Inj 20 mg Fe/mL, 2.5, 5, 10 mL vials **SE:** Muscle cramps, N/V, strange taste in the mouth, diarrhea, constipation, HA, cough, back/jt pain, dizziness, swelling of the arms/legs **Notes:** Safety in peds not established

Isoniazid (INH) **Uses:** *Rx & prophylaxis of TB* **Acts:** Bactericidal; interferes w/ mycolic acid synth, disrupts cell wall **Dose:** *Adults. Active TB:* 5 mg/kg/24 h PO or IM (usually 300 mg/d) or *DOT:* 15 mg/kg (max 900 mg) 3×/wk. *Prophylaxis:* 300 mg/d PO for 6–12 mo or 900 mg 2×/wk. *Peds. Active TB:* 10–15 mg/kg/d daily-bid PO or IM 300 mg/d max. *Prophylaxis:* 10 mg/kg/24 h PO; ↓ in hepatic/renal dysfunction **W/P:** [C, +] Liver Dz, dialysis; avoid EtOH **CI:** Acute liver Dz, Hx INH hep **Disp:** Tabs 100, 300 mg; syrup 50 mg/5 mL; Inj 100 mg/mL **SE:** Hep, peripheral neuropathy, GI upset, anorexia, dizziness, skin Rxn **Notes:** Use w/ 2–3 other drugs for active TB, based on INH resistance patterns when TB acquired & sensitivity results; prophylaxis usually w/ INH alone. IM rarely used. ↓ Peripheral neuropathy w/ pyridoxine 50–100 mg/d. See CDC guidelines (http://www.cdc.gov/tb/) for current TB recommendations

Isoproterenol (Isuprel) **Uses:** *Shock, cardiac arrest, AV nodal block* **Acts:** β_1- & β_2-receptor stimulant **Dose:** *Adults.* 2–10 mcg/min IV Inf; titrate; 2–10 mcg/min titrate (*ECC 2005*) *Peds.* 0.2–2 mcg/kg/min IV Inf; titrate **W/P:** [C, ?] **CI:** Angina, tachyarrhythmias (digitalis-induced or others) **Disp:** 0.02 mg/mL, 0.2 mg/mL **SE:** Insomnia, arrhythmias, HA, trembling, dizziness **Notes:** Pulse > 130 BPM may induce arrhythmias

Isosorbide Dinitrate (Isordil, Sorbitrate, Dilatrate-SR) **Uses:** *Rx & prevent angina*, CHF (w/ hydralazine) **Acts:** Relaxes vascular smooth muscle

Dose: *Acute angina:* 5–10 mg PO (chew tabs) q2–3h or 2.5–10 mg SL PRN q5–10 min; do not give > 3 doses in a 15–30-min period. *Angina prophylaxis:* 5–40 mg PO q6h; do not give nitrates on a chronic q6h or qid basis > 7–10 d; tolerance may develop; provide 10–12-h drug-free intervals; *dose in CHF:* initial 20 mg 3–4×/d,target 120–160 mg/d **W/P:** [C, ?] **CI:** Severe anemia, NAG, postural ↓ BP, cerebral hemorrhage, head trauma (can ↑ ICP), w/ sildenafil, tadalafil, vardenafil **Disp:** Tabs 5, 10, 20, 30; SR tabs 40 mg; SL tabs 2.5, 5 mg; SR caps 40 mg **SE:** HA, ↓ BP, flushing, tachycardia, dizziness **Notes:** Higher PO dose needed for same results as SL forms

Isosorbide Mononitrate (Ismo, Imdur) Uses: *Prevention/Rx of angina pectoris* **Acts:** Relaxes vascular smooth muscle **Dose:** 5–10 mg PO bid, w/ the 2 doses 7 h apart or XR (Imdur) 30–60 mg/d PO, max 240 mg **W/P:** [C, ?] **CI:** Head trauma/cerebral hemorrhage (can ↑ ICP), w/ sildenafil, tadalafil, vardenafil **Disp:** Tabs 10, 20 mg; XR 30, 60, 120 mg **SE:** HA, dizziness, ↓ BP

Isotretinoin [13-*cis* Retinoic Acid] (Accutane, Amnesteem, Claravis, Sotret) **BOX:** Must not be used by PRG females; can induce severe birth defects; pt must be capable of complying w/ mandatory contraceptive measures; prescribed according to product-specific risk management system. Because of teratogenicity, is approved for marketing only under a special restricted distribution FDA program called iPLEDGE Uses: *Refractory severe acne* **Acts:** Retinoic acid derivative **Dose:** 0.5–2 mg/kg/d PO ÷ bid; ↓ in hepatic Dz, take w/ food **W/P:** [X, –] Avoid tetracyclines **CI:** Retinoid sensitivity, PRG **Disp:** Caps 10, 20, 30, 40 mg **SE:** *Rare:* Depression, psychosis, suicidal thoughts; derm sensitivity, xerostomia, photosens, ↑ LFTs, & triglycerides **Notes:** Risk management program requires 2 (–) PRG tests before Rx & use of 2 forms of contraception 1 mo before, during, & 1 mo after Rx; to prescribe isotretinoin, the prescriber must access the iPLEDGE system via the Internet (www.ipledgeprogram.com); monitor LFTs & lipids

Isradipine (DynaCirc) Uses: *HTN* **Acts:** CCB **Dose:** *Adults.* 2.5–5 mg PO bid. **W/P:** [C, ?] **CI:** Severe heart block, sinus bradycardia, CHF, dosing w/in several hours of IV β-blockers **Disp:** Caps 2.5, 5 mg; tabs CR 5, 10 mg **SE:** HA, edema, flushing, fatigue, dizziness, palpitations

Itraconazole (Sporanox) **BOX:** CI w/ cisapride, pimozide, quinidine, dofetilide, or levacetylmethadol. Serious CV events (e.g., ↑ QT, torsades de pointes, ventricular tachycardia, cardiac arrest, and/or sudden death) reported w/ these meds and other CYP3A4 inhib. Do not use for onychomycosis w/ ventricular dysfunction Uses: *Fungal Infxns (aspergillosis, blastomycosis, histoplasmosis, candidiasis)* **Acts:** Azole antifungal, ↓ ergosterol synth **Dose:** 200 mg PO daily-bid (caps w/ meals or cola/grapefruit juice); PO soln on empty stomach; avoid antacids **W/P:** [C, ?] Numerous interactions **CI:** See Box; PRG or considering PRG; ventricular dysfunction **Disp:** Caps 100 mg; soln 10 mg/mL **SE:** N/V, rash, hepatotoxic, ↓ K+, CHF, ↑ BP, neuropathy **Notes:** soln & caps not interchangeable; useful in pts who cannot take amphotericin B; follow LFTs

Ixabepilone Kit (Ixempra)   **BOX:** CI in combo w/ capecitabine w/ AST/ALT > 2.5× ULN or bili > 1× ULN d/t ↑ tox and neutropenia-related death **Uses:** *Metastatic/locally advanced breast CA after failure of an anthracycline, a taxane, and capecitabine* **Acts:** Microtubule inhib **Dose:** 40 mg/m² IV over 3 h q3wk **W/P:** [D, ?/–] **CI:** Hypersens to Cremophor EL; baseline ANC < 1500 cells/mm³ or plt < 100,000 cells/mm³; AST/ or ALT > 2.5× ULN, bili > 1× ULN **Disp:** Inj 15, 45 mg (use supplied diluent) **SE:** neutropenia, leukopenia, anemia, thrombocytopenia, peripheral sensory neuropathy, fatigue/asthenia, myalgia/arthralgia, alopecia, N/V/D, stomatitis/mucositis **Notes:** Substrate CYP3A4, adjust dose w/ strong CYP3A4 inhib/inducers

Japanese Encephalitis Vaccine, Inactivated, Adsorbed (Ixiaro, Je-Vax)   **Uses:** *Prevent Japanese encephalitis* **Action:** Inactivated vaccine **Dose:** *Adults.*0.5 mL IM, repeat 28 days later *Peds.* Use Je-Vax, 1–3 y: Three 0.5 mL SQ doses day 0, 7, 30; > 3 y: Three 1 mL SQ doses on day 0, 7, 30 **W/P:** [B (Ixiaro)/C (Je-Vax), ?] **SE:** HA, fatigue, inj site pain, flu-like syndrome, hypersens Rxns **Notes:** Abbrev admin schedules of 3 doses on day 0, 7, and 14; booster dose recommended after 2 y. Avoid EtOH 48 h after dose

Ketamine (Ketalar) [C-III]   Uses: *Induction/maintenance of anesthesia* (in combo w/ sedatives), sedation, analgesia **Action** Dissociative anesthesia; IV onset 30 s, duration 5–10 min **Dose:** *Adults.* 1–4.5 mg/kg IV, typical 2 mg/kg; 3–8 mg/kg IM *Peds.* 0.5–2 mg/kg IV; 0.5–1 mg/kg for minor procedures(also IM/PO regimens) **W/P:** w/ CAD, ↑ BP, tachycardia, EtOH use/abuse [C, ?/–] **CI:** When ↑ BP hazardous **Disp:** Soln 10, 50, 100 mg/mL **SE:** Arrhythmia, ↑/↓ HR, ↑/↓ BP, N/V, resp depression, emergence Rxn, ↑ CSF pressure. CYP2B6 inhibs w/ ↓ metabolism **Notes:** Used in RSI protocols; street drug of abuse

Ketoconazole (Nizoral)   **BOX:** (Oral use) Risk of fatal hepatotox. Concomitant terfenadine, astemizole, and cisapride are CI d/t serious CV adverse events **Uses:** *Systemic fungal Infxns (Candida, blastomycosis, histoplasmosis, etc); refractory topical dermatophyte Infxn*; PCa when rapid ↓ testosterone needed or hormone refractory **Acts:** Azole, ↓ fungal cell wall synth; high dose blocks P450, to ↓ testosterone production **Dose:** *PO:* 200 mg PO daily; ↑ to 400 mg PO daily for serious Infxn. *PCa:* 400 mg PO tid w/hydrocortisone 20–40 mg ÷ bid; best on empty stomach **W/P:** [C, +/–] w/ Any agent that ↑ gastric pH (↓ absorption); may enhance anticoagulants; w/ EtOH (disulfiram-like Rxn); numerous interactions including statins, niacin; do not use w/ clopidogrel (↓ effect) **CI:** CNS fungal infxns, w/ astemizole, triazolam **Disp:** Tabs 200 mg **SE:** N, rashes, hair loss, HA, ↑ wgt gain, dizziness, disorientation, fatigue, impotence, hepatox, adrenal suppression, acquired cutaneous adherence ("sticky skin synd") **Notes:** Monitor LFTs; can rapidly ↓ testosterone level

Ketoconazole, Topical (Extina, Kuric, Nizoral A-D Shampoo, Xolegel) [Shampoo—OTC]   Uses: *Topical for seborrheic dermatitis, shampoo for dandruff* local fungal infxns d/t dermatophytes & yeast **Acts:** azole, ↓ fungal cell wall synth **Dose:** *Topical:* Apply q day-bid **W/P:** [C, +/–] **CI:** Broken/

inflamed skin **Disp:** Topical cream 2%; (*Xolegel*) gel 2%, (*Extina*) foam 2%, shampoo 1% & 2% **SE:** Irritation, pruritus, stinging **Notes:** Do not dispense foam into hands

Ketoprofen (Orudis, Oruvail) **BOX:** May ↑ risk of CV events & GI bleeding; CI for perioperative pain in CABG surgery **Uses:** *Arthritis (RA/OA), pain* **Acts:** NSAID; ↓ prostaglandins **Dose:** 25–75 mg PO tid-qid, 300 mg/d/max; SR 200 mg/d; w/ food; ↓ w/ hepatic/renal impair, elderly **W/P:** [C (D 3rd tri), –] w/ ACE, diuretics; ↑ warfarin, Li, MTX **CI:** NSAID/ASA sensitivity **Disp:** Caps 50, 75 mg; caps, SR 200 mg **SE:** GI upset, peptic ulcers, dizziness, edema, rash, ↑ BP, ↑ LFTs, renal dysfunction

Ketorolac (Toradol) **BOX:** For short-term (≤5 d) Rx of mod–severe acute pain; CI w/ PUD, GI bleed, post CABG, anticipated major surgery, severe renal Insuff, bleeding diathesis, labor & delivery, nursing, and w/ ASA/NSAIDs. NSAIDs may cause ↑ risk of CV/thrombotic events (MI, stroke). PO CI in peds < 16 y **Uses:** *Pain* **Acts:** NSAID; ↓ prostaglandins **Dose:** *Adults.* 15–30 mg IV/IM q6h; 10 mg PO qid only as continuation of IM/IV; max IV/IM 120 mg/d, max PO 40 mg/d. *Peds 2–16 y.* 1 mg/kg IM × 1 dose; 30 mg max; IV: 0.5 mg/kg, 15 mg max; do not use for > 5 d; ↓ if > 65 y, elderly, w/ renal impair, < 50 kg **W/P:** [C (D 3rd tri), –] w/ ACE inhib, diuretics, BP meds, warfarin **CI:** See Box **Disp:** Tabs 10 mg; Inj 15 mg/mL, 30 mg/mL **SE:** Bleeding, peptic ulcer Dz, ↑ Cr & LFTs, ↑ BP, edema, dizziness, allergy

Ketorolac, Nasal (Sprix) **BOX:** For short-term (5 d) use; CI w/ PUD, GI bleed, suspected bleeding risk, post-op CABG, advanced renal Dz or risk of renal failure w/ vol depletion; risk CV thrombotic events (MI, stroke). **Uses:** *Short-term (< 5 d) Rx pain requiring opioid level analgesia* **Acts:** NSAID; ↓ prostaglandins **Dose:** < 65 y: 31.5 mg (one 15.75 mg spray each nostril) q6–8h; max 126 mg/d. ≥65 y, w/ renal impair or < 50 kg: 15.75 mg (one 15.75 mg spray in only one nostril) q6–8h; max 63 mg/d **W/P:** [C (D 3rd tri), –] do not use w/ other NSAIDs; can cause severe skin Rxns; do not use w/ critical bleeding risk; w/ CHF **CI:** See Box; prophylactic to major surgery/L&D, w/ Hx allergy to other NSAIDs **Disp:** Nasal spray 15.75 mg ketorolac/100 mcL spray (8 sprays/bottle) **SE:** nasal discomfort/rhinitis, ↑ lacrimation, throat irritation, oliguria, rash, ↓ HR, ↓ urine output, ↑ ALT/AST, ↑ BP **Notes:** Not for peds; discard open bottle after 24 h

Ketorolac Ophthalmic (Acular, Acular LS, Acular PF) **Uses:** *Ocular itching w/ seasonal allergies; inflammation w/ cataract extraction*; pain/photophobia w/ incisional refractive surgery (Acular PF); pain w/ corneal refractive surgery (Acular LS) **Acts:** NSAID **Dose:** 1 gtt qid **W/P:** [C, +] Possible cross-sensitivity to NSAIDs, ASA **CI:** Hypersens **Disp:** *Acular LS:* 0.4% 5 mL; *Acular:* 0.5% 3, 5, 10 mL; *Acular PF:* Soln 0.5% **SE:** Local irritation, ↑ bleeding ocular tissues, hyphemas, slow healing, keratitis **Notes:** Do not use w/ contacts

Ketotifen (Alaway, Zaditor) [OTC] **Uses:** *Allergic conjunctivitis* **Acts:** Antihistamine H_1-receptor antagonist, mast cell stabilizer **Dose:** *Adults & Peds > 3 y.*

1 gtt in eye(s) q8–12h **W/P:** [C, ?/–] **Disp:** Soln 0.025%/5 & 10 mL **SE:** Local irritation, HA, rhinitis, keratitis, mydriasis **Notes:** Wait 10 min before inserting contacts

Kunecatechins [Sinecatechins] (Veregen) **Uses:** *External genital/perianal warts* **Acts:** Unknown; green tea extract **Dose:** Apply 0.5-cm ribbon to each wart 3×/d until all warts clear; not > 16 wk **W/P:** [C, ?] **Disp:** Oint 15% **SE:** Erythema, pruritus, burning, pain, erosion/ulceration, edema, induration, rash, phimosis **Notes:** Wash hands before/after use; not necessary to wipe off prior to next use; avoid on open wounds

Labetalol (Trandate) **Uses:** *HTN* & hypertensive emergencies (IV) **Acts:** α- & β-Adrenergic blocker **Dose:** *Adults.* HTN: Initial, 100 mg PO bid, then 200–400 mg PO bid. *Hypertensive emergency:* 20–80 mg IV bolus, then 2 mg/min IV Inf, titrate up to 300 mg; *ECC 2010.* 10 mg IV over 1–2 min; repeat or double dose q10min (150 mg max); or initial bolus, then 2–8 mg/min. **Peds.** PO: 1–3 mg/kg/d in ÷ doses, 1200 mg/d max. *Hypertensive emergency:* 0.4–1.5 mg/kg/h IV cont Inf **W/P:** [C (D in 2nd or 3rd tri), +] **CI:** Asthma/COPD, cardiogenic shock, uncompensated CHF, heart block, sinus brady **Disp:** Tabs 100, 200, 300 mg; Inj 5 mg/mL **SE:** Dizziness, N, ↓ BP, fatigue, CV effects

Lacosamide (Vimpat) **BOX:** Antiepileptics associated w/ ↑ risk of suicide ideation **Uses:** *Adjunct in partial-onset Szs* **Action:** Anticonvulsant **Dose:** *Initial:* 50 mg IV or PO BID, ↑ weekly; *Maint:* 200–400 mg/d; 300 mg/d max if CrCl < 30 mL/min or mild/mod hepatic Dz **W/P:** [C, ?] **CI:** None **Disp:** IV: 200 mg/mL; Tabs: 50, 100, 150, 200 mg; oral soln 10 mg/mL **SE:** Dizziness, N/V, ataxia **Notes:** ✓ ECG before dosing; may ↑ PR interval

Lactic Acid & Ammonium Hydroxide [Ammonium Lactate] (Lac-Hydrin) **Uses:** *Severe xerosis & ichthyosis* **Acts:** Emollient moisturizer, humectant **Dose:** Apply bid **W/P:** [B, ?] **Disp:** Cream, lotion, lactic acid 12% w/ ammonium hydroxide **SE:** Local irritation, photosens **Notes:** Shake well before use

Lactobacillus (Lactinex Granules) [OTC] **Uses:** *Control of D*, especially after antibiotic Rx **Acts:** Replaces nl intestinal flora, lactase production; *Lactobacillus acidophilus* and *Lactobacillus helveticus.* **Dose:** *Adults & Peds > 3 y.* 1 packet, 1–2 caps, or 4 tabs q day-qid **W/P:** [A, +] Some products may contain whey **CI:** Milk/lactose allergy **Disp:** Tabs, caps; granules in packets (all OTC) **SE:** Flatulence **Notes:** May take granules on food

Lactulose (Constulose, Generlac, Enulose, Others) **Uses:** *Hepatic encephalopathy; constipation* **Acts:** Acidifies the colon, allows ammonia to diffuse into colon; osmotic effect to ↑ peristalsis **Dose:** *Acute hepatic encephalopathy:* 30–45 mL PO q1h until soft stools, then tid-qid, adjust 2–3 stool/d. *Constipation:* 15–30 mL/d, ↑ to 60 mL/d 1–2 ÷ doses, adjust to 2–3 stools. *Rectally:* 200 g in 700 mL of H₂O PR, retain 30–60 min q4–6h. *Peds Infants.* 2.5–10 mL/24 h ÷ tid-qid. *Other Peds.* 40–90 mL/24 h ÷ tid-qid. *Peds Constipation:* 5 g (7.5 mL) PO after breakfast **W/P:** [B, ?] **CI:** Galactosemia **Disp:** Syrup 10 g/15 mL, soln 10 g/15 mL, 10, 20 g/packet **SE:** Severe D, N/V, cramping, flatulence; life-threatening electrolyte disturbances

Lamivudine (Epivir, Epivir-HBV, 3TC [Many Combo Regimens])
BOX: Lactic acidosis & severe hepatomegaly w/ steatosis reported w/ nucleoside analogs **Uses:** *HIV Infxn, chronic hep B* **Acts:** NRTI, ↓ HIV RT & hep B viral polymerase, causes viral DNA chain termination **Dose:** *HIV: Adults & Peds > 16 y.* 150 mg PO bid or 300 mg PO daily. *Peds able to swallow pills. 14–21 kg:* 75 mg bid; *22–29 kg:* 75 mg q A.M., 150 mg P.M.; *> 30 kg:* 150 mg bid. *Neonates < 30 d:* 2 mg/kg bid. *Epivir-HBV: Adults.* 100 mg/d PO. *Peds 2–17 y.* 3 mg/kg/d PO, 100 mg max; ↓ w/ CrCl < 50 mL/min **W/P:** [C, –] w/ Interferon-α and ribavirin may cause liver failure; do not use w/ zalcitabine or w/ ganciclovir/valganciclovir **Disp:** Tabs 100 mg (Epivir-HBV) 150 mg, 300 mg; soln 5 mg/mL (Epivir-HBV), 10 mg/mL **SE:** Malaise, fatigue, N/V/D, HA, pancreatitis, lactic acidosis, peripheral neuropathy, fat redistribution, rhabdomyolysis hyperglycemia, nasal Sxs **Notes:** Differences in formulations; do not use Epivir-HBV for hep in pt w/ unrecognized HIV d/t rapid emergence of HIV resistance

Lamotrigine (Lamictal) **BOX:** Serious rashes requiring hospitalization & D/C of Rx reported; rash less frequent in adults; ↑ suicidality risk for antiepileptic drug, higher for those w/ epilepsy vs. those using drug for psychological indications **Uses:** *Partial Szs, tonic-clonic Szs, bipolar disorder, Lennox-Gastaut synd* **Acts:** Phenyltriazine antiepileptic, ↓ glutamate, stabilize neuronal membrane **Dose:** *Adults. Szs:* Initial 50 mg/d PO, then 50 mg PO bid × 1–2 wk, maint 300–500 mg/d in 2 ÷ doses. *Bipolar:* Initial 25 mg/d PO × 1–2 wk, 50 mg PO daily for 2 wk, 100 mg PO daily for 1 wk, maint 200 mg/d. *Peds.* 0.6 mg/kg in 2 ÷ doses for wk 1 & 2, then 1.2 mg/kg for wk 3 & 4, q1–2wk to maint 5–15 mg/kg/d (max 400 mg/d) 1–2 ÷ doses; ↓ in hepatic Dz or if w/ enzyme inducers or valproic acid **W/P:** [C, –] Interactions w/ other antiepileptics, estrogen, rifampin **Disp:** Tabs 25, 100, 150, 200 mg; chew tabs 2, 5, 25 mg (color-coded for those on interacting meds) **SE:** Photosens, HA, GI upset, dizziness, diplopia, blurred vision, blood dyscrasias, ataxia, rash (may be much more life-threatening to peds than to adults), aseptic meningitis **Notes:** Value of therapeutic monitoring uncertain, taper w/ D/C

Lamotrigine, Extended-Release (Lamictal XR) **BOX:** Life-threatening serious rashes, including Stevens-Johnson syndrome and toxic epidermal necrolysis, and/or rash-related death reported; D/C at first sign of rash **Uses:** *Adjunct primary generalized tonic-clonic Sz, conversion to monotherapy in pt > 13 y w/ partial Szs* **Acts:** Phenyltriazine antiepileptic, ↓ glutamate, stabilize neuronal membrane **Dose:** Adjunct target 200–600 mg/d; monotherapy conversion target dose 25–300 mg/d *Adults. w/ Valproate:* wk 1–2 25 mg qod, wk 3–4, 25 mg qd, wk 5 50 mg qd, wk 6 100 mg qdwk 7 150 mg qd, then maint 200–250 mg qd. *w/o Carbamazepine, Phenytoin, Phenobarbital, Primidone, or Valproate:* wk 1–2 25 mg qd, wk 3–4 50 mg qd, wk 5 100 mg qd, wk 6 150 mg qd, wk 7 200 mg qd, then maint 300–400 mg qd. *Convert IR to ER tabs:* Initial dose = total daily dose of IR. *Convert adjunctive to monotherapy:* Maint: 250–300 mg qd. Refer to PI for specifics.

w/ *Estrogen-containing OCP*: See insert. *Peds > 13 y.* See adult **W/P:** [C, –] Interactions w/ other antiepileptics, estrogen (OCP), rifampin; valproic acid ↑ levels at least 2×; ↑ suicidal ideation; withdrawal Szs **SE:** Component hypersensitivity (see Box) **Disp:** Tabs 25, 100, 150, 200 mg **SE:** Dizziness, tremor/intention tremor, V, and diplopia. Rash (may be much more life-threatening to peds than to adults), aseptic meningitis, blood dyscrasias **Notes:** Taper over 2 wk w/d

Lansoprazole (Prevacid, Prevacid IV, Prevacid 24HR [OTC]) **Uses:** *Duodenal ulcers, prevent & Rx NSAID gastric ulcers, active gastric ulcers, *H. pylori* Infxn, erosive esophagitis, & hypersecretory conditions, GERD* **Acts:** Proton pump inhib **Dose:** 15–30 mg/d PO; *NSAID ulcer prevention:* 15 mg/d PO × 12 wk. *NSAID ulcers:* 30 mg/d PO × 8 wk; *hypersecretory condition:* 60 mg/d before food; 30 mg IV daily = 7 d change to PO for 6–8 wk; ↓ w/ severe hepatic impair **W/P:** [B, ?/–] w/ clopidogrel **Disp:** *Prevacid:* DR Caps 15, 30 mg; *Prevacid 24HR* [OTC] 15 mg; *Prevacid SoluTab* (ODT) 15 mg (contains phenylalanine); IV 30 mg **SE:** N/V, Abd pain, HA, fatigue **Notes:** For IV provided inline filter must be used; do not crush/chew; granules can be given w/applesauce or apple juice (NG tube) only; ? ↑ risk of fractures w/ all PPI; caution w/ ODT in feeding tubes; risk of hypomagnesemia w/ long-term use; monitor

Lanthanum Carbonate (Fosrenol) **Uses:** *Hyperphosphatemia in renal Dz* **Acts:** Phosphate binder **Dose:** 750–1500 mg PO daily ÷ doses, w/ or immediately after meal; titrate q2–3wk based on PO$_4^{2-}$ levels **W/P:** [C, ?/–] No data in GI Dz; not for peds **Disp:** Chew tabs 250, 500, 750, 1000 mg **SE:** N/V, graft occlusion, HA, ↓ BP **Notes:** Chew tabs before swallowing; separate from meds that interact w/ antacids by 2 h

Lapatinib (Tykerb) **Uses:** *Advanced breast CA w/ capecitabine w/ tumors that over express HER2 and failed w/ anthracycline, taxane, & trastuzumab* **Acts:** TKI **Dose:** Per protocol, 1250 mg PO days 1–21 w/ capecitabine 2000 mg/m^2/d ÷ 2 doses/d on days 1–14; ↓ w/ severe cardiac or hepatic impair **W/P:** [D,:?] Avoid CYP3A4 inhib/inducers **CI:** w/ Phenothiazines **Disp:** Tabs 250 mg **SE:** N/V/D, anemia, ↓ plt, neutropenia, ↑ QT interval, hand-foot synd, ↑ LFTs, rash, ↓ left ventricular ejection fraction, interstitial lung Dz and pneumonitis **Notes:** Consider baseline LVEF & periodic ECG

Latanoprost (Xalatan) **Uses:** *Open-angle glaucoma, ocular HTN* **Acts:** Prostaglandin, ↑ outflow of aqueous humor **Dose:** 1 gtt eye(s) hs **W/P:** [C, ?] **Disp:** 0.005% soln **SE:** May darken light irides; blurred vision, ocular stinging, & itching, ↑ number & length of eyelashes **Notes:** Wait 15 min before using contacts; separate from other eye products by 5 min

Leflunomide (Arava)   **BOX:** PRG must be excluded prior to start of Rx **Uses:** *Active RA, orphan drug for organ rejection* **Acts:** DMARD, ↓ pyrimidine synth **Dose:** Initial 100 mg/d PO for 3 d, then 10–20 mg/d **W/P:** [X, –] w/ Bile acid sequestrants, warfarin, rifampin, MTX **CI:** PRG **Disp:** Tabs 10, 20, 100 mg **SE:** D, Infxn, HTN, alopecia, rash, N, joint pain, hep, interstitial lung Dz, immunosuppression

Notes: Monitor LFTs, CBC, PO$^+$ during initial Rx; vaccine should be up-to-date, do not give w/ live vaccines

Lenalidomide (Revlimid) **BOX:** Significant teratogen; pt must be enrolled in RevAssist risk-reduction program; hematologic tox, DVT & PE risk **Uses:** *MDS, combo w/ dexamethasone in multiple myeloma in pt failing one prior Rx* **Acts:** Thalidomide analog, immune modulator **Dose:** *Adults.* 10 mg PO daily; swallow whole w/ water; multiple myeloma 25 mg/d days 1–21 of 28-d cycle w/ protocol dose of dexamethasone **W/P:** [X, –] w/ Renal impair **Disp:** Caps 5, 10, 15, 25 mg **SE:** D, pruritus, rash, fatigue, night sweats, edema, nasopharyngitis, ↓ BM (plt, WBC), ↑ K$^+$, ↑ LFTs, thromboembolism **Notes:** Monitor CBC and for thromboembolism, hepatotox; routine PRG tests required; Rx only in 1-mo increments; limited distribution network; males must use condom and not donate sperm; use at least 2 forms contraception > 4 wk beyond D/C

Lepirudin (Refludan) **Uses:** *HIT* **Acts:** Direct thrombin inhib **Dose:** *Bolus:* 0.4 mg/kg IV, then 0.15 mg/kg/h Inf; if > 110 kg 44 mg of Inf 16.5 mg/h max; ↓ dose & Inf rate w/ if CrCl < 60 mL/min or if used w/ thrombolytics **W/P:** [B, ?/–] Hemorrhagic event, or severe HTN **CI:** Active bleeding **Disp:** Inj 50 mg **SE:** Bleeding, anemia, hematoma, anaphylaxis **Notes:** Adjust based on aPTT ratio, maintain aPTT 1.5–2 × control

Letrozole (Femara) **Uses:** *Breast CA:* Adjuvant w/postmenopausal hormone receptor positive early Dz; adjuvant in postmenopausal women with early breast CA w/prior adjuvant tamoxifen therapy; 1st/2nd-line in postmenopausal w/ hormone receptor positive or unknown dx* **Acts:** Nonsteroidal aromatase inhib **Dose:** 2.5 mg/d PO; q other day w/ severe liver Dz or cirrhosis **W/P:** [D, ?] **CI:** PRG, premenopausal **Disp:** Tabs 2.5 mg **SE:** Anemia, N, hot flashes, arthralgia **Notes:** Monitor CBC, thyroid Fxn, lytes, LFTs, & SCr

Leucovorin (Wellcovorin) **Uses:** *OD of folic acid antagonist; megaloblastic anemia, augment 5-FU impaired MTX elimination; w/ 5-FU in colon CA* **Acts:** Reduced folate source; circumvents action of folate reductase inhib (e.g., MTX) **Dose:** *Leucovorin rescue:* 10 mg/m^2 PO/IM/IV q6h; start w/in 24 h after dose or 15 mg PO/IM/IV q6h, 25 mg/dose max PO; *Folate antagonist OD (e.g., Pemetrexed)* 100 mg/m^2 IM/IV × 1 then 50 mg/m^2 IM/IV q6h × 8 d; *5-FU adjuvant tx, colon CA per protocol; low dose:* 20 mg/m^2/d IV × 5 d w/ 5-FU 425 mg/m^2/d IV × 5 d, repeat q4–5wk × 6; *high dose:* 500 mg/m^2 IV q wk × 6, w/ 5-FU 500 mg/m^2 IV q wk × 6 wk, repeat after 2 wk off × 4; *Megaloblastic anemia:* 1 mg IM/IV daily **W/P:** [C, ?/–] **CI:** Pernicious anemia **Disp:** Tabs 5, 10, 15, 25 mg; Inj 50, 100, 200, 350, 500 mg **SE:** Allergic Rxn, N/V/D, fatigue, wheezing, ↑ plt **Notes:** Monitor Cr, methotrexate levels q24h w/ leucovorin rescue; do not use intrathecally/intraventricularly; w/ 5-FU CBC w/ diff, plt, LFTs, lytes

Leuprolide (Lupron, Lupron DEPOT, Lupron DEPOT-Ped, Viadur, Eligard) **Uses:** *Advanced PCa (all except Depot-Ped), endometriosis (*Lupron*), uterine fibroids (*Lupron*), & precocious puberty (*Lupron-Ped*)* **Acts:** LHRH agonist;

paradoxically ↓ release of GnRH w/ ↓ LH from anterior pituitary; in men ↓ testosterone **Dose: *Adults. PCa: Lupron DEPOT:*** 7.5 mg IM q28d or 22.5 mg IM q3mo or 30 mg IM q4mo or 45 mg IM q4mo. *Eligard:* 7.5 mg IM q28d or 22.5 mg SQ q3mo or 30 mg SQ q4mo or 45 mg SQ 6 mo. *Endometriosis (Lupron DEPOT):* 3.75 mg IM q mo × 6 or 11.25 IM q3mo × 2. *Fibroids:* 3.75 mg IM q mo × 3 or 11.25 mg IM × 1. **Peds.** *CPP (Lupron DEPOT-Ped):* 50 mcg/kg/d SQ Inj; ↑ by 10 mcg/kg/d until total downregulation achieved. *Lupron DEPOT: < 25 kg:* 7.5 mg IM q4wk; *> 25–37.5 kg:* 11.25 mg IM q4wk; *> 37.5 kg:* 15 mg IM q4wk, ↑ by 3.75 mg q4wk until response **W/P:** [X, −] w/ Impending cord compression in PCa **CI:** AUB, implant in women/pegs; **PRG Disp:** Inj 5 mg/mL; *Lupron DEPOT:* 3.75 mg (1 mo for fibroids, endometriosis); *Lupron DEPOT* for PCa: 7.5 mg (1 mo), 11.25 (3 mo), 22.5 (3 mo), 30 (4 mo), 45 mg (6 mo); *Eligard depot* for PCA: 7.5 (1 mo); 22.5 (3 mo), 30 (4 mo), 45 (6 mo); *Viadur* 65 mg 12-mo SQ implant (unavailable to new Rx), Lupron DEPOT-Ped: 7.5, 11.25, 15 mg **SE:** Hot flashes, gynecomastia, N/V, alopecia, anorexia, dizziness, HA, insomnia, paresthesias, depression exacerbation, peripheral edema, & bone pain (transient "flare Rxn" at 7–14 d after the 1st dose [LH/testosterone surge before suppression]); ↓ BMD w/ > 6 mo use, bone loss possible **Notes:** Nonsteroidal antiandrogen (e.g., bicalutamide) may block flare in men w/ PCa

Levalbuterol (Xopenex, Xopenex HFA) **Uses:** *Asthma (Rx & prevention of bronchospasm)* **Acts:** Sympathomimetic bronchodilator; *R*-isomer of albuterol **Dose:** Based on NIH Guidelines 2007 **Adults.** Acute–severe exacerbation Xopenex HFA 4–8 puffs q20min up to 4 h, the q1–4h PRN or nebulizer 1/25–2.5 mg q20min × 3, then 1.25–5 mg q1–4h PRN; *Peds < 4 y.* Quick relief 0.31–1.25 mg q4–6h PRN, severe 1.25 mg q20min × 3, then 0.075–0.15 mg/kg q1–4h PRN, 5 mg max. **5–11 y:** Acute–severe exacerbation 1.25 mg q20min × 3, then 0.075–0.15 mg/kg q1–4h PRN, 5 mg max. **> 11 y:** 0.63–1.25 mg nebulizer q6–8h **W/P:** [C, ?] w/ Non–K+-sparing diuretics, CAD, HTN, arrhythmias, ↓ K+ **CI:** w/ Phenothiazines & TCAs, MAOI w/in 14 d **Disp:** Multidose inhaler (Xopenex HFA) 45 mcg/puff (15 g); soln nebulizer Inh 0.31, 0.63, 1.25 mg/3 mL; concentrate 1.25 mg/0.5 mL **SE:** Paradox bronchospasm, anaphylaxis, angioedema, tachycardia, nervousness, V, ↓ K+ **Notes:** May ↓ CV SEs compared w/ albuterol; do not mix w/ other nebs or dilute

Levetiracetam (Keppra) **Uses:** *Adjunctive PO Rx in partial onset Sz (adults & peds ≥4 y), myoclonic Szs (adults & peds ≥12 y) w/ juvenile myoclonic epilepsy (JME), primary generalized tonic-clonic (PGTC) Szs (adults & peds ≥6 y) w/ idiopathic generalized epilepsy. Adjunctive Inj Rx partial-onset Szs in adults w/ epilepsy; and myoclonic Szs in adults w/ JME. Inj alternative for adults (≥16 y) when PO not possible* **Acts:** Unknown **Dose: Adults & Peds > 16 y.** 500 mg PO bid, titrate q2wk, may ↑ 3000 mg/d max. **Peds 4–15 y.** 10–20 mg/kg/d ÷ in 2 doses, 60 mg/kg/d max (↓ in renal Insuff) **W/P:** [C, ?/−] Elderly, w/ renal impair, psychological disorders; ↑ suicidality risk for antiepileptic drugs, higher for those w/ epilepsy vs. those using drug for psychological indications; Inj not for < 16 y **CI:** Component allergy **Disp:** Tabs 250, 500, 750, 1000 mg, soln 100 mg/mL; Inj 100 mg/mL **SE:** Dizziness, somnolence, HA, N/V, hostility, aggression, hallucinations, myelosuppression, impaired coordination **Notes:** Do not D/C abruptly; postmarket hepatic failure and pancytopenia reported

Levobunolol (A-K Beta, Betagan) **Uses:** *Open-angle glaucoma, ocular HTN* **Acts:** β-Adrenergic blocker **Dose:** 1 gtt daily-bid **W/P:** [C, ?] w/ Verapamil or systemic β-blockers **CI:** Asthma, COPD, sinus bradycardia, heart block (2nd-, 3rd-degree) CHF **Disp:** Soln 0.25, 0.5% **SE:** Ocular stinging/burning, ↓ HR, ↓ BP **Notes:** Possible systemic effects if absorbed

Levocetirizine (Xyzal) **Uses:** *Perennial/seasonal allergic rhinitis, chronic urticaria* **Acts:** Antihistamine **Dose:** *Adults.* 5 mg q day *Peds 6–11 y.* 2.5 mg q day **W/P:** [B, ?] ↓ Adult dose w/ renal impair, CrCl 50–80 mL/min 2.5 mg daily, 30–50 mL/min 2.5 mg q other day 10–30 mL/min 2.5 mg 2×/wk **CI:** Peds 6–11 y w/ renal impair, adults w/ ESRD **Disp:** Tab 5 mg, soln 0.5 mL/min (150 mL) **SE:** CNS depression, drowsiness, fatigue, xerostomia **Notes:** Take in evening

Levofloxacin (Levaquin, Generic) **BOX:** ↑ Risk Achilles tendon rupture and tendonitis **Uses:** *Skin/skin structure Infxn (SSSI), UTI, chronic bacterial prostatitis, acute pyelo, acute bacterial sinusitis, acute bacterial exacerbation of chronic bronchitis, CAP, including multidrug-resistant S. pneumoniae, nosocomial pneumonia; Rx inhalational anthrax in adults & peds ≥6 mo* **Acts:** Quinolone, ↓ DNA gyrase. *Spectrum:* Excellent gram(+) except MRSA & E. faecium; excellent gram(−) except Stenotrophomonas maltophilia & Acinetobacter sp; poor anaerobic **Dose:** *Adults ≥18 y:* IV/PO: *Bronchitis:* 500 mg q day × 7 d. *CAP:* 500 mg q day × 7–14 d or 750 mg q day × 5 d. *Sinusitis:* 500 mg q day × 10–14 d or 750 mg q day × 5 d. *Prostatitis:* 500 mg q day × 28 d. *Uncomp SSSI:* 500 mg q day × 7–10 d. *Comp SSSI/Nosocomial Pneumonia:* 750 mg q day × 7–14 d. *Anthrax:* 500 mg q day × 60 d. *Uncomp UTI:* 250 mg q day × 3 d. *Comp UTI/Acute Pyelo:* 250 mg q day × 10 d or 750 mg q day × 5 d. CrCl 10–19 mL/min: 250 mg, then 250 mg q48h or 750 mg, then 500 mg q48h. *Hemodialysis:* 750 mg, then 500 mg q48h. *Peds ≥ 6 mo. Anthrax only > 50 kg:* 500 mg q 24h × 60 d, < 50 kg 8 mg/kg (250 mg/dose max) q12h for 60 d ↓ w/ renal impair avoid antacids w/ PO; oral soln 1 h before, 2 h after meals **W/P:** [C, −] w/ Cation-containing products (e.g., antacids), w/ drugs that ↑ QT interval **CI:** Quinolone sensitivity **Disp:** Tabs 250, 500, 750 mg; premixed IV 250, 500, 750 mg, Inj 25 mg/mL; Leva-Pak 750 mg × 5 d **SE:** N/D, dizziness, rash, GI upset, photosens, CNS stimulant w/ IV use, C. difficile enterocolitis; rare fatal hepatox **Notes:** Use w/ steroids ↑ tendon risk; only for anthrax in peds

Levofloxacin Ophthalmic (Quixin, Iquix) **Uses:** *Bacterial conjunctivitis* **Acts:** See levofloxacin **Dose:** *Ophthal:* 1–2 gtt in eye(s) q2h while awake × 2 d, then q4h while awake × 5 d **W/P:** [C, −] **CI:** Quinolone sensitivity **Disp:** 25 mg/mL ophthal soln 0.5% (Quixin), 1.5% (Iquix) **SE:** Ocular burning/ pain, ↓ vision, fever, foreign body sensation, HA, pharyngitis, photophobia

Levonorgestrel (Next Choice, Plan B One-Step) Uses: *Emergency contraceptive ("morning-after pill")* Prevents PRG if taken < 72 h after unprotected sex/contraceptive failure Acts: Progestin, alters tubal transport & endometrium to implantation Dose: *Adults & Peds (postmenarche females).* w/in 72 h of unprotected intercourse: *Next Choice* 0.75 mg q12h × 2; *Plan B One-Step* 1.5 mg × 1 W/P: [X, +] w/ AUB; may ↑ ectopic PRG risk CI: Known/suspected PRG Disp: *Next Choice* tab, 0.75 mg, 2 blister pack; *Plan B One-Step* tab, 1.5 mg, 1 blister pack SE: N/V/D, abd pain, fatigue, HA, menstrual changes, dizziness, breast changes Notes: Will not induce abortion; OTC ("behind the counter") if > 17 y, RX if < 17 y but varies by state

Levonorgestrel IUD (Mirena) Uses: *Contraception, long-term* Acts: Progestin, alters endometrium, thicken cervical mucus, inhibits ovulation and implantation Dose: Up to 5 y, insert w/in 7 d menses onset or immediately after 1st tri abortion; wait 6 wk if postpartum; replace any time during menstrual cycle W/P: [C, ?] CI: PRG, w/active hepatic Dz or tumor, uterine anomaly, breast CA, acute/Hx of PID, postpartum endometriosis, infected abortion last 3 mo, gynecological neoplasia, abnormal Pap, AUB, untreated cervicitis/vaginitis, multiple sex partners, ↑ susceptibility to Infxn Disp: 52 mg IUD SE: Failed insertion, ectopic PRG, sepsis, PID, infertility, PRG comps w/ IUD left in place, abortion, embedment, ovarian cysts, perforation uterus/cervix, intestinal obst/perforation, peritonitis, N, Abd pain, ↑ BP, acne, HA Notes: Inform pt does not protect against STD/HIV; see PI for insertion instructions; reexamine placement after 1st menses; 80% PRG w/in 12 mo of removal

Levorphanol (Levo-Dromoran) [C-II] Uses: *Mod–severe pain; chronic pain* Acts: Narcotic analgesic, morphine derivative Dose: 2–4 mg PO PRN q6–8h; ↓ in hepatic impair W/P: [B/D (prolonged use/high doses at term), ?/–] w/ ↑ ICP, head trauma, adrenal Insuff CI: Component allergy Disp: Tabs 2 mg SE: Tachycardia, ↑ BP, drowsiness, GI upset, constipation, resp depression, pruritus

Levothyroxine (Synthroid, Levoxyl, Others) BOX: Not for obesity or wgt loss; tox w/ high doses, especially when combined w/ sympathomimetic amines Uses: *Hypothyroidism, pituitary thyroid-stimulating hormone (TSH) suppression, myxedema coma* Acts: T_4 supl l-thyroxine Dose: Adults. *Hypothyroid* titrate until euthyroid > 50 y w/o heart Dz or < 50 w/ heart Dz 25–50 mcg/d, ↑ q6–8wk; > 50 y w/o heart Dz 12.5–25 mcg/d, ↑ q6–8wk; usual 100–200 mcg/d. *Myxedema:* 200–500 mcg IV, then 100–300 mcg/d. Peds. *Hypothyroid:* 0–3 mo: 10–15 mcg/kg/24 h PO; *3–6 mo:* 8–10 mcg/kg/d PO; *6–12 mo:* 6–8 mcg/kg/d PO; *1–5 y:* 5–6 mcg/kg/d PO; *6–12 y:* 4–5 mcg/kg/d PO; > 12 y: 2–3 mcg/kg/d PO; if growth and puberty complete 1.7 mcg/kg/d; ↓ dose by 50% if IV; titrate based on response & thyroid tests; dose can ↑ rapidly in young/middle-aged; best on empty stomach W/P: [A, +] w/ warfarin monitor INR CI: Recent MI, uncorrected adrenal Insuff; many drug interactions; in elderly w/ CV Dz Disp: Tabs 25, 50, 75, 88, 100, 112, 125, 137, 150, 175, 200, 300 mcg; Inj 200, 500 mcg SE: Insomnia, wgt loss,

N/V/D, ↑ LFTs, irregular periods, ↓ BMD, alopecia, arrhythmia **Notes:** Take w/ full glass of water (prevents choking); PRG may ↑ need for higher doses; takes 6 wk to see effect on TSH; wait 6 wk before checking TSH after dose change

Linagliptin (Tradjenta) Uses: *Type 2 DM alone or combo (w/ metformin or glimepiride)* **Acts:** ↑ insulin release; blocks enzyme dipeptidyl peptidase-4 **Dose:** 5 mg/d w/wo food **W/P:** [B, ?] Not for type 1 DM; w/ insulin secretagogue (e.g., sulfonylurea) ↑ secretagogue dose **CI:** N **Disp:** Tabs 5 mg **SE:** URI, stuffy nose, sore throat, muscle pain, HA

Lidocaine, Systemic (Xylocaine, Others) Uses: *Rx cardiac arrhythmias* **Acts:** Class IB antiarrhythmic **Dose:** *Adults. Antiarrhythmic, ET:* 5 mg/kg; follow w/ 0.5 mg/kg in 10 min if effective. *IV load:* 1 mg/kg/dose bolus over 2–3 min; repeat in 5–10 min; 200–300 mg/h max; cont Inf 20–50 mcg/kg/min or 1–4 mg/min; *ECC 2010. Cardiac arrest from VF/VT refractory VF: Initial:* 1–1.5 mg/kg IV/IO, additional 0.5–0.75 mg/kg IV push, repeat in 5–10 min, max total 3 mg/kg. ET: 2–4 mg/kg as last resort. *Reperfusing stable VT, wide complex tachycardia, or ectopy:* Doses of 0.5–0.75 mg/kg to 1–1.5 mg/kg may be used initially; repeat 0.5–0.75 mg/kg q5–10min; max dose 3 mg/kg. *Peds. ECC 2010. VF/pulseless VT, wide-complex tach (w/ pulses):* 1 mg/kg IV/IO, then maint 20–50 mcg/kg/min (repeat bolus if inf started > 15 min after initial dose); RSI: 1–2 mg/kg IV/IO **W/P:** [B, +] Corn allergy **CI:** Adams-Stokes synd; heart block **Disp:** *Inj IV:* 1% (10 mg/mL), 2% (20 mg/mL); admixture 4, 10, 20%. *IV Inf:* 0.2, 0.4% **SE:** Dizziness, paresthesias, & convulsions associated w/ tox **Notes:** 2nd line to amiodarone in ECC; dilute ET dose 1–2 mL w/ NS; for IV forms, ↓ w/ liver Dz or CHF; *Systemic levels:* steady state 6–12 h; *Therapeutic:* 1.2–5 mcg/mL; *Toxic:* > 6 mcg/mL; *1/2-life:* 1.5 h

Lidocaine; Lidocaine w/ Epinephrine (Anestacon Topical, Xylocaine, Xylocaine Viscous, Xylocaine MPF, Others) Uses: *Local anesthetic, epidural/caudal anesthesia, regional nerve blocks, topical on mucous membranes (mouth/pharynx/urethra)* **Acts:** Anesthetic; stabilizes neuronal membranes; inhibits ionic fluxes required for initiation and conduction **Dose:** *Adults. Local Inj anesthetic:* 4.5 mg/kg max total dose or 300 mg; w/ epi 7 mg/kg or total 500 mg max dose. *Oral:* 15 mL viscous swish and spit or *pharyngeal* gargle and swallow, do not use < 3-h intervals or > 8 × in 24 h. *Urethra:* 10–15 mL (200–300 mg) jelly in men, 5 mL female urethra; 600 mg/24 h max. *Peds. Topical:* Apply max 3 mg/kg/dose. *Local Inj anesthetic:* Max 4.5 mg/kg (Table 1, p 282) **W/P:** [B, +] Corn allergy; epi-containing soln may interact w/ TCA or MAOI and cause severe ↑ BP **CI:** Do not use lidocaine w/ epi on digits, ears, or nose (vasoconstriction & necrosis) **Disp:** *Inj local:* 0.5, 1.5, 1, 1.5, 2, 4, 10, 20%; *Inj w/ epi* 0.5%/1:200,000, 1%/1:100,000, 2%/1:100,000; (MPF) 1%/1:200,000, 1.5%/1:200,000, 2%/1:200,000; *(Dental formulations)* 2%/1:50,000, 2%/1:100,000; cream 2%; gel 2, 2.5%; oint 2.5, 5%; liq 2.5%; soln 2, 4%; viscous 2% **SE:** Dizziness, paresthesias, & convulsions associated w/ tox **Notes:** See Table 1, p 282

Lidocaine Powder Intradermal Injection System (Zingo) Uses:
Local anesthesia before venipuncture or IV in peds 3–18 y **Acts:** Local amide
anesthetic **Dose:** Apply 3 min before procedure **W/P:** [N/A, N/A] only on intact
skin **CI:** Lidocaine allergy **Disp:** 6.5-Inch device to administer under pressure 0.5
mg lidocaine powder in 2-cm area, single use **SE:** Skin Rxn, edema, petechiae

Lidocaine/Prilocaine (EMLA, LMX) Uses: *Topical anesthetic for intact
skin or genital mucous membranes; adjunct to phlebotomy or dermal procedures*
Acts: Amide local anesthetics **Dose:** *Adults. EMLA cream, anesthetic disc
(1 g/10 cm²):* Thick layer 2–2.5 g to intact skin, cover w/ occlusive dressing (e.g.,
Tegaderm) for at least 1 h. *Anesthetic disc:* 1 g/10 cm² for at least 1 h. *Peds. Max
dose: < 3 mo or < 5 kg:* 1 g/10 cm² for 1 h. *3–12 mo & > 5 kg:* 2 g/20 cm² for 4 h.
1–6 y & > 10 kg: 10 g/100 cm² for 4 h. *7–12 y & > 20 kg:* 20 g/200 cm² for 4 h
W/P: [B, +] Methemoglobinemia **CI:** Use on mucous membranes, broken skin,
eyes; allergy to amide-type anesthetics **Disp:** Cream 2.5% lidocaine/2.5% prilo-
caine; anesthetic disc (1 g); periodontal gel 2.5/2.5% **SE:** Burning, stinging, methemoglobinemia **Notes:** Longer contact time ↑ effect

Lindane (Kwell, Others) BOX: Only for pts intolerant/failed 1st-line Rx w/
safer agents. Szs and deaths reported w/ repeat/prolonged use. Caution d/t increased
risk of neurotox in infants, children, elderly, w/ other skin conditions, and if < 50 kg.
Instruct pts on proper use and inform that itching occurs after successful killing of
scabies or lice Uses: *Head lice, pubic "crab" lice, body lice, scabies* **Acts:**
Ectoparasiticide & ovicide **Dose:** *Adults & Peds. Cream or lotion:* Thin layer to
dry skin after bathing, leave for 8–12 h, rinse; also use on laundry. *Shampoo:* Apply
30 mL to dry hair, develop a lather w/ warm water for 4 min, comb out nits **W/P:**
[C, +/–] **CI:** Premature infants, uncontrolled Sz disorders open wounds **Disp:**
Lotion 1%; shampoo 1% **SE:** Arrhythmias, Szs, local irritation, GI upset, ataxia,
alopecia, N/V, aplastic anemia **Notes:** Caution w/ overuse (may be absorbed); may
repeat Rx in 7 d; try OTC first w/ pyrethrins (Pronto, Rid, others)

Linezolid (Zyvox) Uses: *Infxns caused by gram(+) bacteria (including VRE),
pneumonia, skin Infxns* **Acts:** Unique, binds ribosomal bacterial RNA; bacteriocidal
for streptococci, bacteriostatic for enterococci & staphylococci. *Spectrum:* Excellent
gram(+) including VRE & MRSA **Dose:** *Adults.* 400–600 mg IV or PO q12h. *Peds.*
10 mg/kg IV or PO q8h (q12h in preterm neonates) **W/P:** [C, ?/–] w/ MAOI (may
cause serotonin syndrome when used with these psych meds), avoid foods w/ tyramine
& cough/cold products w/ pseudoephedrine; w/ ↓ BM **Disp:** Inj 200, 600 mg; tabs
600 mg; susp 100 mg/5 mL **SE:** Lactic acidosis, peripheral/optic neuropathy, HTN,
N/D, HA, insomnia, GI upset, ↓ BM, tongue discoloration **Notes:** ✓ weekly CBC; not
for gram(–) Infxn, ↑ deaths in catheter-related Infxns; MAOI activity

Liothyronine (Cytomel, Triostat, T₃) BOX: Not for obesity or wgt loss
Uses: *Hypothyroidism, nontoxic goiter, myxedema coma, thyroid suppression Rx*
Acts: T₃ replacement **Dose:** *Adults.* Initial 25 mcg/24 h, titrate q1–2wk to response
& TFT; maint of 25–100 mcg/d PO. *Myxedema coma:* 25–50 mcg IV. *Myxedema:*

5 mcg/d, PO ↑ 5–10 mcg/d q1–2wk; maint 50–100 mcg/d. *Nontoxic goiter:* 5 mcg/d PO, ↑ 5–10 mcg/d q1–2wk, usual dose 75 mcg/d. *T_3 suppression test:* 75–100 mcg/d × 7d. **Peds.** Initial 5 mcg/24 h, titrate by 5-mcg/24-h increments at q3–4d intervals; maint peds 1–3 yrs: 50 mcg/d. **Infants–12 mo:** 20 mcg/d > *3 y:* Adult dose; ↓ in elderly & CV Dz **W/P:** [A, +] **CI:** Recent MI, uncorrected adrenal Insuff, uncontrolled HTN, thyrotoxicosis, artificial rewarming **Disp:** Tabs 5, 25, 50 mcg; Inj 10 mcg/mL mcg **SE:** Alopecia, arrhythmias, CP, HA, sweating, twitching, ↑ HR, ↑ BP, MI, CHF, fever **Notes:** Monitor TFT; separate antacids by 4 h; monitor glucose w/ DM meds; when switching from IV to PO, taper IV slowly

Liraglutide, Recombinant (Victoza) **BOX:** CI w/ personal or fam Hx of medullary thyroid CA (MTC) or w/ multiple endocrine neoplasia synd type 2 (MEN2) **Uses:** *Type 2 DM* **Acts:** Glucagon-like peptide-1 receptor agonist **Dose:** 1.8 mg/d; begin 0.6 mg/d any time of day SQ (abd/thigh/upper arm), ↑ to 1.2 mg after 1 wk, may ↑ to 1.8 mg after **W/P:** [C, ?/–] **CI:** See Box **Disp:** Multidose pens, 0.6, 1.2, 1.8 mg/dose, 6 mg/mL **SE:** pancreatitis, MTC, ↓ glucose w/ sulfonylurea, HA, N/D **Notes:** Delays gastric emptying

Lisdexamfetamine Dimesylate (Vyvanse) [C-II] **BOX:** Amphetamines have high potential for abuse; prolonged administration may lead to dependence; misuse may cause sudden death and serious CV events **Uses:** *ADHD* **Acts:** CNS stimulant **Dose: *Adults & Peds 6–12 y.*** 30 mg daily, ↑ q wk 10–20 mg/d, 70 mg/d max **W/P:** [C, ?/–] w/ Potential for drug dependency in pt w/ psychological or Sz disorder, Tourette synd, HTN **CI:** Severe arteriosclerotic CV Dz, mod–severe ↑ BP, ↑ thyroid, sensitivity to sympathomimetic amines, NAG, agitated states, Hx drug abuse, w/ or w/in 14 d of MAOI **Disp:** Caps 30, 50, 70 mg **SE:** Headache, insomnia, decreased appetite **Notes:** AHA statement April 2008: All children diagnosed w/ ADHD who are candidates for stimulant meds should undergo CV assessment prior to use

Lisinopril (Prinivil, Zestril) **BOX:** ACE inhib can cause fetal injury/death in 2nd/3rd tri; D/C w/ PRG **Uses:** *HTN, CHF, prevent DN & AMI* **Acts:** ACE inhib **Dose:** 5–40 mg/24 h PO daily-bid, CHF target 40 mg/d. *AMI:* 5 mg w/in 24 h of MI, then 5 mg after 24 h, 10 mg after 48 h, then 10 mg/d; ↓ in renal insuff; use low dose, ↑ slowly in elderly **W/P:** [D, –] w/ aortic stenosis/cardiomyopathy **CI:** Bilateral RAS, PRG, ACE inhib sensitivity (angioedema) **Disp:** Tabs 2.5, 5, 10, 20, 30, 40 mg **SE:** Dizziness, HA, cough, ↓ BP, angioedema, ↑ K^+, ↑ Cr, rare ↓ BM **Notes:** To prevent DN, start when urinary microalbuminuria begins; ✓ K, BUN, Cr, K^+, WBC

Lisinopril and Hydrochlorothiazide (Prinzide, Zestoretic, Generic) **BOX:** ACE inhib can cause fetal injury/death in 2nd/3rd tri; D/C w/ PRG **Uses:** *HTN* **Acts:** ACE inhib w/ diuretic (HCTZ) **Dose:** Initial 10 mg lisinopril/12.5mg HCTZ, titrate upward to effect; > 80 mg/d lisinopril or > 50 mg/day HCTZ are not recommended; ↓ in renal insuff; use low dose, ↑ slowly in elderly **W/P:** [C 1st tri, D after, –] w/ aortic stenosis/cardiomyopathy **CI:** Bilateral RAS, PRG, ACE inhib sensitivity (angioedema) **Disp:** Tabs (mg lisinopril/mg HCTZ) 10/12.5, 20/12.5; Zestoretic also available as 20/25 **SE:** Anaphylactoid Rxn (rare), dizziness, HA, cough, fatigue, ↓ BP, angioedema, ↑/↓ K+, ↑ Cr, rare ↓ BM/cholestatic jaundice **Notes:** Use only when monotherapy fails; ✓ K, BUN, Cr, K+, WBC

Lithium Carbonate (Eskalith, Lithobid, Others) **BOX:** Li tox related to serum levels and can be seen at close to therapeutic levels **Uses:** *Manic episodes of bipolar Dz*, augment antidepressants, aggression, posttraumatic stress disorder **Acts:** ?, Effects shift toward intraneuronal metabolism of catecholamines **Dose:** *Adults. Bipolar, acute mania:* 1800 mg/d PO in 2–3 ÷ doses (target serum 1–1.5 mEq/L ✓ 2×/wk until stable). *Bipolar maint:* 900–1200 /d PO in 2–3 ÷ doses (target serum 0.6–1.2 mEq/L). *Peds ≥12 y.* See Adults; ↓ in renal Insuff, elderly **W/P:** [D, –] Many drug interactions; avoid ACE inhib or diuretics; thyroid Dz **CI:** Severe renal impair or CV Dz, lactation **Disp:** Caps 150, 300, 600 mg; tabs 300 mg; SR tabs 300 mg, CR tabs 450 mg; syrup & soln 300 mg/5 mL **SE:** Polyuria, polydipsia, nephrogenic DI, long-term may affect renal conc ability and cause fibrosis; tremor; Na+ retention or diuretic use may ↑ tox; arrhythmias, dizziness, alopecia, goiter ↓ thyroid, N/V/D, ataxia, nystagmus, ↓ BP **Notes:** Levels: *Trough:* just before next dose: *Therapeutic:* 0.8–1.2 mEq/mL; *Toxic:* > 1.5 mEq/mL *1/2-life:* 18–20 h. Follow levels q1–2mo on maint

Lodoxamide (Alomide) **Uses:** *Vernal conjunctivitis/keratitis* **Acts:** Stabilizes mast cells **Dose:** *Adults & Peds > 2 y.* 1–2 gtt in eye(s) qid = 3 mo **W/P:** [B, ?] **Disp:** Soln 0.1% **SE:** Ocular burning, stinging, HA **Notes:** Do not use soft contacts during use

Loperamide (Diamode, Imodium) [OTC] **Uses:** *Diarrhea* **Acts:** Slows intestinal motility **Dose:** *Adults.* Initial 4 mg PO, then 2 mg after each loose stool, up to 16 mg/d. *Peds 2–5 y, 13–20 kg:* 1 mg PO tid; *6–8 y, 20–30 kg:* 2 mg PO bid; *8–12 y, > 30 kg:* 2 mg PO tid **W/P:** [C, –] Not for acute D caused by *Salmonella, Shigella,* or *C. difficile;* w/ HIV may cause toxic megacolon **CI:** Pseudomembranous colitis, bloody D, Abd pain w/o D, < 2 y **Disp:** Caps 2 mg; tabs 2 mg; liq 1 mg/5 mL, 1 mg/7.5 mL (OTC) **SE:** Constipation, sedation, dizziness, Abd cramp, N

Lopinavir/Ritonavir (Kaletra) **Uses:** *HIV Infxn* **Acts:** Protease inhib **Dose:** *Adults.* TX naïve: 800/200 mg PO daily or 400/100 mg PO bid; *TX Tx-experienced pt:* 400/100 mg PO bid (↑ dose if w/ amprenavir, efavirenz, fosamprenavir, nelfinavir, nevirapine); do not use q day dosing w/ concomitant Rx. *Peds 7–15 kg:* 12/3 mg/kg PO bid. *15–40 kg:* 10/2.5 mg/kg PO bid. > *40 kg:* Adult dose; w/ food **W/P:** [C, ?/–] Numerous interactions, w/ hepatic impair; do not use w/salmeterol, colchicine (w/renal/hepatic failure); adjust dose w/ bosentan, tadalafil for PAH **CI:** w/ Drugs dependent on CYP3A/CYP2D6 (Table 10, p 301), statins, St. John's wort, fluconazole; w/ alpha 1-adrenoreceptor antagonist (alfuzosin); w/ PDE5 inhibitor sildenafil **Disp:** (mg lopinavir/mg ritonavir) Tab 100/25, 200/50, soln 400/100/5 mL **SE:** Avoid disulfiram (soln has EtOH), metronidazole; GI upset, asthenia, ↑ cholesterol/triglycerides, pancreatitis; protease metabolic synd

Loratadine (Claritin, Alavert) Uses: *Allergic rhinitis, chronic idiopathic urticaria* **Acts:** Nonsedating antihistamine **Dose:** *Adults.* 10 mg/d PO. *Peds 2–5 y.* 5 mg PO daily. *> 6 y:* Adult dose; on empty stomach; ↓ in hepatic Insuff; q other day dose w/ CrCl < 30 mL/min **W/P:** [B, +/–] **CI:** Component allergy **Disp:** Tabs 10 mg (OTC); rapidly disintegrating RediTabs 10 mg; chew tabs 5 mg; syrup 1 mg/mL **SE:** HA, somnolence, xerostomia, hyperkinesis in pts

Lorazepam (Ativan, Others) [C-IV] Uses: *Anxiety & anxiety w/ depression; sedation; control status epilepticus*; EtOH withdrawal; antiemetic **Acts:** Benzodiazepine; antianxiety agent; works via postsynaptic GABA receptors **Dose:** *Adults.* Anxiety: 1–10 mg/d PO in 2–3 ÷ doses. *Pre-op:* 0.05 mg/kg to 4 mg max IM 2 h before or 0.044 mg/kg to 2 mg dose max IV 15–20 min before surgery. *Insomnia:* 2–4 mg PO hs. *Status epilepticus:* 4 mg/dose slow over 2–5 min IV PRN q10–15min; usual total dose 8 mg. *Antiemetic:* 0.5–2 mg IV or PO q4–6h PRN. *EtOH withdrawal:* 2–5 mg IV or 1–2 mg PO initial depending on severity; titrate. **Peds.** Status epilepticus: 0.05–0.1 mg/kg/dose IV over 2–5 min, repeat at 1–20-min intervals × 2 PRN. Antiemetic, 2–15 y: 0.05 mg/kg (to 2 mg/dose) prechemotherapy; ↓ in elderly; do not administer IV > 2 mg/min or 0.05 mg/kg/min w/P: [D, ?/–] w/ Hepatic impair, other CNS depression, COPD; ↓ dose by 50% w/ valproic acid and probenecid **CI:** Severe pain, severe ↓ BP, sleep apnea, NAG, allergy to propylene glycol or benzyl alcohol **Disp:** Tabs 0.5, 1, 2 mg; soln, PO conc 2 mg/mL; Inj 2, 4 mg/mL **SE:** Sedation, memory impair, EPS, dizziness, ataxia, tachycardia, ↓ BP, constipation, resp depression **Notes:** ~10 min for effect if IV; IV Inf requires inline filter

Losartan (Cozaar) BOX: Can cause fatal injury and death if used in 2nd & 3rd trimesters. D/C Rx if PRG detected Uses: *HTN, DN, prevent CVA in HTN and LVH* **Acts:** Angiotensin II receptor antagonist **Dose:** *Adults.* 25–50 mg PO daily-bid, max 100 mg; ↓ in elderly/hepatic impair. *Peds ≥6 y. HTN:* Initial 0.7 mg/kg q day, ↑ to 50 mg/d PRN; 1.4 mg/kg/d or 100 mg/d max **W/P:** [C (1st tri, D 2nd & 3rd tri), ?/–] w/ NSAIDs; w/ K⁺-sparing diuretics, supl may cause ↑ K⁺; w/ RAS, hepatic impair **CI:** PRG, component sensitivity **Disp:** Tabs 25, 50, 100 mg **SE:** ↓ BP in pts on diuretics; ↑ K⁺; GI upset, facial/ angioedema, dizziness, cough, weakness, ↓ renal fxn

Lovastatin (Mevacor, Altoprev) Uses: *Hypercholesterolemia to ↓ risk of MI, angina* **Acts:** HMG-CoA reductase inhib **Dose:** *Adults.* 20 mg/d PO w/ P.M. meal; may ↑ at 4-wk intervals to 80 mg/d max or 60 mg ER tab; take w/ meals. *Peds 10–17 y (at least 1-y postmenarchal). Familial ↑ cholesterol:* 10 mg PO q day, ↑ q4wk PRN to 40 mg/d max (immediate release w/ P.M. meal) **W/P:** [X, –] Avoid w/ grapefruit juice, gemfibrozil; dose escalation w/ renal impair **CI:** Active liver Dz, PRG, lactation **Disp:** Tabs generic 10, 20, 40 mg; *Mevacor* 20,40 mg; *Altoprev* ER tabs 20, 40, 60 mg **SE:** HA & GI intolerance common; promptly report any unexplained muscle pain, tenderness, or weakness (myopathy) **Notes:** Maintain cholesterol-lowering diet; LFTs q12wk × 1 y, then q6mo; may alter TFT

Lubiprostone (Amitiza) Uses: *Chronic idiopathic constipation in adults, IBS w/ constipation in females > 18 y* Acts: Selective Cl⁻ channel activator; ↑ intestinal motility Dose: *Adults.* Constipation: 24 mcg PO bid w/ food. *IBS:* 8 mcg bid; w/ food CI: Mechanical GI obst W/P: [C, ?/–] Severe D, severe renal or mod–severe hepatic impair Disp: Gelcaps 8, 24 mcg SE: N/D, HA, GI distention, Abd pain Notes: Not approved in males; requires (–) PRG test before; use contraception; periodically reassess drug need; not for chronic use; may experience severe dyspnea w/in 1 h of dose, usually resolves w/in 3 h

Lurasidone (Latuda) BOX: Elderly w/ dementia-related psychosis at ↑ death risk. Not approved for dementia-related psychosis. Uses: *Schizophrenia* Acts: Atypical antipsychotic: central DA type 2 (D2) and serotonin type 2 (5HT2A) receptor antagonist Dose: 40–80 mg/d PO; 40 mg max w/ CrCl 10–49 mL/min OR mod–severe hepatic impair W/P: [B, –] CI: w/ Strong CYP3A4 inhib/inducer Disp: Tabs 40, 80 mg SE: Somnolence, agitation, tardive dyskinesia, akathisia, parkinsonism, stroke, TIAs, Sz, orthostatic hypotension, syncope, dysphagia, neuroleptic malignant syndrome, body temp dysregulation, N, ↑ wgt, type 2 DM, ↑ lipids, hyperprolactinemia, ↓ WBC Notes: w/ DM risk ✓ glucose

Lutropin Alfa (Luveris) Uses: *Infertility w/ profound LH deficiency* Acts: Recombinant LH Dose: 75 units SQ w/ 75–150 units FSH, 2 separate Inj max 14 d W/P: [X, ?/M] Potential for arterial thromboembolism CI: Primary ovarian failure, uncontrolled thyroid/adrenal dysfunction, intracranial lesion, AUB, hormone-dependent GU tumor, ovarian cyst, PRG Disp: Inj 75 units SE: HA, N, ovarian hyperstimulation synd, ovarian torsion, Abd pain d/t ovarian enlargement, breast pain, ovarian cysts; ↑ risk of multiple births Notes: Rotate Inj sites; do not exceed 14 d duration unless signs of imminent follicular development; monitor ovarian ultrasound and serum estradiol; specific pt information packets given

Lymphocyte Immune Globulin [Antithymocyte Globulin, ATG] (Atgam) BOX: Should only be used by physician experienced in immunosuppressive therapy or management of solid-organ and/or bone marrow transplant pts. Adequate lab and supportive resources must be readily available Uses: *Allograft rejection in renal transplant pts; aplastic anemia if not candidates for BMT *, prevent rejection of other solid-organ transplants, GVHD after BMT Acts: ↓ Circulating antigen-reactive T lymphocytes; human, & equine product Dose: *Adults.* Prevent rejection: 15 mg/kg/d IV × 14 d, then q other day × 14 d; initial w/in 24 h before/after transplant. Rx rejection: Same but use 10–15 mg/kg/d; max 21 doses in 28 d, Q day 1st 14 days. Aplastic anemia: 10–20 mg/kg/d × 8–14 d, then q other day × 7 doses for total 21 doses in 28 d. **Peds.** Prevent renal allograft rejection: 5–25 mg/kg/d IV; aplastic anemia 10–20 mg/kg/d IV W/P: [C, –] CI: Hx previous Rxn or Rxn to other equine γ-globulin prep, ↓ plt and WBC Disp: Inj 50 mg/mL SE: D/C w/ severe ↓ plt and WBC; rash, fever, chills, ↓ BP, HA, CP, edema, N/V/D, lightheadedness Notes: Test dose: 0.1 mL 1:1000 dilution in NS, a systemic Rxn precludes use; give via central line; pretreat w/ antipyretic, antihistamine, and/or steroids; monitor WBC, plt; plt counts usually return to nl w/o D/C Rx

Magaldrate (Riopan-Plus) [OTC] Uses: *Hyperacidity associated w/ peptic ulcer, gastritis, & hiatal hernia* Acts: Low-Na⁺ antacid Dose: 5–10 mL PO between meals & hs, on empty stomach W/P: [C, ?/+] CI: Ulcerative colitis, diverticulitis, appendicitis, ileostomy/colostomy, renal Insuff (d/t Mg²⁺ content) Disp: Susp magalrate/simethicone 540/20 mg & 1080/40 mg/5 mL (OTC) SE: ↑ Mg²⁺, ↓ PO₄, white flecked feces, constipation, N/V/D Notes: < 0.3 mg Na¹⁺/tab or tsp

Magnesium Citrate (Citroma, Others) [OTC] Uses: *Vigorous bowel prep*; constipation Acts: Cathartic laxative Dose: Adults. 120–300 mL PO PRN. Peds. 0.5 mL/kg/dose, q4–6h to 200 mL PO max; w/ a beverage W/P: [B, +] w/ Neuromuscular Dz CI: Severe renal Dz, heart block, N/V, rectal bleeding intestinal obst/perforation/impaction, colostomy, ileostomy, UC, diverticulitis Disp: soln 290 mg/5 mL (300 mL); 100 mg tabs SE: Abd cramps, gas, ↓ BP, ↑ Mg²⁺, resp depression Notes: Only for occasional use w/ constipation

Magnesium Hydroxide (Milk of Magnesia) [OTC] Uses: *Constipation, hyperacidity, Mg²⁺ replacement* Acts: NS laxative Dose: Adults. Antacid: 5–15 mL (400 mg/5 mL) or 2–4 tabs (311 mg) PO PRN up to qid. Mg²⁺ replacement: 2–4 (500 mg) tabs PO qhs or ÷ doses. Laxative: 30–60 mL (400 mg/5 mL) or 15–30 mL (800 mg/5 mL) or 8 tabs (311 mg) PO qhs or ÷ doses. Peds. Antacid and Mg²⁺ replacement: < 12 y not OK. Laxative: < 2 y not OK. 2–5 y: 5–15 mL (400 mg/5 mL) PO qhs or ÷ doses. 6–11 y: 15–30 mL (400 mg/5 mL) or 7.5–15 mL (800 mg/5 mL) PO qhs or ÷ doses. 3–5 y: 2 (311 mg) tabs PO qhs or ÷ doses. 6–11 y: 4 (311 mg) tabs PO qhs or ÷ doses W/P: [B, +] w/ Neuromuscular Dz or renal impair CI: Renal Insuff, intestinal obst, ileostomy/colostomy Disp: Chew tabs 311, 500 mg; liq 400, 800 mg/5 mL (OTC) SE: D, Abd cramps Notes: For occasional use in constipation

Magnesium Oxide (Mag-Ox 400, Others) [OTC] Uses: *Replace low Mg²⁺ levels* Acts: Mg²⁺ supl Dose: 400–800 mg/d or ÷ w/ food in full glass of H₂O; ↓ w/ renal impair W/P: [B, +] w/ Neuromuscular Dz & renal impair, w/ bisphosphonates, calcitriol, CCBs, neuromuscular blockers, tetracyclines, quinolones CI: UC, diverticulitis, ileostomy/colostomy, heart block Disp: Caps 140 250, 500, 600 mg; tabs 400 mg (OTC) SE: D, N

Magnesium Sulfate (Various) Uses: *Replace low Mg²⁺; preeclampsia, eclampsia, & premature labor; cardiac arrest, AMI arrhythmias, cerebral edema, barium poisoning, Szs, pediatric acute nephritis*; refractory ↓ K⁺ & ↓ Ca²⁺ Acts: Mg²⁺ supl, bowel evacuation, ↓ acetylcholine in nerve terminals, ↓ rate of sinoatrial node firing Dose: Adults. 3 g PO q6h × 4 PRN; Supl: 1–2 g IM or IV; repeat PRN. Preeclampsia/premature labor: 4-g load then 1–4 g/h IV Inf. ECC 2010. VF/ pulseless VT arrest w/ torsade de pointes: 1–2 g IV push (2–4 mL 50% solution) in 10 mL D5W. If pulse present, then 1–2 g in 50–100 mL D5W over 5–60 min. Peds. 25–50 mg/kg/dose IM, IV, IO q4–6h for 3–4 doses; repeat PRN; q8–12h in neonates; max 2 g single dose; *ECC 2010. Pulseless VT w/ torsades:* 25–50 mg/kg IV/IO bolus; max dose 2 g; *Pulseless VT w/ torsades or hypomagnesemia:* 25–50 mg/kg IV/IO over 10–20 min; max dose 2 g; *Status asthmaticus:* 25–50 mg/kg IV/ IO over 15–30 min **W/P:** [A/C (manufacturer specific), +] w/ Neuromuscular Dz; interactions see Magnesium Oxide and aminoglycosides **CI:** Heart block, renal failure ; ↓ dose w/ low urinary output or renal insuff **Disp:** Premix Inj: 10, 20, 40, 80 mg/mL; Inj 125, 500 mg/mL; oral/topical powder 227, 454, 480, 1810, 1920, 2721 g **SE:** CNS depression, D, flushing, heart block, ↓ BP, vasodilation **Notes:** different formulation may contain Al^{2+}

Mannitol (Various) **Uses:** *Cerebral edema, ↑ IOP, renal impair, poisonings, GU irrigation* **Acts:** Osmotic diuretic **Dose:** *Test dose:* 0.2 g/kg/dose IV over 3–5 min; if no diuresis w/in 2 h, D/C. *Oliguria:* 50–100 g IV over 90 min ↑ *IOP:* 0.5–2 g/kg IV over 30 min. *Cerebral edema:* 0.25–1.5 g/kg/dose IV > 30 min **W/P:** [C, ?/M] w/ CHF or vol overload, w/ nephrotoxic drugs & lithium **CI:** Anuria, dehydration, heart failure, PE **Disp:** Inj 5, 10, 15, 20, 25%; GU soln 5% **SE:** May exacerbate CHF, N/V/D, ↓/↑ BP, ↑ HR **Notes:** Monitor for vol depletion

Maraviroc (Selzentry) **BOX:** Possible drug-induced hepatotox **Uses:** *Tx of CCR5-tropic HIV Infxn* **Acts:** Antiretroviral, CCR5 coreceptor antagonist **Dose:** 300 mg bid **W/P:** [B, −] w/ Concomitant CYP3A inducers/inhib **CI:** None **Disp:** Tab 150, 300 mg **SE:** Fever, URI, cough, rash

Measles, Mumps, & Rubella Vaccine Live [MMR] (M-M-R II) **Uses:** *Vaccination against measles, mumps, & rubella 12 mo and older* **Acts:** Active immunization, live attenuated viruses **Dose:** 1 (0.5-mL) SQ Inj, 1st dose 12 mo 2nd dose 4–6 y, at least 3 mo between doses (28 d if > 12 y), adults born after 1957 unless CI, Hx measles & mumps or documented immunity and childbearing age women w/ rubella immunity documented **W/P:** [C, ?/M] Hx of cerebral injury, Szs, fam Hx Szs (febrile Rxn), ↓ plt **CI:** Component and gelatin sensitivity, Hx anaphylaxis to neomycin, blood dyscrasia, lymphoma, leukemia, malignant neoplasias affecting BM, immunosuppression, fever, PRG, Hx of active untreated TB **Disp:** Inj, single dose **SE:** Fever, febrile Szs (5–12 days after vaccination), Inj site Rxn, rash, ↓ plt **Notes:** Per FDA, CDC ↑ of febrile Sz (2×) w/ MMRV vs. MMR and varicella separately; preferable to use 2 separate vaccines; allow 1 mo between Inj & any other measles vaccine or 3 mo between any other varicella vaccine; limited avail of MMRV; avoid those who have not been exposed to varicella for 6 wk post-Inj; may contain albumin or trace egg antigen; avoid salicylates for 6 wks postvaccination; avoid PRG for 3 mo following vaccination; do not give w/in 3 mo of transfusion or immune globulin

Measles, Mumps, Rubella, & Varicella Virus Vaccine Live [MMRV] (ProQuad) **Uses:** *Vaccination against measles, mumps, rubella, & varicella* **Acts:** Active immunization, live attenuated viruses **Dose:** 1 (0.5-mL) vial SQ Inj 12 mo–12 y or for 2nd dose of measles, mumps, & rubella (MMR)*, at least 3 mos between doses (28 days if > 12 y) **W/P:** [C, ?/M] Hx of cerebral injury or Szs & fam Hx Szs (febrile Rxn), ↓ plt **CI:** Component and gelatin sensitivity, Hx anaphylaxis to neomycin, blood dyscrasia, lymphoma, leukemia, malignant neoplasias affecting BM, immunosuppression, fever, active untreated TB, PRG **Disp:** Inj **SE:** Fever, febrile Szs, (5–12 days after vaccination), Inj site Rxn, rash, ↓ plt, **Notes:** Per FDA, CDC ↑ of febrile Sz (2 × risk) w/ combo vaccine (MMRV) vs. MMR and varicella vaccine); preferable to use 2 separate vaccines; allow 1 mo between Inj & any other measles vaccine or 3 mo between any other varicella vaccine; limited avail of MMRV; substitute MMR II and/or Varivax; avoid those who have not been exposed to varicella for 6 wk post-Inj; may contain albumin or trace egg antigen; avoid salicylates

Mecasermin (Increlex, Iplex) **Uses:** *Growth failure in severe primary IGF-1 deficiency or human growth hormone (HGH) antibodies* **Acts:** Human IGF-1 (recombinant DNA origin) **Dose:** *Peds.* 0.04–0.08 mg/kg SQ bid; may ↑ by 0.04 mg/kg per dose to 0.12 mg/kg bid; take w/in 20 min of meal d/t insulin-like hypoglycemic effect **W/P:** [C, ?/M] Contains benzyl alcohol **CI:** Closed epiphysis, neoplasia, not for IV **Disp:** Vial 40 mg **SE:** Tonsillar hypertrophy, ↑ AST, ↑ LDH, HA, Inj site Rxn, V, hypoglycemia **Notes:** Rapid dose ↑ may cause hypoglycemia; initial funduscopic exam and during Tx; consider monitoring glucose until dose stable; limited distribution; rotate Inj site

Mechlorethamine (Mustargen) **BOX:** Highly toxic, handle w/ care, limit use to experienced physicians; avoid exposure during PRG; vesicant **Uses:** *Hodgkin Dz (stages III, IV), cutaneous T-cell lymphoma (mycosis fungoides), lung CA, CML, malignant pleural effusions, CLL, polycythemia vera,* psoriasis **Acts:** Alkylating agent, nitrogen analog of sulfur mustard **Dose:** Per protocol; 0.4 mg/kg single dose or 0.1 mg/kg/d for 4 d, repeat at 4–6-wk intervals; 6 mg/m² IV on days 1 & 8 of 28-d cycle; *Intracavitary:* 0.2–0.4 mg/kg × 1, may repeat PRN; *Topical:* 0.01–0.02% soln, lotion, oint **W/P:** [D, ?/–] **CI:** PRG, known infect Dz, severe myelosuppression **Disp:** Inj 10 mg; topical soln, lotion, oint **SE:** ↓ BM, thrombosis, thrombophlebitis at site; tissue damage w/ extrav (Na thiosulfate used topically to Rx); N/V/D, skin rash/allergic dermatitis w/ contact, amenorrhea, sterility (especially in men), secondary leukemia if treated for Hodgkin Dz, chromosomal alterations, hepatotox, peripheral neuropathy **Notes:** Highly volatile and emetogenic; give w/in 30–60 min of prep

Meclizine (Antivert) (Bonine, Dramamine [OTC]) **Uses:** *Motion sickness, vertigo* **Acts:** Antiemetic, anticholinergic, & antihistaminic properties **Dose:** *Adults & Peds > 12 y. Motion Sickness:* 12.5–25 mg PO 1 h before travel, repeat PRN q12–24h. *Vertigo:* 25–100 mg/d ÷ doses **W/P:** [B, ?/–] NAG, BPH, BOO, elderly, asthma **Disp:** Tabs 12.5, 25, 50 mg; chew tabs 25 mg; caps 25, 30 mg (OTC) **SE:** Drowsiness, xerostomia, blurred vision, thickens bronchial secretions

Medroxyprogesterone (Provera, Depo Provera, Depo-Sub Q Provera) **BOX:** Do not use in the prevention of CV Dz or dementia; ↑ risk MI, stroke, breast CA, PE, & DVT in postmenopausal women (50–79 y). ↑ Dementia risk in postmenopausal women (≥65 y). Risk of sig bone loss **Uses:** *Contraception; secondary amenorrhea; endometrial CA, ↓ endometrial hyperplasia* AUB caused by hormonal imbalance **Acts:** Progestin supl **Dose:** *Contraception:* 150 mg IM q3mo depo or 104 mg SQ q3mo (depo SQ). *Secondary amenorrhea:* 5–10 mg/d PO for 5–10 d. *AUB:* 5–10 mg/d PO for 5–10 d beginning on the 16th or 21st d of menstrual cycle. *Endometrial CA:* 400–1000 mg/wk IM. *Endometrial hyperplasia:* 5–10 mg/d × 12–14 d on day 1 or 16 of cycle; ↓ in hepatic Insuff **W/P:** *Provera* [X, −] *Depo Provera* [X, +] **CI:** Thrombophlebitis/embolic disorders, cerebral apoplexy, ↑ LFTs, CA breast/genital organs, undiagnosed vag bleeding, missed abortion, PRG, as a diagnostic test for PRG **Disp:** Provera tabs 2.5, 5, 10 mg; depot Inj 150, 400 mg/mL; depo SQ Inj 104 mg/10.65 mL **SE:** Breakthrough bleeding, spotting, altered menstrual flow, breast tenderness, galactorrhea, depression, insomnia, jaundice, N, wgt gain, acne, hirsutism, vision changes **Notes:** Perform breast exam & Pap smear before contraceptive Rx; obtain PRG test if last Inj > 3 mo

Megestrol Acetate (Megace, Megace-ES) **Uses:** *Breast/endometrial CAs; appetite stimulant in cachexia (CA & HIV)* **Acts:** Hormone; anti-leutenizing; progesterone analog **Dose:** *CA:* 40–320 mg/d PO in ÷ doses. *Appetite:* 800 mg/d PO ÷ dose or Megace ES 625 mg/d **W/P:** [X, −] Thromboembolism; handle w/ care **CI:** PRG **Disp:** Tabs 20, 40 mg; susp 40 mg/mL, Megace ES 125 mg/mL **SE:** DVT, edema, menstrual bleeding, photosens, N/V/D, HA, mastodynia, ↑ CA, ↑ glucose, insomnia, rash, ↓ BM, ↑ BP, CP, palpitations, **Notes:** Do not D/C abruptly; Megace ES not equivalent to others mg/mg; Megace ES approved only for anorexia

Meloxicam (Mobic) **BOX:** May ↑ risk of cardiovascular CV events & GI bleeding; CI in post-op CABG **Uses:** *OA, RA, JRA* **Acts:** NSAID w/ ↑ COX-2 activity **Dose:** *Adults.* 7.5–15 mg/d PO. *Peds > 2 y.* 0.125 mg/kg/d, max 7.5 mg; ↓ in renal Insuff; take w/ food **W/P:** [C, D (3rd tri), ?/−] w/ Severe renal Insuff, CHF, ACE inhib, diuretics, Li²⁺, MTX, warfarin **CI:** Peptic ulcer, NSAID, or ASA sensitivity, PRG, post-op coronary artery bypass graft **Disp:** Tabs 7.5, 15 mg; susp. 7.5 mg/5 mL **SE:** HA, dizziness, GI upset, GI bleeding, edema, ↑ BP, renal impair, rash (SJS), ↑ LFTs

Melphalan [L-PAM] (Alkeran) **BOX:** Administer under the supervision of a qualified physician experienced in the use of chemotherapy; severe BM depression, leukemogenic, & mutagenic **Uses:** *Multiple myeloma, ovarian CAs*, breast & testicular CA, melanoma; allogenic & ABMT (high dose), neuroblastoma, rhabdomyosarcoma **Acts:** Alkylating agent, nitrogen mustard **Dose:** *Adults. Multiple myeloma:* 16 mg/m² IV q2wk × 4 doses then at 4-wk intervals after tox resolves; w/ renal impair ↓ IV dose 50% or 6 mg PO q day × 2–3 wk, then D/C up to 4 wk, follow counts then 2 mg q day. *Ovarian CA:* 0.2 mg/kg q day × 5 d, repeat q4–5wk based on counts. *Peds. Off-label rhabdomyosarcoma:* 10–35 mg/m²/dose IV q21–28d. *w/ BMT for Neuroblastoma:* 100–220 mg/m²/dose IV × 1 or ÷ 2–5 daily doses; Inf over 60 min; ↓ in renal Insuff **W/P:** [D, ?/−] w/ Cisplatin, digitalis, live vaccines **CI:** Allergy or resistance **Disp:** Tabs 2 mg; Inj 50 mg **SE:** N/V, secondary malignancy, AF, ↓ LVEF, ↓ BM, secondary leukemia, alopecia, dermatitis, stomatitis, pulm fibrosis; rare allergic Rxns **Notes:** Take PO on empty stomach, false(+) direct Coombs test

Memantine (Namenda, Namenda XR) Uses: *Mod/severe Alzheimer Dz*, mild–mod vascular dementia, mild cognitive impair **Acts:** *N*-methyl-D-aspartate (NMDA) receptor antagonist **Dose:** *Namenda* Target 20 mg/d, start 5 mg/d, ↑ 5 mg/d to 20 mg/d, wait > 1 wk before ↑ dose; use ÷ doses if > 5 mg/d. *Vascular dementia:* 10 mg PO bid; *Namenda XR* (Alzheimer) 7 mg inital 1× QD, ↑ each week to maint 28 mg/d × 1; ↓ to 14 mg w/ severe renal impair **W/P:** [B, ?/–] Hepatic/mod renal impair; Sx disorders **Disp:** *Namenda* Tabs 5, 10 mg, combo pack: 5 mg × 28 + 10 mg × 21; soln 2 mg/mL. *Namenda XR* 7, 14, 21, 28 mg **CI:** Component hypersens **SE:** Dizziness, HA, D **Notes:** Renal clearance ↓ by alkaline urine (↓ 80% at pH 8)

Meningococcal Conjugate Vaccine [Quadrivalent, MCV4] (Menactra, Menveo) Uses: *Immunize against N. meningitidis* (meningococcus) high-risk 2–10 and 19–55 y and everyone 11–18* high-risk (college freshmen, military recruits, travel to endemic areas, terminal complement deficiencies, asplenia); if given age 11–12, give booster at 16, should have booster w/in 5 y of college **Acts:** Active immunization; *N. meningitidis* A, C, Y, W-135 polysaccharide conjugated to diphtheria toxoid (*Menactra*) or lyophilized conjugate component (*Menveo*) **Dose:** *Adults 18–55 y & Peds > 2 y.* 0.5 mL IM × 1 **W/P:** [C, ?/–] w/ immunosuppression (↓ response) and bleeding disorders **CI:** Allergy to class/diphtheria toxoid/compound/latex; Hx Guillain-Barré **Disp:** Inj site Rxns, HA, N/V/D, anorexia, fatigue, irritability, arthralgia, Guillain-Barré **Notes:** IM only, reported accidental SQ; keep epi available for Rxns; use polysaccharide *Menomune* (MPSV4) if > 55 y; do not confuse w/ *Menactra, Menveo*; ACIP rec: MCV4 for 2–55 y, ↑ local Rxn compared to *Menomune* (MPSV4) but ↑ ab titers; peds 2–10, ab levels ↓ 3 y w/ MPSV4, revaccinate in 2–3 y, use MCV4 revaccination

Meningococcal Polysaccharide Vaccine [MPSV4] (Menomune A/C/Y/W-135) Uses: *Immunize against N. meningitidis* (meningococcus)* in high-risk (college freshmen, military recruits, travel to endemic areas, terminal complement deficiencies, asplenia) **Acts:** Active immunization **Dose:** *Adults & Peds > 2 y.* 0.5 mL SQ only; may repeat in 3–5 y if high risk; repeat in 2–3 y if 1st dose given 2–4 y **W/P:** [C, ?/–] if immunocompromised (↓ response) **CI:** Thimerosal/latex sensitivity; w/ pertussis or typhoid vaccine, < 2 y **Disp:** Inj **SE:** Peds 2–10 y: Inj site Rxns, drowsiness, irritability 11–55 y: Inj site Rxns, HA, fatigue, malaise, fever, D **Notes:** Keep epi (1:1000) available for Rxns. Recommended > 55 y, but also alternative to MCV4 in 2–55 y if no MCV4 available (MCV4 is preferred). Active against serotypes A, C, Y, & W–135 but not group B; antibody levels ↓ 3 y; high risk: revaccination q3–5y (use MCV4)

Meperidine (Demerol, Meperitab) [C–II] Uses: *Mod–severe pain*, postoperative shivering, rigors from amphotericin B **Acts:** Narcotic analgesic **Dose:** *Adults.* 50–150 mg PO or IV/IM/SQ q3–4h PRN. *Peds.* 1–1.5 mg/kg/dose PO or IM/SQ q3–4h PRN, up to 100 mg/dose; ↓ in elderly/hepatic impair, avoid in renal impair **W/P:** [C/D (prolonged use or high dose at term), +] ↓ Sz threshold, adrenal Insuff, head injury, ↑ ICP, hepatic impair, not OK in sickle cell Dz **CI:** w/ MAOIs, renal failure, PRG **Disp:** Tabs 50, 100 mg; syrup/soln 50 mg/5 mL; Inj 10, 25, 50, 75, 100 mg/mL **SE:** Resp/CNS depression, Szs, sedation, constipation, ↓ BP, rash N/V, biliary and urethral spasms, dyspnea **Notes:** Analgesic effects potentiated w/ hydroxyzine; 75 mg IM = 10 mg morphine IM; not best in elderly; do not use oral for acute pain; not ok for repetitive use in ICU setting

Meprobamate (Various) [C-IV] **Uses:** *Short-term relief of anxiety* muscle spasm, TMJ relief **Acts:** Mild tranquilizer; antianxiety **Dose:** *Adults.* 400 mg PO tid-qid, max 2400 mg/d. *Peds 6–12 y.* 100–200 mg PO bid-tid; ↓ in renal/liver impair **W/P:** [D, +/–] Elderly, Sz Dz **CI:** NAG, porphyria, PRG **Disp:** Tabs 200, 400 mg **SE:** Drowsiness, syncope, tachycardia, edema, rash (SJS), N/V/D, ↓ WBC, agranulocytosis **Notes:** Do not abruptly D/C

Mercaptopurine [6-MP] (Purinethol) **Uses:** *ALL* 2nd-line Rx for CML & NHL, maint ALL in children, immunosuppressant w/ autoimmune Dzs (Crohn Dz, ulcerative colitis) **Acts:** Antimetabolite, mimics hypoxanthine **Dose:** *Adults. ALL induction:* 1.5–2.5 mg/kg/d; *maint* 80–100 mg/m²/d or 2.5–5 mg/kg/d; w/ allopurinol use 67–75% ↓ dose of 6-MP (interference w/ xanthine oxidase metabolism). *Peds. ALL induction:* 2.5–5 mg/kg/d PO or 70–100 mg/m²/d; *maint* 1.5–2.5 mg/kg/d PO or 50–75 mg/m²/d q day; ↓ w/ renal/hepatic Insuff; take on empty stomach **W/P:** [D, ?] w/ Allopurinol, immunosuppression, TMP-SMX, warfarin, salicylates **CI:** Prior resistance, severe hepatic Dz, BM suppression, PRG **Disp:** Tabs 50 mg **SE:** Mild hematotoxicity, mucositis, stomatitis, D, rash, fever, eosinophilia, jaundice, hep, hyperuricemia, hyperpigmentation, alopecia **Notes:** Handle properly; limit use to experienced physicians; ensure adequate hydration; for ALL, evening dosing may ↓ risk of relapse; low emetogenicity

Meropenem (Merrem) **Uses:** *Intra-Abd Infxns, bacterial meningitis, skin Infxn* **Acts:** Carbapenem; ↓ cell wall synth. **Spectrum:** Excellent gram(+) (except MRSA, methicillin-resistant *S. epidermidis* [MRSE] & *E. faecium*) excellent gram(–) including extended-spectrum β-lactamase producers; good anaerobic **Dose:** *Adults. Abd Infxn:* 1–2 g IV q8h. *Skin Infxn:* 50 mg IV q8h. *Meningitis:* 2 g IV q8h. *Peds > 3 mo, < 50 kg. Abd Infxn:* 20 mg/kg IV q8h. *Skin Infxn:* 50 mg/kg IV q8h. *Meningitis:* 40 mg/kg IV q8h; *Peds > 50 kg.* Use adult dose; max 2 g IV q8h; ↓ in renal Insuff (see PI) **W/P:** [B, ?] w/ Probenecid, VPA **CI:** β-Lactam sensitivity **Disp:** Inj 1 g, 500 mg **SE:** Less Sz potential than imipenem; *C. difficile* enterocolitis, D, ↓ plt **Notes:** Overuse ↑ bacterial resistance

Mesalamine (Asacol, Canasa, Lialda, Pentasa, Rowasa) **Uses:** *Rectal: mild–mod distal ulcerative colitis, proctosigmoiditis, proctitis; oral: treat/maint of mild–mod ulcerative colitis* **Acts:** 5-ASA derivative, may inhibit prostaglandins, may ↓ leukotrienes and TNF-α **Dose:** *Rectal:* 60 mL qhs, retain 8 h (enema), 500 mg bid-tid or 1000 mg qhs (supp) *PO:* Caps: 1 g PO qid; tab: 1.6–2.4 g/d ÷ doses (tid-qid); DR 2.4–4.8 g PO daily 8 wk max, do not cut/crush/chew w/ food; ↓ initial dose in elderly **W/P:** [B, M] w/ Digitalis, PUD, pyloric stenosis, renal Insuff, elderly **CI:** Salicylate sensitivity **Disp:** Tabs ER (*Asacol*) 400, 800 mg; ER caps (*Pentasa*) 250, 500 mg; DR tab (*Lialda*) 1.2 g; supp 500, (*Canasa*) 1000 mg; (*Rowasa*) rectal susp 4 g/60 mL **SE:** Yellow-brown urine, HA, malaise, Abd pain, flatulence, rash, pancreatitis, pericarditis, dizziness, rectal pain, hair loss, intolerance synd (bloody D) **Notes:** Retain rectally 1–3 h; ✓ CBC, Cr, BUN; Sx may ↑ when starting

Mesna (Mesnex) Uses: *Prevent hemorrhagic cystitis d/t ifosamide or cyclophosphamide* **Acts:** Antidote, reacts w/ acrolein and other metabolites to form stable compounds **Dose:** Per protocol; dose as % of ifosamide or cyclophosphamide dose. *IV bolus:* 20% (e.g., 10–12 mg/kg) IV at 0, 4, & 8 h, then 40% at 0, 1, 4, & 7 h; *IV Inf:* 20% prechemotherapy, 50–100% w/ chemotherapy, then 25–50% for 12 h following chemotherapy; *Oral:* 100% ifosamide dose given as 20% IV at hour 0 then 40% PO at hours 4 & 8; if PO dose vomited repeat or give dose IV; mix PO w/ juice **W/P:** [B; ?/–] **CI:** Thiol sensitivity **Disp:** Inj 100 mg/mL; tabs 400 mg **SE:** ↓ BP, ↓ plt, ↑ HR, ↑ RR allergic Rxns, HA, GI upset, taste perversion **Notes:** Hydration helps ↓ hemorrhagic cystitis; higher dose for BMT; IV contains benzyl alcohol

Metaproterenol (Alupent, Metaprel) Uses: *Asthma & reversible bronchospasm, COPD* **Acts:** Sympathomimetic bronchodilator **Dose:** *Adults. Nebulized:* 5% 2.5 mL q4–6h or PRN. *MDI:* 1–3 Inh q3–4h, 12 Inh max/24 h; wait 2 min between Inh. *PO:* 20 mg q6–8h. *Peds ≥12 y. MDI:* 2–3 Inh q3–4h, 12 Inh/d max. *Nebulizer:* 2.5 mL (soln 0.4%, 0.6%) tid-qid, up to q4h. *Peds > 9 y or > 60 lbs.* 20 mg PO tid-qid; *6–9 y or < 60 lbs:* 10 mg PO tid-qid; ↓ in elderly **W/P:** [C, ?/–] w/ MAOI, TCA, sympathomimetics; avoid w/ β-blockers **CI:** Tachycardia, other arrhythmias **Disp:** Aerosol 0.65 mg/Inh; soln for Inh 0.4%, 0.6%; tabs 10, 20 mg; syrup 10 mg/5 mL **SE:** Nervousness, tremor, tachycardia, HTN, ↑ glucose, ↓ K⁺, ↑ IOP **Notes:** Fewer β₁ effects than isoproterenol & longer acting, but not a 1st-line β-agonist. Use w/ face mask < 4 y; oral ↑ ADR; contains ozone-depleting CFCs; will be gradually removed from US market

Metaxalone (Skelaxin) Uses: *Painful musculoskeletal conditions* **Acts:** Centrally acting skeletal muscle relaxant **Dose:** 800 mg PO tid-qid **W/P:** [C, ?/–] w/ Elderly, EtOH & CNS depression, anemia **CI:** Severe hepatic/renal impair; drug-induced, hemolytic, or other anemias **Disp:** Tabs 800 mg **SE:** N/V, HA, drowsiness, hep

Metformin (Glucophage, Glucophage XR) **BOX:** Associated w/ lactic acidosis, risk ↑ w/ sepsis, dehydration, renal/hepatic impair, ↑ alcohol, acute CHF; Sxs include myalgias, malaise, resp distress, abd pain, somnolence; Labs: ↓ pH, ↑ anion gap, ↑ blood lactate; D/C immediately & hospitalize if suspected Uses: *Type 2 DM*, polycystic ovary synd (PCOS), HIV lipodystrophy **Acts:** Biguanide; ↓ hepatic glucose production & intestinal absorption of glucose; ↑ insulin sensitivity **Dose:** *Adults.* Initial: 500 mg PO bid; or 850 mg daily, titrate 1–2-wk intervals may ↑ to 2550 mg/d max; take w/ A.M. & P.M. meals; can convert total daily dose to daily dose of XR. *Peds 10–16 y.* 500 mg PO bid, ↑ 500 mg/wk to 2000 mg/d max in ÷ doses; do not use XR formulation in peds **W/P:** [B, +/–] Avoid EtOH; hold dose before & 48 h after ionic imaging contrast; hepatic impair, elderly **CI:** SCr > 1.4 mg/dL in females or > 1.5 mg/dL in males; hypoxemic conditions (e.g., acute CHF/sepsis); metabolic acidosis **Disp:** Tabs 500, 850, 1000 mg; XR tabs 500, 750, 1000 mg; soln 100 mg/mL **SE:** Anorexia, N/V/D, flatulence, weakness, myalgia, rash

Methadone (Dolophine, Methadose) [C-II]   **BOX:** Deaths reported during initiation and conversion of pain pts to methadone Rx from Rx w/ other opioids. Resp depression and QT prolongation, arrhythmias observed. Only dispensed by certified opioid Tx programs for addiction. Analgesic use must outweigh risks **Uses:** *Severe pain not responsive to non-narcotics; detox w/ maint of narcotic addiction* **Acts:** Narcotic analgesic **Dose:** *Adults.* 2.5–10 mg IM/IV/SQ q8–12h or 5–15 mg PO q8h; titrate as needed; see PI for conversion from other opioids. *Peds.* (Not FDA approved) 0.1 mg/kg q4–12h IV; ↑ slowly to avoid resp depression; ↓ in renal impair **W/P:** [C, –] Avoid w/ severe liver Dz **CI:** Resp depression, acute asthma, ileus **Disp:** Tabs 5, 10 mg; tab dispersible 40 mg; PO soln 5, 10 mg/5 mL; PO conc 10 mg/mL; Inj 10 mg/mL **SE:** Resp depression, sedation, constipation, urinary retention, ↑ QT interval, arrhythmias, ↓ HR, syncope, ↓ K$^+$, ↓ Mg^{2+} **Notes:** Parenteral:oral 1:2; Equianalgesic w/ parenteral morphine; longer 1/2; resp depression occurs later and lasts longer than analgesic effect, use w/ caution to avoid iatrogenic OD

Methenamine Hippurate (Hiprex), Methenamine Mandelate (UROQUID-Acid No. 2)   **Uses:** *Suppress recurrent UTI long-term. Use only after infxn cleared by antibiotics* **Acts:** Converted to formaldehyde & ammonia in acidic urine; nonspecific bacteriacidal action **Dose:** *Adults.* Hippurate: 1 g PO bid. *Mandelate:* initial 1 g qid PO pc & hs, maint 1–2 g/d. *Peds 6–12 y.* Hippurate: 0.5–1 g PO bid PO ÷ bid. *> 2 y.* Mandelate: 50–75 mg/kg/d PO ÷ qid; take w/ food, ascorbic acid w/ hydration **W/P:** [C, +] **CI:** Renal Insuff, severe hepatic Dz, & severe dehydration **Disp:** *Methenamine hippurate* (Hiprex, Urex): Tabs 1 g. *Methenamine mandelate:* 500 mg, 1 g EC tabs **SE:** Rash, GI upset, dysuria, ↑ LFTs, superinfection w/ prolonged use, *C. difficile*-associated diarrhea. **Notes:** Use w/ sulfonamides may precipitate in urine. Hippurate not indicated in peds < 6 y. Not for pts w/ indwelling catheters as dwell time in bladder required for action

Methenamine, Phenyl Salicylate, Methylene Blue, Benzoic Acid, Hyoscyamine (Prosed)   **Uses:** *Lower urinary tract discomfort* **Acts:** Methenamine in acid urine releases formaldehyde (antiseptic), phenyl salicylate mild analgesic methylene blue/benzoic acid mild antiseptic, hyoscyamine parasympatholytic ↓ muscle spasm **Dose:** *Adults Peds > 12 y.* 1 tabs PO qid **W/P:** [C, ?/–] avoid w/ sulfonamides **CI:** NAG, pyloric/duodenal obst, BOO, coronary artery spasm **Disp:** Tabs **SE:** Rash, dry mouth, flushing, ↑ pulse, dizziness, blurred vision, urine/feces discoloration, voiding difficulty/retention **Notes:** Take w/ plenty of fluid, can cause crystalluria

Methimazole (Tapazole) Uses: *Hyperthyroidism, thyrotoxicosis*, prep for thyroid surgery or radiation **Acts:** Blocks T_3 & T_4 formation, but does not inactivate circulating T_3, T_4 **Dose: Adults.** Initial based on severity: 15–60 mg/d PO q8h. *Maint:* 5–15 mg PO daily. *Peds. Initial:* 0.4–0.7 mg/kg/24 h PO q8h. *Maint:* 1/3–2/3 of initial dose PO daily; take w/ food **W/P:** [D, –] w/ Other meds **CI:** Breast-feeding **Disp:** Tabs 5, 10, 20 mg **SE:** GI upset, dizziness, blood dyscrasias, dermatitis, fever, hepatic Rxns, lupus-like synd **Notes:** Follow clinically & w/ TFT, CBC w/ diff

Methocarbamol (Robaxin) Uses: *Relief of discomfort associated w/ painful musculoskeletal conditions* **Acts:** Centrally acting skeletal muscle relaxant **Dose: Adults & Peds > 16 y.** 1.5 g PO qid for 2–3 d, then 1-g PO qid maint. *Tetanus:* 1–2 g IV q6h × 3 d, then use PO. *< 16 y:* 15 mg/kg/dose or 500 mg/m² IV, may repeat PRN (tetanus only), max 1.8 g/m²/d × 3 d **W/P:** Sz disorders [C, +] **CI:** MyG, renal impair w/IV **Disp:** Tabs 500, 750 mg; Inj 100 mg/mL **SE:** Can discolor urine, lightheadedness, drowsiness, GI upset, ↓ HR, ↓ BP **Note:** Tabs can be crushed and added to NG, do not operate heavy machinery

Methotrexate (Rheumatrex Dose Pack, Trexall) **BOX:** Administration only by experienced physician; do not use in women of childbearing age unless absolutely necessary (teratogenic); impaired elimination w/ impaired renal Fxn, ascites, pleural effusion; severe ↓ BM w/ NSAIDs; hepatotoxic, occasionally fatal; can induce life-threatening pneumonitis; D and ulcerative stomatitis require D/C; lymphoma risk; may cause tumor lysis synd; can cause severe skin Rxn, opportunistic infxns; w/ RT can ↑ tissue necrosis risk. Preservatives make this agent unsuitable for intrathecal IT or higher dose use Uses: *ALL, AML, leukemic meningitis, trophoblastic tumors (choriocarcinoma, hydatidiform mole), breast, lung, head, & neck CAs, Burkitt lymphoma, mycosis fungoides, osteosarcoma, Hodgkin Dz & NHL, psoriasis, RA, JRA, SLE*, chronic Dz **Acts:** ↓ Dihydrofolate reductase-mediated prod of tetrahydrofolate, causes ↓ DNA synth **Dose: Adults.** *CA:* Per protocol. *RA:* 7.5 mg/kg PO 1/wk or 2.5 mg q12h PO for 3 doses/wk. *Psoriasis:* 2.5–5 mg PO q12h × 3d/wk or 10–25 mg PO/IM q wk. *Chronic:* 15–25 mg IM/SQ q wk, then 15 mg/wk. *Peds.* 10 mg/m² PO/IM q wk, then 5–14 mg/m² × 1 or as 3 divided doses 12 h apart; ↓ elderly, w/ renal/hepatic impair **W/P:** [D, –] w/ Other nephro-/hepatotoxic meds, multiple interactions, w/ Sz, profound ↓ BM other than CA related **CI:** Severe renal/hepatic impair; PRG/lactation **Disp:** Dose pack 2.5 mg in 8, 12, 16, 20, or 24 doses; tabs 2.5, 5, 7.5, 10, 15 mg; Inj 25 mg/mL; Inj powder 20 mg, 1 g **SE:** ↓ BM, N/V/D, anorexia, mucositis, hepatotox (transient & reversible; may progress to atrophy, necrosis, fibrosis, cirrhosis), rashes, dizziness, malaise, blurred vision, alopecia, photosens, renal failure, pneumonitis; rare pulm fibrosis; chemical arachnoiditis & HA w/ IT delivery **Notes:** Monitor CBC, LFTs, Cr, MTX levels & CXR; "high dose" > 500 mg/m² requires leucovorin rescue to ↓ tox; w/ IT, use preservative-/alcohol-free soln; systemic levels: *Therapeutic:* > 0.01 micromole; *Toxic:* > 10 micromoles over 24 h

Methyldopa (Aldomet) Uses: *HTN* Acts: Centrally acting antihypertensive, ↓ sympathetic outflow Dose: *Adults.* 250–500 mg PO bid-tid (max 2–3 g/d) or 250 mg–1 g IV q6–8h. *Peds Neonates.* 2.5–5 mg/kg PO/IV q8h. *Other peds.* 10 mg/kg/24 h PO in 2–3 ÷ doses or 5–10 mg/kg/dose IV q6–8h to max 65 mg/kg/24 h; ↓ in renal Insuff/elderly W/P: [B(PO), C(IV), +] CI: Liver Dz, w/ MAOIs, bisulfate allergy Disp: Tabs 250, 500 mg; Inj 50 mg/mL SE: Discolors urine; initial transient sedation/drowsiness, edema, myocardial ischemia, hepatic disorders, fevers, nightmares Notes: Tolerance may occur, false(+) Coombs test

Methylene Blue (Urolene Blue, Various) Uses: *Methemoglobinemia, vasoplegic syndrome, ifosfamide-induced encephalopathy, cyanide poisoning, dye in therapeutics/diagnosis* Acts: Low IV dose converts methemoglobin to hemoglobin; excreted, appears in urine as green/green blue color; MAOI activity Dose: 0.1–0.2 mL/kg body weight IV; direct instillation into fistulous tract W/P: [D, –] CI: w/ psych meds such as SSRI, SNRI, TCAs (may cause serotonin syndrome) Disp: 1, 10 mL Inj SE: IV use: N, abdominal, chest pain, sweating Notes: Component of other medications; stains tissue blue, limits repeat use in surgical visualization

Methylergonovine (Methergine) Uses: *Postpartum bleeding (atony, hemorrhage)* Acts: Ergotamine derivative, rapid and sustained uterotonic effect Dose: 0.2 mg IM after anterior shoulder delivery or puerperium, may repeat in 2–4-h intervals or 0.2–0.4 mg PO q6–12h for 2–7 d W/P: [C, ?] w/ Sepsis, obliterative vascular Dz, hepatic/renal impair, w/ CYP3A4 inhib (Table 10, p 301) CI: HTN, PRG, toxemia Disp: Inj 0.2 mg/mL; tabs 0.2 mg SE: HTN, N/V, CP, ↓ BP, Sz Notes: Give IV only if absolutely necessary over > 1 min w/ BP monitoring

Methylnaltrexone Bromide (Relistor) Uses: *Opioid-induced constipation in pt w/ advanced illness such as CA* Acts: Peripheral opioid antagonist Dose: *Adults. Wgt-based < 38 kg:* 0.15 mg/kg SQ; *38–61 kg:* 8 mg SQ; *62–114 kg:* 12 mg SQ, dose q other day PRN, max 1 dose q24h W/P: [B, NR] w/ CrCl < 30 mL/min ↓ dose 50% Disp: Inj 12 mg/0.6 mL SE: N/D, Abd pain, dizziness Notes: Does not affect opioid analgesic effects or induce withdrawal

Methylphenidate, Oral (Concerta, Metadate CD, Methylin, Ritalin, Ritalin LA, Ritalin SR, Others) [C-II] BOX: w/ Hx of drug or alcohol dependence, avoid abrupt D/C; chronic use can lead to dependence or psychotic behavior; observe closely during withdrawal of drug Uses: *ADHD, narcolepsy*, depression Acts: CNS stimulant, blocks reuptake of norepinephrine and DA Dose: *Adults. Narcolepsy:* 10 mg PO 2–3×/d, 60 mg/d max. *Depression:* 2.5 mg q A.M.; ↑ slowly, 20 mg/d max, ÷ bid 7 A.M. & 12 P.M.; use regular release only. *Adults and Peds > 6 y. ADHD: IR:* 5 mg PO bid, ↑ 5–10 mg/d to 60 mg/d, max (2 mg/kg/d), *ER/SR* use total IR dose q day. *CD/LA* 20 mg PO q day, ↑ 10–20 mg q wk to 60 mg/d max. *Concerta:* 18 mg PO q A.M. Rx naïve or already on 20 mg/d, 36 mg PO q A.M. if on 30–45 mg/d, 54 mg PO q A.M. if on 40–60 mg/d, 72 mg PO q A.M. W/P: [C, +/–] w/ Hx EtOH/drug abuse, CV Dz, HTN, bipolar Dz, Sz; separate from MAOIs by 14 d Disp: Chew tabs 2.5, 5, 10 mg; tabs scored IR (Ritalin) 5, 10, 20 mg; *Caps ER*

(Ritalin LA) 10, 20, 30, 40 mg *Caps ER (Metadate CD)* 10, 20, 30, 40, 50, 60 mg *(Methylin ER)* 10, 20 mg. *Tabs SR (Ritalin SR)* 20 mg; ER tabs *(Concerta)* 18, 27, 36, 54 mg. Oral soln 5, 10 mg/5 mL **SE:** CV/CNS stimulation, growth retard, GI upset, pancytopenia, ↑ LFTs **CI:** Marked anxiety, tension, agitation, NAG, motor tics, family Hx or diagnosis of Tourette synd, severe HTN, angina, arrhythmias, CHF, recent MI, ↑ thyroid; w/ or w/in 14 d of MAOI **Notes:** See also transdermal form; titrate dose; take 30–45 min ac; do not chew or crush; *Concerta* "ghost tablet" in stool, avoid w/ GI narrowing; Metadate contains sucrose, avoid w/ lactose/galactose problems. Do not use these meds w/ halogenated anesthetics; abuse and diversion concerns; AHA recommends: all ADHD peds need CV assessment and consideration for ECG before Rx

Methylphenidate, Transdermal (Daytrana) [C-II] **BOX:** w/ Hx of drug or alcohol dependence; chronic use can lead to dependence or psychotic behavior; observe closely during withdrawal of drug **Uses:** *ADHD in children 6–17 y* **Acts:** CNS stimulant, blocks reuptake of norepinephrine and DA **Dose:** *Adults & Peds ≥6 y.* Apply to hip in A.M. (2 h before desired effect), remove 9 h later; titrate 1st wk 10 mg/9 h, 2nd wk 15 mg/9 h, 3rd wk 20 mg/9 h, 4th wk 30 mg/9 h **W/P:** [C, +/–] See methylphenidate, oral sensitization may preclude subsequent use of oral forms; abuse and diversion concerns **CI:** significant anxiety, agitation; component allergy; glaucoma; w/ or w/in 14 d of MAOI; tics, or family Hx Tourette synd **Disp:** Patches 10, 15, 20, 30 mg **SE:** Local Rxns, N/V, nasopharyngitis, ↓ wgt, ↓ appetite, lability, insomnia, tic **Notes:** Titrate dose weekly; effects last hours after removal; evaluate BP, HR at baseline and periodically; avoid heat exposure to patch, may cause OD, AHA rec: all ADHD peds need CV assessment and consideration for ECG before Rx

Methylprednisolone (Solu-Medrol) [See Steroids, p 244, and Table 2, p 283] *Peds. ECC 2010. Status asthmaticus, anaphylactic shock:* 2 mg/kg IV/IO/IM (max 60 mg). *Maint:* 0.5 mg/kg IV q6h or 1 mg/kg q12h to 120 mg/d

Metoclopramide (Metozolv, Reglan, Generic) **BOX:** Chronic use may cause tardive dyskinesia; D/C if Sxs develop; avoid prolonged use (> 12 wks) **Uses:** *Diabetic gastroparesis, symptomatic GERD; chemo & post-op N/V, facilitate small-bowel intubation & upper GI radiologic exam*, *GERD, diabetic gastroparesis (Metozolv)* stimulate gut in prolonged post-op ileus* **Acts:** ↑ Upper GI motility; blocks dopamine in chemoreceptor trigger zone, sensitized tissues to ACH **Dose:** *Adults. Gastroparesis (Reglan):* 10 mg PO 30 min ac & hs for 2–8 wk PRN, or same dose IM/IV for 10 d, then PO. *Reflux:* 10–15 mg PO 30 min ac & hs. *Chemo antiemetic:* 1–3 mg/kg/dose IV 30 min before chemo, then 2 mg/kg/dose, then q3h × 3 doses. *Post-op:* 10–20 mg IV/IM q4–6h PRN. *Adults & Peds > 14 y. Intestinal intubation:* 10 mg IV × 1 over 1–2 min. *Peds. Reflux:* 0.1 mg/kg/dose PO 30 min ac & hs, max 0.3–0.75 mg/kg/d × 2 wk–6 mo. *Chemo antiemetic:* 1–2 mg/kg/dose IV as adults. *Post-op:* 0.25 mg/kg/dose IV q6–8h PRN. *Peds. Intestinal intubation:*

6–14 y: 2.5–5 mg IV × 1 over 1–2 min; *< 6 y:* use 0.1 mg/kg IV × 1 **W/P:** [B, –] Drugs w/ extrapyramidal ADRs, MAOIs, TCAs, sympathomimetics **CI:** w/ EPS meds, GI bleeding, pheochromocytoma, Sz disorders, GI obst **Disp:** Tabs 5, 10 mg; syrup 5 mg/5 mL; ODT *(Metzolv)* 5, 10 g; Inj 5 mg/mL **SE:** Dystonic Rxns common w/ high doses (Rx w/IV diphenhydramine), fluid retention, restlessness, D, drowsiness **Notes:** ↓ w/ renal impair/elderly; ✓ baseline Cr

Metolazone (Zaroxolyn)   **Uses:** *Mild–mod essential HTN & edema of renal Dz or cardiac failure* **Acts:** Thiazide-like diuretic; ↓ distal tubule Na reabsorption **Dose:** *HTN:* 2.5–5 mg/d PO maint 5–20 mg PO q day *Edema:* 2.5–20 mg/d PO. **W/P:** [D, +] Avoid w/ Li, gout, digitalis, SLE, many interactions **CI:** Anuria, hepatic coma or precoma. **Disp:** Tabs 2.5, 5, 10 mg **SE:** Monitor fluid/lytes; dizziness, ↓ BP, ↓ K^+, ↑ HR, ↑ uric acid, CP, photosens

Metoprolol Tartrate (Lopressor) Metoprolol Succinate (Toprol XL)   **BOX:** Do not acutely stop Rx as marked worsening of angina can result; taper over 1–2 wk **Uses:** *HTN, angina, AMI, CHF (XL form)* **Acts:** β_1-Adrenergic receptor blocker **Dose:** *Adults. Angina:* 50–200 mg PO bid max 400 mg/d; ER form dose q day. *HTN:* 50–200 mg PO bid max 450 mg/d, ER form dose q day. *AMI:* 5 mg IV q2min × 3 doses, then 50 mg PO q6h × 48 h, then 100 mg PO bid. *CHF: (XL form preferred)* 12.5–25 mg/d PO × 2 wk, ↑ 2-wk intervals, 200 mg/max, use low dose w/ greatest severity; *ECC 2010.* AMI: 5 mg slow IV q5min, total 15 mg; then 50 mg PO, titrate to effect. *Peds 1–17 y. HTN* IR form 1–2 mg/kg/d PO, max 6 mg/kg/d (200 mg/d). *≥6 y: HTN* ER form 1 mg/kg/d PO, initial max 50 mg/d, ↑ PRN to 2 mg/kg/d max; ↓ w/ hepatic failure; take w/ meals **W/P:** [C, +] Uncompensated CHF, ↓ HR, heart block, hepatic impair, MyG, PVD, Raynaud, thyrotoxicosis **CI:** For HTN/angina SSS (unless paced), severe PVD, pheochromocytoma. For MI sinus brady < 45 BPM, 1st-degree block (PR > 0.24 s), 2nd-, 3rd-degree block, SBP < 100 mm Hg, severe CHF, cardiogenic shock **Disp:** Tabs 25, 50, 100 mg; ER tabs 25, 50, 100, 200 mg; Inj 1 mg/mL **SE:** Drowsiness, insomnia, ED, ↓ HR, bronchospasm **Notes:** IR:ER 1:1 daily dose but ER/XL is q day. OK to split XL tab but do not crush/chew

Metronidazole (Flagyl, MetroGel)   **BOX:** Carcinogenic in rats **Uses:** *Bone/joint, endocarditis, intra-Abd, meningitis, & skin infxns; amebiasis and amebic liver abscess; trichominiasis in pt and partner; bacterial vaginosis; PID; giardiasis; antibiotic associated pseudomembranous colitis (C. difficile), eradicate H. pylori w/ combo Rx, rosacea, prophylactic in post-op colorectal surgery* **Acts:** Interferes w/ DNA synth. *Spectrum:* Excellent anaerobic, *C. difficile* **Dose:** *Adults. Anaerobic* Infxns: 500 mg IV q6–8h. *Amebic dysentery:* 500–750 mg/d PO q8h × 5–10 d. *Trichomonas:* 250 mg PO tid for 7 d or 2 g PO × 1 (Rx partner). *C. difficile:* 500 mg PO or IV q8h for 7–10 d (PO preferred; IV only if pt NPO), if no response, change to PO vancomycin. *Vaginosis:* 1 applicator intravag q day or bid × 5 d, or 500 mg PO bid × 7 d or 750 mg PO q day × 7 d. *Acne rosacea/skin:* Apply bid. *Giardia:* 500 mg PO bid × 5–7 d. *H. pylori:* 250–500 mg PO w/ meals & hs ×

14 d, combine w/ other antibiotic & a proton pump inhib or H₂ antagonist. **Peds.** 30 mg/kg PO/IV/d ÷ q6H, 4 g/d max ÷. *Amebic dysentery:* 35–50 mg/kg/24 h PO in 3 ÷ doses for 5–10 d; Rx 7–10 d for *C. difficile. Trichomonas:* 15–30 mg/kg/d PO ÷ q8h × 7 d. *C. difficile:* 20 mg/kg/d PO ÷ q6h × 10 d, max 2 g/d; ↓ w/ severe hepatic/renal impair **W/P:** [B, +/–] Avoid EtOH, w/ warfarin, CYP3A4 substrates (Table 10, p 301), ↑ Li levels **CI:** First tri of PRG **Disp:** Tabs 250, 500 mg; XR tabs 750 mg; caps 375 mg; IV 500 mg/100 mL; lotion 0.75%; gel 0.75, 1%; intra-vag gel 0.75% (5 g/applicator 37.5 mg in 70-g tube), cream 0.75,1% **SE:** Disulfiram-like Rxn; dizziness, HA, GI upset, anorexia, urine discoloration, flushing, metallic taste **Notes:** For trichomonas, Rx pt's partner; no aerobic bacteria activity; use in combo w/ serious mixed Infxns; wait 24 h after 1st dose to breast-feed or 48 h if extended Rx, take ER on empty stomach

Mexiletine (Mexitil) BOX: Mortality risks noted for flecainide and/or encainide (class I antiarrhythmics). Reserve for use in pts w/ life-threatening ventricular arrhythmias **Uses:** *Suppress symptomatic vent arrhythmias* **DN Acts:** Class IB antiarrhythmic (Table 9, p 300) **Dose:** *Adults.* 200–300 mg PO q8h. Initial 200 mg q8h, can load w/ 400 mg if needed, ↑ q2–3d, 1200 mg/d max. **W/P:** [C, +] CHF, may worsen severe arrhythmias; interacts w/ hepatic inducers & suppressors **CI:** Cardiogenic shock or 2nd-/3rd-degree AV block w/o pacemaker **Disp:** Caps 150, 200, 250 mg **SE:** Light-headedness, dizziness, anxiety, incoordination, GI upset, ataxia, hepatic damage, blood dyscrasias, PVCs, N/V, tremor **Notes:** ✓ LFTs, CBC, false(+) ANA

Miconazole (Monistat 1 Combo, Monistat 3, Monistat 7) [OTC] (Monistat-Derm) Uses: *Candidal Infxns, dermatomycoses (tinea pedis/tinea cruris/tinea corporis/tinea versicolor/Candidiasis)* **Acts:** Azole antifungal, alters fungal membrane permeability **Dose:** *Intravag:* 100 mg supp or 2% cream intravag qhs × 7 d or 200 mg supp or 4% cream intravag qhs × 3 d. *Derm:* Apply bid, A.M./P.M.. *Tinea versicolor:* Apply q day. Treat tinea pedis for 1 mo and other infxns for 2 wk. *Peds ≥12 y.* 100 mg supp or 2% cream intravag qhs × 7 d or 200 mg supp or 4% cream intravag qhs × 3 d. **W/P:** [C, ?] Azole sensitivity **Disp:** *Monistat-Derm:* (Rx) cream 2%; *Monistat 1 Combo:* (2% cream w/ 1200 mg supp, *Monistat 3:* Vag cream 4%, supp 200 mg; *Monistat 7:* cream 2%, supp 100 mg; lotion 2%; powder 2%; effervescent tab 2%, oint 2%, spray 2%; vag supp 100, 200, 1200 mg; vag cream 2%, 4%; [OTC] **SE:** Vag burning; on skin contact dermatitis, irritation, burning **Notes:** May interfere w/ condom and diaphragm, do not use w/ tampons

Miconazole, Buccal (Oravig) Uses: *Oropharyngeal candidiasis* **Acts:** Azole antifungal, alters fungal membrane permeability **Dose:** *Adults.* Apply one 50 mg buccal tab to gum once daily × 14 d; do not crush/chew/swallow tab **W/P:** [C, ?/–] allergic Rxns may occur; may ↑ effect of warfarin (monitor INR) **CI:** Hypersens to milk protein or components **Disp:** Tabs buccal 50 mg **SE:** HA, N/V/D, upper abd pain, dysgeusia

Miconazole/Zinc Oxide/Petrolatum (Vusion) **Uses:** *Candidal diaper rash* **Acts:** Combo antifungal **Dose:** *Peds > 4 wk.* Apply at each diaper change × 7 d **W/P:** [C, ?] **CI:** None **Disp:** Miconazole/zinc oxide/petrolatum oint 0.25/15/81.35%, 50-, 90-g tube **SE:** None **Notes:** Keep diaper dry, not for prevention

Midazolam (Various) [C-IV] **BOX:** Associated w/ resp depression and resp arrest especially when used for sedation in noncritical care settings. Reports of airway obst, desaturation, hypoxia, and apnea w/ other CNS depressants. Cont monitoring required **Uses:** *Pre-op sedation, conscious sedation for short procedures & mechanically ventilated pts, induction of general anesthesia* **Acts:** Short-acting benzodiazepine **Dose:** *Adults.* 1–5 mg IV or IM or 0.02–0.35 mg/kg based on indication; titrate to effect. *Peds. Pre-op: > 6 mo:* 0.25–1 mg/kg PO, 20 mg max. *Conscious sedation:* 0.08 mg/kg × 1. *> 6 mo:* 0.1–0.15 mg/kg IM × 1 max 10 mg. *General anesthesia:* 0.025–0.1 mg/kg IV q2min for 1–3 doses PRN to induce anesthesia (↓ in elderly, w/ narcotics or CNS depressants) **W/P:** [D, +/–] w/ CYP3A4 substrate (Table 9, p 300), multiple drug interactions **CI:** NAG; w/ fosamprenavir, atazanavir, nelfinavir, ritonavir **Disp:** Inj 1, 5 mg/mL; syrup 2 mg/mL **SE:** Resp depression; ↓ BP w/ conscious sedation, N **Notes:** Reversal w/ flumazenil; monitor for resp depression; not for epidural/intrathecal IT use

Midodrine (Proamatine) **Uses:** *Tx orthostatic hypotension* **Acts:** Vasopressor/antihypotensive; α_1-agonist **Dose:** 10 mg PO tid when pt plans to be upright **W/P:** [C, ?] **CI:** Pheochromocytoma, renal Dz, thyrotoxicosis, severe heart Dz, urinary retention **Disp:** Tabs 2.5, 5, 10 mg **SE:** Supine HTN, paresthesia, urinary retention **Notes:** SBP $\geq$ 200 mm Hg in ~13% pts given 10 mg

Mifepristone [RU 486] (Mifeprex) **BOX:** Pt counseling & information required; associated w/ fatal Infxns & bleeding **Uses:** *Terminate intrauterine pregnancies PRGs of < 49 d* **Acts:** Antiprogestin; ↑ prostaglandins, results in uterine contraction **Dose:** Administered w/ 3 office visits: Day 1: 600 mg PO × 1; day 3, unless abortion confirmed, 400 mcg PO of misoprostol (*Cytotec*); about day 14, verify termination of PRG. Surgical termination if Rx fails. **W/P:** [X, –] w/ Infxn, sepsis **CI:** Ectopic PRG, undiagnosed adnexal mass, w/ IUD, adrenal failure, w/ long-term steroid Rx, hemorrhagic Dz, w/ anticoagulants, prostaglandin hypersens. Pts who do not have access to medical facilities or unable to understand treatment or comply. **Disp:** Tabs 200 mg **SE:** Abd pain & 1–2 wk of uterine bleeding, N/V/D, HA **Notes:** Under physician's supervision only, 9–16 d using misoprostol on average after using

Miglitol (Glyset) **Uses:** *Type 2 DM* **Acts:** α-Glucosidase inhib; delays carbohydrate digestion **Dose:** Initial 25 mg PO tid; maint 50–100 mg tid (w/ 1st bite of each meal), titrate over 4–8 wk **W/P:** [B, –] w/ Digitalis & digestive enzymes **CI:** DKA, obstructive/inflammatory GI disorders; SCr > 2 mg/dL **Disp:** Tabs 25, 50, 100 mg **SE:** Flatulence, D, Abd pain **Notes:** Use alone or w/ sulfonylureas

Milnacipran (Savella) **BOX:** Antidepressants associated w/ ↑ risk of suicide ideation in children and young adults **Uses:** *Fibromyalgia* **Action:** Antidepressant, SNRI **Dose:** 50 mg PO bid, max 200 mg/d; ↓ to 25 mg bid w/ CrCl < 30 mL/min

W/P: [C, /?] **CI:** NAG, w/ recent MAOI **Disp:** Tabs: 12.5, 25, 50, 100 mg **SE:** Headache, N/V, constipation, dizziness, ↑ HR, ↑ BP **Notes:** Monitor HR and BP

Milrinone (Primacor) **Uses:** *CHF acutely decompensated*, calcium antagonist intoxication **Acts:** Phosphodiesterase inhib, (+) inotrope & vasodilator; little chronotropic activity **Dose:** 50 mcg/kg, IV over 10 min then 0.375–0.75 mcg/kg/min IV Inf; ↓ w/ renal impair **W/P:** [C, ?] **CI:** Allergy to drug; w/ inamrinone **Disp:** Inj 200 mcg/mL **SE:** Arrhythmias, ↓ BP, HA **Notes:** Monitor fluids, lytes, CBC, Mg^{2+}, BP, HR; not for long-term use

Mineral Oil [OTC] **Uses:** *Constipation, bowel irrigation, fecal impaction* **Acts:** Lubricant laxative **Dose:** *Adults. Constipation:* 15–45 mL PO/d PRN. *Fecal impaction or after barium:* 118 mL rectally × 1. *Peds > 6 y. Constipation:* 5–25 mL PO q day. *2–12 y: Fecal impaction:* 118 mL rectally × 1. **W/P:** [C, ?] w/ N/V, difficulty swallowing, bedridden pts; may ↓ absorption of vit A, D, E, K, warfarin **CI:** Colostomy/ileostomy, appendicitis, diverticulitis, ulcerative colitis **Disp:** All [OTC] liq PO 13.5 mL/15 mL, PO microemulsion 2.5 mL/5 mL, rectal enema 118 mL **SE:** Lipid pneumonia (aspiration of PO), N/V, temporary anal incontinence **Notes:** Take PO upright, do not use PO in peds < 6 y

Mineral Oil-Pramoxine HCl-Zinc Oxide (Tucks Ointment, [OTC]) **Uses:** *Temporary relief of anorectal disorders (itching, etc)* **Acts:** Topical anesthetic **Dose:** *Adults & Peds ≥12 y.* Cleanse, rinse, & dry, apply externally or into anal canal w/ tip 5×/d × 7 d max. **W/P:** [?, ?] Do not place into rectum **CI:** None **Disp:** Oint 30-g tube **SE:** Local irritation **Notes:** D/C w/ or if rectal bleeding occurs or if condition worsens or does not improve w/in 7 d

Minocycline (Dynacin, Minocin, Solodyn) **Uses:** *Mod–severe nonnodular acne (Solodyn)*, anthrax, rickettsiae, skin Infxn, URI, UTI, nongonococcal urethritis, amebic dysentery, asymptomatic meningococcal carrier, *Mycobacterium marinum* **Acts:** Tetracycline, bacteriostatic, ↓ protein synth **Dose:** *Adults & Peds > 12 y. Usual:* 200 mg, then 100 mg q12h or 100–200 mg, then 50 mg qid. *Gonococcal urethritis, men:* 100 mg q12h × 5 d. *Syphilis:* Usual dose × 10–15 d. *Meningococcal carrier:* 100 mg q12h × 5 d. *M. marinum:* 100 mg q12h × 6–8 wk. *Uncomp urethral, endocervical, or rectal Infxn:* 100 mg q12h × 7 d minimum. *Adults & Peds > 12 y. Acne: (Solodyn)* 1 mg/kg PO q day × 12 wk. > *8 y:* 4 mg/kg initially then 2 mg/kg q12h w/ food to ↓ irritation, hydrate well, ↓ dose or extend interval w/ renal impair. **W/P:** [D, –] Associated w/ pseudomembranous colitis, w/ renal impair, may ↓ OCP, or w/ warfarin may ↑ INR **CI:** Allergy, women of childbearing potential **Disp:** Tabs 50, 75, 100 mg; tabs ER *(Solodyn)* 45, 55, 65, 80, 90, 105, 115, 135 mg, caps *(Minocin)* 50, 100 mg, susp 50 mg/mL **SE:** D, HA, fever, rash, joint pain, fatigue, dizziness, photosens, hyperpigmentation, SLE synd, pseudotumor cerebri **Notes:** Do not cut/crush/chew; keep away from children, tooth discoloration in < 8 y or w/ use last half of PRG

Minoxidil, Oral **BOX:** May cause pericardial effusion, occasional tamponade, and angina pectoris may be exacerbated. Only for non-responders to max doses of 2 other antihypertensivs and a diuretic. Administer under supervision w/ a β-blocker and diuretic. Monitor for ↓ BP in those receiving guanethidine w/ malignant HTN **Uses:** *Severe HTN* **Acts:** Peripheral vasodilator **Dose:** *Adults & Peds > 12 y.* 5 mg PO ÷ daily, titrate q3d, 100 mg/d max. *Peds.* 0.2–1 mg/kg/24 h ÷ PO q12–24h, titrate q3d, max 50 mg/d; ↓ w/ elderly, renal insuff **W/P:** [C, +] **CI:** Pheochromocytoma, component allergy, CHF, renal impair **Disp:** Tabs 2.5, 10 mg **SE:** Pericardial effusion & vol overload w/ PO use; hypertrichosis w/ chronic use, edema, ECG changes, wgt gain **Note:** Avoid for 1 mo after MI

Minoxidil, Topical (Theroxidil, Rogaine) [OTC]   **Uses:** *Male & female pattern baldness* **Acts:** Stimulates vertex hair growth **Dose:** Apply 1 mL bid to area, D/C if no growth in 4 mo. **W/P:** [?, ?] **CI:** Component allergy **Disp:** Soln & aerosol foam 5% **SE:** Changes in hair color/texture **Note:** requires chronic use to maintain hair

Mirtazapine (Remeron, Remeron SolTab)   **BOX:** ↑ Risk of suicidal thinking and behavior in children, adolescents, and young adults w/ major depression and other psychological disorders. Not for peds **Uses:** *Depression* **Acts:** α$_2$-Antagonist antidepressant, ↑ norepinephrine & 5-HT **Dose:** 15 mg PO hs, up to 45 mg/d hs **W/P:** [C, ?] Hx anticholesterol effects, w/ Sz, clonidine, CNS depressant use, CYP1A2, CYP3A4 inducers/inhib **CI:** MAOIs w/in 14 d **Disp:** Tabs 15, 30, 45 mg; rapid dispersion tabs (SolTab) 15, 30, 45 mg **SE:** Somnolence, ↑ cholesterol, constipation, xerostomia, wgt gain, agranulocytosis, ↓ BP, edema, musculoskeletal pain **Notes:** Do not ↑ dose < q1–2wk; handle rapid tabs w/ dry hands, do not cut or chew

Misoprostol (Cytotec)   **BOX:** Use in PRG can cause abortion, premature birth, or birth defects; do not use to ↓ decrease ulcer risk in women of childbearing age; must comply w/ birth control measures **Uses:** *Prevent NSAID-induced gastric ulcers; medical termination of PRG < 49 d w/ mifepristone*; induce labor (cervical ripening); incomplete & therapeutic abortion **Acts:** Prostaglandin (PGE-1); antisecretory & mucosal protection; induces uterine contractions **Dose:** *Ulcer prevention:* 200 mcg PO qid w/ meals; in females, start 2nd/3rd d of next nl period. *Induction of labor (term):* 25–50 mcg intravag. *PRG termination:* 400 mcg PO on day 3 of mifepristone; take w/ food **W/P:** [X, –] **CI:** PRG, component allergy **Disp:** Tabs 100, 200 mcg **SE:** Miscarriage w/ severe bleeding; HA, D, Abd pain, constipation. **Note:** Not used for induction of labor w/ previous C-section or major uterine surgery

Mitomycin (Mutamycin)   **BOX:** Administer by physician experienced in chemotherapy; myelosuppressive; can induce hemolytic uremic synd w/ irreversible renal failure **Uses:** *Stomach, pancreas*, breast, colon CA; squamous cell carcinoma of the anus; NSCLC, head & neck, cervical; bladder CA (intravesically) **Acts:** Alkylating agent; generates oxygen-free radicals w/ DNA strand breaks **Dose:** (Per protocol) 20 mg/m^2 q6–8wk IV or 10 mg/m^2 combo w/ other myelosuppressive drugs q6–8wk. *Bladder CA:* 20–40 mg in 40 mL NS via a urethral catheter once/wk × 8 wk, followed by monthly × 12 mo for 1 y; ↓ in renal/hepatic impair **W/P:** [D, –] **CI:** ↓ Plt, ↓ WBC, coagulation disorders, Cr > 1.7 mg/dL,

↑ cardiac tox w/ vinca alkaloids/doxorubicin **Disp:** Inj 5, 20, 40 mg **SE:** ↓ BM (persists for 3–8 wk, may be cumulative; minimize w/ lifetime dose < 50–60 mg/m^2), N/V, anorexia, stomatitis, renal tox, microangiopathic hemolytic anemia w/ renal failure (hemolytic–uremic synd), venoocclusive liver Dz, interstitial pneumonia, alopecia, extrav Rxns, contact dermatitis; CHF

Mitoxantrone (Novantrone) **BOX:** Administer only by physician experienced in chemotherapy; except for acute leukemia, do not use w/ ANC count of < 1500 cells/mm^3; severe neutropenia can result in Infxn, follow CBC; cardiotoxic (CHF), secondary AML reported **Uses:** *AML (w/ cytarabine), ALL, CML, PCA, MS, lung CA*, breast CA, & NHL **Acts:** DNA-intercalating agent; ↓ DNA synth by interacting w/ topoisomerase II **Dose:** Per protocol; ↓ w/ hepatic impair, leukopenia, thrombocytopenia **W/P:** [D, –] Reports of secondary AML, w/ MS ↑ CV risk, do not treat MS pt w/ low LVEF **CI:** PRG, sig ↓ in LVEF **Disp:** Inj 2 mg/mL **SE:** ↓ BM, N/V, stomatitis, alopecia (infrequent), cardiotox, urine discoloration, secretions & scleras may be blue-green **Notes:** Maintain hydration; baseline CV evaluation w/ ECG & LVEF; cardiac monitoring prior to each dose; not for intrathecal use

Modafinil (Provigil) [C-IV] **Uses:** *Improve wakefulness in pts w/ excess daytime sleepiness (narcolepsy, sleep apnea, shift work sleep disorder)* **Acts:** Alters dopamine & norepinephrine release, ↓ GABA-mediated neurotransmission **Dose:** 200 mg PO q A.M.; ↓ dose 50% w/ elderly/hepatic impair **W/P:** [C, ?/–] CV Dz; ↑ effects of warfarin, diazepam, phenytoin; ↓ OCP, cyclosporine, & theophylline effects **CI:** Component allergy **Disp:** Tabs 100, 200 mg **SE:** Serious rash including SJS, HA, N, D, paresthesias, rhinitis, agitation, psychological Sx **Notes:** CV assessment before using

Moexipril (Univasc) **BOX:** ACE inhib can cause fatal injury/death in 2nd/3rd tri; D/C w/ PRG **Uses:** *HTN, post-MI*, DN **Acts:** ACE inhib **Dose:** 7.5–30 mg in 1–2 ÷ doses 1 h ac ↓ in renal impair **W/P:** [C (1st tri), D (2nd & 3rd tri), ?] **CI:** ACE inhib sensitivity **Disp:** Tabs 7.5, 15 mg; **SE:** ↓ BP, edema, angioedema, HA, dizziness, cough, ↑ K$^+$

Molindone (Moban) **Uses:** *Schizophrenia* **Acts:** Piperazine phenothiazine **Dose:** *Adults.* 50–75 mg/d PO, ↑ to max 225 mg/d q3–4d PRN. *Peds 3–5 y.* 1–2.5 mg/d PO in 4 ÷ doses. *5–12 y.* 0.5–1.0 mg/kg/d in 4 ÷ doses **W/P:** [C, ?] NAG **CI:** Drug/EtOH CNS depression, coma **Disp:** Tabs 5, 10, 25, 50 mg scored; **SE:** Drowsiness, extrapyramidal Rxns, ↓ BP, tachycardia, arrhythmias, EPS, neuroleptic malignant synd, Szs, constipation, xerostomia, blurred vision. **Notes:** ✓ lipid profile, fasting glucose, HgA$_{1c}$; may ↑ prolactin

Mometasone and Formoterol (DULERA) **BOX:** Increased risk of worsening wheezing or asthma-related death w/ long-acting β$_2$-adrenergic agonists; use only if asthma not controlled on agent such as inhaled steroid **Uses:** *Maint Rx for asthma* **Acts:** Corticosteroid (mometasone) w/ LA bronchodilator β$_2$ agonist (formoterol) **Dose:** *Adults & Peds > 12 y.* 2 Inh q12h **W/P:** [C, M] w/ P450 3A4 inhib (e.g., ritonavir), adrenergic/beta blockers, meds that ↑ QT interval; candida infection of mouth/throat; immunosuppression, adrenal suppression, ↓ bone density, w/ glaucoma/cataracts, may ↑ glucose, ↓ K; other LABA should not be used **CI:** Acute asthma attack; component hypersensitivity **Disp:** MDI 120 inhal/canister (mcg mometasone/mcg formoterol) 100/5, 200/5 **SE:** Nasopharyngitis, sinusitis, HA, palpitations, chest pain, rapid heart rate, tremor or nervousness **Notes:** For pts not controlled on other meds (e.g., low-medium dose Inh steroids) or whose Dz severity warrants 2 maint therapies

Mometasone, Inhaled (Asmanex Twisthaler) Uses: *Maint Rx for asthma* **Acts:** Corticosteroid **Dose:** *Adults & Peds > 11 y. On bronchodilators alone or inhaled steroids:* 220 mcg × 1 q P.M. (max 440 mcg/d). *On oral steroids:* 440 mcg bid (max 880 mcg/d) with slow oral taper. *Peds 4–11 y.* 110 mcg × 1 q P.M. (max 110 mcg/d) **W/P:** [C, M] candida infection of mouth/throat; hypersens Rxns possible; may worsen certain Infxn (TB, fungal, etc); monitor for ↑/↓ cortisol Sxs; ↓ bone density; ↓ growth in peds; monitor for NAG or cataracts; may ↑ glucose **CI:** Acute asthma attack; component hypersens/milk proteins **Disp:** MDI inhal mometasone 110 mcg *Twisthaler* delivers 100 mcg/actuation; 220 mcg *Twisthaler* delivers 200 mcg/actuation **SE:** HA, allergic rhinitis, pharyngitis, URI, sinusitis, oral candidiasis, dysmenorrhea, musculoskeletal/back pain, dyspepsia **Notes:** Rinse mouth after use; treat paradoxical bronchospasm w/ inhaled bronchodilator

Mometasone, Nasal (Nasonex) Uses: *Nasal Sx allergic/seasonal rhinitis; prophylaxis of seasonal allergic rhinitis; nasal polyps in adults* **Acts:** Corticosteroid **Dose:** *Adults & Peds > 12 y. Rhinitis:* 2 sprays/each nostril QD. **Adults.** *Nasal polyps:* 2 sprays/each nostril BID *Peds 2–11 y.* 1 spray/each nostril qd **W/P:** [C, M] monitor for adverse effects on nasal mucosa (bleeding, candidal Infxn, ulceration, perf); may worsen existing Infxns; monitor for NAG, cataracts; monitor for ↑/↓ cortisol Sxs; ↓ growth in peds **CI:** component hypersens **Disp:** 50 mcg mometasone/spray **SE:** Viral infection, pharyngitis, epistaxis, HA

Montelukast (Singulair) Uses: *Prevent/chronic Rx asthma ≥12 mo; seasonal allergic rhinitis ≥2 y; perennial allergic rhinitis ≥6 mo; prevent exercise induced bronchoconstriction (EIB) ≥15 y; prophylaxis & Rx of chronic asthma, seasonal allergic rhinitis* **Acts:** Leukotriene receptor antagonist **Dose:** *Asthma: Adults & Peds > 15 y.* 10 mg/d PO in P.M. *6–23 mo:* 4-mg pack granules q day. *2–5 y:* 4 mg/d PO q P.M. *6–14 y:* 5 mg/d PO q P.M. **W/P:** [B, M] **CI:** Component allergy **Disp:** Tabs 10 mg; chew tabs 4, 5 mg; granules 4 mg/pack **SE:** HA, dizziness, fatigue, rash, GI upset, Churg-Strauss synd, flu, cough, neuropsych events (agitation, restlessness, suicidal ideation) **Notes:** Not for acute asthma; use w/in 15 min of opening package

Morphine and Naltrexone (Embeda) [C-II] **BOX:** For mod–severe chronic pain; do not use as prn analgesic; swallow whole or sprinkle contents of cap on applesauce; do not crush/dissolve, chew caps—rapid release & absorption of morphine may be fatal & of naltrexone may lead to withdrawal in opioid-tolerant pts; do not consume EtOH or EtOH-containing products; 100/4 mg caps for opioid-tolerant pts only **Uses:** *Chronic mod–severe pain* **Acts:** Mu-opioid receptor agonist & antagonist **Dose:** *Adult.* Individualize PO q12–24h; if opioid intolerant start 20/0.8 mg q24h; titrate q48h; ↓ start dose in elderly, w/ hepatic/renal insuf; taper to D/C **W/P:** [C, ?/–] w/ EtOH, CNS depress, muscle relaxants, use w/in 14 days of D/C of MAOI **CI:** Resp depression, acute/severe asthma/hypercarbia, ileus, hypersens **Disp:** Caps ER (morphine mg/naltrexone mg) 20/0.8, 30/1.2, 50/2, 60/2.4, 80/3.2, 100/4 **SE:** N/V/D, constipation, somnolence, dizziness, HA, ↓ BP, pruritus, insomnia, anxiety, respiratory depression, seizures, MI, apnea, withdrawal with abrupt D/C, anaphylaxis, biliary spasm

Morphine (Avinza XR, Astramorph/PF, Duramorph, Infumorph, MS Contin, Kadian SR, Oramorph SR, Roxanol) [C-II] BOX: Do not crush/chew SR/CR forms; 100 and 200 mg SR formulation for opioid-tolerant pt only; controlled release; not to be crushed or chewed **Uses:** *Rx severe pain* AMI, acute pulmonary edema **Acts:** Narcotic analgesic; SR/CR forms for chronic use **Dose:** *Adults. Short-term use PO:* 5–30 mg q4h PRN; *IV/IM:* 2.5–15 mg q2–6h; *supp:* 10–30 mg q4h. SR formulations 15–60 mg q8–12h (do not chew/crush). *IT/epidural* (Duramorph, Infumorph, Astramorph/PF): Per protocol in Inf device. *ECC 2010.* STEMI: 2–4 mg IV (over 1–5 min), then give 2–8 mg IV q5–15min as needed. NSTEMI: 1–5 mg slow IV if Sxs unrelieved by nitrates or recur; use w/ caution; can be reversed with 0.4–2 mg IV naloxone. *Peds > 6 mo.* 0.1–0.2 mg/kg/dose IM/IV q2–4h PRN to 15 mg/dose max; 0.2–0.5 mg/kg PO q4–6h PRN; 0.3–0.6 mg/kg SR tabs PO q12h; 2–4 mg IV (over 1–5 min) q5–30 min *(ECC 2005)* **W/P:** [C, +/–] Severe resp depression possible; w/ head injury; chewing delayed release forms can cause severe rapid release of morphine **CI:** Severe asthma, resp depression, GI obst **Disp:** IR tabs 15, 30 mg; soln 10, 20, 100 mg/5 mL; supp 5, 10, 20, 30 mg; Inj 2, 4, 5, 8, 10, 15, 25, 50 mg/mL; *MS Contin CR* tabs 15, 30, 60, 100, 200 mg; *Oramorph SR* tabs 15, 30, 60, 100 mg; *Kadian SR caps* 10, 20, 30, 50, 60, 80, 100 mg; *Avinza XR* caps 30, 60, 90, 120 mg; *Duramorph/Astramorph PF:* Inj 0.5, 1 mg/mL; *Infumorph* 10, 25 mg/mL, **SE:** Narcotic SE (resp depression, sedation, constipation, N/V, pruritus, diaphoresis, urinary retention, biliary colic), granulomas w/ IT **Notes:** May require scheduled dosing to relieve severe chronic pain

Morphine Liposomal (DepoDur) **Uses:** *Long-lasting epidural analgesia* **Acts:** ER morphine analgesia **Dose:** 10–20 mg lumbar epidural Inj (C-section 10 mg after cord clamped) **W/P:** [C, +/–] Elderly, biliary Dz (sphincter of Oddi spasm) **CI:** Ileus, resp depression, asthma, obstructed airway, suspected/known head injury ↑ ICP, allergy to morphine **Disp:** Inj 10 mg/mL **SE:** Hypoxia, resp depression, ↓ BP, retention, N/V, constipation, flatulence, pruritus, pyrexia, anemia, HA, dizziness, tachycardia, insomnia, ileus **Notes:** Effect = 48 h; not for IT/IV/IM

Moxifloxacin (Avelox)   **BOX:** ↑ risk of tendon rupture and tendonitis; ↑ risk w/ age > 60, transplant pts; may ↑ sx of MG. **Uses:** *Acute sinusitis & bronchitis, skin/soft-tissue/intra-Abd Infxns, conjunctivitis, CAP* TB, anthrax, endocarditis **Acts:** 4th-gen quinolone; ↓ DNA gyrase. *Spectrum:* Excellent gram(+) except MRSA & *E. faecium;* good gram(−) except *P. aeruginosa, Stenotrophomonas maltophilia,* & *Acinetobacter* sp; good anaerobic **Dose:** 400 mg/d PO/IV daily; avoid cation products, antacids. tid **W/P:** [C, ?/−] Quinolone sensitivity; interactions w/ Mg^{2+}, Ca^{2+}, Al^{2+}, Fe^{2+} containing products, & class IA & III antiarrhythmic agents (Table 9, p 300) **CI:** Quinolone/component sensitivity **Disp:** Tabs 400 mg, ABC Pak 5 tabs, Inj **SE:** Dizziness, N, QT prolongation, Szs, photosens

Moxifloxacin, Ophthalmic (Moxeza, Vigamox)   **Uses:** *Bacterial conjunctivitis* **Acts:** See Moxifloxacin **Dose:** Instill into affected eye/s: Moxeza 1 gtt BID × 7 d; Vigamox 1 gtt tid × 7 d **W/P:** [C, ?/−] not well studied in Peds < 12 mo **CI:** Quinolone/component sensitivity **Disp:** ophthal sol 0.5% **SE:** ↓ Visual acuity, ocular pain, itching, tearing, conjunctivitis; prolonged use may result in fungal overgrowth; do not wear contacts w/ conjunctivitis

Multivitamins, Oral [OTC] (See Table 12, p 304)

Mupirocin (Bactroban, Bactroban Nasal)   **Uses:** *Impetigo (oint); skin lesion infect w/ S. aureus or S. pyogenes;* eradicate MRSA in nasal carriers* **Acts:** ↓ Bacterial protein synth **Dose:** *Topical:* Apply small amount 3×/d × 5–14 d. *Nasal:* Apply 1/2 single-use tube bid in nostrils × 5 d **W/P:** [B, ?] Do not use w/ other nasal products **Disp:** Oint 2%; cream 2%; nasal oint 2% 1-g single-use tubes **SE:** Local irritation, rash **Notes:** Pt to contact health care provider if no improvement in 3–5 d

Muromonab-CD3 (Orthoclone OKT3)   **BOX:** Can cause anaphylaxis; monitor fluid status; cytokine release synd **Uses:** *Acute rejection following organ transplantation* **Acts:** Murine Ab, blocks T-cell Fxn **Dose:** Per protocol *Adults.* 5 mg/d IV for 10–14 d. *Peds < 30 kg.* 2.5 mg/d. > *30 kg:* 5 mg/d IV for 10–14 d **W/P:** [C, ?/−] w/ Hx of Szs, PRG, uncontrolled HTN **CI:** Murine sensitivity, fluid overload **Disp:** Inj 5 mg/5 mL **SE:** Anaphylaxis, pulm edema, fever/chills w/ 1st dose (premedicate w/ steroid/APAP/antihistamine); cytokine release synd (↓ BP, fever, rigors) **Notes:** Monitor during Inf; use 0.22-micron filter

Mycophenolic Acid (Myfortic)   **BOX:** ↑ Risk of infxns, lymphoma, other CA's, progressive multifocal leukoencephalopathy (PML), risk of PRG loss and malformation, female of childbearing potential must use contraception **Uses:** *Prevent rejection after renal transplant* **Acts:** Cytostatic to lymphocytes **Dose:** *Adults.* 720 mg PO bid. *Peds. BSA 1.19–1.58 m^2:* 540 mg bid. *BSA > 1.8 m^2:* Adult dose; used w/ steroids & cyclosporine ↓ w/ renal Insuff/neutropenia; take on empty stomach **W/P:** [D, ?/−] **CI:** Component allergy **Disp:** Delayed release tabs 180, 360 mg **SE:** N/V/D, GI bleed, pain, fever, HA, Infxn, HTN, anemia, leukopenia, pure red cell aplasia, edema

Mycophenolate Mofetil (CellCept) **BOX:** ↑ Risk of infxns, lymphoma, other CAs, progressive multifocal leukoencephalopathy (PML); risk of PRG loss and malformation; female of childbearing potential must use contraception **Uses:** *Prevent organ rejection after transplant* **Acts:** Cytostatic to lymphocytes **Dose:** *Adults.* 1 g PO bid. *Peds. BSA 1.2–1.5 m^2:* 750 mg PO bid. *BSA > 1.5 m^2:* 1 g PO bid; may taper up to 600 mg/m² PO bid; used w/ steroids & cyclosporine; ↓ in renal Insuff or neutropenia. *IV:* Infuse over > 2 h. *PO:* Take on empty stomach, do not open caps **W/P:** [D, ?/–] **CI:** Component allergy; IV use in polysorbate 80 allergy **Disp:** Caps 250, 500 mg; susp 200 mg/mL, Inj 500 mg **SE:** N/V/D, pain, fever, HA, Infxn, HTN, anemia, leukopenia, edema

Nabilone (Cesamet) [C-II] **BOX:** Psychotomimetic Rxns, may persist for 72 h following D/C; caregivers should be present during initial use or dosage modification; pts should not operate heavy machinery; avoid alcohol, sedatives, hypnotics, other psychoactive substances **Uses:** *Refractory chemotherapy-induced emesis* **Acts:** Synthetic cannabinoid **Dose:** *Adults.* 1–2 mg PO bid 1–3 h before chemotherapy, 6 mg/d max; may continue for 48 h beyond final chemotherapy dose **W/P:** [C, ?/–] Elderly, HTN, heart failure, w/ psychological illness, substance abuse; high protein binding w/ 1st-pass metabolism may lead to drug interactions **Disp:** Caps 1 mg **SE:** Drowsiness, vertigo, xerostomia, euphoria, ataxia, HA, difficulty concentrating, tachycardia, ↓ BP **Notes:** May require initial dose evening before chemotherapy; Rx only quantity for single treatment cycle

Nabumetone (Relafen) **BOX:** May ↑ risk of CV events & GI bleeding, perforation; CI w/ post-op coronary artery bypass graft **Uses:** *OA and RA*, pain **Acts:** NSAID; ↓ prostaglandins **Dose:** 1000–2000 mg/d ÷ daily-bid w/ food **W/P:** [C, –] Severe hepatic Dz **CI:** w/ Peptic ulcer, NSAID sensitivity, after coronary artery bypass graft surgery **Disp:** Tabs 500, 750 mg **SE:** Dizziness, rash, GI upset, edema, peptic ulcer, ↑ BP

Nadolol (Corgard) **Uses:** *HTN & angina* migraine prophylaxis **Acts:** Competitively blocks β-adrenergic receptors ($β_1$, $β_2$) **Dose:** 40–80 mg/d; ↑ to 240 mg/d (angina) or 320 mg/d (HTN) at 3–7-d intervals; ↓ in renal Insuff & elderly **W/P:** [C (1st tri; D if 2nd or 3rd tri), +] **CI:** Uncompensated CHF, shock, heart block, asthma **Disp:** Tabs 20, 40, 80, 120, 160 mg **SE:** Nightmares, paresthesias, ↓ BP, ↓ HR, fatigue

Nafcillin (Nallpen, Unipen) **Uses:** *infxns d/t susceptible strains of Staphylococcus & Streptococcus* **Acts:** Bactericidal; β-lactamase-resistant PCN; ↓ cell wall synth **Spectrum:** Good gram(+) except MRSA & enterococcus; no gram(–), poor anaerobe **Dose:** *Adults.* 1–2 g IV q4–6h. *Peds.* 50–200 mg/kg/d ÷ q4–6h **W/P:** [B, ?] **CI:** PCN allergy **Disp:** Inj powder 1, 2 g **SE:** Interstitial nephritis, N/D, fever, rash, allergic Rxn **Notes:** No adjustment for renal Fxn

Naftifine (Naftin) **Uses:** *Tinea pedis, cruris, & corporis* **Acts:** Allylamine antifungal, ↓ cell membrane ergosterol synth **Dose:** Apply daily (cream) or bid (gel) **W/P:** [B, ?] **CI:** Component sensitivity **Disp:** 1% cream; gel **SE:** Local irritation

Nalbuphine (Nubain) Uses: *Mod–severe pain; pre-op & obstetric analgesia* Acts: Narcotic agonist–antagonist; ↓ ascending pain pathways Dose: *Adults. Pain:* 10 mg/70 kg IV/IM/SQ q3–6h; adjust PRN; 20 mg/dose or 160 mg/d max. *Anesthesia: Induction:* 0.3–3 mg/kg IV over 10–15 min; maint 0.25–0.5 mg/kg IV. *Peds.* 0.2 mg/kg IV or IM, 20 mg max; ↓ w/ renal/in hepatic impair W/P: [B, M] w/ Opiate use CI: Component sensitivity Disp: Inj 10, 20 mg/mL SE: CNS depression, drowsiness; caution, ↓ BP

Naloxone (Generic) Uses: *Opioid addiction (diagnosis) & OD* Acts: Competitive narcotic antagonist Dose: *Adults.* 0.4–2 mg IV, IM, or SQ q2–3 min; total dose 10 mg max. *Peds.* 0.01–0.1 mg/kg/dose IV, IM, or SQ; repeat IV q3min × 3 doses PRN; *ECC 2010. Total reversal of narcotic effects:* 0.1 mg/kg q2min PRN; max dose 2 mg; smaller doses (1–5 mcg/kg may be used); cont inf 2–160 mcg/kg/h W/P: [B, ?] May precipitate acute withdrawal in addicts Disp: Inj 0.4, 1 mg/mL SE: ↑ BP, tachycardia, irritability, GI upset, pulm edema Notes: If no response after 10 mg, suspect nonnarcotic cause

Naltrexone (Depade, ReVia, Vivitrol) BOX: Can cause hepatic injury, CI w/ active liver Dz Uses: *EtOH & narcotic addiction* Acts: Antagonizes opioid receptors Dose: *EtOH/narcotic addiction:* 50 mg/d PO; must be opioid-free for 7–10 d; *EtOH dependence:* 380 mg IM q4wk (*Vivitrol*) W/P: [C, M] Monitor for inj site reactions (*Vivitrol*) CI: Acute hep, liver failure, opioid use Disp: Tabs 50 mg; Inj 380 mg (*Vivitrol*) SE: Hepatotox; insomnia, GI upset, joint pain, HA, fatigue

Naphazoline (Albalon, Naphcon, Others), Naphazoline, & Pheniramine Acetate (Naphcon A, Visine A) Uses: *Relieve ocular redness & itching caused by allergy* Acts: Sympathomimetic (α-adrenergic vasoconstrictor) & antihistamine (pheniramine) Dose: 1–2 gtt up to qid, 3 d max W/P: [C, +] CI: NAG, in children, w/ contact lenses, component allergy SE: CV stimulation, dizziness, local irritation Disp: Ophthal 0.012, 0.025, 0.1%/15 mL; naphazoline & pheniramine 0.025%/0.3% soln

Naproxen and Esomeprazole (Vimovo) BOX: ↑ risk MI, stroke, PE; CI, CABG surgery pain; ↑ risk GI bleed, gastric ulcer, gastric/duodenal perforation Uses: *Pain and/or swelling, RA, OA, ankylosing spondylitis, ↓ risk NSAID assoc gastric ulcers* Acts: NSAID; ↓ prostaglandins & PPI, ↓ gastric acid Dose: 375/20 mg (naproxen/esomeprazole) to 500/20 mg PO bid W/P: [C 1st, 2nd trimester; D 3rd; –] CI: PRG 3rd trimester; asthma, urticaria from ASA or NSAID; mod–severe hepatic/renal Disp: Tabs (naproxen/esomeprazole) DR 375/20 mg; 500/20 mg SE: N/D, Abd pain, gastritis, ulcer, ↑ BP, CHF, edema, serious skin rash (eg, Stevens-Johnson, etc), ↓ renal fxn, papillary necrosis Notes: Risk of GI adverse events elderly; atrophic gastritis w/ long-term PPI use; possible ↑ risk of fractures w/ all PPI; may ↑ Li levels; may cause MTX toxicity; may ↑ INR on warfarin; may ↓ effect BP meds; may ↓ absorption drugs requiring acid environment

Naproxen (Aleve [OTC], Naprosyn, Anaprox) BOX: May ↑ risk of CV events & GI bleeding Uses: *Arthritis & pain* Acts: NSAID; ↓ prostaglandins Dose: *Adults & Peds > 12 y.* 200–500 mg bid-tid to 1500 mg/d max. > *2 y: JRA* 5 mg/kg/dose bid; ↓ in hepatic impair W/P: [C, (D 3rd tri), –] CI: NSAID or ASA triad sensitivity, peptic ulcer, post coronary artery bypass graft pain, 3rd tri PRG Disp: *Tabs:* 220, 250, 375, 500 mg; *DR:* 375 mg, 500 mg; *CR:* 375 mg, 550 mg; susp 125 mL/5 mL SE: Dizziness, pruritus, GI upset, peptic ulcer, edema Note: Take w/ food to ↓ GI upset

Naratriptan (Amerge) Uses: *Acute migraine* Acts: Serotonin 5-HT$_1$ receptor agonist Dose: 1–2.5 mg PO once; repeat PRN in 4 h; 5 mg/24 h max; ↓ in mild renal/hepatic Insuff, take w/ fluids W/P: [C, M] CI: Severe renal/hepatic impair, avoid w/ angina, ischemic heart Dz, uncontrolled HTN, cerebrovascular synds, & ergot use Disp: Tabs 1, 2.5 mg SE: Dizziness, sedation, GI upset, paresthesias, ECG changes, coronary vasospasm, arrhythmias

Natalizumab (Tysabri) BOX: PML reported Uses: *Relapsing MS to delay disability and ↓ recurrences, Crohn Dz* Acts: Integrin receptor antagonist Dose: *Adults.* 300 mg IV q4wk; 2nd-line Tx only CI: PML; immune compromise or w/ immunosuppressant W/P: [C, ?/–] Baseline MRI to rule out PML Disp: Vial 300 mg SE: Infxn, immunosuppression; Inf Rxn precluding subsequent use; HA, fatigue, arthralgia Notes: Give slowly to ↓ Rxns; limited distribution (TOUCH Prescribing program); D/C immediately w/ signs of PML (weakness, paralysis, vision loss, impaired speech, cognitive ↓); evaluate at 3 and 6 mo, then q6mo thereafter

Nateglinide (Starlix) Uses: *Type 2 DM* Acts: ↑ Pancreatic insulin release Dose: 120 mg PO tid 1–30 min ac; ↓ to 60 mg tid if near target HbA$_{1c}$ W/P: [C, –] w/ CYP2C9 metabolized drug (Table 10, p 301) CI: DKA, type 1 DM Disp: Tabs 60, 120 mg SE: Hypoglycemia, URI; salicylates, nonselective β-blockers may enhance hypoglycemia

Nebivolol (Bystolic) Uses: *HTN* Acts: β$_1$-Selective blocker Dose: *Adults.* 5 mg PO daily, ↑ q2wk to 40 mg/d max, ↓ w/ CrCl < 30 mL/min W/P: [D, +/–] w/ Bronchospastic Dz, DM, heart failure, pheochromocytoma, w/ CYP2D6 inhib CI: ↓ HR, cardiogenic shock, decompensated CHF, severe hepatic impair Disp: tabs 5, 10 mg SE: HA, fatigue, dizziness

Nefazodone BOX: Fatal hep & liver failure possible, D/C if LFTs > 3× ULN, do not retreat; closely monitor for worsening depression or suicidality, particularly in ped pts Uses: *Depression* Acts: ↓ Neuronal uptake of serotonin & norepinephrine Dose: Initial 100 mg PO bid; usual 300–600 mg/d in 2 ÷ doses W/P: [C, M] CI: w/ MAOIs, pimozide, carbamazepine, alprazolam; active liver Dz Disp: Tabs 50, 100, 150, 200, 250 mg SE: Postural ↓ BP & allergic Rxns; HA, drowsiness, xerostomia, constipation, GI upset, liver failure Notes: Monitor LFTs, HR, BP

Nelarabine (Arranon) BOX: Fatal neurotox possible Uses: *T-cell ALL or T-cell lymphoblastic lymphoma unresponsive > 2 other regimens* Acts: Nucleoside (deoxyguanosine) analog **Dose:** *Adults.* 1500 mg/m^2 IV over 2 h days 1, 3, 5 of 21-d cycle. *Peds.* 650 mg/m^2 IV over 1 h days 1–5 of 21-d cycle **W/P:** [D, ?/–] **Disp:** Vial 250 mg **SE:** Neuropathy, ataxia, Szs, coma, hematologic tox, GI upset, HA, blurred vision **Notes:** Prehydration, urinary alkalinization, allopurinol before dose; monitor CBC

Nelfinavir (Viracept) **Uses:** *HIV Infxn, other agents* **Acts:** Protease inhib causes immature, noninfectious virion production **Dose:** *Adults.* 750 mg PO tid or 1250 mg PO bid. *Peds.* 25–35 mg/kg PO tid or 45–55 mg/kg bid; take w/ food **W/P:** [B, –] Many drug interactions; do not use w/salmeterol, colchicine (w/renal/ hepatic failure); adjust dose w/ bosentan, tadalafil for PAH **CI:** Phenylketonuria, w/ triazolam/midazolam use or drug dependent on CYP3A4 (Table 10, p 301); w/ alpha 1-adrenoreceptor antagonist (alfuzosin), PDE5 inhibitor sildenafil **Disp:** Tabs 250, 625 mg; powder 50 mg/g; **SE:** Food ↑ absorption; interacts w/ St. John's wort; dyslipidemia, lipodystrophy, D, rash **Notes:** PRG registry; tabs can be dissolved in water

Neomycin, Bacitracin, & Polymyxin B (Neosporin Ointment) (See Bacitracin, Neomycin, & Polymyxin B Topical, p 57)

Neomycin, Colistin, & Hydrocortisone (Cortisporin-TC Otic Drops); Neomycin, Colistin, Hydrocortisone, & Thonzonium (Cortisporin-TC Otic Susp) **Uses:** *Otitis externa*, infxns of mastoid/fenestration cavities **Acts:** Antibiotic w/ anti-inflammatory **Dose:** *Adults.* 5 gtt in ear(s) tid-qid. *Peds.* 3–4 gtt in ear(s) tid-qid **CI:** component allergy; HSV, vaccinia, varicella **W/P:** [B, ?] **Disp:** Otic gtt & susp **SE:** Local irritation, rash **Notes:** Shake well, limit use to 10 d to minimize hearing loss

Neomycin & Dexamethasone (AK-Neo-Dex Ophthalmic, Neo-Decadron Ophthalmic) **Uses:** *Steroid-responsive inflammatory conditions of the cornea, conjunctiva, lid, & anterior segment* **Acts:** Antibiotic w/ anti-inflammatory corticosteroid **Dose:** 1–2 gtt in eye(s) q3–4h or thin coat tid-qid until response, then ↓ to daily **W/P:** [C, ?] **Disp:** Cream: neomycin 0.5%/dexamethasone 0.1%; oint: neomycin 0.35%/dexamethasone 0.05%; soln: neomycin 0.35%/dexamethasone 0.1% **SE:** Local irritation **Notes:** Use under ophthalmologist's supervision

Neomycin & Polymyxin B (Neosporin Cream) [OTC] **Uses:** *Infxn in minor cuts, scrapes, & burns* **Acts:** Bactericidal **Dose:** Apply bid-qid **W/P:** [C, ?] **CI:** Component allergy **Disp:** Cream: neomycin 3.5 mg/polymyxin B 10,000 units/g **SE:** Local irritation **Notes:** Different from *Neosporin oint*

Neomycin, Polymyxin B, & Dexamethasone (Maxitrol) **Uses:** *Steroid-responsive ocular conditions w/ bacterial Infxn* **Acts:** Antibiotic w/ anti-inflammatory corticosteroid **Dose:** 1–2 gtt in eye(s) q3–4h; apply oint in eye(s) tid-qid **CI:** Component allergy; viral, fungal, TB eye Dz **W/P:** [C, ?] **Disp:** Oint: neomycin sulfate 3.5 mg/polymyxin B sulfate 10,000 units/dexamethasone 0.1%/g; susp: identical/5 mL **SE:** Local irritation **Notes:** Use under supervision of ophthalmologist

Neomycin-Polymyxin Bladder Irrigant [Neosporin GU Irrigant]
Uses: *Cont irrigant prevent bacteriuria & gram(−) bacteremia associated w/ indwelling catheter* Acts: Bactericidal; not for *Serratia* sp or streptococci Dose: 1 mL irrigant in 1 L of 0.9% NaCl; cont bladder irrigation w/ 1 L of soln/24 h 10 d max W/P: [D] CI: Component allergy Disp: Soln neomycin sulfate 40 mg & polymyxin B 200,000 units/mL; amp 1, 20 mL SE: Rash, neomycin ototox or nephrotox (rare) Notes: Potential for bacterial/fungal super-Infxn; not for Inj; use only 3-way catheter for irrigation

Neomycin, Polymyxin, & Hydrocortisone Ophthalmic (Generic)
Uses: *Ocular bacterial Infxns* Acts: Antibiotic w/ anti-inflammatory Dose: Apply a thin layer to the eye(s) or 1 gtt daily-qid W/P: [C, ?] Disp: Ophthal soln; ophthal oint SE: Local irritation

Neomycin, Polymyxin, & Hydrocortisone Otic (Cortisporin Otic Solution, Generic Susp) Uses: *Otitis externa and infected mastoidectomy and fenestration cavities* Acts: Antibiotic & anti-inflammatory Dose: *Adults*. 3–4 gtt in the ear(s) tid-qid *Peds > 2 y.* 3 gtt in the ear(s) tid-qid CI: Viral Infxn, hypersens to components W/P: [C, ?] Disp: Otic susp (generic); otic soln (Cortisporin) SE: Local irritation

Neomycin, Polymyxin B, & Prednisolone (Poly-Pred Ophthalmic)
Uses: *Steroid-responsive ocular conditions w/ bacterial Infxn* Acts: Antibiotic & anti-inflammatory Dose: 1–2 gtt in eye(s) tid-qid; apply oint in eye(s) tid-qid W/P: [C, ?] Disp: Susp neomycin/polymyxin B/prednisolone 0.5%/mL SE: Irritation Notes: Use under supervision of ophthalmologist

Neomycin Sulfate (Neo-Fradin, Generic) BOX: Systemic absorption of oral route may cause neuro-/oto-/nephrotox; resp paralysis possible w/ any route of administration Uses: *Hepatic coma, bowel prep* Acts: Aminoglycoside, poorly absorbed PO; ↓ GI bacterial flora Dose: *Adults.* 3–12 g/24 h PO in 3–4 ÷ doses. *Peds.* 50–100 mg/kg/24 h PO in 3–4 ÷ doses W/P: [C, ?/−] Renal failure, neuromuscular disorders, hearing impair CI: Intestinal obst Disp: Tabs 500 mg; PO soln 125 mg/5 mL SE: Hearing loss w/ long-term use; rash, N/V Notes: Do not use parenterally (↑ tox); part of the Condon bowel prep; also topical form

Nepafenac (Nevanac) Uses: *Inflammation postcataract surgery* Acts: NSAID Dose: 1 gtt in eye(s) tid 1 d before, and continue 14 d after surgery CI: NSAID/ASA sensitivity W/P: [C, ?/−] May ↑ bleeding time, delay healing, causes keratitis Disp: Susp 3 mL SE: Capsular opacity, visual changes, foreign-body sensation, ↑ IOP Notes: Prolonged use ↑ risk of corneal damage; shake well before use; separate from other drops by > 5 min

Nesiritide (Natrecor) Uses: *Acutely decompensated CHF* Acts: Human B-type natriuretic peptide Dose: 2 mcg/kg IV bolus, then 0.01 mcg/kg/min IV W/P: [C, ?/−] When vasodilators are not appropriate CI: SBP < 90 mm Hg, cardiogenic shock Disp: Vials 1.5 mg SE: ↓ BP, HA, GI upset, arrhythmias, ↑ Cr Notes: Requires cont BP monitoring; some studies indicate ↑ in mortality

Nevirapine (Viramune) BOX: Reports of fatal hepatotox even w/ short-term use; severe life-threatening skin Rxns (SJS, toxic epidermal necrolysis, & allergic Rxns); monitor closely during 1st 18 wk of Rx **Uses:** *HIV Infxn* **Acts:** Nonnucleoside RT inhib **Dose:** *Adults.* Initial 200 mg/d PO × 14 d, then 200 mg bid. *Peds* > 15 days: 150 mg/m² PO daily ×14 d, then 150 mg/m² PO bid (w/o regard to food) **W/P:** [B, –] OCP **Disp:** Tabs 200 mg; tabs ER 400 mg; susp 50 mg/5 mL **SE:** Life-threatening rash; HA, fever, D, neutropenia, rash **Notes:** HIV resistance when used as monotherapy; use in combo w/ at least 2 additional antiretroviral agents. Restart once daily dosing ×14 d if stopped > 7 d. Not recommended if CD4 > 250 mcL in women or > 400 mcL in men unless benefit > risk of hepatotox

Niacin (Nicotinic Acid) (Niaspan, Slo-Niacin, Niacor, Nicolar) [Some OTC Forms] Uses: *Sig hyperlipidemia/hypercholesteremia, nutritional supl* **Acts:** Vit B₃; ↓ lipolysis; ↓ esterification of triglycerides; ↑ lipoprotein lipase **Dose:** *Hypercholesterolemia:* Start 500 mg PO qhs, ↑ 500 mg q4wk, maint 1–2 g/d; 2 g/d max; qhs w/ low fat snack; do not crush/chew; niacin supl 1 ER tab PO q day or 100 mg PO q day; *Pellagra:* Up to 500 mg/d **W/P:** [C, +] **CI:** Liver Dz, peptic ulcer, arterial hemorrhage **Disp:** ER tabs *(Niaspan)* 500, 750, 1000 mg & *(Slo-Niacin)* 250, 500, 750 mg; tab 500 mg (Niacor); many OTC: tab 50, 100, 250, 500 mg, ER caps 125, 250, 400 mg, ER tab 250, 500 mg, elixir 50 mg/5 mL **SE:** Upper body/facial flushing & warmth; hepatox; GI upset, flatulence, exacerbate peptic ulcer, HA, paresthesias, liver damage, gout, altered glucose control in DM **Notes:** ASA/NSAID 30–60 min prior to ↓ flushing; ✓ cholesterol, LFTs, if on statins (e.g., Lipitor, etc) also ✓ CPK and K⁺; *RDA adults:* male 16 mg/d, female 14 mg/d

Niacin & Lovastatin (Advicor) Uses: *Hypercholesterolemia* **Acts:** Combo antilipemic agent, w/ HMG-CoA reductase inhib **Dose:** *Adults.* Niacin 500 mg/ lovastatin 20 mg, titrate q4wk, max niacin 2000 mg/lovastatin 40 mg **W/P:** [X, –] See individual agents, D/C w/ LFTs > 3× ULN **CI:** PRG **Disp:** Niacin mg/lovastatin mg: 500/20, 750/20, 1000/20, 1000/40 tabs **SE:** Flushing, myopathy/rhabdomyolysis, N, Abd pain, ↑ LFTs **Notes:** ↓ Flushing by taking ASA or NSAID 30 min before

Niacin & Simvastatin (Simcor) Uses: *Hypercholesterolemia* **Acts:** Combo antilipemic agent w/ HMG-CoA reductase inhib **Dose:** *Adults* Niacin 500 mg/simvastatin 20 mg, titrate q4wk not to exceed niacin 2000 mg/simvastatin 40 mg; max 1000 mg/20 mg/d w/ amlodipine and ranolazine **W/P:** [X, –] See individual agents, discontinue Rx if LFTs > 3× ULN **CI:** PRG **Disp:** Niacin mg/simvastatin mg: 500/20, 500/40, 750/20, 1000/20, 1000/40 tabs **SE:** Flushing, myopathy/rhabdomyolysis, N, Abd pain, ↑ LFTs **Notes:** ↓ Flushing by taking ASA or NSAID 30 min before

Nicardipine (Cardene) Uses: *Chronic stable angina & HTN*; prophylaxis of migraine **Acts:** CCB **Dose:** *Adults.* *PO:* 20–40 mg PO tid. *SR:* 30–60 mg PO bid. *IV:* 5 mg/h IV cont Inf; ↑ by 2.5 mg/h q15min to max 15 mg/h. **Peds.** (Not established) *PO:* 20–30 mg PO q8h. *IV:* 0.5–5 mcg/kg/min; ↓ in renal/hepatic impair **W/P:** [C, ?/–] Heart block, CAD **CI:** Cardiogenic shock, aortic stenosis **Disp:** Caps 20, 30 mg; SR caps 30, 45, 60 mg; Inj 2.5 mg/mL **SE:** Flushing, tachycardia, ↓ BP, edema, HA **Notes:** *PO-to-IV conversion:* 20 mg tid = 0.5 mg/h, 30 mg tid = 1.2 mg/h, 40 mg tid = 2.2 mg/h; take w/ food (not high fat)

Nicotine Gum (Nicorette, Others) [OTC]
Uses: *Aid to smoking cessation, relieve nicotine withdrawal* **Acts:** Systemic delivery of nicotine **Dose:** Wk 1–6 one piece q1–2h PRN; wk 7–9 one piece q2–4h PRN; wk 10–12 one piece q4–8h PRN; max 24 pieces/d **W/P:** [C, ?] **CI:** Life-threatening arrhythmias, unstable angina **Disp:** 2 mg, 4 mg/piece; mint, orange, original flavors **SE:** Tachycardia, HA, GI upset, hiccups **Notes:** Must stop smoking & perform behavior modification for max effect; use at least 9 pieces 1st 6 wk; > 25 cigarettes/d use 4 mg; < 25 cigarettes/d use 2 mg

Nicotine Nasal Spray (Nicotrol NS)
Uses: *Aid to smoking cessation, relieve nicotine withdrawal* **Acts:** Systemic delivery of nicotine **Dose:** 0.5 mg/actuation; 1–2 doses/h, 5 doses/h max; 40 doses/d max **W/P:** [D, M] **CI:** Life-threatening arrhythmias, unstable angina **Disp:** Nasal inhaler 10 mg/mL **SE:** Local irritation, tachycardia, HA, taste perversion **Notes:** Must stop smoking & perform behavior modification for max effect; 1 dose = 1 spray each nostril = 1 mg

Nicotine Transdermal (Habitrol, NicoDerm CQ [OTC], Others)
Uses: *Aid to smoking cessation; relief of nicotine withdrawal* **Acts:** Systemic delivery of nicotine **Dose:** Individualized; 1 patch (14–21 mg/d) & taper over 6 wk **W/P:** [D, M] **CI:** Life-threatening arrhythmias, unstable angina **Disp:** *Habitrol* & *NicoDerm CQ:* 7, 14, 21 mg of nicotine/24 h **SE:** Insomnia, pruritus, erythema, local site Rxn, tachycardia, vivid dreams **Notes:** Wear patch 16–24 h; must stop smoking & perform behavior modification for max effect; > 10 cigarettes/d start w/ 21-mg patch; < 10 cigarettes/d 14-mg patch

Nifedipine (Procardia, Procardia XL, Adalat CC)
Uses: *Vasospastic or chronic stable angina & HTN*; tocolytic **Acts:** CCB **Dose:** *Adults.* SR tabs 30–90 mg/d. *Tocolysis:* per local protocol. *Peds.* 0.25–0.9 mg/kg/24 h ÷ tid-qid **W/P:** [C, +] Heart block, aortic stenosis **CI:** IR preparation for urgent or emergent HTN; acute MI **Disp:** Caps 10, 20 mg; SR tabs 30, 60, 90 mg **SE:** HA common on initial Rx; reflex tachycardia may occur w/ regular-release dosage forms; peripheral edema, ↓ BP, flushing, dizziness **Notes:** Adalat CC & Procardia XL not interchangeable; SL administration not OK

Nilotinib (Tasigna)
BOX: May ↑ QT interval; sudden deaths reported, use w/ caution in hepatic failure; administer on empty stomach **Uses:** *Ph(+) CML, refractory or at first diagnosis* **Acts:** TKI **Dose:** *Adults.* 400 mg bid, on empty stomach 1 h prior or 2 h post meal. **W/P:** [D, ?/–] Avoid w/ CYP3A4 inhib/inducers (Table 10, p 301), adjust w/ hepatic impair, heme tox, QT ↑, avoid QT-prolonging agents, w/ Hx pancreatitis, ↓ absorption w/gastrectomy **CI:** Bilirubin > 3× ULN, AST/ALT > 5× ULN, resume at 400 mg/d once levels return to normal **Disp:** 200 mg

caps **SE:** ↓ WBC, ↓ plt, anemia, N/V/D, rash, edema, ↑ lipase **Notes:** Use chemotherapy precautions when handling

Nilutamide (Nilandron) **BOX:** Interstitial pneumonitis possible; most cases in 1st 3 mo; check CXR before and during Rx **Uses:** *Combo w/ surgical castration for metastatic PCa* **Acts:** Nonsteroidal antiandrogen **Dose:** 300 mg/d PO in ÷ doses × 30 d, then 150 mg/d **W/P:** [Not used in females] **CI:** Severe hepatic impair, resp Insuff **Disp:** Tabs 150 mg **SE:** Interstitial pneumonitis, hot flashes, ↓ libido, impotence, N/V/D, gynecomastia, hepatic dysfunction **Notes:** May cause Rxn when taken w/ EtOH, follow LFTs

Nimodipine (Nimotop) **BOX:** Do not give IV or by other parenteral routes; can cause death **Uses:** *Prevent vasospasm following subarachnoid hemorrhage* **Acts:** CCB **Dose:** 60 mg PO q4h for 21 d; ↓ in hepatic failure **W/P:** [C, ?] **CI:** Component allergy **Disp:** Caps 30 mg **SE:** ↓ BP, HA, constipation **Notes:** Give via NG tube if caps cannot be swallowed whole

Nisoldipine (Sular) **Uses:** *HTN* **Acts:** CCB **Dose:** 8.5–34 mg/d PO; take on empty stomach; ↓ start doses w/ elderly or hepatic impair **W/P:** [C, –] **Disp:** ER tabs 8.5, 17, 25.5, 34 mg **SE:** Edema, HA, flushing, ↓ BP

Nitazoxanide (Alinia) **Uses:** *Cryptosporidium* or *Giardia lamblia*-induced D* **Acts:** Antiprotozoal interferes w/ pyruvate ferredoxin oxidoreductase. *Spectrum: Cryptosporidium, Giardia* **Dose:** *Adults.* 500 mg PO q12h × 3 d. *Peds 1–3 y.* 100 mg PO q12h × 3 d. *4–11 y:* 200 mg PO q12h × 3 d. *> 12 y:* 500 mg q12h × 3 d; take w/ food **W/P:** [B, ?] Not effective in HIV or immunocompromised **Disp:** 100 mg/5 mL PO susp, 500 tab **SE:** Abd pain **Notes:** Susp contains sucrose, interacts w/ highly protein-bound drugs

Nitrofurantoin (Furadantin, Macrodantin, Macrobid) **BOX:** Pulm fibrosis possible **Uses:** *Prophylaxis & Rx UTI* **Acts:** Bacteriocidal; interferes w/ carbohydrate metabolism. *Spectrum:* Some gram(+) & (−) bacteria; *Pseudomonas, Serratia,* & most *Proteus* resistant **Dose:** *Adults. Prophylaxis:* 50–100 mg/d PO. *Rx:* 50–100 mg PO qid × 7 d; *Macrobid* 100 mg PO bid × 7 d. *Peds. Prophylaxis:* 1–2 mg/ kg/d ÷ 1–2 doses, max 100 mg/d. *Rx:* 5–7 mg/kg/24 h in 4 ÷ doses (w/ food/milk/antacid) **W/P:** [B, +/not OK if child < 1 mo] Avoid w/ CrCl < 60 mL/min **CI:** Renal failure, infants < 1 mo, PRG at term **Disp:** Caps 25, 50, 100 mg; susp 25 mg/5 mL **SE:** GI effects, dyspnea, various acute/chronic pulm Rxns, peripheral neuropathy, hemolytic anemia w/ G6PD deficiency, rare aplastic anemia **Notes:** Macrocrystals (Macrodantin) < N than other forms; not for comp UTI; may turn urine brown

Nitroglycerin (Nitrostat, Nitrolingual, Nitro-Bid Ointment, Nitro-Bid IV, Nitrodisc, Transderm-Nitro, NitroMist, Others) **Uses:** *Angina pectoris, acute & prophylactic Rx, CHF, BP control* **Acts:** Relaxes vascular smooth muscle, dilates coronary arteries **Dose:** *Adults. SL:* 1 tab q5min SL PRN for 3 doses. *Translingual:* 1–2 metered-doses sprayed onto PO mucosa q3–5min, max 3 doses. *PO:* 2.5–9 mg tid. *IV:* 5–20 mcg/min, titrated to effect. *Topical:* Apply 1/2 inch of oint to chest wall tid, wipe off at night. *Transdermal:* 0.2–0.4 mg/h/patch daily; *Aerosol:* 1 spray at 5-min intervals, max 3 doses *ECC 2010.* IV bolus: 12.5–25 mcg (if no spray or SL dose given); inf: Start 10 mcg/min, ↑ by 10 mcg/min q3–5min until desired effect; ceiling dose typically 200 mcg/min. SL: 0.3–0.4 mg, repeat q5min. *Aerosol spray:* Spray 0.5–1 s at 5-min intervals. *Peds.* 0.25–0.5 mcg/kg/min IV, titrate; *ECC 2010. Heart failure, HTN emergency, pulm HTN:* Cont inf 0.25–0.5 mcg/kg/min initial, titrate 1 mcg/kg/min q15–20min (typical dose 1–5 mcg/kg/min) **W/P:** [B, ?] Restrictive cardiomyopathy **CI:** w/ Sildenafil, tadalafil, vardenafil, head trauma, NAG, pericardial tamponade, constrictive pericarditis. **Disp:** SL tabs 0.3, 0.4, 0.6 mg; translingual spray 0.4 mg/dose; SR caps 2.5, 6.5, 9 mg; Inj 0.1, 0.2, 0.4 mg/mL (premixed); 5 mg/mL Inj soln; oint 2%; transdermal patches 0.1, 0.2, 0.4, 0.6 mg/h; aerosol (*NitroMist*) 0.4 mg/spray **SE:** HA, ↓ BP, light-headedness, GI upset **Notes:** Nitrate tolerance w/ chronic use after 1–2 wk; minimize by providing 10–12 h nitrate-free period daily, using shorter-acting nitrates tid, & removing LA patches & oint before sleep to ↓ tolerance

Nitroprusside (Nipride, Nitropress) Uses: *Hypertensive crisis, CHF, controlled ↓ BP periop (↓ bleeding)*, aortic dissection, pulm edema **Acts:** ↓ Systemic vascular resistance **Dose:** *Adults & Peds.* 0.5–10 mcg/kg/min IV Inf, titrate; usual dose 3 mcg/kg/min. *ECC 2010.* 0.1 mcg/kg/min start, titrate (max dose 5–10 mcg/kg/min). *Peds. ECC 2010. Cardiogenic shock, severe HTN:* 0.3–1 mcg/kg/min, then titrate to 8 mcg/kg/min PRN **W/P:** [C, ?] ↓ cerebral perfusion **CI:** High output failure, compensatory HTN **Disp:** Inj 50 mg/mL **SE:** Excessive hypotensive effects, palpitations, HA **Notes:** Thiocyanate (metabolite w/ renal excretion) w/ tox at 5–10 mg/dL, more likely if used for > 2–3 d; w/ aortic dissection use w/ β-blocker

Nizatidine (Axid, Axid AR [OTC]) Uses: *Duodenal ulcers, GERD, heartburn*** Acts:** H_2-receptor antagonist **Dose:** *Adults. Active ulcer:* 150 mg PO bid or 300 mg PO hs; maint 150 mg PO hs. *GERD:* 150 mg PO bid. *Heartburn:* 75 mg PO bid. *Peds. GERD:* 10 mg/kg PO bid in ÷ doses, 150 mg bid max; ↓ in renal impair **W/P:** [B, ?] **CI:** H_2-receptor antagonist sensitivity **Disp:** Tab 75 mg [OTC]; caps 150, 300 mg; soln 15 mg/mL **SE:** Dizziness, HA, constipation, D

Norepinephrine (Levophed) Uses: *Acute ↓ BP, cardiac arrest (adjunct)* **Acts:** Peripheral vasoconstrictor of arterial/venous beds **Dose:** *Adults.* 8–30 mcg/min IV, titrate. *Peds.* 0.05–0.1 mcg/kg/min IV, titrate **W/P:** [C, ?] **CI:** ↓ BP d/t hypovolemia, vascular thrombosis, do not use w/ cyclopropane/halothane anesthetics **Disp:** Inj 1 mg/mL **SE:** ↓ HR, arrhythmia **Notes:** Correct vol depletion as much as possible before vasopressors; interaction w/ TCAs leads to severe HTN; use large vein to avoid extrav; phentolamine 5–10 mg/10 mL NS injected locally for extrav

Norethindrone Acetate/Ethinyl Estradiol Tablets (FemHRT) (See Estradiol/ Norethindrone Acetate)

Norfloxacin (Noroxin, Chibroxin, Ophthalmic) **BOX:** Use associated w/ tendon rupture and tendonitis (pending) Uses: *Comp & uncomp UTI d/t gram(−)

bacteria, prostatitis, gonorrhea*, infectious D, conjunctivitis **Acts:** Quinolone, ↓ DNA gyrase, bactericidal *Spectrum:* Broad gram(+) and (−) *E. faecalis, E. coli, K. pneumoniae, P. mirabilis, P. aeruginosa, S. epidermidis, S. saprophyticus* **Dose:** *Uncomp UTI (E. coli, K. pneumoniae, P. mirabilis):* 400 mg PO bid × 3 d; other uncomp UTI Rx × 7–10 d. *Comp UTI:* 400 mg PO q12h for 10–21 d. *Gonorrhea:* 800 mg × 1 dose. *Prostatitis:* 400 mg PO bid × 28 d. *Gastroenteritis, traveler's D:* 400 mg PO bid × 1–3 d; take 1 h ac or 2 h pc. *Adults & Peds > 1 y.* Ophthal: 1 gtt each eye qid for 7 d; CrCl < 30 mL/min use 400 mg q day **W/P:** [C, −] Quinolone sensitivity, w/ some antiarrhythmics **CI:** Hx allergy or tendon problems **Disp:** Tabs 400 mg; ophthal 3 mg/mL **SE:** Photosens, HA, dizziness, asthenia, GI upset, pseudomembranous colitis; ocular burning w/ ophthal **Notes:** Interactions w/ antacids, theophylline, caffeine; good conc in the kidney & urine, poor blood levels; not for urosepsis; CDC suggests do not use for GC

Nortriptyline (Pamelor) **BOX:** ↑ Suicide risk in pts < 24 y w/ major depressive/other psychological disorders especially during 1st month of Tx; risk ↓ pts > 65 y; observe all pts for clinical Sxs; not for ped use **Uses:** *Endogenous depression* **Acts:** TCA; ↑ synaptic CNS levels of serotonin &/or norepinephrine **Dose:** *Adults.* 25 mg PO tid-qid; > 150 mg/d not OK. *Elderly:* 10–25 mg hs. *Peds 6–7 y.* 10 mg/d. *8–11 y:* 10–20 mg/d. *> 11 y:* 25–35 mg/d, ↓ w/ hepatic Insuff **W/P:** [D, −] NAG, CV Dz **CI:** TCA allergy, use w/ MAOI **Disp:** Caps 10, 25, 50, 75 mg; soln 10 mg/5 mL **SE:** Anticholinergic (blurred vision, retention, xerostomia, sedation) **Notes:** Max effect may take > 2–3 wk

Nystatin (Mycostatin) **Uses:** *Mucocutaneous *Candida* Infxns (oral, skin, vag)* **Acts:** Alters membrane permeability. *Spectrum:* Susceptible *Candida* sp **Dose:** *Adults & Peds.* **PO:** 400,000–600,000 units PO "swish & swallow" qid. *Vaginal:* 1 tab vaginally hs × 2 wk. *Topical:* Apply bid-tid to area. *Peds Infants.* 200,000 units PO q6h. **W/P:** [B (C PO), +] **Disp:** PO susp 100,000 units/mL; PO tabs 500,000 units; troches 200,000 units; vag tabs 100,000 units; topical cream/oint 100,000 units/g, powder 100,000 units/g **SE:** GI upset, SJS **Notes:** Not absorbed PO; not for systemic Infxns

Octreotide (Sandostatin, Sandostatin LAR) **Uses:** *↓ Severe D associated w/ carcinoid & neuroendocrine GI tumors (e.g., vasoactive intestinal peptide-secreting tumor [VIPoma], ZE synd), acromegaly*; bleeding esophageal varices **Acts:** LA peptide; mimics natural somatostatin **Dose:** *Adults.* 100–600 mcg/d SQ/IV in 2–4 ÷ doses; start 50 mcg daily-bid. *Sandostatin LAR (depot):* 10–30 mg IM q4wk. *Peds.* 1–10 mcg/kg/24 h SQ in 2–4 ÷ doses **W/P:** [B, +] Hepatic/renal impair **Disp:** Inj 0.05, 0.1, 0.2, 0.5, 1 mg/mL; 10, 20, 30 mg/5 mL LAR depot **SE:** N/V, Abd discomfort, flushing, edema, fatigue, cholelithiasis, hyper-/hypoglycemia, hep, hypothyroidism **Notes:** Stabilize for at least 2 wk before changing to LAR form

Ofatumumab (Arzerra) **BOX:** Administer only by physician experienced in chemotherapy. Do not give IV push d/t severe Inf Rxn **Uses:** *Rx refractory CLL* **Action:** MoAb, binds CD20 molecule on B-lymphocytes w/ cell lysis **Dose:**

Adults. 300 mg (0.3 mg/mL) IV week one, then 2000 mg (2 mg/mL) weekly × 7 doses, then 2000 mg q4wks × 4 doses. Titrate Inf; start 12 mL/h × 30 min, ↑ 25 mL/h for 30 min, ↑ to 50 mL/h × 30 min, ↑ to 100 mL/h × 30 min, then 200 mL/h for duration. **W/P:** [C, ?] **Disp:** Inj 20 mg/mL (5 mL) **SE:** Infusion Rxns (bronchospasm, pulmonary edema, ↑/↓ BP, syncope, cardiac ischemia, angioedema), ↑ WBC, anemia, fever, fatigue, rash, N/D, pneumonia, Infxns **Notes:** Premed w/ acetaminophen, antihistamine, and IV steroid

Ofloxacin (Floxin) **BOX:** Use associated w/ tendon rupture and tendonitis **Uses:** *Lower resp tract, skin, & skin structure, & UTI, prostatitis, uncomp gonorrhea, & Chlamydia Infxns* **Acts:** Bactericidal; ↓ DNA gyrase. *Broad spectrum gram(+) & (−): S. pneumoniae, S. aureus, S. pyogenes, H. influenzae, P. mirabilis, N. gonorrhoeae, C. trachomatis, E. coli* **Dose:** *Adults.* 200–400 mg PO bid or IV q12h. ↓ in renal impair, take on empty stomach **W/P:** [C, −] ↓ Absorption w/ antacids, sucralfate, Al^{2+}, Ca^{2+}, Mg^{2+}, Fe^{2+}, Zn^+-containing drugs, Hx Szs **CI:** Quinolone allergy **Disp:** Tabs 200, 300, 400 mg; Inj 20, 40 mg/mL; ophthal & otic 0.3% **SE:** N/V/D, photosens, insomnia, HA, local irritation

Ofloxacin, Ophthalmic (Ocuflox Ophthalmic) **Uses:** *Bacterial conjunctivitis, corneal ulcer* **Acts:** See Ofloxacin **Dose:** *Adults & Peds > 1 y.* 1–2 gtt in eye(s) q2–4h × 2 d, then qid × 5 more d **W/P:** [C, +/−] **CI:** Quinolone allergy **Disp:** Ophthal 0.3% soln **SE:** Burning, hyperemia, bitter taste, chemosis, photophobia

Ofloxacin, Otic (Floxin Otic, Floxin Otic Singles) **Uses:** *Otitis externa; chronic suppurative otitis media w/ perf drums; otitis media in peds w/ tubes* **Acts:** See Ofloxacin **Dose:** *Adults & Peds > 13 y. Otitis externa:* 10 gtt in ear(s) daily × 7 d. *Peds 1–12 y. Otitis media* 5 gtt in ear(s) bid × 10 d **W/P:** [C, −] **CI:** Quinolone allergy **Disp:** Otic 0.3% soln 5/10 mL bottles; singles 0.25 mL foil pack **SE:** Local irritation **Notes:** W/ tubes/perforated drums; 10 gtt = 0.5 mL

Olanzapine (Zyprexa, Zydis) **BOX:** ↑ Mortality in elderly w/ dementia-related psychosis **Uses:** *Bipolar mania, schizophrenia*, psychotic disorders, acute agitation in schizophrenia **Acts:** Dopamine & serotonin antagonist; atypical antipsychotic. **Dose:** *Bipolar/schizophrenia:* 5–10 mg/d, weekly PRN, 20 mg/d max. *Agitation;* atypical antipsychotic 5–10 mg IM q2–4h PRN, 30 mg d/max **W/P:** [C, −] **Disp:** Tabs 2.5, 5, 7.5, 10, 15, 20 mg; PO disintegrating tabs (Zyprexa, Zydis) 5, 10, 15, 20 mg; Inj 10 mg **SE:** HA, somnolence, orthostatic ↓ BP, tachycardia, dystonia, xerostomia, constipation, hyperglycemia; ↑ wgt, ↑ prolactin levels; and sedation may be ↑ in peds **Notes:** Takes wk to titrate dose; smoking ↓ levels; may be confused w/ *Zyrtec* or *Zyprexa Relprevv*

Olanzapine, LA Parenteral (Zyprexa Relprevv) **BOX:** ↑ risk for severe sedation/coma following parenteral injection; observe closely for 3 h in appropriate facility; restricted distribution; ↑ mortality in elderly w/ dementia-related psychosis; not approved for dementia-related psychosis **Uses:** * Schizophrenia* **Acts:**

See Olanzapine **Dose:** IM: 150 mg/2 wk, 300 mg/4 wk, 210 mg/2 wk, 405 mg/4 wk, or 300 mg/2 wk **W/P:** [C, –] IM only, do not confuse w/ *Zyprexa* IM; can cause neuroleptic malignant synd, ↑ glucose/lipids/prolactin, ↓ BP, tardive dyskinesia, cognitive impair, ↓ WBC **CI:** None **Disp:** Vials, 210, 300, 405 mg **SE:** HA, sedation, ↑ wgt, cough, N/V/D, ↑ appetite, dry mouth, nasopharyngitis, somnolence **Notes:** ✓ glucose/lipids/CBC baseline and periodically

Olmesartan, Olmesartan, & Hydrochlorothiazide (Benicar, Benicar HCT) **BOX:** Use in PRG 2nd/3rd trimesters can harm fetus; D/C when PRG detected **Uses:** *Hypertension, alone or in combo* **Acts:** *Benicar* angiotensin II receptor blocker (ARB); *Benicar HCT* ARB w/ diuretic HCTZ **Dose:** *Adults. Benicar* 20–40 mg qd; *Benicar HCT* 20–40 mg olmesartan w/ 12.5–25 mg HCTZ based on effect *Peds 6–16 y. Benicar:* < 35 kg start 10 mg PO, range 10-20 mg qd; ≥ 35 kg start 20 mg PO qd, target 20–40 mg qd **W/P:** [C 1st tri, D 2nd, 3rd, ?/–] *Benicar HCT* not rec w/ CrCl < 30 mL/min; follow closely if volume depleted with start of med **CI:** Component allergy **Disp:** *Benicar* tabs mg olmesartan 5, 20, 40. *Benicar HCT* mg olmesartan/mg HCTZ 20/12.5, 40/12.5, 40/25 **SE:** Dizziness, ↓ K⁺ w/ HCTZ product (may require replacement) **Notes:** If *Benicar* does not control BP a diuretic can be added or *Benicar HCT* used

Olmesartan, Amlodipine, & Hydrochlorothiazide (Tribenzor) **Uses:** *Hypertension* **Acts:** Combo angiotensin II receptor blocker, CCB, thiazide diuretic **Dose:** begin w/ 20/5/12.5 olmesartan/amlodipine/HCTZ, ↑ to max 40/10/25 mg **W/P:** [C 1st tri, D 2nd, 3rd; –] **CI:** Anuria; sulfa allergy; PRG, neonate exposure, CrCl < 30 mg/min, age > 75 y, severe liver dx **Disp:** Tabs (olmesartan mg/amlodipine mg/HCTZ mg) 20/5/12.5, 40/5/12.5, 40/5/25, 40/10/12.5, 40/10/25 **SE:** Edema, HA, fatigue, N/D, muscle spasms, jt swelling, URI, syncope **Notes:** Avoid w/ volume depletion; thiazide diuretics may exacerbate SLE, associated NA glaucoma

Olopatadine, Nasal (Patanase) **Uses:** *Seasonal allergic rhinitis* **Acts:** H₁-receptor antagonist **Dose:** 2 sprays each nostril bid **W/P:** [C, ?] **Disp:** 0.6% 240-Spray bottle **SE:** Epistaxis, bitter taste somnolence, HA, rhinitis

Olopatadine, Ophthalmic (Patanol, Pataday) **Uses:** *Allergic conjunctivitis* **Acts:** H₁-receptor antagonist **Dose:** *Patanol:* 1–2 gtt in eye(s) bid; *Pataday:* 1 gtt in eye(s) q day **W/P:** [C, ?] **Disp:** *Patanol:* Soln 0.1% 5 mL *Pataday:* 0.2% 2.5 mL **SE:** Local irritation, HA, rhinitis **Notes:** Wait 10 min after to insert contacts

Olsalazine (Dipentum) **Uses:** *Maintain remission in UC* **Acts:** Topical anti-inflammatory **Dose:** 500 mg PO bid (w/ food) **W/P:** [C, –] **CI:** Salicylate sensitivity **Disp:** Caps 250 mg **SE:** D, HA, blood dyscrasias, hep

Omalizumab (Xolair) **BOX:** Reports of anaphylaxis 2–24 h after administration, even in previously treated pts **Uses:** *Mod–severe asthma in ≥ 12 y w/ reactivity to an allergen & when Sxs inadequately controlled w/ inhaled steroids* **Acts:** Anti-IgE Ab **Dose:** 150–375 mg SQ q2–4wk (dose/frequency based on serum IgE level & body wgt; see PI) **W/P:** [B, ?/–] **CI:** Component allergy, acute bronchospasm **Disp:** 150-mg single-use 5-mL vial **SE:** Site Rxn, sinusitis, HA, anaphylaxis reported in 3 pts **Notes:** Continue other asthma meds as indicated

Omega-3 Fatty Acid [Fish Oil] (Lovaza) Uses: *Rx hypertriglyceridemia* **Acts:** Omega-3 acid ethyl esters, ↓ thrombus inflammation & triglycerides **Dose:** *Hypertriglyceridemia:* 4 g/d ÷ in 1–2 doses **W/P:** [C, –], Fish hypersens; PRG, risk factor w/ anticoagulant use, w/ bleeding risk **CI:** Hypersens to components **Disp:** 1000-mg gel caps **SE:** Dyspepsia, N, GI pain, rash, flu-like synd **Notes:** Only FDA-approved fish oil supl; not for exogenous hypertriglyceridemia (type 1 hyperchylomicronemia); many OTC products (p 277). D/C after 2 mo if triglyceride levels do not ↓; previously called "Omacor"

Omeprazole (Prilosec, Prilosec OTC) Uses: *Duodenal/gastric ulcers (adults), GERD and erosive gastritis (adults and children)*, prevent NSAID ulcers, ZE synd, *H. pylori* Infxns **Acts:** PPI **Dose:** *Adults.* 20–40 mg PO daily-bid × 4–8 wk; *H. pylori* 20 mg PO bid × 10 d w/ amoxicillin & clarithromycin or 40 mg PO × 14 d w/ clarithromycin; pathologic hypersecretory cond 60 mg/d (varies); 80 mg/d max. *Peds (1–16 y) 5–10 kg.* 5 mg/d; *10–20 kg:* 10 mg PO q day. > *20 kg:* 20 mg PO q day; 40 mg/d max **W/P:** [C, –/+] w/ drugs that rely on gastric pH (e.g., ampicillin); avoid w/ atazanavir and nelfinavir; caution w/ warfarin, diazepam, phenytoin; do not use w/ clopidogrel (↓ effect); response does not R/O malignancy **Disp:** OTC tabs 20 mg; *Prilosec* DR caps 10, 20, 40 mg; *Prilosec* DR susp 2.5, 10 mg **SE:** HA, abd pain, N/V/D, flatulence **Notes:** Combo w/ antibiotic Rx for *H. pylori*; ? ↑ risk of fractures, *C. difficile*, CAP w/ all PPI; risk of hypomagnesemia w/ long-term use, monitor

Omeprazole and Sodium Bicarbonate (Zegerid, Zegerid OTC) Uses: *Duodenal/gastric ulcers, GERD and erosive gastritis, ZE synd, prevent NSAID ulcers (in critically ill patients)*, prevent NSAID ulcers, ZE synd, *H. pylori* Infxns **Acts:** PPI w/ sodium bicarb **Dose:** *Duodenal ulcer:* 20 PO daily-bid × 4–8 wk; *Gastric ulcer:* 40 PO daily-bid × 4–8 wk; *GERD no erosions* 20 mg PO daily × 4 wks, *w/erosions* treat 4–6 wk; *UGI bleed prevention:* 40 mg q6–8h then 40 mg/d × 14 d **W/P:** [C, –/+] w/ drugs that rely on gastric acid (e.g., ampicillin); avoid w/ atazanavir and nelfinavir; w/ warfarin, diazepam, phenytoin; do not use w/ clopidogrel (↓ effect); response does not R/O malignancy **Disp:** Omeprazole mg/sodium bicarb mg: *Zegerid* 20/1100; *Zegerid* 20/1100, mg 40/1100; *Zegerid powder packet* for oral susp 20/1680, 40/1680 **SE:** HA, abd pain, N/V/D, flatulence **Notes:** Not approved in peds; take 1 h ac; mix powder in small cup w/ 2 tbsp H_2O (not food or other liq) refill and drink; do not open caps; possible ↑ risk of fractures, *C. difficile*, CAP w/ all PPI; risk of hypomagnesemia w/ long-term use, monitor

Omeprazole, Sodium Bicarbonate, & Magnesium Hydroxide (Zegerid With Magnesium Hydroxide) Uses: *Duodenal or gastric ulcer, GERD, maintenance esophagitis* **Acts:** PPI w/ acid buffering; **Dose:** 20–40 mg omeprazole daily, empty stomach 1 h pc; *Duodenal ulcer, GERD:* 20 mg 4–8 wk;

Gastric ulcer: 40 mg 4–8 wk; *Esophagitis maint:* 20 mg **W/P:** [C, ?/–] w/ resp alkalosis, ↓ K^+, ↓ Ca^{+2}; ↑ drug levels metabolized by cytochrome P450; may ↑ INR w/ warfarin; may ↓ absorption drugs requiring acid environment **CI:** ↓ renal Fxn; **Disp:** Chew tabs, 20, 40 mg omeprazole; w/ 600 mg $NaHCO_3$; 700 mg $MgOH_2$ **SE:** N, V, D, abd pain, HA **Notes:** atrophic gastritis w/ long-term PPI; ? ↑ risk of fractures, *C. difficile,* CAP w/ all PPI; long-term use + Ca^{+2} → milk-alkali syndrome

Ondansetron (Zofran, Zofran ODT) Uses: *Prevent chemotherapy-associated & post-op N/V* **Acts:** Serotonin receptor ($5-HT_3$) antagonist **Dose:** *Adults & Peds. Chemotherapy:* 0.15 mg/kg/dose IV prior to chemotherapy, then 4 & 8 h after 1st dose or 4–8 mg PO tid; 1st dose 30 min prior to chemotherapy & give on schedule, not PRN. *Adults. Post-operation:* 4 mg IV immediately preanesthesia or post-operation. *Peds. Post-operation:* < *40 kg:* 0.1 mg/kg. > *40 kg:* 4 mg IV; ↓ w/ hepatic impair **W/P:** [B, +/–] arrhythmia risk, may ↑ QT interval **Disp:** Tabs 4, 8, 24 mg, soln 4 mg/5 mL, Inj 2 mg/mL, 32 mg/50 mL; *Zofran ODT* tabs 4, 8 mg; **SE:** D, HA, constipation, dizziness

Ondansetron, Oral Soluble Film (Zuplenz) Uses: *Prevent chemotherapy/ RT-associated & post-op N/V* **Acts:** Serotonin receptor ($5-HT_3$) antagonist **Dose:** *Adults. Highly emetogenic chemo:* 24 mg (8 mg film × 3) 30 min pre-chemo; *RT N & V:* 8 mg film tid. *Adults & Peds > 12 y. Mod emetogenic chemo:* 8 mg film 30 min pre-chemo, then 8 mg in 8 h; 8 mg film bid × 1–2 d after chemo. *Adults. Post-op: 16 mg (8 mg film × 2) 1 h pre-op;* ↓ w/ hepatic impair **W/P:** [B, +/–] **CI:** w/ apomorphine (↓ *BP, LOC*). **Disp:** oral soluble film 4, 8 mg **SE:** HA, malaise/ fatigue, constipation, D **Notes:** Use with dry hands, do not chew/swallow; place on tongue, dissolves in 4–20 s

Oprelvekin (Neumega) BOX: Allergic Rxn w/ anaphylaxis reported; D/C w/ any allergic Rxn Uses: *Prevent ↓ plt w/ chemotherapy* **Acts:** ↑ Proliferation & maturation of megakaryocytes (IL-11) **Dose:** *Adults.* 50 mcg/kg/d SQ for 10–21 d. *Peds > 12 y.* 75–100 mcg/kg/d SQ for 10–21 d. < *12 y:* Use only in clinical trials; ↓ w/ CrCl < 30 mL/min 25 mcg/kg. **W/P:** [C, ?/–] **Disp:** 5 mg powder for Inj **SE:** Tachycardia, palpitations, arrhythmias, edema, HA, dizziness, visual disturbances, papilledema, insomnia, fatigue, fever, N, anemia, dyspnea, allergic Rxns including anaphylaxis

Oral Contraceptives (See Table 5, p 288) BOX: Cigarette smoking ↑ risk of serious CV SEs; ↑ risk w/ > 15 cigarettes/d, > 35 y; strongly advise women on OCP to not smoke. Pt should be counseled that these products do not protect against HIV and other STD Uses: *Birth control; regulation of anovulatory bleeding; dysmenorrhea; endometriosis; polycystic ovaries; acne* (Note: FDA approvals vary widely, see PI) **Acts:** *Birth control:* Suppresses LH surge, prevents ovulation; progestins thicken cervical mucus; ↓ fallopian tubule cilia, ↓ endometrial thickness to ↓ chances of fertilization. *Anovulatory bleeding:* Cyclic hormones mimic body's natural cycle & regulate endometrial lining, results in regular bleeding q28d; may ↓ uterine bleeding & dysmenorrhea **Dose:** Start day 1 menstrual cycle or 1st

Sunday after onset of menses; 28-d cycle pills take daily; 21-d cycle pills take daily, no pills during last 7 d of cycle (during menses); some available as transdermal patch **W/P:** [X, +] Migraine, HTN, DM, sickle cell Dz, gallbladder Dz; monitor for breast Dz; w/ drospirenone containing OCP ✓ K^+ if taking drugs w/ ↑ K^+ risk; drospirenone implicated in ↑ VTE risk. **CI:** AUB, PRG, estrogen-dependent malignancy, ↑ hypercoagulation/liver Dz, hemiplegic migraine, smokers > 35 y; drospirenone has mineralocorticoid effect; do not use w/ renal/liver/adrenal problems. **Disp:** See Table 5, p 288. 28-d cycle pills (21 active pills + 7 placebo or Fe or folate supl); 21-d cycle pills (21 active pills) **SE:** Intra-menstrual bleeding, oligomenorrhea, amenorrhea, ↑ appetite/wgt gain, ↓ libido, fatigue, depression, mood swings, mastalgia, HA, melasma, ↑ vag discharge, acne/greasy skin, corneal edema, N **Notes:** Taken correctly, up to 99.9% effective for contraception; no STDs prevention instruct in use of condoms to reduce STD use additional barrier contraceptive; long-term, can ↓ risk of ectopic PRG, benign breast Dz, ovarian & uterine CA. Suggestions for OCP prescribing and/or regimen changes are noted below. Listing of other forms of Rx birth control can be found on p 24.

- *Rx menstrual cycle control:* Start w/ monophasic × 3 mo before switching to another brand; w/ continued bleeding change to pill w/ ↑ estrogen
- *Rx birth control:* Choose pill w/lowest SE profile for particular pt; SEs numerous; d/t estrogenic excess or progesterone deficiency; each pill's SE profile can be unique (see PI); newer extended-cycle combos have shorter/fewer hormone-free intervals, ? ↓ PRG risk; OCP troubleshooting SE w/ suggested OCP.
  - *Absent menstrual flow:* ↑ Estrogen, ↓ progestin: Brevicon, Necon 1/35, Norinyl 1/35, Modicon, Necon 1/50, Norinyl 1/50, Ortho-Cyclen, Ortho-Novum 1/50, Ortho-Novum 1/35, Ovcon 35
  - *Acne:* Use ↑ estrogen, ↓ androgenic: Brevicon, Ortho-Cyclen, Demulen 1/50, Estrostep, Ortho Tri-Cyclen, Mircette, Modicon, Necon, Ortho Evra, Yasmin, Yaz
  - *Break-through bleed:* ↑ Estrogen, ↑ progestin, ↓ androgenic: Demulen 1/50, Desogen, Estrostep, Loestrin 1/20, Ortho-Cept, Ovcon 50, Yasmin, Zovia 1/50
  - *Breast tenderness or ↑ wgt:* ↓ Estrogen, ↓ progestin: Use ↓ estrogen pill rather than current; Alesse, Levlite, Loestrin 1/20 Fe, Ortho Evra, Yasmin, Yaz
  - *Depression:* ↓ Progestin: Alesse, Brevicon, Levlite, Modicon, Necon, Ortho Evra, Ovcon 35, Ortho-Cyclen, Ortho Tri-Cyclen Tri-Levlen, Triphasil, Trivora
  - *Endometriosis:* ↓ Estrogen, ↓ progestin: Demulen 1/35, Loestrin 1.5/30, Loestrin 1/20 Fe, Lo Oval, Levlen, Levora, Nordette, Zovia 1/35; cont w/o placebo pills or w/ 4 d of placebo pills
  - *HA:* ↓ Estrogen, ↓ progestin: Alesse, Levlite, Ortho Evra
  - *Moodiness &/or irritability:* ↓ Progestin: Alesse, Brevicon, Levlite, Modicon, Necon 1/35, Ortho Evra, Ortho-Cyclen, Ortho Tri-Cyclen, Ovcon 35, Tri-Levlen, Triphasil, Trivora
  - *Severe menstrual cramping:* ↑ Progestin: Demulen 1/50, Desogen, Loestrin 1.5/30, Mircette, Ortho-Cept, Yasmin, Yaz, Zovia 1/50E, Zovia 1/35E

Orlistat (Xenical, Alli [OTC]) Uses: *Manage obesity w/ body mass index ≥30 kg/m^2 or ≥27 kg/m^2 w/ other risk factors; type 2 DM, dyslipidemia* Acts: Reversible inhib of gastric & pancreatic lipases. Dose: 120 mg PO tid w/ a fat-containing meal; Alli (OTC) 60 mg PO tid w/ fat-containing meals W/P: [B, ?] May ↓ cyclosporine & warfarin dose requirements; severe liver injury reported CI: Cholestasis, malabsorption, organ transplant Disp: *Xenical* caps 120 mg; *Alli OTC* caps 60 mg SE: Abd pain/discomfort, fatty stools, fecal urgency Notes: Do not use if meal contains no fat; GI effects ↑ w/ higher-fat meals; supl w/ fat-soluble vits; tell patients about S/Sx of liver injury (including itching, yellow eyes or skin, etc)

Orphenadrine (Norflex) Uses: *Discomfort associated w/ painful musculoskeletal conditions* Acts: Central atropine-like effect; indirect skeletal muscle relaxation, euphoria, analgesia Dose: 100 mg PO bid, 60 mg IM/IV q12h W/P: [C, +/−] CI: NAG, GI/ or bladder obst, cardiospasm, MyG Disp: SR tabs 100 mg; Inj 30 mg/mL SE: Drowsiness, dizziness, blurred vision, flushing, tachycardia, constipation

Oseltamivir (Tamiflu) Uses: *Prevention & Rx influenza A & B* Acts: ↓ Viral neuraminidase Dose: *Adults. Tx:* 75 mg PO bid for 5 d; *Prophylaxis:* 75 mg PO daily × 10 d. *Peds. Tx:* dose BID × 5 days: *< 15 kg:* 30 mg. *15–23 kg:* 45 mg. *23–40 kg:* 60 mg. *> 40 kg:* adult dose. *Prophylaxis:* Same dosing but once daily for 10 days ↓ w/ renal impair W/P: [C, ?/−] CI: Component allergy Disp: Caps 30, 45, 75 mg, powder 6 mg/mL for suspension (Note: 12 mg/mL dose is being phased out due to dosing concerns) SE: N/V, insomnia, reports of neuropsychological events in children (self-injury, confusion, delirium) Notes: Start w/in 48 h of Sx onset or exposure; 2009 H1N1 strains susceptible; ✓ CDC updates http://www.cdc.gov/h1n1flu/guidance/

Oxacillin (Prostaphlin) Uses: *Infxns d/t susceptible S. aureus & Streptococcus* Acts: Bactericidal; ↓ cell wall synth. *Spectrum:* Excellent gram(+), poor gram(−) Dose: *Adults.* 250–500 mg (2 g severe) IM/IV q4–6h. *Peds.* 150–200 mg/kg/d IV ÷ q4–6h W/P: [B, M] CI: PCN sensitivity Disp: Powder for Inj 500 mg, 1, 2, 10 g SE: GI upset, interstitial nephritis, blood dyscrasias

Oxaliplatin (Eloxatin) BOX: Administer w/ supervision of physician experienced in chemotherapy. Appropriate management is possible only w/ adequate diagnostic & Rx facilities. Anaphylactic-like Rxns reported Uses: *Adjuvant Rx stage III colon CA (primary resected) & metastatic colon CA w/ 5-FU* Acts: Metabolized to platinum derivatives, crosslinks DNA Dose: Per protocol; see PI. *Premedicate:* Antiemetic w/ or w/o dexamethasone W/P: [D, −] See Box CI: Allergy to components or platinum Disp: Inj 50, 100 mg SE: Anaphylaxis, granulocytopenia, paresthesia, N/V/D, stomatitis, fatigue, neuropathy, hepatotox, pulm tox Notes: 5-FU & leucovorin are given in combo; epi, corticosteroids, & antihistamines alleviate severe Rxns

Oxandrolone (Oxandrin) [C-III] BOX: Risk of peliosis hepatis, liver cell tumors, may ↑ risk atherosclerosis Uses: *Wt ↑ after wt ↓ from severe trauma, extensive surgery* Acts: Anabolic steroid; ↑ lean body mass Dose: *Adults.* 2.5–20 mg/d PO ÷ bid-qid *Peds.* ≤0.1 mg/kg/d ÷ bid-qid W/P: [X, ?/–] ↑ INR w/ warfarin CI: PRG, prostate CA, male breast CA, breast CA w/ hypercalcemia, nephrosis Disp: Tabs 2.5, 10 mg SE: Acne, hepatotox, dyslipidemia Notes: ✓ lipids & LFTs; Use judiciously 2–4 wk typical

Oxaprozin (Daypro, Daypro ALTA) BOX: May ↑ risk of cardiovascular CV events & GI bleeding Uses: *Arthritis & pain* Acts: NSAID; ↓ prostaglandin synth Dose: *Adults.* 600–1200 mg/daily (÷ dose helps GI tolerance); ↓ w/ renal/hepatic impair *Peds. JRA (Daypro): 22–31 kg:* 600 mg/d. *32–54 kg:* 900 mg/d W/P: [C (D 3rd tri), ?] Peptic ulcer, bleeding disorders CI: ASA/NSAID sensitivity, perioperative pain w/ CABG Disp: *Daypro ALTA:* tabs 600 mg; caplets 600 mg SE: CNS inhibition, sleep disturbance, rash, GI upset, peptic ulcer, edema, renal failure, anaphylactoid Rxn w/ "ASA triad" (asthmatic w/ rhinitis, nasal polyps and bronchospasm w/ NSAID use)

Oxazepam [C-IV] Uses: *Anxiety, acute EtOH withdrawal*, anxiety w/ depressive Sxs Acts: Benzodiazepine; diazepam metabolite Dose: *Adults.* 10–15 mg PO tid-qid; severe anxiety & EtOH withdrawal may require up to 30 mg qid. *Peds.* 1 mg/kg/d ÷ doses W/P: [D, ?/–] CI: Component allergy, NAG Disp: Caps 10, 15, 30 mg; tabs 15 mg SE: Sedation, ataxia, dizziness, rash, blood dyscrasias, dependence Notes: Avoid abrupt D/C

Oxcarbazepine (Trileptal) Uses: *Partial Szs*, bipolar disorders Acts: Blocks voltage-sensitive Na⁺ channels, stabilization of hyperexcited neural membranes Dose: *Adults.* 300 mg PO bid, ↑ weekly to target maint 1200–2400 mg/d. *Peds.* 8–10 mg/kg bid, 600 mg/d max, ↑ weekly to target maint dose; ↓ w/ renal Insuff W/P: [C, –] Carbamazepine sensitivity; CI: Component sensitivity Disp: Tabs 150, 300, 600 mg; susp 300 mg/5 mL SE: ↓ Na⁺, HA, dizziness, fatigue, somnolence, GI upset, diplopia, concentration difficulties, fatal skin/multiorgan hypersens Rxns Notes: Do not abruptly D/C, ✓ Na⁺ if fatigued; advise about SJS and topic epidermal necrolysis

Oxiconazole (Oxistat) Uses: *Tinea cruris, tinea corporis, tinea pedis, tinea versicolor* Acts: ? ↓ Ergosterols in fungal cell membrane. *Spectrum:* Most *Epidermophyton floccosum, Trichophyton mentagrophytes, Trichophyton rubrum, Malassezia furfur* Dose: Apply thin layer daily-bid W/P: [B, M] CI: Component allergy Disp: Cream, lotion 1% SE: Local irritation

Oxybutynin (Ditropan, Ditropan XL) Uses: *Symptomatic relief of urgency, nocturia, incontinence w/ neurogenic or reflex neurogenic bladder* Acts: Anticholinergic, relaxes bladder smooth muscle, ↑ bladder capacity Dose: *Adults.* 5 mg bid-tid, 5 mg qid max. XL 5–10 mg/d, 30 mg/d max. *Peds > 5 y.* 5 mg PO bid-tid; 15 mg/d max. *Peds 1–5 y.* 0.2 mg/kg/dose bid-qid (syrup 5 mg/5 mL); 15 mg/d max; ↓ in elderly; periodic drug holidays OK W/P: [B, ?] CI: NAG, MyG, GI/GU obst, ulcerative colitis, megacolon **Disp:** Tabs 5 mg; XL tabs 5, 10, 15 mg; syrup 5 mg/5 mL **SE:** Anticholinergic (drowsiness, xerostomia, constipation, tachycardia), ↑ QT interval, memory impair; ER form empty shell expelled in stool

Oxybutynin, Topical (Gelnique) **Uses:** *OAB* **Acts:** Anticholinergic, relaxes bladder smooth muscle, ↑ bladder capacity **Dose:** 1 g sachet qd to dry skin (abd/shoulders/thighs/upper arms) **W/P:** [B, ?/–] **CI:** Gastric or urinary retention; NAG **Disp:** Gel 10%, 1 g sachets (100 mg oxybutynin) **SE:** Anticholinergic (lethargy, xerostomia, constipation, blurred vision, ↑ HR); rash, pruritus, redness, pain at site; UTI **Notes:** Cover w/ clothing, skin-to-skin transfer can occur; gel is flammable; after applying wait 1 h before showering

Oxybutynin Transdermal System (Oxytrol) **Uses:** *Rx OAB* **Acts:** Anticholinergic, relaxes bladder smooth muscle, ↑ bladder capacity **Dose:** One 3.9 mg/d system apply 2×/wk (q3–4d) to abd, hip, or buttock **W/P:** [B, ?/–] **CI:** GI/GU obst, NAG **Disp:** 3.9 mg/d transdermal patch **SE:** Anticholinergic, itching/redness at site **Notes:** Do not apply to same site w/in 7 d

Oxycodone [Dihydro Hydroxycodone] (OxyContin, Roxicodone) [C-II] **BOX:** High abuse potential; controlled release only for extended chronic pain, not for PRN use; 60, 80-mg tab for opioid-tolerant pts; do not crush, break, or chew **Uses:** *Mod–severe pain, usually in combo w/ nonnarcotic analgesics* **Acts:** Narcotic analgesic **Dose:** *Adults.* 5 mg PO q6h PRN (IR). *Mod–severe chronic pain:* 10–160 mg PO q12h (ER). *Peds 6–12 y.* 1.25 mg PO q6h PRN. *> 12 y:* 2.5 mg q6h PRN; ↓ w/ severe liver/renal Dz, elderly; w/ food **W/P:** [B (D if prolonged use/near term), M] **CI:** Allergy, resp depression, acute asthma, ileus w/ microsomal morphine **Disp:** IR caps (OxyIR) 5 mg; CR Roxicodone tabs 15, 30 mg; ER (OxyContin) 10, 15, 20, 30, 40, 60, 80 mg; liq 5 mg/5 mL; soln conc 20 mg/mL **SE:** ↓ BP, sedation, resp depression, dizziness, GI upset, constipation, risk of abuse **Notes:** *OxyContin* for chronic CA pain; do not crush/chew/cut ER product; sought after as drug of abuse; reformulated *OxyContin* is intended to prevent the opioid medication from being cut, broken, chewed, crushed, or dissolved to release more medication

Oxycodone & Acetaminophen (Percocet, Tylox) [C-II] **Uses:** *Mod–severe pain* **Acts:** Narcotic analgesic **Dose:** *Adults.* 1–2 tabs/caps PO q4–6h PRN (acetaminophen max dose 4 g/d). *Peds.* Oxycodone 0.05–0.15 mg/kg/dose q 4–6h PRN, 5 mg/dose max **W/P:** [C (D prolonged use or near term), M] **CI:** Allergy, paralytic ileus, resp depression **Disp:** Percocet tabs, mg oxycodone/mg APAP: 2.5/325, 5/325, 7.5/325, 10/325, 7.5/500, 10/650; Tylox caps 5 mg oxycodone, 500 mg APAP; soln 5 mg oxycodone & 325 mg APAP/5 mL **SE:** ↓ BP, sedation, dizziness, GI upset, constipation **Notes:** See Acetaminophen note p 34

Oxycodone & Aspirin (Percodan) [C-II] **Uses:** *Mod–severe pain* **Acts:** Narcotic analgesic w/ NSAID **Dose:** *Adults.* 1–2 tabs/caps PO q4–6h PRN. *Peds.* Oxycodone 0.05–0.15 mg/kg/dose q 4–6h PRN, up to 5 mg/dose; ↓ in severe hepatic failure **W/P:** [D, –] w/peptic ulcer, CNS depression, elderly, Hx Szs **CI:** Component allergy, children (< 16 y) w/ viral Infxn (Reyes synd), resp depression, ileus, hemophilia **Disp:** *Generics:* 4.83 mg oxycodone hydrochloride, 0.38 mg oxycodone terephthalate, 325 mg ASA; *Percodan* 4.83 mg oxycodone hydrochloride, 325 mg ASA **SE:** Sedation, dizziness, GI upset/ulcer, constipation, allergy **Notes:** monitor for possible drug abuse

Oxycodone/Ibuprofen (Combunox) [C-II] BOX: May ↑ risk of serious CV events; CI in perioperative coronary artery bypass graft pain; ↑ risk of GI events such as bleeding **Uses:** *Short-term (not > 7 d) management of acute mod–severe pain* **Acts:** Narcotic w/ NSAID **Dose:** 1 tab q6h PRN 4 tab max/24 h; 7 d max **W/P:** [C, –] w/ Impaired renal/hepatic Fxn; COPD, CNS depression, avoid in PRG CI: Paralytic ileus, 3rd tri PRG, allergy to ASA or NSAIDs, where opioids are CI **Disp:** Tabs 5 mg oxycodone/400 mg ibuprofen **SE:** N/V, somnolence, dizziness, sweating, flatulence, ↑ LFTs **Notes:** ✓ renal Fxn; abuse potential w/ oxycodone

Oxymorphone (Opana, Opana ER) [C-II] BOX: *(Opana ER)* Abuse potential, controlled release only for chronic pain; do not consume EtOH-containing beverages, may cause fatal OD **Uses:** *Mod/severe pain, sedative* **Acts:** Narcotic analgesic **Dose:** 10–20 mg PO q4–6h PRN if opioid-naïve or 1–1.5 mg SQ/IM q4–6h PRN or 0.5 mg IV q4–6h PRN; starting 20 mg/dose max PO; *Chronic pain:* ER 5 mg PO q12h; if opioid-naïve ↑ PRN 5–10 mg PO q12h q3–7d; take 1 h pc or 2 h ac; ↓ dose w/ elderly, renal/hepatic impair **W/P:** [B, ?] **CI:** ↑ ICP, severe resp depression, w/ EtOH or liposomal morphine, severe hepatic impair **Disp:** Tabs 5, 10 mg; ER 5, 10, 20, 40 mg **SE:** ↓ BP, sedation, GI upset, constipation, histamine release **Notes:** Related to hydromorphone

Oxytocin (Pitocin) **Uses:** *Induce labor, control postpartum hemorrhage* **Acts:** Stimulate muscular contractions of the uterus **Dose:** 0.0005–0.001 units/min IV Inf; titrate 0.001–0.002 units/min q30–60min **W/P:** [Uncategorized, +/–] **CI:** Where vag delivery not favorable, fetal distress **Disp:** Inj 10 units/mL **SE:** Uterine rupture, fetal death; arrhythmias, anaphylaxis, H_2O intoxication **Notes:** Monitor vital signs; nasal form for breast-feeding only

Paclitaxel (Taxol, Abraxane) BOX: Administration only by physician experienced in chemotherapy; fatal anaphylaxis and hypersens possible; severe myelosuppression possible **Uses:** *Ovarian & breast CA, PCa*, Kaposi sarcoma, NSCLC **Acts:** Mitotic spindle poison; promotes microtubule assembly & stabilization against depolymerization **Dose:** Per protocols; use glass or polyolefin containers (e.g., nitroglycerin tubing set); PVC sets leach plasticizer; ↓ in hepatic failure **W/P:** [D, –] **CI:** Neutropenia < 1500 WBC/mm^3; solid tumors, component allergy **Disp:** Inj 6 mg/mL, 5 mg/mL albumin bound (Abraxane) **SE:** ↓ BM, peripheral neuropathy, transient ileus, myalgia, ↓ HR, ↓ BP, mucositis, N/V/D, fever, rash, HA, phlebitis; hematologic tox schedule-dependent; leukopenia dose-limiting by 24-h Inf; neurotox limited w/ short (1–3 h) Inf; allergic Rxns (dyspnea, ↓ BP, urticaria, rash) **Notes:** Maintain hydration; allergic Rxn usually w/in 10 min of Inf; minimize w/ corticosteroid, antihistamine pretreatment

Palifermin (Kepivance) Uses: *Oral mucositis w/ BMT* Acts: Synthetic keratinocyte GF Dose: *Phase 1:* 60 mcg/kg IV daily × 3, 3rd dose 24–48 h before chemotherapy. *Phase 2:* 60 mcg/kg IV daily × 3, immediately after stem cell Inf W/P: [C, ?/–] CI: N/A Disp: Inj 6.25 mg SE: Unusual mouth sensations, tongue thickening, rash, ↑ amylase & lipase Notes: *E. coli*–derived; separate phases by 4 d; safety unknown w/ nonhematologic malignancies

Paliperidone (Invega, Invega Sustenna) BOX: Not for dementia-related psychosis Uses: *Schizophrenia* Acts: Risperidone metabolite, antagonizes dopamine, and serotonin receptors Dose: *Invega:* 6 mg PO q A.M., 12 mg/d max; CrCl 50–79 mL/min: 6 mg/d max; CrCl 10–49 mL/min: 3 mg/d max. *Invega Sustenna:* 234 mg day 1, 156 mg one week later IM (deltoid), then 117 mg maint (deltoid or gluteal); range 39–234 mg/mo W/P: [C, ?/–] w/ ↓ HR, ↓ K⁺/Mg²⁺, renal/hepatic impair; w/ phenothiazines, ranolazine, ziprasidone, prolonged QT, Hx arrhythmia CI: Risperidone/paliperidone hypersens Disp: *Invega:* ER tabs 1.5, 3, 6, 9 mg; *Invega Sustenna:* Prefilled syringes 39, 78, 117, 156, 234 mg SE: Impaired temp regulation, ↑ QT & HR, HA, anxiety, dizziness, N, dry mouth, fatigue, EPS Notes: Do not chew/cut/crush pill; determine tolerability to oral risperidone or paliperidone before using injectable

Palivizumab (Synagis) Uses: *Prevent RSV Infxn* Acts: MoAb Dose: *Peds.* 15 mg/kg IM monthly, typically Nov–Apr W/P: [C, ?] Renal/hepatic dysfunction CI: Component allergy Disp: Vials 50, 100 mg SE: hypersens Rxn, URI, rhinitis, cough, ↑ LFTs, local irritation

Palonosetron (Aloxi) BOX: May ↑ QTc interval Uses: *Prevention acute & delayed N/V w/ emetogenic chemotherapy; prevent postoperative N/V* Acts: 5-HT₃-receptor antagonist Dose: *Chemotherapy:* 0.25 mg IV 30 min prior to chemotherapy. *Postoperative N/V:* 0.75 mg immediately before induction W/P: [B, ?] CI: Component allergy Disp: 0.25 mg/5 mL vial SE: HA, constipation, dizziness, Abd pain, anxiety

Pamidronate (Aredia) Uses: *Hypercalcemia of malignancy, Paget Dz, palliate symptomatic bone metastases* Acts: Bisphosphonate; ↓ nl & abnormal bone resorption Dose: *Hypercalcemia:* 60–90 mg IV over 2–24 h or 90 mg IV over 24 h if severe; may repeat in 7 d. *Paget Dz:* 30 mg/d IV slow Inf over 4 h × 3 d. *Osteolytic bone mets in myeloma:* 90 mg IV over 4 h q mo. *Osteolytic bone mets breast CA:* 90 mg IV over 2 h q3–4wk; 90 mg/max single dose. W/P: [D, ?/–] Avoid invasive dental procedures w/ use CI: PRG, bisphosphonate sensitivity Disp: Inj 30, 60, 90 mg SE: Fever, malaise, convulsions, Inj site Rxn, uveitis, fluid overload, HTN, Abd pain, N/V, constipation, UTI, bone pain, ↓ K⁺, ↓ Ca²⁺, ↓ Mg²⁺, hypophosphatemia; jaw osteonecrosis (mostly CA pts; avoid dental work), renal tox Notes: Perform dental exam pretherapy; follow Cr, hold dose if Cr ↑ by 0.5 mg/dL w/ nl baseline or by 1 mg/dL w/ abnormal baseline; restart when Cr returns w/in 10% of baseline; may ↑ atypical subtrochanteric femur fractures

Pancrelipase (Pancrease, Cotazym, Creon, Ultrase) Uses: *Exocrine pancreatic secretion deficiency (e.g., CF, chronic pancreatitis, pancreatic Insuff), steatorrhea of malabsorption* Acts: Pancreatic enzyme supl Dose: 1–3 caps (tabs) w/ meals & snacks; ↑ to 8 caps (tabs); do not crush or chew EC products; dose dependent on digestive requirements of pt; avoid antacids W/P: [C, ?/–] CI: Pork product allergy, acute pancreatitis Disp: Caps, tabs SE: N/V, Abd cramps Notes: Individualize Rx

Pancuronium (Pavulon) BOX: Should only be administered by adequately trained individuals Uses: *Paralysis w/ mechanical ventilation* Acts: Nondepolarizing neuromuscular blocker Dose: *Adults & Peds > 1 mo.* Initial 0.06–0.1 mg/kg; maint 0.01 mg/kg 60–100 min after, then 0.01 mg/kg q25–60min PRN; ↓ w/ renal/hepatic impair; intubate pt & keep on controlled ventilation; use adequate sedation or analgesia W/P: [C, ?/–] CI: Component or bromide sensitivity Disp: Inj 1, 2 mg/mL SE: Tachycardia, HTN, pruritus, other histamine Rxns

Panitumumab (Vectibix) BOX: Derm tox common (89%) and severe in 12%; can be associated w/ Infxn (sepsis, abscesses requiring I&D); w/ severe derm tox, hold or D/C and monitor for Infxn; severe inf Rxns (anaphylactic Rxn, bronchospasm, fever, chills, hypotension) in 1%; w/ severe Rxns, immediately D/C inf and possibly permanent D/C Uses: *Rx EGFR-expressing metastatic colon CA* Acts: Anti-EGFR MoAb Dose: 6 mg/kg IV Inf over 60 min for doses < 1000 mg over 90 min ↓ Inf rate by 50% w/ grade 1–2 Inf Rxn, D/C permanently w/ grade 3–4 Rxn. For derm tox, hold until < grade 2 tox. If improves < 1 mo, restart 50% original dose. If tox recurs or resolution > 1 mo permanently D/C. If ↓ dose tolerated, ↑ dose by 25% W/P: [C, –] D/C nursing care, 2 mo after Disp: Vial 20 mg/mL SE: Rash, acneiform dermatitis, pruritus, paronychia, ↓ Mg²⁺, Abd pain, N/V/D, constipation, fatigue, dehydration, photosens, conjunctivitis, ocular hyperemia, ↑ lacrimation, stomatitis, mucositis, pulm fibrosis, severe derm tox, inf Rxns Notes: May impair female fertility; ✓ lytes; wear sunscreen/hats, limit sun exposure

Pantoprazole (Protonix) Uses: *GERD, erosive gastritis*, ZE synd, PUD Acts: Proton pump inhib Dose: 40 mg/d PO; do not crush/chew tabs; 40 mg IV/d (not > 3 mg/min, use Protonix filter) W/P: [B, ?/–] do not use w/ clopidogrel (↓ effect) Disp: Tabs, DR 20, 40 mg; 40 mg powder for oral susp (mix in applesauce or juice, give immediately); Inj 40 mg SE: Chest pain, anxiety, GI upset, ↑ LFTs Notes: ? ↑ risk of fractures w/ all PPI; risk of hypomagnesemia w/ long-term use, monitor

Paregoric [Camphorated Tincture of Opium] [C-III] Uses: *D*, pain & neonatal opiate withdrawal synd Acts: Narcotic Dose: *Adults.* 5–10 mL PO daily–qid PRN. *Peds.* 0.25–0.5 mL/kg daily–qid. *Neonatal withdrawal:* 3–6 gtt PO q3–6h PRN to relieve Sxs × 3–5 d, then taper over 2–4 wk W/P: [B (D w/ prolonged use/high dose near term, +] CI: Toxic D; convulsive disorder, morphine sensitivity Disp: Liq 2 mg morphine = 20 mg opium/5 mL SE: ↓ BP, sedation, constipation Notes: Contains anhydrous morphine from opium; short-term use only

Paroxetine (Paxil, Paxil CR, Pexeva) **BOX:** Closely monitor for worsening depression or emergence of suicidality, particularly in children, adolescents, and young adults; not for use in peds **Uses:** *Depression, OCD, panic disorder, social anxiety disorder*, PMDD **Action:** SSRI **Dose:** 10–60 mg PO single daily dose in A.M.; CR 25 mg/d PO; ↑ 12.5 mg/wk (max range 26–62.5 mg/d) **W/P:** [D, ?/] ↑ Bleeding risk **CI:** w/ MAOI, thioridazine, pimozide, linezolid, methylthioninium chloride (methylene blue) **Disp:** Tabs 10, 20, 30, 40 mg; susp 10 mg/5 mL; CR 12.5, 25, 37.5 mg **SE:** HA, somnolence, dizziness, GI upset, N/D, ↓ appetite, sweating, xerostomia, tachycardia, ↓ libido, ED, anorgasmia

Pazopanib Hydrochloride (Votrient) **BOX:** Administer only by physician experienced in chemotherapy. Severe and fatal hepatotoxicity observed. **Uses:** *Rx advanced RCC* **Action:** TKI **Dose:** *Adults.* 800 mg po once daily, ↓ to 200 mg daily if moderate hepatic impair, not recommended in severe hepatic disease (bili > 3× ULN) **W/P:** [D, –] Avoid w/ CYP3A4 inducers/inhibitors and QTc prolonging drugs, all SSRI. **CI:** Severe hepatic disease **Disp:** 200 mg tablet **SE:** ↑ BP, N/V/D, GI perf, anorexia, hair depigmentation, ↓ WBC, ↓ plt, ↑ bleeding, ↑ AST/ALT/bili, ↓ Na, chest pain, ↑ QT **Notes:** Hold for surgical procedures

Pegfilgrastim (Neulasta) **Uses:** *↓ Frequency of Infxn in pts w/ nonmyeloid malignancies receiving myelosuppressive anti-CA drugs that cause febrile neutropenia* **Acts:** Granulocyte and macrophage-stimulating factor **Dose:** *Adults.* 6 mg SQ × 1/chemotherapy cycle. **W/P:** [C, M] w/ Sickle cell **CI:** Allergy to *E. coli*-derived proteins or filgrastim **Disp:** Syringes: 6 mg/0.6 mL **SE:** Splenic rupture, HA, fever, weakness, fatigue, dizziness, insomnia, edema, N/V/D, stomatitis, anorexia, constipation, taste perversion, dyspepsia, Abd pain, granulocytopenia, neutropenic fever, ↑ LFTs & uric acid, myalgia, bone pain, ARDS, alopecia, worsen sickle cell Dz **Notes:** Never give between 14 d before & 24 h after dose of cytotoxic chemotherapy

Peginterferon Alfa-2a [Pegylated Interferon] (Pegasys) **BOX:** Can cause or aggravate fatal or life-threatening neuropsychological, autoimmune, ischemic, and infectious disorders. Monitor pts closely **Uses:** *Chronic hep C w/ compensated liver Dz* **Acts:** Immune modulator **Dose:** 180 mcg (1 mL) SQ q wk × 48 wk; ↓ in renal impair **W/P:** [C, /?–] **CI:** Autoimmune hep, decompensated liver Dz **Disp:** 180 mcg/mL Inj **SE:** Depression, insomnia, suicidal behavior, GI upset, ↓ WBC and plt, alopecia, pruritus

Peginterferon Alfa-2b [Pegylated Interferon] (PegIntron) **BOX:** Can cause or aggravate fatal or life-threatening neuropsychological, autoimmune, ischemic, and infectious disorders; monitor pts closely **Uses:** *Rx hep C* **Acts:** Immune modulator **Dose:** 1 mcg/kg/wk SQ; 1.5 mcg/kg/wk combo w/ ribavirin **W/P:** [C, ?/–] w/ Psychological disorder Hx **CI:** Autoimmune hep, decompensated liver Dz, hemoglobinopathy **Disp:** Vials 50, 80, 120, 150 mcg/0.5 mL; Redipen 50, 80, 120, 150 mcg/5 mL; reconstitute w/ 0.7 mL w/ sterile water **SE:** Depression, insomnia, suicidal behavior, GI upset, neutropenia, thrombocytopenia, alopecia, pruritus **Notes:** Give hs or w/ APAP to ↓ flu-like Sxs; monitor CBC/plt; use immediately or store in refrigerator × 24 h; do not freeze

Pegloticase (Krystexxa)   **BOX:** Anaphylaxis/infusion Rxns reported; admin in settings prepared to manage these Rxns; pre-med w/ antihistamines and corticosteroids **Uses:** *Refractory gout* **Acts:** PEGylated recombinant urate-oxidase enzyme **Dose:** 8 mg IV q2wk (in 250 mL NS/½NS over 120 mins) pre-med w/ antihistamines and corticosteroids **W/P:** [C, –] **CI:** G6PD deficiency **Disp:** Inj **SE:** Inf Rxn (anaphylaxis, urticaria, pruritis, erythema, chest pain, dyspnea); may cause gout flare, N **Notes:** ✓ uric acid level before each infusion, consider D/C if 2 consecutive levels > 6 mg/dL; do not IV push

Pemetrexed (Alimta)   **Uses:** *w/ Cisplatin in nonresectable mesothelioma*, NSCLC **Acts:** Antifolate antineoplastic **Dose:** 500 mg/m² IV over 10 min q3wk; hold if CrCl < 45 mL/min; give w/ vit B₁₂ (1000 mcg IM q9wk) & folic acid (350–1000 mcg PO daily); start 1 wk before; dexamethasone 4 mg PO bid × 3, start 1 d before each Rx **W/P:** [D, –] w/ Renal/hepatic/BM impair **CI:** Component sensitivity **Disp:** 500-mg vial **SE:** Neutropenia, thrombocytopenia, N/V/D, anorexia, stomatitis, renal failure, neuropathy, fever, fatigue, mood changes, dyspnea, anaphylactic Rxns **Notes:** Avoid NSAIDs, follow CBC/plt; ↓ dose w/ grade 3–4 mucositis

Pemirolast (Alamast)   **Uses:** *Allergic conjunctivitis* **Acts:** Mast cell stabilizer **Dose:** 1–2 gtt in each eye qid **W/P:** [C, ?/–] **Disp:** 0.1% (1 mg/mL) in 10-mL bottles **SE:** HA, rhinitis, cold/flu Sxs, local irritation **Notes:** Wait 10 min before insert-ting contacts

Penbutolol (Levatol)   **Uses:** *HTN* **Acts:** β-Adrenergic receptor blocker, β₁, β₂ **Dose:** 20–40 mg/d; ↓ in hepatic Insuff **W/P:** [C 1st tri; D if 2nd/3rd tri, M] **CI:** Asthma, cardiogenic shock, cardiac failure, heart block, ↓ HR, COPD, pulm edema **Disp:** Tabs 20 mg **SE:** Flushing, ↓ BP, fatigue, hyperglycemia, GI upset, sexual dysfunction, bronchospasm

Penciclovir (Denavir)   **Uses:** *Herpes simplex (herpes labialis/cold sores)* **Acts:** Competitive inhib of DNA polymerase **Dose:** Apply at 1st sign of lesions, then q2h while awake × 4 d **W/P:** [B, ?/–] **CI:** Allergy, previous Rxn to famciclovir **Disp:** Cream 1% **SE:** Erythema, HA **Notes:** Do not apply to mucous membranes

Penicillin G, Aqueous (Potassium or Sodium) (Pfizerpen, Pentids) **Uses:** *Bacteremia, endocarditis, pericarditis, resp tract Infxns, meningitis, neurosyphilis, skin/skin structure Infxns* **Acts:** Bactericidal; ↓ cell wall synth. *Spectrum:* Most gram(+) (not staphylococci), streptococci, *N. meningitidis,* syphilis, clostridia, & anaerobes (not *Bacteroides*) **Dose:** *Adults.* Based on indication range 0.6–24 mill units/d in ÷ doses q4h. *Peds Newborns < 1 wk.* 25,000–50,000 units/kg/dose IV q12h. *Infants 1 wk–< 1 mo:* 25,000–50,000 units/kg/dose IV q8h. *Children:* 100,000–300,000 units/kg/24h IV ÷ q4h; ↓ in renal impair **W/P:** [B, M] **CI:** Allergy **Disp:** Powder for Inj **SE:** Allergic Rxns; interstitial nephritis, D, Szs **Notes:** Contains 1.7 mEq of K⁺/mill units

Penicillin G Benzathine (Bicillin) Uses: *Single-dose regimen for strepto-coccal pharyngitis, rheumatic fever, glomerulonephritis prophylaxis, & syphilis* Acts: Bactericidal; ↓ cell wall synth. Spectrum: See Penicillin G Dose: Adults. 1.2–2.4 mill units deep IM Inj q2–4wk. Peds. 50,000 units/kg/dose, 2.4 mill units/dose max; deep IM Inj q2–4 wk W/P: [B, M] CI: Allergy Disp: Inj 300,000, 600,000 units/mL; Bicillin L-A benzathine salt only; Bicillin C-R combo of benza-thine & procaine (300,000 units procaine w/ 300,000 units benzathine/mL or 900,000 units benzathine w/ 300,000 units procaine/2 mL) SE: Inj site pain, acute interstitial nephritis, anaphylaxis Notes: IM use only; sustained action, w/ levels up to 4 wk; drug of choice for non-congenital syphilis

Penicillin G Procaine (Wycillin, Others) Uses: *Infxns of resp tract, skin/soft tissue, scarlet fever, syphilis* Acts: Bactericidal; ↓ cell wall synth. Spec-trum: PCN G-sensitive organisms that respond to low, persistent serum levels Dose: Adults. 0.6–4.8 mill units/d in ÷ doses q12–24h; give probenecid at least 30 min prior to PCN to prolong action. Peds. 25,000–50,000 units/kg/d IM ÷ daily-bid W/P: [B, M] CI: Allergy Disp: Inj 300,000, 500,000, 600,000 units/mL SE: Pain at Inj site, interstitial nephritis, anaphylaxis Notes: LA parenteral PCN; levels up to 15 h

Penicillin V (Pen-Vee K, Veetids, Others) Uses: Susceptible streptococcal infxns, otitis media, URIs, skin/soft-tissue Infxns (PCN-sensitive staphylococci) Acts: Bactericidal; ↓ cell wall synth. Spectrum: Most gram(+), including strepto-cocci Dose: Adults. 250–500 mg PO q6h, q8h, q12h. Peds. 25–50 mg/kg/25h PO in 4 doses; ↓ in renal impair; take on empty stomach W/P: [B, M] CI: Allergy Disp: Tabs 125, 250, 500 mg; susp 125, 250 mg/5 mL SE: GI upset, interstitial nephritis, anaphylaxis, convulsions Notes: Well-tolerated PO PCN; 250 mg = 400,000 units of PCN G

Pentamidine (Pentam 300, NebuPent) Uses: *Rx & prevention of PCP* Acts: ↓ DNA, RNA, phospholipid, & protein synth Dose: Rx: Adults & Peds. 4 mg/kg/24 h IV daily × 14–21 d. Prevention: Adults & Peds > 5 y. 300 mg once q4wk, give via Respirgard II nebulizer; ↓ IV w/ renal impair W/P: [C, ?] CI: Component allergy, use w/ didanosine Disp: Inj 300 mg/vial; aerosol 300 mg SE: Pancreatic cell necrosis w/ hyperglycemia; pancreatitis, CP, fatigue, dizziness, rash, GI upset, renal impair, blood dyscrasias (leukopenia, thrombocytopenia) Notes: Follow CBC, glucose, pancreatic Fxn monthly for 1st 3 mo; monitor for ↓ BP fol-lowing IV dose; prolonged use may ↑ Infxn risk

Pentazocine (Talwin, Talwin Compound, Talwin NX) [C-IV] BOX: Oral use only; severe and potentially lethal Rxns from misuse by Inj Uses: *Mod–se-vere pain* Acts: Partial narcotic agonist–antagonist Dose: Adults. 30 mg IM or IV; 50–100 mg PO q3–4h PRN. Peds 5–8 y. 15 mg IM q4h PRN. 8–14 y: 30 mg IM q4h PRN; ↓ in renal/hepatic impair W/P: [C (1st tri, D w/ prolonged use/high dose near term), +/–] CI: Allergy, ↑ ICP (unless ventilated) Disp: Talwin Compound tab 12.5 mg + 325 mg ASA; Talwin NX 50 mg + 0.5 mg naloxone; Inj 30 mg/mL

SE: Considerable dysphoria; drowsiness, GI upset, xerostomia, Szs **Notes:** 30–60 mg IM = 10 mg of morphine IM; Talwin NX has naloxone to curb abuse by nonoral route

Pentobarbital (Nembutal, Others) [C-II] **Uses:** *Insomnia (short-term), convulsions*, sedation, induce coma w/ severe head injury **Acts:** Barbiturate **Dose:** *Adults.* *Sedative:* 150–200 mg IM × 1100 mg IV, repeat PRN to 500 mg/max. *Hypnotic:* 100–200 mg PO or PR hs PRN. *Induced coma:* Load 5–10 mg/kg IV, w/ maint 1–3 mg/kg/h IV. *Peds. Induced coma:* As adult **W/P:** [D, +/–] Severe hepatic impair **CI:** Allergy **Disp:** Caps 50, 100 mg; elixir 18.2 mg/5 mL (= 20 mg pentobarbital); supp 30, 60, 120, 200 mg; Inj 50 mg/mL **SE:** Resp depression, ↓ BP w/ aggressive IV use for cerebral edema; ↓ HR, ↓ BP, sedation, lethargy, resp ↓, hangover, rash, SJS, blood dyscrasias **Notes:** Tolerance to sedative–hypnotic effect w/in 1–2 wk

Pentosan Polysulfate Sodium (Elmiron) **Uses:** *Relieve pain/discomfort w/ interstitial cystitis* **Acts:** Bladder wall buffer **Dose:** 100 mg PO tid; on empty stomach w/ H$_2$O 1 h ac or 2 h pc **W/P:** [B, ?/–] **CI:** Allergy **Disp:** Caps 100 mg **SE:** Alopecia, N/D, HA, ↑ LFTs, anticoagulant effects, ↓ plts, rectal bleed **Notes:** Reassess after 3 mo

Pentoxifylline (Trental) **Uses:** *Rx Sxs of peripheral vascular Dz* **Acts:** ↓ Blood cell viscosity, restores RBC flexibility **Dose:** *Adults.* 400 mg PO tid pc; Rx min 8 wk for effect; ↓ to bid w/ GI/CNS SEs **W/P:** [C, +/–] **CI:** Cerebral/retinal hemorrhage, methylxanthine (caffeine) intolerance **Disp:** Tabs CR 400 mg; Tabs ER 400 mg **SE:** Dizziness, HA, GI upset

Perindopril Erbumine (Aceon) **BOX:** ACE inhib can cause death to developing fetus; D/C immediately w/ PRG **Uses:** *HTN*, CHF, DN, post-MI **Acts:** ACE inhib **Dose:** 4–8 mg/d ÷ dose; 16 mg/d max; avoid w/ food; ↓ w/ elderly/renal impair **W/P:** [C (1st tri), D 2nd & 3rd tri), ?/–] ACE inhib-induced angioedema **CI:** Bilateral RAS, primary hyperaldosteronism **Disp:** Tabs 2, 4, 8 mg **SE:** Weakness, HA, ↓ BP, dizziness, GI upset, cough **Notes:** OK w/ diuretics

Permethrin (Nix, Elimite) [OTC] **Uses:** *Rx lice/scabies* **Acts:** Pediculicide **Dose:** *Adults & Peds.* *Lice:* Saturate hair & scalp; allow 10 min before rinsing. *Scabies:* Apply cream head to toe; leave for 8–14 h, wash w/ H$_2$O **W/P:** [B, ?/–] **CI:** Allergy **Disp:** Topical lotion 1%; cream 5% **SE:** Local irritation **Notes:** Sprays available (Rid, A200, Nix) to disinfect clothing, bedding, combs, & brushes; lotion not OK in peds < 2 y; may repeat after 7 d

Perphenazine (Trilafon) **Uses:** *Psychotic disorders, severe N*, intractable hiccups **Acts:** Phenothiazine, blocks brain dopaminergic receptors **Dose:** *Adults.* *Antipsychotic:* 4–16 mg PO tid; max 64 mg/d. *Hiccups:* 5 mg IM q6h PRN or 1 mg IV at intervals not < 1–2 mg/min, 5 mg max. *Peds 1–6 y.* 4–6 mg/d PO in ÷ doses. *6–12 y:* 6 mg/d PO in ÷ doses. > *12 y:* 4–16 mg PO bid-qid; ↓ in hepatic Insuff **W/P:** [C, ?/–] NAG, severe ↑/↓ BP **CI:** Phenothiazine sensitivity, BM depression, severe liver or cardiac Dz **Disp:** Tabs 2, 4, 8, 16 mg; PO conc 16 mg/5 mL; Inj 5 mg/mL **SE:** ↓ BP, ↑/↓ HR, EPS, drowsiness, Szs, photosens, skin discoloration, blood dyscrasias, constipation

Phenazopyridine (Pyridium, Azo-Standard, Urogesic, Many Others)
Uses: *Lower urinary tract irritation* **Acts:** Anesthetic on urinary tract mucosa **Dose:** *Adults.* 100–200 mg PO tid; 2 d max w/ antibiotics for UTI; ↓ w/ renal Insuff **W/P:** [B, ?] Hepatic Dz **CI:** Renal failure **Disp:** Tabs 100, 200 mg **SE:** GI disturbances, red-orange urine color (can stain clothing, contacts), HA, dizziness, acute renal failure, methemoglobinemia, tinting of sclera/skin **Notes:** Take w/ food

Phenelzine (Nardil) **BOX:** Antidepressants ↑ risk of suicidal thinking and behavior in children and adolescents w/ major depressive disorder and other psychological disorders; not for peds use **Uses:** *Depression*, bulimia **Acts:** MAOI **Dose:** *Adults.* 15 mg PO tid, ↑ to 60–90 mg/d ÷ doses. *Elderly:* 15–60 mg/d ÷ doses **W/P:** [C, –] Interacts w/ SSRI, ergots, triptans **CI:** CHF, Hx liver Dz, pheochromocytoma **Disp:** Tabs 15 mg **SE:** Postural ↓ BP; edema, dizziness, sedation, rash, sexual dysfunction, xerostomia, constipation, urinary retention **Notes:** 2–4 wk for effect; avoid tyramine-containing foods (e.g., cheeses)

Phenobarbital [C-IV] **Uses:** *Sz disorders*, insomnia, anxiety **Acts:** Barbiturate **Dose:** *Adults. Sedative–hypnotic:* 30–120 mg/d PO or IM PRN. *Anticonvulsant:* Load 10–12 mg/kg in 3 ÷ doses, then 1–3 mg/kg/24 h PO, IM, or IV. *Peds. Sedative–hypnotic:* 2–3 mg/kg/24 h PO or IM hs PRN. *Anticonvulsant:* Load 15–20 mg/kg ÷ in 2 equal doses 4 h apart, then 3–5 mg/kg/24h PO ÷ in 2–3 doses; ↓ w/ CrCl < 10 mL/min **W/P:** [D, M] **CI:** Porphyria, hepatic impair, dyspnea, airway obst **Disp:** Tabs 15, 16, 30, 32, 60, 65, 100 mg; elixir 15, 20 mg/5 mL; Inj 30, 60, 65, 130 mg/mL **SE:** ↓ HR, ↓ BP, hangover, SJS, blood dyscrasias, resp depression **Notes:** Tolerance develops to sedation; paradoxic hyperactivity seen in ped pts; long 1/2-life allows single daily dosing. Levels: *Trough:* Just before next dose. *Therapeutic: Trough:* 15–40 mcg/mL; *Toxic: Trough:* > 40 mcg/mL *1/2-life:* 40–120 h

Phenylephrine, Nasal (Neo-Synephrine Nasal) (OTC) **BOX:** Not for use in Peds < 2 y **Uses:** *Nasal congestion* **Acts:** α-Adrenergic agonist **Dose:** *Adults.* 1–2 sprays/nostril q4h (usual 0.25%) PRN. *Peds 2–6 y.* 0.125% 1 drop/ nostril q2–4h. *6–12 y:* 1–2 sprays/nostril q4h 0.25% 2–3 drops **W/P:** [C, +/–] HTN, acute pancreatitis, hep, coronary Dz, NAG, hyperthyroidism **CI:** ↓ HR, arrhythmias **Disp:** Nasal soln 0.125, 0.25, 0.5, 1%; liq 7.5 mg/5 mL; drops 2.5 mg/mL **SE:** Arrhythmias, HTN, nasal irritation, dryness, sneezing, rebound congestion w/ prolonged use, HA **Notes:** Do not use > 3 d

Phenylephrine, Ophthalmic (Neo-Synephrine Ophthalmic, AK-Dilate, Zincfrin [OTC]) **Uses:** *Mydriasis, ocular redness [OTC], perioperative mydriasis, posterior synechiae, uveitis w/ posterior synechiae* **Acts:** α-Adrenergic agonist **Dose:** *Adults. Redness:* 1 gtt 0.12% q3–4h PRN. *Exam mydriasis:* 1 gtt 2.5% (15 min–1 h for effect). *Pre-op:* 1 gtt 2.5–10% 30–60 min pre-op. *Ocular disorders:* 1 gtt 2.5–10% daily-tid *Peds.* As adult, only use 2.5% for exam, pre-op, and ocular conditions **W/P:** [C, May cause late-term fetal anoxia/↓ HR, +/–] HTN, w/ elderly w/ CAD **CI:** NAG **Disp:** Ophthal soln 0.12%

(Zincfrin OTC), 2.5, 10% **SE:** Tearing, HA, irritation, eye pain, photophobia, arrhythmia, tremor

Phenylephrine, Oral (Sudafed PE, SudoGest PE, Nasop, Lusonal, AH-chew D, Sudafed PE Quick Dissolve) (OTC) **BOX:** Not for use in peds < 2 y **Uses:** *Nasal congestion* **Acts:** α-Adrenergic agonist **Dose:** *Adults.* 10–20 mg PO q4h PRN, max 60 mg/d. *Peds.* 5 mg PO q4h PRN, max 60 mg/d **W/P:** [C, +/–] HTN, acute pancreatitis, hep, coronary Dz, NAG, hyperthyroidism **CI:** MAOI w/in 14 d, NAG, severe ↑ BP or CAD, urinary retention **Disp:** Liq 7.5 mg/5 mL; drops 2.5 mg/mL; tabs 5, 10 mg; chew tabs 10 mg; tabs once daily 10 mg; strips 10 mg **SE:** Arrhythmias, HTN, HA, agitation, anxiety, tremor, palpitations

Phenylephrine, Systemic (Neo-Synephrine) **BOX:** Prescribers should be aware of full prescribing information before use **Uses:** *Vascular failure in shock, allergy, or drug-induced ↓ BP* **Acts:** α-Adrenergic agonist **Dose:** *Adults. Mild–mod* ↓ BP: 2–5 mg IM or SQ ↑ BP for 2 h; 0.1–0.5 mg IV elevates BP for 15 min. *Severe* ↓ *BP/shock:* Cont Inf at 100–180 mcg/min; after BP stable, maint 40–60 mcg/min. *Peds.* ↓ *BP:* 5–20 mcg/kg/dose IV q10–15min or 0.1–0.5 mcg/kg/min IV Inf, titrate to effect **W/P:** [C, +/–] HTN, acute pancreatitis, hep, coronary Dz, NAG, hyperthyroidism **CI:** ↓ HR, arrhythmias **Disp:** Inj 10 mg/mL **SE:** Arrhythmias, HTN, peripheral vasoconstriction ↑ w/ oxytocin, MAOIs, & TCAs; HA, weakness, necrosis, ↓ renal perfusion **Notes:** Restore blood vol if loss has occurred; use large veins to avoid extrav; phentolamine 10 mg in 10–15 mL of NS for local Inj to Rx extrav

Phenytoin (Dilantin) **Uses:** *Sz disorders* **Acts:** ↓ Sz spread in the motor cortex **Dose:** *Adults & Peds. Load:* 15–20 mg/kg IV, 50 mg/min max or PO in 400-mg doses at 4-h intervals; *Adults. Maint:* Initial 200 mg PO or IV bid or 300 mg hs then follow levels; alternatively 5–7 mg/kg/d based on IBW ÷ daily-tid, *Peds. Maint:* 4–7 mg/kg/24h PO or IV ÷ daily-bid; avoid PO susp (erratic absorption) **W/P:** [D, +] **CI:** Heart block, sinus bradycardia **Disp:** *Dilantin Infatab:* chew 50 mg. *Dilantin/Phenytek:* caps 100 mg; caps, ER 30, 100, 200, 300 mg; susp 125 mg/5 mL; Inj 50 mg/mL. **SE:** Nystagmus/ataxia early signs of tox; gum hyperplasia w/ long-term use. *IV:* ↓ BP, ↓ HR, arrhythmias, phlebitis; peripheral neuropathy, rash, blood dyscrasias, SJS **Notes:** Levels: *Trough:* Just before next dose. *Therapeutic:* 10–20 mcg/mL *Toxic:* > 20 mcg/mL Phenytoin albumin bound, levels = bound & free phenytoin; w/ ↓ albumin & azotemia, low levels may be therapeutic (nl free levels); do not change dosage at intervals < 7–10 d; hold tube feeds 1 h before and after dose if using oral susp; avoid large dose ↑

Physostigmine (Antilirium) **Uses:** *Antidote for TCA, atropine, & scopolamine OD; glaucoma* **Acts:** Reversible cholinesterase inhib **Dose:** *Adults.* 0.5–2 mg IV or IM q20 min *Peds.* 0.01–0.03 mg/kg/dose IV q5–10 min up to 2 mg total PRN **W/P:** [C, ?] **CI:** GI/GU obst, CV Dz, asthma **Disp:** Inj 1 mg/mL **SE:** Rapid IV administration associated w/ Szs; cholinergic SEs; sweating, salivation, lacrimation, GI upset, asystole, changes in HR **Notes:** Excessive readministration can result in cholinergic crisis; crisis reversed w/ atropine

Phytonadione [Vitamin K] (AquaMEPHYTON, Others) Uses: *Coagulation disorders d/t faulty formation of factors II, VII, IX, X*; hyperalimentation **Acts:** Cofactor for production of factors II, VII, IX, & X **Dose:** *Adults & Peds. Anticoagulant-induced prothrombin deficiency:* 1–10 mg PO or IV slowly. *Hyperalimentation:* 10 mg IM or IV q wk. *Infants:* 0.5–1 mg/dose IM, SQ, or PO **W/P:** [C, +] **CI:** Allergy **Disp:** Tabs 5 mg; Inj 2, 10 mg/mL **SE:** Anaphylaxis from IV dosage; give IV slowly; GI upset (PO), Inj site Rxns **Notes:** w/ Parenteral Rx, 1st change in PT/INR usually seen in 12–24 h; use makes re-warfarinization more difficult

Pimecrolimus (Elidel) BOX: Associated w/ rare skin malignancies and lymphoma, limit to area, not for age < 2 y Uses: *Atopic dermatitis* refractory, severe perianal itching **Acts:** Inhibits T-lymphocytes **Dose:** *Adults & Peds > 2 y.* Apply bid; use at least 1 wk following resolution **W/P:** [C, ?/–] w/ Local Infxn, lymphadenopathy; immunocompromised; avoid in pts < 2 y **CI:** Allergy component, < 2 y **Disp:** Cream 1% **SE:** Phototox, local irritation/burning, flu-like Sxs, may ↑ malignancy **Notes:** Use on dry skin only; wash hands after; 2nd-line/short-term use only

Pimozide (Orap) BOX: ↑ Mortality in elderly w/ dementia-related psychosis Uses: * Tourette Dz* agitation, psychosis **Action:** typical antipsychotic, dopamine antagonist **Dose:** 10 mg PO q day, ↓ to 5 mg w/ SE or hepatic impair **W/P:** [D, /–] NAG, elderly, hepatic impair, neurologic Dz, **CI:** compound hypersens, CNS depression, coma, dysrhythmia, ↑ QT syndrome, w/ QT prolonging drugs, ↓ K, ↓ Mg, w/ CYP3A4 inhib (Table 10, p 301) **Disp:** Tabs 1, 2 mg **SE:** CNS (somnolence, agitation, others), rash, xerostomia, weakness, rigidity, visual changes, constipation, ↑ salivation, akathisia, tardive dyskinesia, neuroleptic malignant syndrome, ↑ QT **Notes:** ✓ ECG

Pindolol (Visken) Uses: *HTN* **Acts:** β-Adrenergic receptor blocker, β₁, β₂, ISA **Dose:** 5–10 mg bid, 60 mg/d max; ↓ in hepatic/renal failure **W/P:** [B (1st tri; D 2nd/3rd tri), +/–] **CI:** Uncompensated CHF, cardiogenic shock, ↓ HR, heart block, asthma, COPD **Disp:** Tabs 5, 10 mg **SE:** Insomnia, dizziness, fatigue, edema, GI upset, dyspnea; fluid retention may exacerbate CHF

Pioglitazone (Actos) BOX: May cause or worsen CHF Uses: *Type 2 DM* **Acts:** ↑ Insulin sensitivity, a thiazolidinedione **Dose:** 15–45 mg/d PO **W/P:** [C, –] w/ Hx bladder CA; do not use w/ active bladder CA **CI:** CHF, hepatic impair **Disp:** Tabs 15, 30, 45 mg **SE:** Wgt gain, myalgia, URI, HA, hypoglycemia, edema, ↑ fracture risk in women; may ↑ bladder CA risk

Pioglitazone/Metformin (ACTOplus Met, ACTOplus MET XR) BOX: Metformin can cause lactic acidosis, fatal in 50% of cases; pioglitazone may cause or worsen CHF Uses: *Type 2 DM as adjunct to diet and exercise* **Acts:** Combined ↑ insulin sensitivity w/ ↓ hepatic glucose release **Dose:** Initial 1 tab PO daily or bid, titrate; max daily pioglitazone 45 mg & metformin 2550 mg; XR: 1 tab PO daily w/ evening meal; max daily pioglitazone 45 mg & metformin XR 2550 mg, metformin ER 2000 mg; give w/ meals **W/P:** [C, –] Stop w/ radiologic IV contrast agents; w/ Hx bladder CA; do not use w/ active bladder CA **CI:** CHF, renal impair, acidosis **Disp:** Tabs (pioglitazone mg/metformin): 15/500, 15/850; Tabs XR (pioglitazone mg/metformin ER mg) 15/1000, 30/1000 mg **SE:** Lactic acidosis, CHF, ↓ glucose, edema, wgt gain, myalgia, URI, HA, GI upset, liver damage **Notes:** Follow LFTs; ↑ fracture risk in women receiving pioglitazone; may ↑ bladder CA risk

Piperacillin (Pipracil) **Uses:** *Infxns of skin, bone, resp, & urinary tract, abd, sepsis* **Acts:** 4th-Gen PCN; bactericidal; ↓ cell wall synth. *Spectrum:* Primarily gram(+), better *Enterococcus, H. influenzae,* not staphylococci; gram(−) *E. coli, Proteus, Shigella, Pseudomonas,* not β-lactamase producing **Dose:** *Adults.* 2–4 g IV q4–6h. *Peds.* 200–300 mg/kg/d IV + q4–6h; ↓ in renal failure **W/P:** [B, M] **CI:** PCN/β-lactam sensitivity **Disp:** Powder for Inj: 2, 3, 4, 40 g **SE:** ↓ Plt aggregation, interstitial nephritis, renal Insuff, anaphylaxis, hemolytic anemia **Notes:** Often used w/ aminoglycoside

Piperacillin–Tazobactam (Zosyn) **Uses:** *Infxns of skin, bone, resp & urinary tract, abd, sepsis* **Acts:** 4th-Gen PCN plus β-lactamase inhib; bactericidal; ↓ cell wall synth. *Spectrum:* Good gram(+), excellent gram(−); anaerobes & β-lactamase producers **Dose:** *Adults.* 3.375–4.5 g IV q6h; ↓ in renal Insuff **W/P:** [B, M] **CI:** PCN or β-lactam sensitivity **Disp:** *Powder for Inj:* Frozen, premix Inj 3.25, 3.375, 4.5 g **SE:** D, HA, insomnia, GI upset, serum sickness-like Rxn, pseudomembranous colitis **Notes:** Often used in combo w/ aminoglycoside

Pirbuterol (Maxair) **Uses:** *Prevention & Rx reversible bronchospasm* **Acts:** β₂-Adrenergic agonist **Dose:** 2 Inh q4–6h; max 12 Inh/d **W/P:** [C, ?/–] **Disp:** Aerosol 0.2 mg/actuation (contains ozone-depleting CFCs; will be gradually removed from US market) **SE:** Nervousness, restlessness, trembling, HA, taste changes, tachycardia **Note:** Teach pt proper inhaler technique

Piroxicam (Feldene) **BOX:** May ↑ risk of cardiovascular CV events & GI bleeding **Uses:** *Arthritis & pain* **Acts:** NSAID; ↓ prostaglandins **Dose:** 10–20 mg/d **W/P:** [B (1st tri; D if 3rd tri or near term), +] GI bleeding **CI:** ASA/ NSAID sensitivity **Disp:** Caps 10, 20 mg **SE:** Dizziness, rash, GI upset, edema, acute renal failure, peptic ulcer

Pitavastatin (Livalo) **Uses:** *Reduce elevated total cholesterol* **Action:** Statin, inhibits HMG-CoA reductase **Dose:** 1–4 mg once/d w/o regard to meals; Cr Cl 30–60 mg/min start 1 mg w/ 2 mg max **W/P:** [X, –/] May cause myopathy and rhabdomyolysis **CI:** Active liver Dz, w/ lopinavir/ritonavir/cyclosporine, severe renal impair not on dialysis **Disp:** Tabs 1, 2, 4 mg **SE:** Muscle pain, back pain, joint pain, and constipation, ↑ LFTs **Notes:** ✓ LFTs; OK w/ grapefruit

Plasma Protein Fraction (Plasmanate, Others) **Uses:** *Shock & ↓ BP* **Acts:** Plasma vol expander **Dose:** *Adults. Initial:* 250–500 mL IV (not > 10 mL/min); subsequent Inf based on response. *Peds.* 10–15 mL/kg/dose IV; subsequent Inf based on response **W/P:** [C, +] **CI:** Renal Insuff, CHF, cardiopulmonary bypass **Disp:** Inj 5% **SE:** ↓ BP w/ rapid Inf; hypocoagulability, metabolic acidosis, PE **Notes:** 130–160 mEq Na⁺²/L; not substitute for RBC

Plerixafor (Mozobil) **Uses:** *Mobilize stem cells for ABMT in lymphoma and myeloma in combo w/ G-CSF* **Action:** Hematopoietic stem cell mobilizer **Dose:** 0.24 mg/kg SQ daily; max 40 mg/d); CrCl < 50 mL/min: 0.16 mg/kg, max

27 mg/d) **W/P:** [D, /?] **CI: Disp:** IV: 20 mg/mL (1.2 mL) **SE:** HA, N/V/D, Inj site rxns, ↑ WBC, ↓ plt **Notes:** Give w/ filgrastim 10 mcg/kg

Pneumococcal 13-Valent Conjugate Vaccine (Prevnar 13)   Uses:
Immunization against pneumococcal Infxns in infants & children **Acts:** Active immunization **Dose:** 0.5 mL IM/dose; series of 4 doses; 1st dose age 2 mo; then 4 mo, 6 mo, and 12–15 mo; if previous *Prevnar* switch to *Prevnar 13*; if completed *Prevnar* series, supplemental dose *Prevnar 13* at least 8 wk after last *Prevnar* dose **W/P:** [C, +] w/ ↓ plt **CI:** Sensitivity to components/diphtheria toxoid, febrile illness **Disp:** Inj **SE:** Local Rxns, anorexia, fever, irritability, ↑/↓ sleep, V, D **Notes:** Keep epi (1:1000) available for Rxns; replaces *Prevnar* (has additional spectrum); does not replace *Pneumovax-23* in age > 24 mo w/ immunosuppression

Pneumococcal Vaccine, Polyvalent (Pneumovax-23)   Uses:
Immunization against pneumococcal Infxns in pts at high risk (all pts > 65 y, also asplenia, sickle cell Dz, HIV, and other immunocompromised and w/ chronic illnesses) **Acts:** Active immunization **Dose:** 0.5 mL IM or SQ **W/P:** [C, ?] **CI:** Do not vaccinate during immunosuppressive Rx **Disp:** Inj 0.5 mL **SE:** Fever, Inj site Rxn also hemolytic anemia w/ other heme conditions, ↓ plt w/ stable ITP, anaphylaxis, Guillain-Barré synd **Notes:** Keep epi (1:1000) available for Rxns. Revaccinate q3–5 y if very high risk (e.g., asplenia, nephrotic synd), consider revaccination if > 6 y since initial or if previously vaccinated w/ 14-valent vaccine

Podophyllin (Podocon-25, Condylox Gel 0.5%, Condylox)   Uses:
Topical Rx of benign growths (genital & perianal warts [condylomata acuminata], papillomas, fibromas) **Acts:** Direct antimitotic effect; exact mechanism unknown **Dose:** *Condylox gel & Condylox:* Apply bid for 3 consecutive d/wk for 4 wk; 0.5 mL/d max; *Podocon-25:* Use sparingly on the lesion, leave on for 1–4 h, thoroughly wash off **W/P:** [X, ?] Immunosuppression **CI:** DM, bleeding lesions **Disp:** *Podocon-25* (w/ benzoin) 15-mL bottles; *Condylox gel* 0.5% 35-g clear gel; *Condylox soln* 0.5% 35-g clear **SE:** Local Rxns, sig absorption; anemias, tachycardia, paresthesias, GI upset, renal/hepatic damage **Notes:** Podocon-25 applied by the clinician; do not dispense directly to pt

Polyethylene Glycol [PEG]-Electrolyte Soln (GoLYTELY, Colyte)
Uses: *Bowel prep prior to examination or surgery* **Acts:** Osmotic cathartic **Dose:** **Adults.** Following 3–4-h fast, drink 240 mL of soln q10min until 4 L consumed or until BMs are clear. **Peds.** 25–40 mL/kg/h for 4–10 h **W/P:** [C, ?] **CI:** GI obst, bowel perforation, megacolon, ulcerative colitis **Disp:** Powder for recons to 4 L **SE:** Cramping or N, bloating **Notes:** 1st BM should occur in approximately 1 h; chilled soln more palatable

Polyethylene Glycol [PEG] 3350 (MiraLAX [OTC])   Uses: *Occasional
constipation* **Acts:** Osmotic laxative **Dose:** 17-g powder (1 heaping tsp) in 8 oz (1 cup) of H$_2$O & drink; max 14 d **W/P:** [C, ?] Rule out bowel obst before use **CI:** GI obst, allergy to PEG **Disp:** Powder for reconstitution; bottle cap holds 17 g **SE:** Upset

stomach, bloating, cramping, gas, severe D, hives **Notes:** Can add to H_2O, juice, soda, coffee, or tea

Polymyxin B & Hydrocortisone (Otobiotic Otic) **Uses:** *Superficial bacterial infxns of external ear canal* **Acts:** Antibiotic/anti-inflammatory combo **Dose:** 4 gtt in ear(s) tid-qid **W/P:** [B, ?] **CI:** Component sensitivity **Disp:** Soln polymyxin B 10,000 units/hydrocortisone 0.5%/mL **SE:** Local irritation **Notes:** Useful in neomycin allergy

Posaconazole (Noxafil) **Uses:** *Prevent Aspergillus and Candida infxns in severely immunocompromised; Rx oropharyngeal candida* **Acts:** ↓ Cell membrane ergosterol synth **Dose:** *Adults.* Invasive fungal prophylaxis: 200 mg PO bid. *Oropharyngeal candidiasis:* 100 mg PO daily × 13 d, if refractory 400 mg PO bid *Peds > 13 y.* 200 mg PO tid; take w/ meal **W/P:** [C, ?] Multiple drug interactions; ↑ QT, cardiac Dzs, severe renal/liver impair **CI:** Component hypersens; w/ many drugs including alfuzosin, astemizole, alprazolam, phenothiazines, terfenadine, triazolam, others **Disp:** Soln 40 mg/mL **SE:** ↑ QT, ↑ LFTs, hepatic failure, fever, N/V/D, HA, Abd pain, anemia, ↓ plt, ↓ K⁺ rash, dyspnea, cough, anorexia, fatigue **Notes:** Monitor LFTs, CBC, lytes

Potassium Citrate (Urocit-K) **Uses:** *Alkalinize urine, prevention of urinary stones (uric acid, calcium stones if hypocitraturic)* **Acts:** Urinary alkalinizer **Dose:** 1 packet dissolved in H_2O or 15–30 mL pc & hs 10–20 mEq PO tid w/ meals, max 100 mEq/d **W/P:** [A, +] **CI:** Severe renal impair, dehydration, ↑ K⁺, peptic ulcer; w/ K⁺-sparing diuretics, salt substitutes **Disp:** 540, 1080 mg tabs **SE:** GI upset, ↓ Ca²⁺, ↑ K⁺, metabolic alkalosis **Notes:** Tabs 540 mg = 5 mEq, 1080 mg = 10 mEq

Potassium Citrate & Citric Acid (Polycitra-K) **Uses:** *Alkalinize urine, prevent urinary stones (uric acid, CA stones if hypocitraturic)* **Acts:** Urinary alkalinizer **Dose:** 10–20 mEq PO tid w/ meals, max 100 mEq/d **W/P:** [A, +] **CI:** Severe renal impair, dehydration, ↑ K⁺, peptic ulcer; w/ use of K⁺-sparing diuretics or salt substitutes **Disp:** Soln 10 mEq/5 mL; powder 30 mEq/packet **SE:** GI upset, ↓ Ca²⁺, ↑ K⁺, metabolic alkalosis

Potassium Iodide [Lugol's Soln] (Iosat, SSKI, Thyro-Block, Thyro-Safe, ThyroShield) [OTC] **Uses:** *Thyroid storm*, ↓ vascularity before thyroid surgery, block thyroid uptake of radioactive iodine (nuclear scans or nuclear emergency), thin bronchial secretions **Acts:** Iodine supl **Dose:** *Adults & Peds > 2 y.* *Pre-op thyroidectomy:* 50–250 mg PO tid (2–6 gtt strong iodine soln); give 10 d pre-op. *Protection:* 130 mg/d. *Peds. Protection:* < 1 y: 16.25 mg q day. *1 mo–3y:* 32.5 mg q day. *3–12 y:* 1/2 adult dose **W/P:** [D, +] ↑ K⁺, TB, PE, bronchitis, renal impair **CI:** Iodine sensitivity **Disp:** Tabs 65, 130 mg; soln (saturated soln of potassium iodide [SSKI]) 1 g/mL; Lugol Soln, strong iodine 100 mL/1 g; syrup 325 mg/5 mL **SE:** Fever, HA, urticaria, angioedema, goiter, GI upset, eosinophilia **Notes:** w/ Nuclear radiation emergency, give until radiation exposure no longer exists

Potassium Supplements (Kaon, Kaochlor, K-Lor, Slow-K, Micro-K, Klorvess, Others) **Uses:** *Prevention or Rx of ↓ K⁺* (e.g., diuretic use) **Acts:**

K$^+$ supl **Dose: *Adults.*** 20–100 mEq/d PO ÷ daily-bid; IV 10–20 mEq/h, max 40 mEq/h & 150 mEq/d (monitor K$^+$ levels frequently and in presence of continuous ECG monitoring w/ high-dose IV). ***Peds.*** Calculate K$^+$ deficit; 1–3 mEq/kg/d PO ÷ daily–qid; IV max dose 0.5–1 mEq/kg/× 1-2 h **W/P:** [A, +] Renal Insuff, use w/ NSAIDs & ACE inhib **CI:** ↑ K$^+$ **Disp:** PO forms (Table 6, p 296); Inj **SE:** GI irritation; ↓ HR, ↑ K$^+$, heart block **Notes:** Mix powder & liq w/ beverage (unsalted tomato juice, etc); swallow SR tabs must be swallowed whole; follow monitor K$^+$; Cl$^-$ salt OK w/ alkalosis; w/ acidosis use acetate, bicarbonate, citrate, or gluconate salt; Do not administer IV K$^+$ undiluted

Pralatrexate (Folotyn) **BOX:** Administer only by physician experienced in chemotherapy. **Uses:** *Tx refractory T-cell lymphoma* **Action:** Folate analogue metabolic inhibitor; ↓ dihydrofolate reductase **Dose: *Adults.*** IV push over 3–5 min: 30 mg/m^2 once weekly for 6 wks **W/P:** [D, –] **Disp:** Inj 20 mg/mL (1 mL, 2mL) **SE:** ↓ plt, anemia, ↓ WBC, mucositis, N/V/D, edema, fever, fatigue, rash **Notes:** Give folic acid supplements prior to and during therapy

Pramipexole (Mirapex, Mirapex ER) **Uses:** *Parkinson Dz (Mirapex, Mirapex ER)*, restless leg synd *(Mirapex)* **Acts:** Dopamine agonist **Dose:** *Mirapex:* 1.5–4.5 mg/d PO, initial 0.375 mg/d in 3 ÷ doses; titrate slowly; *RLS:* 0.125–0.5 mg PO q P.M. *Mirapex ER:* Start 0.375 PO daily, ↑ dose every 5–7 d to 0.75, then by 0.75 mg to max 4.5 mg/d **W/P:** [C, ?/–] Daytime falling asleep, ↓ BP **CI:** None **Disp:** *Mirapex:* Tabs 0.125, 0.25, 0.5, 0.75, 1, 1.5 mg; *Mirapex ER:* 0.375, 0.75, 1.5, 3, 4.5 mg **SE:** Somnolence, N, constipation, dizziness, fatigue, hallucinations, dry mouth, muscle spasms, edema

Pramoxine (Anusol Ointment, ProctoFoam-NS, Others) **Uses:** *Relief of pain & itching from hemorrhoids, anorectal surgery*; topical for burns & dermatosis **Acts:** Topical anesthetic **Dose:** Apply freely to anal area q3h **W/P:** [C, ?] **Disp:** [OTC] All 1%; foam *(ProctoFoam-NS)*, cream, oint, lotion, gel, pads, spray **SE:** Contact dermatitis, mucosal thinning w/ chronic use

Pramoxine + Hydrocortisone (Enzone, ProctoFoam-HC) **Uses:** *Relief of pain & itching from hemorrhoids* **Acts:** Topical anesthetic, anti-inflammatory **Dose:** Apply freely to anal area tid-qid **W/P:** [C, ?/–] **Disp:** *Cream:* pramoxine 1% acetate 0.5/1%; *foam:* pramoxine 1% hydrocortisone 1%; *lotion:* pramoxine 1% hydrocortisone 0.25/1/2.5%, pramoxine 2.5% & hydrocortisone 1% **SE:** Contact dermatitis, mucosal thinning w/ chronic use

Prasugrel Hydrochloride (Effient) **BOX:** Can cause significant, sometimes fatal, bleeding; do not use w/ planned CABG, w/ active bleeding, Hx TIA or stroke or pts > 75 y **Uses:** *↓ thrombotic CV events (e.g., stent thrombosis)*, administer ASAP in ECC setting w/ high-risk ST depression or T-wave inversion w/ planned PCI **Acts:** ↓ Plt aggregation **Dose:** 10 mg/d; wgt < 60 kg, consider 5 mg/d; 60 mg PO loading dose in ECC; 2009 ACCF/AHA/SCAI joint STEMI/PCI guidelines: use at least 12 mo w/ cardiac stent (bare or drug eluting); consider > 15 mo w/ drug eluting stent **W/P:** [B, ?] Active bleeding; ↑ bleed risk; w/ CYP3A4 substrates

CI: Coag disorders, active intracranial bleeding or PUD; Hx TIA/stroke **Disp:** Tabs 5, 10 mg **SE:** ↑ bleeding time, ↑ BP, GI intolerance, HA, dizziness, rash, ↓ WBC **Notes:** Plt aggregation to baseline ~ 7 d after D/C, plt transfusion reverses acutely

Pravastatin (Pravachol) Uses: *↓ Cholesterol* **Acts:** HMG-CoA reductase inhibitor **Dose:** 10–80 mg PO hs; ↓ in sig renal/hepatic impair **W/P:** [X, –] w/ Gemfibrozil **CI:** Liver Dz or persistent LFTs ↑ **Disp:** Tabs 10, 20, 40, 80 mg **SE:** Use caution w/ concurrent gemfibrozil; HA, GI upset, hep, myopathy, renal failure **Note:** OK w/ grapefruit juice

Prazosin (Minipress) Uses: *HTN* **Acts:** Peripherally acting α-adrenergic blocker **Dose:** *Adults.* 1 mg PO tid; can ↑ to 20 mg/d max PRN. *Peds.* 0.05–0.1 mg/kg/d in 3 ÷ doses; max 0.5 mg/kg/d **W/P:** [C, ?] use w/ phosphodiesterase-5 (PDE5) inhib (e.g., sildenafil) can cause ↓ BP **CI:** Component allergy, concurrent use of PDE5 inhib **Disp:** Caps 1, 2, 5 mg; tabs ER 2.5, 5 mg **SE:** Dizziness, edema, palpitations, fatigue, GI upset **Notes:** Can cause orthostatic ↓ BP, take the 1st dose hs; tolerance develops to this effect; tachyphylaxis may result

Prednisolone (See Steroids, p 244, and Table 2, p 283)

Prednisone (See Steroids, p 244, and Table 2, p 283)

Pregabalin (Lyrica) Uses: *DM peripheral neuropathy pain; postherpetic neuralgia; fibromyalgia; adjunct w/ adult partial onset Szs* **Acts:** Nerve transmission modulator, antinociceptive, antiseizure effect; mechanism ?; related to gabapentin **Dose:** *Neuropathic pain:* 50 mg PO tid, ↑ to 300 mg/d w/in 1 wk based on response, 300 mg/d max *Postherpetic neuralgia:* 75–150 mg bid, or 50–100 mg tid; start 75 mg bid or 50 mg tid; ↑ to 300 mg/d w/in 1 wk PRN; if pain persists after 2–4 wk, ↑ to 600 mg/d. *Epilepsy:* Start 150 mg/d (75 mg bid or 50 mg tid) may ↑ to max 600 mg/d; ↓ w/ CrCl < 60; w/ or w/o food **W/P:** [C, –] w/ Sig renal impair (see PI), w/ elderly & severe CHF avoid abrupt D/C w/ PRG **Disp:** Caps 25, 50, 75, 100, 150, 200, 225, 300 mg; soln 20 mg/mL **SE:** Dizziness, drowsiness, xerostomia, edema, blurred vision, wgt gain, difficulty concentrating; suicidal ideation **Notes:** w/ D/C, taper over at least 1 wk

Probenecid (Benemid, Others) Uses: *Prevent gout & hyperuricemia; extends levels of PCNs & cephalosporins* **Acts:** Uricosuric, renal tubular blocker of organic anions **Dose:** *Adults. Gout:* 250 mg bid × 1 wk, then 0.5 g PO bid; can ↑ by 500 mg/mo up to 2–3 g/d. *Antibiotic effect:* 1–2 g PO 30 min before dose. *Peds > 2 y.* 25 mg/kg, then 40 mg/kg/d PO ÷ qid **W/P:** [B, ?] **CI:** High-dose ASA, mod–severe renal impair, age < 2 y **Disp:** Tabs 500 mg **SE:** GI upset, rash, pruritus, dizziness, blood dyscrasias **Notes:** Do not use during acute gout attack

Procainamide (Pronestyl, Pronestyl SR, Procanbid) **BOX:** Positive ANA titer or SLE w/ prolonged use; only use in life-threatening arrhythmias; hematologic tox can be severe, follow CBC Uses: *Supraventricular/ventricular arrhythmias* **Acts:** Class 1A antiarrhythmic (Table 9, p 300) **Dose:** *Adults. Recurrent VF/VT:* 20 mg/min IV (total 17 mg/kg max). *Maint:* 1–4 mg/min. *Stable wide-complex tachycardia of unknown origin, AF w/ rapid rate in WPW:*

20 mg/min IV until arrhythmia suppression, ↓ BP, or QRS widens > 50%, then 1–4 mg/min. *Chronic dosing:* 50 mg/kg/d PO in ÷ doses q4–6h. *Recurrent VF/VT:* 20–50 mg/min IV; max total 17 mg/kg. *ECC 2010. Stable monomorphic VT, refractory reentry SVT, stable wide-complex tachycardia, AFib w/ WPW:* 20 mg/min IV until one of these: arrhythmia stopped, hypotension, QRS widens > 50%, total 17 mg/kg; then maintenance infusion of 1–4 mg/min. **Peds.** *Chronic maint:* 15–50 mg/kg/24 h PO ÷ q3–6h; *ECC 2010. SVT, aflutter, VT (w /pulses):* 15 mg/kg IV/IO over 30–60 min **W/P:** [C, +] in renal/hepatic impair **CI:** Complete heart block, 2nd/3rd-degree heart block w/o pacemaker, torsades de pointes, SLE **Disp:** Tabs & caps 250, 500 mg; SR tabs 500, 750, 1000 mg; Inj 100, 500 mg/mL **SE:** ↓ BP, lupus-like synd, GI upset, taste perversion, arrhythmias, tachycardia, heart block, angioneurotic edema, blood dyscrasias **Notes:** Levels: *Trough:* Just before next dose. *Therapeutic:* 4–10 mcg/mL; *N*-acetyl procainamide (NAPA) + procaine 5–30 mcg/mL *Toxic:* > 10 mcg/mL; NAPA + procaine > 30 mcg/mL *1/2-life:* procaine 3–5 h, NAPA 6–10 h

Procarbazine (Matulane) BOX: Highly toxic; handle w/ care **Uses:** *Hodgkin Dz*, NHL, brain & lung tumors **Acts:** Alkylating agent; ↓ DNA & RNA synth **Dose:** Per protocol **W/P:** [D, ?] w/ EtOH ingestion **CI:** Inadequate BM reserve **Disp:** Caps 50 mg **SE:** ↓ BM, hemolytic Rxns (w/ G6PD deficiency), N/V/D; disulfiram-like Rxn; cutaneous & constitutional Sxs, myalgia, arthralgia, CNS effects, azoospermia, cessation of menses

Prochlorperazine (Compazine) **Uses:** *N/V, agitation, & psychotic disorders* **Acts:** Phenothiazine; blocks postsynaptic dopaminergic CNS receptors **Dose:** **Adults.** *Antiemetic:* 5–10 mg PO tid-qid or 25 mg PR bid or 5–10 mg deep IM q4–6h. *Antipsychotic:* 10–20 mg IM acutely or 5–10 mg PO tid-qid for maint; ↑ doses may be required for antipsychotic effect. **Peds.** 0.1–0.15 mg/kg/dose IM q4–6h or 0.4 mg/kg/24 h PO ÷ tid-qid **W/P:** [C, +/–] NAG, severe liver/cardiac Dz **CI:** Phenothiazine sensitivity, BM suppression; age < 2 y or wgt < 9 kg **Disp:** Tabs 5, 10, 25 mg; caps 10, 15 mg; syrup 5 mg/5 mL; supp 2.5, 5, 25 mg; Inj 5 mg/ mL **SE:** EPS common; Rx w/ diphenhydramine or benztropine

Promethazine (Phenergan) BOX: Do not use in pts < 2 yrs; resp depression risk; tissue damage, including gangrene w/ extravasation. **Uses:** *N/V, motion sickness, adjunct to post op analgesics, sedation, rhinitis* **Acts:** Phenothiazine; blocks CNS postsynaptic mesolimbic dopaminergic receptors **Dose:** **Adults.** 12.5–50 mg PO, PR, or IM bid-qid PRN. *Peds > 2 y* 0.1–0.5 mg/kg/dose PO/ or IM q2–6h PRN **W/P:** [C, +/–] Use w/ agents w/ resp depressant effects **CI:** Component allergy, NAG, age < 2 y **Disp:** Tabs 12.5, 25, 50 mg; syrup 6.25 mg/5 mL, 25 mg/5 mL; supp 12.5, 25, 50 mg; Inj 25, 50 mg/mL **SE:** Drowsiness, tardive dyskinesia, EPS, lowered Sz threshold, ↓ BP, GI upset, blood dyscrasias, photosens, resp depression in children **Notes:** IM/PO preferred route; not SQ or intra-arterial

Propafenone (Rythmol) BOX: Excess mortality or nonfatal cardiac arrest rate possible; avoid use w/ asymptomatic and symptomatic non–life-threatening ventricular arrhythmias **Uses:** *Life-threatening ventricular arrhythmias, AF* **Acts:** Class IC antiarrhythmic (Table 9, p 300) **Dose:** *Adults.* 150–300 mg PO q8h. *Peds.* 8–10 mg/kg/d ÷ in 3–4 doses; may ↑ 2 mg/kg/d, 20 mg/kg/d max **W/P:** [C, ?] w/ Fosamprenavir, ritonavir, MI w/in 2 y, w/ liver/renal impair **CI:** Uncontrolled CHF, bronchospasm, cardiogenic shock, AV block w/o pacer **Disp:** Tabs 150, 225, 300 mg; ER caps 225, 325, 425 mg **SE:** Dizziness, unusual taste, 1st-degree heart block, arrhythmias, prolongs QRS & QT intervals; fatigue, GI upset, blood dyscrasias

Propantheline (Pro-Banthine) Uses: *PUD*, symptomatic Rx of small intestine hypermotility, spastic colon, ureteral spasm, bladder spasm, pylorospasm **Acts:** Antimuscarinic **Dose:** *Adults.* 15 mg PO ac & 30 mg PO hs; ↓ in elderly. *Peds.* 2–3 mg/kg/24 h PO ÷ tid-qid **W/P:** [C, ?] **CI:** NAG, ulcerative colitis, toxic megacolon, GI/GU obst **Disp:** Tabs 7.5, 15 mg **SE:** Anticholinergic (e.g., xerostomia, blurred vision)

Propofol (Diprivan) Uses: *Induction & maint of anesthesia; sedation in intubated pts* **Acts:** Sedative–hypnotic; mechanism unknown; acts in 40 s **Dose:** *Adults. Anesthesia:* 2–2.5 mg/kg (also *ECC 2005*), then 0.1–0.2 mg/kg/min Inf. *ICU sedation:* 5 mcg/kg/min IV × 5 min, ↑ PRN 5–10 mcg/kg/min q5–10 min, 5–50 mcg/kg/min cont Inf. *Peds. Anesthesia:* 2.5–3.5 mg/kg induction; then 125–300 mcg/kg/min; ↓ in elderly, debilitated, ASA II/IV pts **W/P:** [B, +] **CI:** If general anesthesia CI, sensitivity to egg, egg products, soybeans, soybean products **Disp:** Inj 10 mg/mL **SE:** May ↑ triglycerides w/ extended dosing; ↓ BP, pain at site, apnea, anaphylaxis **Notes:** 1 mL has 0.1 g fat

Propoxyphene (Darvon); Propoxyphene & Acetaminophen (Darvocet); Propoxyphene & Aspirin (Darvon Compound-65, Darvon-N + w/ Aspirin) [C-IV] **Note:** In November 2010 the FDA banned all products containing propoxyphene due to the increased risk of abnormal and potentially fatal heart rhythm disturbances.

Propranolol (Inderal) Uses: *HTN, angina, MI, hyperthyroidism, essential tremor, hypertrophic subaortic stenosis, pheochromocytoma; prevents migraines & atrial arrhythmias* **Acts:** β-Adrenergic receptor blocker, β₁, β₂; only β-blocker to block conversion of T₄ to T₃ **Dose:** *Adults. Angina:* 80–320 mg/d PO ÷ bid-qid or 80–160 mg/d SR. *Arrhythmia:* 10–80 mg PO tid-qid or 1 mg IV slowly, repeat q5min, 5 mg max. *HTN:* 40 mg PO bid or 60–80 mg/d SR, ↑ weekly to max 640 mg/d. *Hypertrophic subaortic stenosis:* 20–40 mg PO bid-qid. *MI:* 180–240 mg PO ÷ tid-qid. *Migraine prophylaxis:* 80 mg/d ÷ qid-tid, ↑ weekly 160–240 mg/d ÷ tid-qid max; wean if no response in 6 wk. *Pheochromocytoma:* 30–60 mg/d ÷ tid-qid. *Thyrotoxicosis:* 1–3 mg IV × 1; 10–40 mg PO q6h. *Tremor:* 40 mg PO bid, ↑ PRN 320 mg/d max; *ECC 2010. SVT:* 0.5–1 mg IV given over 1 min; repeat PRN up to 0.1 mg/kg. *Peds. Arrhythmia:* 0.5–1.0 mg/kg/d ÷ tid-qid, ↑ PRN q3–7d to 60 mg/d max; 0.01–0.1 mg/kg IV over 10 min, 1 mg max. *HTN:* 0.5–1.0 mg/kg ÷ bid-qid, ↑ PRN q3–7d to 2 mg/kg/d max; ↓ in renal impair **W/P:** [C (1st tri, D if 2nd or 3rd tri), +] **CI:** Uncompensated CHF, cardiogenic shock, ↓ HR, heart block, PE, severe resp Dz **Disp:** Tabs 10, 20, 40, 80 mg; SR caps 60, 80, 120, 160 mg; oral soln 4, 8, mg/mL; Inj 1 mg/mL **SE:** ↓ HR, ↓ BP, fatigue, GI upset, ED

Propylthiouracil [PTU]   BOX: Severe liver failure reported; use only if pt cannot tolerate methimazole; d/t fetal anomalies w/ methimazole, PTU may be DOC in 1st tri **Uses:** *Hyperthyroidism* **Acts:** ↓ Production of T_3 & T_4 & conversion of T_4 to T_3 **Dose: Adults. Initial:** 100 mg PO q8h (may need up to 1200 mg/d); after pt euthyroid (6–8 wk), taper dose by 1/2 q4–6wk to maint, 50–150 mg/24 h; can usually D/C in 2–3 y; ↓ in elderly. **Peds. Initial:** 5–7 mg/kg/24 h PO ÷ q8h. **Maint:** 1/3–2/3 of initial dose **W/P:** [D, –] See Box **CI:** Allergy **Disp:** Tabs 50 mg **SE:** Fever, rash, leukopenia, dizziness, GI upset, taste perversion, SLE-like synd, ↑ LFT, liver failure **Notes:** Monitor pt clinically; report any S/Sx of hepatic dysfunction, ✓ TFT and LFT

Protamine (Generic)   Uses: *Reverse heparin effect* **Acts:** Neutralize heparin by forming a stable complex **Dose:** Based on degree of heparin reversal; give IV slowly; 1 mg reverses ~100 units of heparin given in the preceding 3–4 h, 50 mg max **W/P:** [C, ?] **CI:** Allergy **Disp:** Inj 10 mg/mL **SE:** Follow coagulants; anticoagulant effect if given w/o heparin; ↓ BP, ↓ HR, dyspnea, hemorrhage **Notes:** ✓ aPTT ~15 min after use to assess response

Pseudoephedrine (Sudafed, Novafed, Afrinol, Others) [OTC]   BOX: Not for use in peds < 2 y **Uses:** *Decongestant* **Acts:** Stimulates α-adrenergic receptors w/ vasoconstriction **Dose: Adults.** 30–60 mg PO q6–8h. **Peds 2–5 y.** 15 mg q 4–6 h, 60 mg/24 h max. **6–12 y:** 30 mg q4–6h, 120 mg/24 h max; ↓ w/ renal Insuff **W/P:** [C, +] **CI:** Poorly controlled HTN or CAD, w/ MAOIs **Disp:** Tabs 30, 60 mg; caps 60 mg; SR tabs 120, 240 mg; liq 7.5 mg/0.8 mL, 15, 30 mg/5 mL **SE:** HTN, insomnia, tachycardia, arrhythmias, nervousness, tremor **Notes:** Found in many OTC cough/cold preparations; OTC restricted distribution

Psyllium (Metamucil, Serutan, Effer-Syllium)   Uses: *Constipation & colonic diverticular Dz* **Acts:** Bulk laxative **Dose:** 1 tsp (7 g) in glass of H_2O PO daily–tid **W/P:** [B, ?] **Effer-Syllium** (effervescent psyllium) usually contains K^+, caution w/ renal failure; phenylketonuria (in products w/ aspartame) **CI:** Suspected bowel obst **Disp:** Granules 4, 25 g/tsp; powder 3.5 g/packet, caps 0.52g (3 g/6 caps), wafers 3.4 g/dose **SE:** D, Abd cramps, bowel obst, constipation, bronchospasm

Pyrazinamide (Generic)   Uses: *Active TB in combo w/ other agents* **Acts:** Bacteriostatic; unknown mechanism **Dose: Adults.** 15–30 mg/kg/24 h PO ÷ tid-qid; max 2 g/d; dosing based on lean body wgt; ↓ dose in renal/hepatic impair. **Peds.** 15–30 mg/kg/d PO ÷ daily-bid; ↓ w/ renal/hepatic impair **W/P:** [C, +/–] **CI:** Severe hepatic damage, acute gout **Disp:** Tabs 500 mg **SE:** Hepatotox, malaise, GI upset, arthralgia, myalgia, gout, photosens **Notes:** Use in combo w/ other anti-TB drugs; consult http://www.cdc.gov/tb/ for latest TB recommendations; dosage regimen differs for "directly observed" Rx

Pyridoxine [Vitamin B₆]   Uses: *Rx & prevention of vit B_6 deficiency* **Acts:** Vit B_6 supl **Dose: Adults. Deficiency:** 10–20 mg/d PO. **Drug-induced neuritis:** 100–200 mg/d; 25–100 mg/d prophylaxis. **Peds.** 5–25 mg/d × 3 wk **W/P:** [A (C if doses exceed RDA), +] **CI:** Component allergy **Disp:** Tabs 25, 50, 100 mg; Inj 100 mg/mL **SE:** Allergic Rxns, HA, N

Quetiapine (Seroquel, Seroquel XR) **BOX:** Closely monitor pts for worsening depression or emergence of suicidality, particularly in ped pts; not for use in peds; ↑ mortality in elderly w/ dementia-related psychosis **Uses:** *Acute exacerbations of schizophrenia* **Acts:** Serotonin & dopamine antagonism **Dose:** 150–750 mg/d; initiate at 25–100 mg bid-tid; slowly ↑ dose; *XR:* 400–800 mg PO q P.M.; start 300 mg/d, ↑ 300 mg/d, 800 mg d max ↓ dose w/ hepatic & geriatric pts **W/P:** [C, –] **CI:** Component allergy **Disp:** Tabs 25, 50, 100, 200, 300, 400 mg; 200, 300, 400 XR **SE:** Confusion w/ nefazodone; HA, somnolence, ↑ wgt, ↓ BP, dizziness, cataracts, neuroleptic malignant synd, tardive dyskinesia, ↑ QT internal

Quinapril (Accupril) **BOX:** ACE inhib used during PRG can cause fetal injury & death **Uses:** *HTN, CHF, DN, post-MI* **Acts:** ACE inhib **Dose:** 10–80 mg PO daily; ↓ in renal impair **W/P:** [D, +] w/ RAS, vol depletion **CI:** ACE inhib sensitivity, angioedema, PRG **Disp:** Tabs 5, 10, 20, 40 mg **SE:** Dizziness, HA, ↓ BP, impaired renal Fxn, angioedema, taste perversion, cough

Quinidine (Quinidex, Quinaglute) **BOX:** Mortality rates increased when used to treat non–life-threatening arrhythmias **Uses:** *Prevention of tachy dysrhythmias, malaria* **Acts:** Class IA antiarrhythmic **Dose:** *Adults. AF/A flutter conversion:* After digitalization, 200 mg q2–3h × 8 doses; ↑ daily to 3–4 g max or nl rhythm. *Peds.* 15–60 mg/kg/24 h PO in 4–5 ÷ doses; ↓ in renal impair **W/P:** [C, +] w/ Ritonavir **CI:** Digitalis tox & AV block; conduction disorders **Disp:** *Sulfate:* Tabs 200, 300 mg; SR tabs 300 mg. *Gluconate:* SR tabs 324 mg; Inj 80 mg/mL **SE:** Extreme ↓ BP w/ IV use; syncope, QT prolongation, GI upset, arrhythmias, fatigue, cinchonism (tinnitus, hearing loss, delirium, visual changes), fever, hemolytic anemia, thrombocytopenia, rash **Notes:** Levels: *Trough:* just before next dose. *Therapeutic:* 2–5 mcg/mL *Toxic:* > 10 mcg/mL *1/2-life:* 6–8h; sulfate salt 83% quinidine; gluconate salt 62% quinidine; use w/ drug that slows AV conduction (e.g., digoxin, diltiazem, β-blocker)

Quinupristin–Dalfopristin (Synercid) **Uses:** *Vancomycin-resistant infxns d/t E. faecium & other gram(+)* **Acts:** ↓ Ribosomal protein synth. *Spectrum:* Vancomycin-resistant *E. faecium,* methicillin-susceptible *S. aureus, S. pyogenes;* not against *E. faecalis* **Dose:** *Adults & Peds.* 7.5 mg/kg IV q8–12h (central line preferred); incompatible w/ NS or heparin; flush IV w/ dextrose; ↓ w/ hepatic failure **W/P:** [B, M] Multiple drug interactions w/ drugs metabolized by CYP3A4 (e.g., cyclosporine) **CI:** Component allergy **Disp:** Inj 500 mg (150 mg quinupristin/350 mg dalfopristin) 600 mg (180 quinupristin/420 mg dalfopristin) **SE:** Hyperbilirubinemia, Inf site Rxns & pain, arthralgia, myalgia

Rabeprazole (AcipHex) **Uses:** *PUD, GERD, ZE* H. pylori **Acts:** Proton pump inhib **Dose:** 20 mg/d; may ↑ to 60 mg/d; *H. pylori* 20 mg PO bid × 7 d (w/ amoxicillin and clarithromycin); do not crush/chew tabs; do not use clopidogrel **W/P:** [B, ?/–] do not use w/ clopidogrel (↓ effect) **Disp:** Tabs 20 mg ER **SE:** HA, fatigue, GI upset **Notes:** ? ↑ risk of fractures, *C. difficile,* CAP w/ all PPI; risk of hypomagnesemia w/ long-term use, monitor

Raloxifene (Evista)   BOX: Increased risk of venous thromboembolism and death from stroke **Uses:** *Prevent osteoporosis, breast CA prevention* **Acts:** Partial antagonist of estrogen, behaves like estrogen **Dose:** 60 mg/d **W/P:** [X, −] **CI:** Thromboembolism, PRG **Disp:** Tabs 60 mg **SE:** Chest pain, insomnia, rash, hot flashes, GI upset, hepatic dysfunction, leg cramps

Raltegravir (Isentress)   BOX: Development of immune reconstitution synd: ↑ CK, myopathy, and rhabdomyolysis **Uses:** *HIV in combo w/ other antiretroviral agents* **Acts:** HIV-integrase strand transfer inhib **Dose:** 400 mg PO bid, 800 mg bid if w/ rifampin; w/ or w/o food **W/P:** [C, −] **CI:** None **Disp:** Tabs 400 mg **SE:** N/D, HA, fever, ↑ cholesterol, paranoia and anxiety **Notes:** Monitor lipid profile; initial therapy may cause immune reconstitution synd (inflammatory response to residual opportunistic infections (e.g., *M. avium, Pneumocystis jiroveci*)

Ramelteon (Rozerem)   Uses: *Insomnia* **Acts:** Melatonin receptor agonist **Dose:** 8 mg PO hs **W/P:** [C, ?/−] w/ CYP1A2 inhibitors **CI:** w/ Fluvoxamine; hypersens **Disp:** Tabs 8 mg **SE:** Somnolence, dizziness **Notes:** Avoid w/ high fat meal

Ramipril (Altace)   BOX: ACE inhib used during PRG can cause fetal injury & death **Uses:** *HTN, CHF, DN, post-MI* **Acts:** ACE inhib **Dose:** 2.5–20 mg/d PO ÷ daily-bid; ↓ in renal failure **W/P:** [D, +] **CI:** ACE inhib-induced angioedema **Disp:** Caps 1.25, 2.5, 5, 10 mg **SE:** Cough, HA, dizziness, ↓ BP, renal impair, angioedema **Notes:** OK in combo w/ diuretics

Ranibizumab (Lucentis)   Uses: *Neovascular "wet" macular degeneration* **Acts:** VEGF inhib **Dose:** 0.5 mg intravitreal Inj q mo **W/P:** [C, ?] Hx thromboembolism **CI:** Periocular Infxn **Disp:** Inj **SE:** Endophthalmitis, retinal detachment/hemorrhage, cataract, intraocular inflammation, conjunctival hemorrhage, eye pain, floaters

Ranitidine Hydrochloride (Zantac, Zantac OTC, Zantac EFFERDose)   Uses: *Duodenal ulcer, active benign ulcers, hypersecretory conditions, & GERD* **Acts:** H_2-receptor antagonist **Dose:** *Adults.* *Ulcer:* 150 mg PO bid, 300 mg PO hs, or 50 mg IV q6–8h; or 400 mg IV/d cont Inf, then maint of 150 mg PO hs. *Hypersecretion:* 150 mg PO bid, up to 600 mg/d. *GERD:* 300 mg PO bid; maint 300 mg PO hs. *Dyspepsia:* 75 mg PO daily-bid. *Peds.* 0.75–1.5 mg/kg/dose IV q6–8h or 1.25–2.5 mg/kg/dose PO q12h; ↓ in renal Insuff/failure **W/P:** [B, +] **CI:** Component allergy **Disp:** Tabs 75 [OTC], 150, 300 mg; caps 150, 300 mg; effervescent tabs 25 mg (contains phenylalanine); syrup 15 mg/mL; Inj 25 mg/mL **SE:** Dizziness, sedation, rash, GI upset **Notes:** PO & parenteral doses differ

Ranolazine (Ranexa)   Uses: *Chronic angina* **Acts:** ↓ Ischemia-related Na^+ entry into myocardium **Dose:** *Adults.* 500 mg bid-1000 mg PO bid **CI:** w/ Hepatic impair, CYP3A inhib (Table 10, p 301); w/ agents that ↑ QT interval; ↓ K^+ **W/P:** [C, ?/−] HTN may develop w/ renal impair **Disp:** SR tabs 500 mg **SE:** Dizziness, HA, constipation, arrhythmias **Notes:** Not 1st line; use w/ amlodipine, nitrates, or β-blockers

Rasagiline Mesylate (Azilect) Uses: *Early Parkinson Dz monotherapy; levodopa adjunct w/ advanced Dz* Acts: MAO B inhib Dose: *Adults. Early Dz:* 1 mg PO daily, start 0.5 mg PO daily w/ levodopa; ↓ w/ CYP1A2 inhib or hepatic impair CI: MAOIs, sympathomimetic amines, meperidine, methadone, tramadol, propoxyphene, dextromethorphan, mirtazapine, cyclobenzaprine, St. John's wort, sympathomimetic vasoconstrictors, general anesthetics, SSRIs W/P: [C, ?] Avoid tyramine-containing foods; mod/severe hepatic impair Disp: Tabs 0.5, 1 mg SE: Arthralgia, indigestion, dyskinesia, hallucinations, ↓ wgt, postural ↓ BP, N/V, constipation, xerostomia, rash, sedation, CV conduction disturbances Notes: Rare melanoma reported; periodic skin exams (skin cancer risk); D/C 14 d prior to elective surgery; initial ↓ levodopa dose OK

Rasburicase (Elitek) BOX: Anaphylaxis possible; do not use in G6PD deficiency and hemolysis; can cause methemoglobinemia; can interfere w/uric acid assays; collect blood samples and store on ice Uses: *Reduce ↑ uric acid d/t tumor lysis* Acts: Catalyzes uric acid Dose: *Adult & Peds.* 0.20 mg/kg IV over 30 min, daily × 5; do not bolus W/P: [C, ?/–] Falsely ↓ uric acid values CI: Anaphylaxis, screen for G6PD deficiency to avoid hemolysis, methemoglobinemia Disp: 1.5, 7.5 mg powder Inj SE: Fever, neutropenia, GI upset, HA, rash Note: Place blood test tube for uric acid level on ice to stop enzymatic Rxn; removed by dialysis

Repaglinide (Prandin) Uses: *Type 2 DM* Acts: ↑ Pancreatic insulin release Dose: 0.5–4 mg ac, PO start 1–2 mg, ↑ to 16 mg/d max; take pc W/P: [C, ?/–] CI: DKA, type 1 DM Disp: Tabs 0.5, 1, 2 mg SE: HA, hyper-/hypoglycemia, GI upset

Repaglinide and Metformin (PrandiMet) BOX: Associated w/ lactic acidosis, risk ↑ w/ sepsis, dehydration, renal/hepatic impair, ↑ alcohol, acute CHF; Sxs include myalgias, malaise, resp distress, abd pain, somnolence; Labs: ↓ pH, ↑ anion gap, ↑ blood lactate; D/C immediately & hospitalize if suspected Uses: *Type 2 DM* Acts: Meglitinide & biguanide (see metformin) Dose: *Adults.* 1/500 mg bid w/in 15 min pc (skip dose w/ skipped meal); max 10/2500 mg/d or 4/1000 mg/meal W/P: [C, –] suspend use w/ iodinated contrast, do not use w/ NPH insulin, use w/ cationic drugs & CYP2C8 & CYP3A4 inhib CI: SCr > 1.4 mg/dL (females) or > 1.5 mg/dL (males); metabolic acidosis; w/ gemfibrozil Disp: Tabs (repaglinide mg/metformin mg) 1/500, 2/500 SE: Hypoglycemia, HA, N/V/D, anorexia, weakness, myalgia, rash, ↓ vit B$_{12}$

Retapamulin (Altabax) Uses: *Topical Rx impetigo in pts > 9 mo* Acts: Pleuromutilin antibiotic, bacteriostatic, ↓ bacteria protein synth; *Spectrum:* S. *aureus* (not MRSA), S. *pyogenes* Dose: Apply bid × 5 d W/P: [B, ?] Disp: 10 mg/1 g SE: Local irritation

Reteplase (Retavase) Uses: *Post-AMI* Acts: Thrombolytic Dose: 10 units IV over 2 min, 2nd dose in 30 min, 10 units IV over 2 min; *ECC 2010.* 10 units IV bolus over 2 min; 30 min later, 10 units IV bolus over 2 min w/ NS flush before and after each dose. W/P: [C, ?/–] CI: Internal bleeding, spinal surgery/

trauma, Hx CNS AVM/CVA, bleeding diathesis, severe uncontrolled ↑ BP, sensitivity to thrombolytics **Disp:** Inj 10.8 units/2 mL **SE:** Bleeding including CNS, allergic Rxns

Ribavirin (Virazole, Copegus, Rebetol)   **BOX:** Monotherapy for chronic hep C ineffective; hemolytic anemia possible, teratogenic and embryocidal; use 2 forms of birth control for up to 6 mo after D/C drug; decrease in resp fxn when used in infants as Inh **Uses:** *RSV Infxn in infants [Virazole]; hep C (in combo w/ peg-interferon α-2b)* **Acts:** Unknown **Dose:** *RSV:* 6 g in 300 mL sterile H$_2$O, inhale over 12–18 h. *Hep C:* See individual product labeling for dosing based on wgt & genotype **W/P:** [X, ?] May accumulate on soft contacts lenses **CI:** PRG, autoimmune hep, CrCl < 50 mL/min **Disp:** Powder for aerosol 6 g; tabs 200, 400, 600 mg, caps 200 mg, soln 40 mg/mL **SE:** Fatigue, HA, GI upset, anemia, myalgia, alopecia, bronchospasm, ↓ HCT; pancytopenia reported **Notes:** Virazole aerosolized by a SPAG, monitor resp Fxn closely; ✓ Hgb/Hct; PRG test monthly; 2 forms birth control hep C viral genotyping may modify dose

Rifabutin (Mycobutin)   **Uses:** *Prevent MAC Infxn in AIDS pts w/ CD4 count < 100 mcL* **Acts:** ↓ DNA-dependent RNA polymerase activity **Dose:** *Adults.* 150–300 mg/d PO. *Peds 1 y.* 15–25 mg/kg/d PO. *2–10 y:* 4.4–18.8 mg/kg/d PO. *14–16 y:* 2.8–5.4 mg/kg/d PO **W/P:** [B, ?/–] WBC < 1000 cells/mm^3 or plts < 50,000 cells/mm^3; ritonavir **CI:** Allergy **Disp:** Caps 150 mg **SE:** Discolored urine, rash, neutropenia, leukopenia, myalgia, ↑ LFTs **Notes:** SE/interactions similar to rifampin

Rifampin (Rifadin)   **Uses:** *TB & Rx & prophylaxis of N. meningitidis, H. influenzae,* or *S. aureus* carriers*; adjunct w/ severe *S. aureus* **Acts:** ↓ DNA-dependent RNA polymerase **Dose:** *Adults. N. meningitidis & H. influenzae carrier:* 600 mg/d PO for 4 d. *TB:* 600 mg PO or IV daily or 2×/wk w/ combo regimen. *Peds.* 10–20 mg/kg/dose PO or IV daily-bid; ↓ in hepatic failure **W/P:** [C, +] w/ Fosamprenavir, multiple drug interactions **CI:** Allergy, active *N. meningitidis* Infxn, w/ saquinavir/ritonavir **Disp:** Caps 150, 300 mg; Inj 600 mg **SE:** Red-orange–colored bodily fluids, ↑ LFTs, flushing, HA **Notes:** Never use as single agent w/ active TB

Rifapentine (Priftin)   **Uses:** *Pulm TB* **Acts:** ↓ DNA-dependent RNA polymerase. *Spectrum: Mycobacterium tuberculosis* **Dose:** *Intensive phase:* 600 mg PO 2×/wk for 2 mo; separate doses by > 3 d. *Continuation phase:* 600 mg/wk for 4 mo; part of 3–4 drug regimen **W/P:** [C, +/– red-orange breast milk] Strong CYP450 inducer, ↓ protease inhib efficacy, antiepileptics, β-blockers, CCBs **CI:** Rifamycins allergy **Disp:** 150-mg tabs **SE:** Neutropenia, hyperuricemia, HTN, HA, dizziness, rash, GI upset, blood dyscrasias, ↑ LFTs, hematuria, discolored secretions **Notes:** Monitor LFTs

Rifaximin (Xifaxan, Xifaxan 550)   **Uses:** *Traveler's D (noninvasive strains of E. coli)* in pts > 12 y (*Xifaxan*); hepatic encephalopathy (*Xifaxan 550*) > 18 y*

Acts: Not absorbed, derivative of rifampicin. *Spectrum: E. coli* **Dose:** Diarrhea (*Xifaxan*): 1 tab PO daily × 3 d; encephalopathy (*Xifaxan 550*) 500 mg PO bid; w/wo food 1 tab PO daily × 3 d **W/P:** [C, ?/–] Hx allergy; pseudomembranous colitis; w/ severe (Child-Pugh C) hepatic impair **CI:** Allergy to rifamycins **Disp:** Tabs: *Xifaxan:* 200 mg; *Xifaxan 550:* 550 mg **SE:** *Xifaxan:* Flatulence, HA, abd pain, rectal tenesmus and urgency, N; *Xifaxan 550:* Edema, N, dizziness, fatigue, ascites, flatulence, HA **Notes:** D/C if D Sx worsen or persist > 24–48h, or w/ fever or blood in stool

Rimantadine (Flumadine) Uses: *Prophylaxis & Rx of influenza A viral Infxns* **Acts:** Antiviral **Dose:** *Adults & Peds > 9 y.* 100 mg PO bid. *Peds 1–9 y.* 5 mg/kg/d PO, 150 mg/d max; daily w/ severe renal/hepatic impair & elderly; initiate w/in 48 h of Sx onset **W/P:** [C, +] w/ Cimetidine; avoid w/ PRG, breast-feeding **CI:** Component & amantadine allergy **Disp:** Tabs 100 mg; syrup 50 mg/5 mL **SE:** Orthostatic ↓ BP, edema, dizziness, GI upset, ↓ Sz threshold **Note:** See CDC (*MMWR*) for current Influenza A guidelines

Rimexolone (Vexol Ophthalmic) Uses: *Post-op inflammation & uveitis* **Acts:** Steroid **Dose:** *Adults & Peds > 2 y. Uveitis:* 1–2 gtt/h daytime & q2h at night, taper to 1 gtt q4h. *Post-op:* 1–2 gtt qid × 2 wk **W/P:** [C, ?/–] Ocular Infxns **Disp:** Susp 1% **SE:** Blurred vision, local irritation **Notes:** Taper dose

Risedronate (Actonel, Actonel W/ Calcium) Uses: *Paget Dz; Rx/ prevention glucocorticoid-induced/postmenopausal osteoporosis, ↑ bone mass in osteoporotic men; w/ calcium only FDA approved for female osteoporosis* **Acts:** Bisphosphonate; ↓ osteoclast-mediated bone resorption **Dose:** *Paget Dz:* 30 mg/d PO for 2 mo. *Osteoporosis Rx/prevention:* 5 mg daily or 35 mg q wk or, 75 mg on 2 consecutive d/month, or 150 mg q month; 30 min before 1st food/drink of the d; stay upright for at least 30 min after dose **W/P:** [C, ?/–] Ca²⁺ supls & antacids ↓ absorption; jaw osteonecrosis, avoid dental work **CI:** Component allergy, ↓ Ca²⁺, esophageal abnormalities, unable to stand/sit for 30 min, CrCl < 30 mL/min **Disp:** Tabs 5, 30, 35, 75, 150 mg; Risedronate 35 mg (4 tabs)/calcium carbonate 1250 mg (24 tabs) **SE:** Back pain, HA, Abd pain, dyspepsia, arthralgia, flu-like Sxs, hypersensitivity (rash, etc), esophagitis, bone pain, eye inflammation **Notes:** Monitor LFTs, Ca²⁺, PO³⁺, K⁺; may ↑ atypical subtrochanteric femur fractures

Risedronate, Delayed-Release (Atelvia) Uses: *Postmenopausal osteoporosis* **Acts:** See Risedronate **Dose:** One 35 mg tab 1 × wk; in A.M. following breakfast w/ 4 oz water; do not lie down for 30 min **W/P:** [C, ?/–] Ca²⁺ & Fe²⁺ supls/ antacids ↓ absorption; do not use w/ Actonel or CrCl < 30 mL/min; jaw osteonecrosis reported, avoid dental work; may ↑ subtrochanteric femur fractures; severe bone/ jt pain **CI:** Component allergy, ↓ Ca²⁺, esophageal abnormalities, unable to stand/sit for 30 min **Disp:** DR Tabs 35 mg **SE:** D, influenza, arthralgia, back/abd pain; rare hypersens, eye inflam **Notes:** Correct ↓ Ca²⁺ before use; ✓ Ca²⁺

Risperidone, Oral (Risperdal, Risperdal M-Tab) **BOX:** ↑ Mortality in elderly w/ dementia-related psychosis Uses: *Psychotic disorders (schizophrenia)*, dementia of the elderly, bipolar disorder, mania, Tourette disorder, autism **Acts:** Benzisoxazole antipsychotic **Dose:** *Adults.* 0.5–6 mg PO bid; *M-Tab:* 1–6 mg/d start 1–2 mg/d, titrate q3–7d. *Peds.* 0.25 mg PO bid, ↑ q5–7d; ↓ start dose w/ elderly, renal/hepatic impair **W/P:** [C, –], ↑ BP w/ antihypertensives, clozapine **CI:** Component allergy **Disp:** Tabs 0.25, 0.5, 1, 2, 3, 4 mg; soln 1 mg/mL, *M-Tab* (ODT) tabs 0.5, 1, 2, 3, 4 mg **SE:** Orthostatic ↓ BP, EPS w/ high dose, tachycardia, arrhythmias, sedation, dystonias, neuroleptic malignant synd, sexual dysfunction, constipation, xerostomia, ↓ WBC, neutropenia and agranulocytosis, cholestatic jaundice **Notes:** Several wk for effect

Risperidone, Parenteral (Risperdal Consta)   **BOX:** Not approved for dementia-related psychosis; ↑ mortality risk in elderly dementia pts on atypical antipsychotics; most deaths d/t CV or infectious events **Uses:** Schizophrenia **Acts:** Benzisoxazole antipsychotic **Dose:** 25 mg q2wk IM may ↑ to max 50 mg q2wk; w/ renal/hepatic impair start PO Risperdal 0.5 mg PO bid × 1 wk titrate weekly **W/P:** [C, –], ↑ BP w/ antihypertensives, clozapine **CI:** Component allergy **Disp:** Inj 25, 37.5, 50 mg/vial **SE:** See Risperidone, oral **Note:** Long-acting Inj

Ritonavir (Norvir)   **BOX:** Life-threatening adverse events when used w/ certain nonsedating antihistamines, sedative hypnotics, antiarrhythmics, or ergot alkaloids d/t inhibited drug metabolism **Uses:** *HIV* **Actions:** Protease inhib; ↓ maturation of immature noninfectious virions to mature infectious virus **Dose:** *Adults.* 300 mg PO bid, titrate over 1 wk to 600 mg PO bid (titration will ↓ GI SE). *Peds > 1 mo.* 250 mg/m² titrate to 400 mg bid (adjust w/ fosamprenavir, indinavir, nelfinavir, & saquinavir); take w/ food **W/P:** [B, +] w/ Ergotamine, amiodarone, bepridil, flecainide, propafenone, quinidine, pimozide, midazolam, triazolam **CI:** Component allergy **Disp:** Caps & tabs 100 mg; soln 80 mg/mL **SE:** ↑ Triglycerides, ↑ LFTs, N/V/D/C, Abd pain, taste perversion, anemia, weakness, HA, fever, malaise, rash, paresthesias **Notes:** Refrigerate

Rivaroxaban (Xarelto)   **BOX:** May ↑ risk of spinal/epidural hematoma w/ paralysis; monitor closely **Uses:** *Prevention DVT in knee/hip replacement surgery* **Acts:** Factor Xa inhibitor **Dose:** 10 mg PO qd × 35 days (hip) or 12 days (knee) w or w/o food **W/P:** [C, –] w/ CYP3A4 inhib/inducers, other anticoagulants or plt inhib; avoid w/CrCl < 30 mL/min or mod/severe hepatic impair **CI:** Active bleeding; component hypersens **Disp:** Tabs 10 mg **SE:** Bleeding

Rivastigmine (Exelon)   **Uses:** *Mild–mod dementia in Alzheimer Dz* **Acts:** Enhances cholinergic activity **Dose:** 1.5 mg bid; ↑ to 6 mg bid, w/ ↑ at 2-wk intervals (take w/ food) **W/P:** [B, ?] w/ β-Blockers, CCBs, smoking, neuromuscular blockade, digoxin **CI:** Rivastigmine or carbamate allergy **Disp:** Caps 1.5, 3, 4.5, 6 mg; soln 2 mg/mL **SE:** Dose-related GI effects, N/V/D, dizziness, insomnia, fatigue, tremor, diaphoresis, HA, wgt loss (in 18–26%) **Notes:** Swallow caps whole, do not break/chew/crush; avoid EtOH

Rivastigmine, Transdermal (Exelon Patch)   **Uses:** *Mild/mod Alzheimer and Parkinson Dz dementia* **Acts:** Acetylcholinesterase inhib **Dose:**

Initial: 4.6-mg patch/d applied to back, chest, upper arm, ↑ 9.5 mg after 4 wk if tolerated **W/P:** [?, ?] Sick sinus synd, conduction defects, asthma, COPD, urinary obst, Szs; death from multiple patches at same time reported **CI:** Hypersens to rivastigmine, other carbamates **Disp:** Transdermal patch 5 cm² (4.6 mg/24 h), 10 cm² (9.5 mg/24 h) **SE:** N/V/D

Rizatriptan (Maxalt, Maxalt MLT) Uses: *Rx acute migraine* **Acts:** Vascular serotonin receptor agonist **Dose:** 5–10 mg PO, repeat in 2 h, PRN, 30 mg/d max **W/P:** [C, M] **CI:** Angina, ischemic heart Dz, ischemic bowel Dz, hemiplegic/basilar migraine, uncontrolled HTN, ergot or serotonin 5-HT₁ agonist use w/in 24 h, MAOI use w/in 14 d **Disp:** Tab 5, 10 mg; *Maxalt MLT:* OD tabs 5, 10 mg. **SE:** Chest pain, palpitations, N, V, asthenia, dizziness, somnolence, fatigue

Rocuronium (Zemuron) Uses: *Skeletal muscle relaxation during rapid-sequence intubation, surgery, or mechanical ventilation* **Acts:** Nondepolarizing neuromuscular blocker **Dose:** *Rapid sequence intubation:* 0.6–1.2 mg/kg IV. *Continuous Inf:* 5–12.5 mcg/kg/min IV; adjust/titrate based on monitoring; ↓ in hepatic impair **W/P:** [C, ?] Aminoglycosides, vancomycin, tetracycline, polymyxins enhance blockade **CI:** Component or pancuronium allergy **Disp:** Inj preservative-free 10 mg/mL **SE:** BP changes, tachycardia

Romidepsin (Istodax) Uses: *Rx cutaneous T-cell lymphoma in pts who have received at least one prior systemic therapy* **Action:** Histone deacetylase (HDAC) inhibitor **Dose:** 14 mg/m² IV over 4h days 1, 8 and 15 of a 28-day cycle; repeat cycles every 28 days if tolerated; treatment d/c or interruption w/ or w/o dose reduction to 10 mg/m² to manage adverse drug reactions **W/P:** [D, ?] risk of ↑QT, hematologic toxicity; strong CYP3A4 inhibitors may ↑ conc **Disp:** Inj 10 mg **SE:** N, V, fatigue, infxn, anorexia, ↓ plt **Notes:** Hazardous agent, precautions for handling and disposal

Romiplostim (Nplate) **BOX:** ↑ Risk for heme malignancies and thromboembolism. D/C may worsen ↓ plt **Uses:** *Rx ↓ plt d/t ITP w/poor response to other therapies)* **Action:** Thrombopoietic, thrombopoietin receptor agonist **Dose:** *Adults.* 1 mcg/kg SQ weekly, adjust 1 mcg/kg/week to plt count > 50,000/mm³; max 10 mcg/kg/wk **W/P:** [C, /?] **CI:** None **Disp:** 500 mcg/mL (250-mcg vial) **SE:** HA, fatigue, dizziness, N/V/D, myalgia, epistaxis **Notes:** ✓ CBC/diff/plt weekly; plt ↑ 4–9 d, peak 12–16 d; D/C if no ↑ plt after 4 wk max dose; ↓ dose w/ plt count > 200,000/mm³

Ropinirole (Requip, Requip XL) Uses: *Rx of Parkinson Dz, restless leg synd (RLS)* **Acts:** Dopamine agonist **Dose:** *Parkinson Dz:* IR initial 0.25 mg PO tid, weekly ↑ 0.25 mg/dose, to 1 mg PO tid (may continue to titrate weekly to max dose of 24 mg/d); ER: 2 mg PO daily, titrate q wk by 2 mg/d to max 24 mg/d **W/P:** [C, ?/–] Severe CV/renal/hepatic impair **CI:** Component allergy **Disp:** Tabs IR 0.25, 0.5, 1, 2, 3, 4, 5 mg; tabs ER 2, 4, 6, 8, 12 mg **SE:** Syncope, postural ↓ BP, N/V, HA, somnolence, dosed-related hallucinations, dyskinesias, dizziness **Notes:** D/C w/ 7-d taper

Rosiglitazone (Avandia) **BOX:** May cause or worsen CHF; may increase myocardial ischemia Uses: *Type 2 DM* **Acts:** Thiazolidinedione; ↑ insulin sensitivity **Dose:** 4–8 mg/d PO or in 2 ÷ doses (w/o regard to meals) **W/P:** [C, –]

w/ ESRD, CHF, edema, **CI:** DKA, severe CHF (NYHA class III), ALT > 2.5 ULN **Disp:** Tabs 2, 4, 8 mg **SE:** May ↑ CV, CHF & ? CA risk; wgt gain, hyperlipidemia, HA, edema, fluid retention, worsen CHF, hyper-/hypoglycemia, hepatic damage w/ ↑ LFTs **Notes:** Not OK in class III, IV heart Dz; ? increased MI risk now requires REMS restricted distribution program

Rosuvastatin (Crestor) **Uses:** *Rx primary hypercholesterolemia & mixed dyslipidemia* **Acts:** HMG-CoA reductase inhib **Dose:** 5–40 mg PO daily; max 5 mg/d w/ cyclosporine, 10 mg/d w/ gemfibrozil or CrCl < 30 mL/min (avoid Al-/Mg-based antacids for 2 h after) **W/P:** [X, ?/–] **CI:** Active liver Dz, unexplained ↑ LFTs **Disp:** Tabs 5, 10, 20, 40 mg **SE:** Myalgia, constipation, asthenia, Abd pain, N, myopathy, rarely rhabdomyolysis **Notes:** May ↑ warfarin effect; monitor LFTs at baseline, 12 wk, then q6mo; ↓ dose in Asian pts; OK w/ grapefruit

Rotavirus Vaccine, Live, Oral, Monovalent (Rotarix) **Uses:** *Prevent rotavirus gastroenteritis in peds* **Acts:** Active immunization w/ live attenuated rotavirus **Dose:** *Peds 6–14 wk.* 1st dose PO at 6 wk of age, wait at least 4 wk then a 2nd dose by 24 wk of age. **W/P:** [C, ?] **CI:** Component sensitivity, uncorrected congenital GI malformation, chronic GI illness, acute mod–severe D illness, fever **Disp:** Single-dose vial **SE:** Irritability, cough, runny nose, fever, ↓ appetite, V **Notes:** Begin series by age 12 wk, conclude by age 24 wk; can be given to infant in house w/ immunosuppressed family member or mother who is breast feeding. Safety and effectiveness not studied in immunocompromised infants.

Rotavirus Vaccine, Live, Oral, Pentavalent (RotaTeq) **Uses:** *Prevent rotavirus gastroenteritis* **Acts:** Active immunization w/ live attenuated rotavirus **Dose:** *Peds 6–14 wk.* Single dose PO at 2, 4, & 6 mo **W/P:** [?, ?] **CI:** Uncorrected congenital GI malformation, chronic GI illness, acute diarrheal illness, fever **Disp:** Oral susp 2-mL single-use tubes **SE:** Fever, D/V **Notes:** Begin series by age 12 wk and conclude by age 32 wk; can be given to infant in house w/ immunosuppressed family member or mother who is breast-feeding. Safety and effectiveness not studied in immunocompromised infants.

Rufinamide (Banzel) **BOX:** Antiepileptics associated w/ ↑ risk of suicide ideation. Severe hypersens Rxns reported **Uses:** *Adjunct Lennox-Gastaut seizures* **Action:** Anticonvulsant **Dose:** *Adults.* Initial: 400–800 mg/d ÷ bid (max 3200 mg/d ÷ bid) *Peds ≥ 4 y.* Initial: 10 mg/kg/day ÷ bid, target 45 mg/kg/d ÷ bid; 3200 mg/d max **W/P:** [C, /–] **CI:** Familial short QT synd **Disp:** Tab: 200, 400 mg **SE:** ↑ QT, HA, somnolence, N/V, ataxia, rash **Notes:** Monitor for rash; use w/ OCP may lead to contraceptive failure

Salmeterol (Serevent Diskus) **BOX:** Long-acting β2-agonists, such as salmeterol, may ↑ risk of asthma-related death. Do not use alone, only as additional Rx for pts not controlled on other asthma meds **Uses:** *Asthma, exercise-induced asthma, COPD* **Acts:** Sympathomimetic bronchodilator, long acting β2-agonist **Dose:** *Adults & Peds > 12 y.* 1 Diskus-dose inhaled bid **W/P:**

[C, ?/–] **CI:** Acute asthma; w/in 14 d of MAOI; w/o concomitant use of inhaled steroid **Disp:** 50 mcg/dose, dry powder discus, metered-dose inhaler, 21 mcg/activation **SE:** HA, pharyngitis, tachycardia, arrhythmias, nervousness, GI upset, tremors **Notes:** Not for acute attacks; must use w/ steroid or short-acting β-agonist

Saquinavir (Fortovase, Invirase) **BOX:** Invirase and Fortovase not bioequivalent/interchangeable; must use Invirase in combo w/ ritonavir, which provides saquinavir plasma levels = to those w/ Fortovase **Uses:** *HIV Infxn* **Acts:** HIV protease inhib **Dose:** 1200 mg PO tid w/in 2 h pc (dose adjust w/ ritonavir, delavirdine, lopinavir, & nelfinavir) **W/P:** [B, +] w/ Ketoconazole, statins, sildenafil **CI:** w/ Rifampin, severe hepatic impair, allergy, sun exposure w/o sunscreen/clothing, triazolam, midazolam, ergots, **Disp:** Caps 200 mg, tabs 500 mg **SE:** Dyslipidemia, lipodystrophy, rash, hyperglycemia, GI upset, weakness **Notes:** Take 2 h after meal, avoid direct sunlight

Sargramostim [GM-CSF] (Leukine) **Uses:** *Myeloid recovery following BMT or chemotherapy* **Acts:** Recombinant GF, activates mature granulocytes & macrophages **Dose:** *Adults & Peds.* 250 mcg/m²/d IV for 21 d (BMT) **W/P:** [C, ?/–] Li, corticosteroids **CI:** > 10% blasts, allergy to yeast, concurrent chemotherapy/RT **Disp:** Inj 250, 500 mcg **SE:** Bone pain, fever, ↓ BP, tachycardia, flushing, GI upset, myalgia **Notes:** Rotate Inj sites; use APAP PRN for pain

Saxagliptin (Onglyza) **Uses:** *Monotherapy/combo for type 2 DM* **Action:** Dipeptidyl peptidase-4 (DDP-4) inhibitor, ↑ insulin synth/release **Dose:** 2.5 or 5 mg once/d w/o regard to meals; 2.5 mg once/d w/ CrCl < 50 mL/min or w/ strong CYP3A4/5 inhibitor (e.g., atazanavir, clarithromycin, indinavir, itraconazole, ketoconazole, nefazodone, nelfinavir, ritonavir, saquinavir, and telithromycin) **W/P:** [B, ?] may ↓ glucose when used w/ insulin secretagogues (e.g., sulfonylureas) **CI:** w/ Insulin or to treat DKA **Disp:** Tabs 2.5, 5 mg **SE:** URI, nasopharyngitis, UTI, HA **Notes:** No evidence for ↑ CV risk

Saxagliptin and Metformin (Kombiglyze XR) **BOX:** Lactic acidosis can occur w/ metformin accumulation; ↑ risk w/ sepsis, vol depletion, CHF, renal/hepatic impair, excess alcohol; if lactic acidosis suspected D/C med and hospitalize **Uses:** *Type 2 DM* **Acts:** Dipeptidyl peptidase-4 (DDP-4) inhibitor, ↑ insulin synth/release & biguanide; ↓ hepatic glucose production & intestinal absorption of glucose; ↑ insulin sens **Dose:** 5/500 mg–5/2000 mg saxagliptin/metformin HCl XR PO daily w/ evening meal **W/P:** [B, ?/–] **CI:** SCr > 1.4 mg/dL (females) or > 1.5 mg/dL (males); met acidosis; radiologic tests w/ iodinated contrast; w/ insulin or to Rx type 1 DM or DKA; vit B₁₂ def; hypoxic states (acute MI, acute CHF, sepsis) **Disp:** Tabs mg saxagliptin/mg metformin XR 5/500, 5/1000, 2.5/1000 **SE:** Lactic acidosis; ↓ vit B₁₂ levels; ↓ glucose w/ insulin secretagogue; N/V/D, anorexia, HA, URI, UTI, urticaria, myalgia **Notes:** Do not exceed 5 mg/2000 mg saxagliptin/metformin HCl XR; do not crush or chew; w/ strong CYP3A4/5 inhibitors do not exceed 2.5 mg saxagliptin/day

Scopolamine (Oral), Scopolamine, Transdermal & Ophthalmic (Scopace, Transderm-Scop) Uses: *Prevent N/V associated w/ motion sickness, anesthesia, opiates; mydriatic*, cycloplegic, Rx uveitis & iridocyclitis Acts: Anticholinergic, inhibits iris & ciliary bodies, antiemetic Dose: 1 mg/72 h, 1 patch behind ear q3d; apply > 4 h before exposure; cycloplegic 1–2 gtt 1 h pre-procedure, uveitis 1–2 gtt up to qid max; ↓ in elderly W/P: [C, +] w/ APAP, levodopa, ketoconazole, digitalis, KCl CI: NAG, GI or GU obst, thyrotoxicosis, paralytic ileus Disp: Patch 1.5 mg, (releases 1 mg over 72 h), ophthal 0.25% SE: Xerostomia, drowsiness, blurred vision, tachycardia, constipation Notes: Do not blink excessively after dose, wait 5 min before dosing other eye; antiemetic activity w/ patch requires several hours

Secobarbital (Seconal) [C-II] Uses: *Insomnia, short-term use*, preanesthetic agent Acts: Rapid-acting barbiturate Dose: *Adults.* 100–200 mg hs, 100–300 mg pre-op. *Peds.* 2–6 mg/kg/dose, 100 mg/max, ↓ in elderly W/P: [D, +] w/ CYP2C9, 3A3/4, 3A5/7 inducer (Table 10, p 301); ↑ tox w/ other CNS depressants CI: Porphyria, w/ voriconazole, PRG Disp: Caps 50, 100 mg SE: Tolerance in 1–2 wk; resp depression, CNS depression, porphyria, photosens

Selegiline, Oral (Eldepryl, Zelapar) BOX: Closely monitor for worsening depression or emergence of suicidality, particularly in ped pts Uses: *Parkinson Dz* Acts: MAOI Dose: 5 mg PO bid; 1.25–2.5 once daily tabs PO q A.M. (before breakfast w/o liq) 2.5 mg/d max; ↓ in elderly W/P: [C, ?] w/ Drugs that induce CYP3A4 (Table 10, p 301) e.g., phenytoin, carbamazepine, nafcillin, phenobarbital, & rifampin); avoid w/ antidepressants CI: w/ Meperidine, MAOI, dextromethorphan, general anesthesia w/in 10 d, pheochromocytoma Disp: Tabs/caps 5 mg; once-daily tabs 1.25 mg SE: N, dizziness, orthostatic ↓ BP, arrhythmias, tachycardia, edema, confusion, xerostomia Notes: ↓ Carbidopa/levodopa if used in combo; see transdermal form

Selegiline, Transdermal (Emsam) BOX: May ↑ risk of suicidal thinking and behavior in children and adolescents w/ major depression disorder Uses: *Depression* Acts: MAOI Dose: *Adults.* Apply patch daily to upper torso, upper thigh, or outer upper arm CI: Tyramine-containing foods w/ 9- or 12-mg doses; serotonin-sparing agents W/P: [C, −] w/ Carbamazepine and oxcarbazepine levels Disp: ER Patches 6, 9, 12 mg SE: Local Rxns requiring topical steroids; HA, insomnia, orthostatic, ↓ BP, serotonin synd, suicide risk Notes: Rotate site; see oral form

Selenium Sulfide (Exsel Shampoo, Selsun Blue Shampoo, Selsun Shampoo) Uses: *Scalp seborrheic dermatitis*, scalp itching & flaking d/t *dandruff*; tinea versicolor Acts: Antiseborrheic Dose: *Dandruff, seborrhea:* Massage 5–10 mL into wet scalp, leave on 2–3 min, rinse, repeat; use 2× wk, then once q1–4wk PRN. *Tinea versicolor:* Apply 2.5% daily on area & lather w/ small amounts of water; leave on 10 min, then rinse W/P: [C, ?] CI: Open wounds Disp: Shampoo [OTC]; 2.5% lotion SE: Dry or oily scalp, lethargy, hair discoloration, local irritation Notes: Do not use more than 2×/wk

Sertaconazole (Ertaczo) Uses: *Topical Rx interdigital tinea pedis* Acts: Imidazole antifungal. *Spectrum: Trichophyton rubrum, Trichophyton mentagrophytes, Epidermophyton floccosum* Dose: *Adults & Peds > 12.* Apply between toes & immediate surrounding healthy skin bid × 4 wk W/P: [C, ?] CI: Component allergy Disp: 2% Cream SE: Contact dermatitis, dry/burning skin, tenderness Notes: Use in immunocompetent pts; not for oral, intravag, ophthal use

Sertraline (Zoloft) BOX: Closely monitor pts for worsening depression or emergence of suicidality, particularly in ped pts Uses: *Depression, panic disorders, OCD, PTSD*, social anxiety disorder, eating disorders, premenstrual disorders Acts: ↓ Neuronal uptake of serotonin Dose: *Adults. Depression:* 50–200 mg/d PO. *PTSD:* 25 mg PO daily × 1 wk, then 50 mg PO daily, 200 mg/d max. *Peds 6–12 y.* 25 mg PO daily. *13–17 y:* 50 mg PO daily W/P: [C, ?/–] w/ Haloperidol (serotonin synd), sumatriptan, linezolid, hepatic impair CI: MAOI use w/in 14 d; concomitant pimozide Disp: Tabs 25, 50, 100, 150, 200 mg; 20 mg/mL oral SE: Activate manic/ hypomanic state, ↓ wgt, insomnia, somnolence, fatigue, tremor, xerostomia, N/D, dyspepsia, ejaculatory dysfunction, ↓ libido, hepatotox

Sevelamer Carbonate (Renvela) Uses: *Control ↑ PO$_4^{3-}$ in ESRD* Acts: Phosphate binder Dose: *Initial:* PO$_4^{3-}$ > 5.5 and < 7.5 mg/dL: 800 mg PO; ≥7.5 mg/ dL: 1600 mg PO tid. *Switching from Sevelamer HCl:* per-g basis; titrate ↑/↓ 1 tab/ meal 2-wk intervals PRN; take w/ food W/P: [C, ?] w/ Swallow disorders, bowel problems, may ↓ absorption of vits D, E, K, ↓ ciprofloxacin & other medicine levels CI: ↓ PO$_4^{3-}$, bowel obst Disp: Tab 800 mg SE: N/V/D, dyspepsia, Abd pain, flatulence, constipation Notes: Separate other meds 1 h before or 3 h after

Sevelamer HCl (Renagel) Uses: *↓ PO$_4^{3-}$ in ESRD* Acts: Binds intestinal PO$_4^{3-}$ Dose: 2–4 caps PO tid w/ meals; adjust based on PO$_4^{3-}$; max 4 g/dose W/P: [C, ?] May ↓ absorption of vits D, E, K, ↓ ciprofloxacin & other medicine levels CI: ↓ PO$_4^{3-}$, bowel obst Disp: Tab 400, 800 mg SE: BP changes, N/V/D, dyspepsia, thrombosis Notes: Do not open/chew caps; separate other meds 1 h before or 3 h after; 800 mg sevelamer = 667 mg Ca acetate

Sildenafil (Viagra, Revatio) Uses: *Viagra:* *ED*; *Revatio:* *Pulm artery HTN* Acts: ↑ Phosphodiesterase type 5 (PDE5) (responsible for cGMP breakdown); ↑ cGMP activity to relax smooth muscles & ↑ flow to corpus cavernosum and pulm vasculature; ? antiproliferative on pulm artery smooth muscle Dose: *ED:* 25–100 mg PO 1 h before sexual activity, max 1/d; ↓ if > 65 y; avoid fatty foods w/ dose; *Revatio: Pulm HTN:* 20 mg PO tid W/P: [B, ?] w/ CYP3A4 inhib (Table 10, p 301), ↓ dose w/ ritonavir; retinitis pigmentosa; hepatic/severe renal impair; w/ sig hypo-/hypertension CI: w/ Nitrates or if sex not advised; w/protease inhibitors for HIV Disp: Tabs *Viagra:* 25, 50, 100 mg, tabs *Revatio:* 20 mg SE: HA; flushing; dizziness; blue haze visual change, hearing loss, priapism Notes: Cardiac events in absence of nitrates debatable; transient global amnesia reports

Silodosin (Rapaflo) Uses: *BPH* Acts: α-blockers of prostatic α$_{1a}$ Dose: 8 mg/d; 4 mg/d w/ CrCl 30–50 mL/min; take w/ food W/P: [B, ?], not for use in females; do not use w/ other α-blockers or w/ cyclosporine; R/O PCa before use; IFIS possible w/ cataract surgery **CI:** Severe hepatic/renal impair (CrCl < 30 mL/min), w/ CYP3A4 inhib (e.g., ketoconazole, clarithromycin, itraconazole, ritonavir) **Disp:** Caps 4, 8 mg **SE:** Retrograde ejaculation, dizziness, D, syncope, somnolence, orthostatic ↓ BP, nasopharyngitis, nasal congestion **Notes:** Not for use as antihypertensive; no effect on QT interval

Silver Nitrate (Dey-Drop, Others) **Uses:** *Removal of granulation tissue & warts; prophylaxis in burns* **Acts:** Caustic antiseptic & astringent **Dose:** *Adults & Peds.* Apply to moist surface 2–3× wk for several wk or until effect **W/P:** [C, ?] **CI:** Do not use on broken skin **Disp:** Topical impregnated applicator sticks, soln 0.5, 10, 25, 50%; ophthal 1% amp; topical ointment 10% **SE:** May stain tissue black, usually resolves; local irritation, methemoglobinemia **Notes:** D/C if redness or irritation develop; no longer used in US for newborn prevention of gonococcus conjunctivitis

Silver Sulfadiazine (Silvadene, Others) **Uses:** *Prevention & Rx of Infxn in 2nd- & 3rd-degree burns* **Acts:** Bactericidal **Dose:** *Adults & Peds.* Aseptically cover the area w/ 1/16-inch coating bid **W/P:** [B unless near term, ?/–] **CI:** Infants < 2 mo, PRG near term **Disp:** Cream 1% **SE:** Itching, rash, skin discoloration, blood dyscrasias, hep, allergy **Notes:** Systemic absorption w/ extensive application

Simethicone (Mylicon, Others) [OTC] **Uses:** *Flatulence* **Acts:** Defoaming, alters gas bubble surface tension action **Dose:** *Adults & Peds > 12 y.* 40–125 mg PO pc & hs PRN; 500 mg/d max. *Peds < 2 y.* 20 mg PO qid PRN. *2–12 y:* 40 mg PO qid PRN **W/P:** [C, ?] **CI:** GI perforation or obst **Disp:** [OTC] Tabs 80, 125 mg; caps 125 mg; softgels 125, 166, 180 mg; susp 40 mg/0.6 mL; chew tabs 80, 125 mg **SE:** N/D **Notes:** Available in combo products OTC

Simvastatin (Zocor) **Uses:** *↓ Cholesterol* **Acts:** HMG-CoA reductase inhib **Dose:** *Adults.* 5–40 mg PO q P.M.; w/ meals; ↓ in renal Insuff; w/o grapefruit. *Peds 10–17 y.* 10 mg, 40 mg/d max **W/P:** [X, –] max 10 mg daily w/ amiodarone, verapamil, diltiazem; max 20 mg daily w/ amlodipine, ranolazine; 80 mg dose restricted to those taking >12 mo w/o muscle tox; w/ Chinese pt on lipid modifying meds **CI:** PRG, liver Dz **Disp:** Tabs 5, 10, 20, 40, 80 mg **SE:** HA, GI upset, myalgia, myopathy (pain, tenderness, weakness w/ creatine kinase 10× ULN) and rhabdomyolysis, hep **Notes:** Combo w/ ezetimibe/simvastatin; follow LFTs

Sipuleucel-T (Provenge) **Uses:** *Asymptomatic/minimally symptomatic metastatic castrate resistant PCa* **Acts:** Autologous (pt specific) cellular immunotherapy **Dose:** 3 weekly doses; pre-med w/ APAP & diphenhydramine **W/P:** [NA, N/A] confirm identity/expir date before inf; acute transfusion Rxn possible; not tested for transmissible Dz **CI:** None **Disp:** 50 mill units autologous CD54+ cells activated w/ PAP GM-CSF, in 250 mL LR **SE:** Chills, fatigue, fever, back pain, N, joint ache, HA **Notes:** Pt must undergo leukophoresis, w/ shipping and autologous cell processing at manufacturing facility before each inf

Sirolimus [Rapamycin] (Rapamune) **BOX:** Use only by physicians experienced in immunosuppression; immunosuppression associated w/ lymphoma,

↑ Infxn risk; do not use in lung transplant (fatal bronchial anastomotic dehiscence) **Uses:** *Prevent organ rejection in new Tx pts* **Acts:** ↓ T-lymphocyte activation **Dose:** *Adults > 40 kg:* 6 mg PO on day 1, then 2 mg/d PO. *Peds < 40 kg & ≥13 y.* 3 mg/m^2 load, then 1 mg/m^2/d (in H$_2$O/orange juice; no grapefruit juice w/ sirolimus); take 4 h after cyclosporine; ↓ in hepatic impair **W/P:** [C, ?/–] Grapefruit juice, ketoconazole **CI:** Component allergy **Disp:** Soln 1 mg/mL, tab 1, 2 mg **SE:** HTN, edema, CP, fever, HA, insomnia, pain, rash, ↑ cholesterol, GI upset, ↑/↓ K$^+$, infxns, blood dyscrasias, arthralgia, tachycardia, renal impair, graft loss & death in liver transplant (hepatic artery thrombosis), ascites, delayed healing **Notes:** Levels: *Trough:* 4–20 ng/mL; varies w/assay method

Sitagliptin (Januvia) Uses: *Monotherapy or combo for type 2 DM*
Action: Dipeptidyl peptidase-4 (DDP-4) inhib, ↑ insulin synth/release **Dose:** 2.5 or 5 mg once/d w/o regard to meals; 2.5 mg once/d w/ CrCl < 50 mL/min or w/ strong CYP3A4/5 inhib (e.g., atazanavir, clarithromycin, indinavir, itraconazole, ketoconazole, nefazodone, nelfinavir, ritonavir, saquinavir, and telithromycin) **W/P:** [?, ?] May cause ↓ blood sugar when used w/ insulin secretagogues such as sulfonylureas **CI:** w/ Insulin or to treat DKA **Disp:** Tabs 2.5, 5 mg **SE:** URI, nasopharyngitis, UTI, HA **Notes:** No evidence for ↑ CV risk

Sitagliptin/Metformin (Janumet) BOX: See metformin, p 179 Uses:
Adjunct to diet and exercise in type 2 DM **Action:** See individual agents **Dose:** 1 tab PO bid, titrate; max 100 mg sitagliptin & 2000 mg metformin/d max; take w/ meals **W/P:** [B, ?/–] **CI:** Type 1 DM, DKA, male Cr > 15; female Cr > 1.4 mg/dL **Disp:** Tabs 50/500, 50 mg/1000 mg **SE:** Nasopharyngitis, N/V/D, flatulence, Abd discomfort, dyspepsia, asthenia, HA **Notes:** Hold w/ contrast study; ✓ Cr, CBC

Smallpox Vaccine (Dryvax) BOX: Acute myocarditis and other infectious
complications possible; CI in immunocompromised, eczema or exfoliative skin conditions, infants < 1 y **Uses:** Immunization against smallpox (variola virus) **Acts:** Active immunization (live attenuated cowpox virus) **Dose:** *Adults (routine nonemergency) or all ages (emergency):* 2–3 Punctures w/ bifurcated needle dipped in vaccine into deltoid, posterior triceps muscle; ✓ site for Rxn in 6–8 d; if major Rxn, site scabs, & heals, leaving scar; if mild/equivocal Rxn, repeat w/ 15 punctures **W/P:** [X, N/A] **CI:** *Nonemergency use:* febrile illness, immunosuppression, Hx eczema & in household contacts. *Emergency:* No absolute CI **Disp:** Vial for reconstitution: 100 mill pock-forming units/mL **SE:** Malaise, fever, regional lymphadenopathy, encephalopathy, rashes, spread of inoculation to other sites; SJS, eczema vaccinatum w/ severe disability **Notes:** Avoid infants for 14 d; intradermal use only; restricted distribution

Sodium Bicarbonate [NaHCO₃] Uses: *Alkalinization of urine, RTA,
metabolic acidosis, ↑ K$^+$, TCA OD **Acts:** Alkalinizing agent **Dose:** *Adults. ECC 2010.* Cardiac arrest w/ good ventilation, hyperkalemia, OD of TCAs, ASA, cocaine, diphenhydramine: 1 mEq/kg IV bolus; repeat 1/2 dose q10min PRN. If rapidly available, use ABG to guide therapy (ABG results unreliable in cardiac

arrest). *Metabolic acidosis:* 2–5 mEq/kg IV over 8 h & PRN based on acid–base status. ↑ K⁺: 1 mg/kg IV over 5 min. *Alkalinize urine:* 4 g (48 mEq) PO, then 1–2 g q4h; adjust based on urine pH; 2 amp (100 mEq/L 1 D₅W at 100–250 mL/h IV, monitor urine pH & serum bicarbonate. *Chronic renal failure:* 1–3 mEq/kg/d. *Distal RTA:* 1 mEq/kg/d PO. **Peds.** Sodium bicarbonate *ECC 2010. Severe metabolic acidosis, hyperkalemia:* 1 mEq/kg IV slow bolus; 4.2% conc in infants < 1 month. *Sodium channel blocker OD:* 1–2 mEq/kg IV/IO bolus until pH > 7.45 (7.50–7.55 severe OD); then inf 150 mEq NaHCO₃/L soln to maint alkalosis. *Chronic renal failure:* See Adults dosage. *Distal RTA:* 2–3 mEq/kg/d PO. *Proximal RTA:* 5–10 mEq/kg/d; titrate based on serum bicarbonate. *Urine alkalinization:* 84–840 mg/kg/d (1–10 mEq/kg/d) in ÷ doses; adjust based on urine pH **W/P:** [C, ?] **CI:** Alkalosis, ↑ Na⁺, severe pulm edema, ↓ Ca²⁺ **Disp:** Powder, tabs; 300 mg = 3.6 mEq; 325 mg = 3.8 mEq; 520 mg = 6.3 mEq; 600 mg = 7.3 mEq; 650 mg = 7.6 mEq; Inj 1 mEq/1 mL, 4.2% (5 mEq/10 mL), 7.5% (8.92 mEq/mL), 8.4% (10 mEq/10 mL) vial or amp **SE:** Belching, edema, flatulence, ↑ Na⁺, metabolic alkalosis **Notes:** 1 g neutralizes 12 mEq of acid; 50 mEq bicarbonate = 50 mEq Na; can make 3 amps in 1 L D₅W to = D₅NS w/ 150 mEq bicarbonate

Sodium Citrate/Citric Acid (Bicitra, Oracit)

Uses: *Chronic metabolic acidosis, alkalinize urine; dissolve uric acid & cysteine stones* **Acts:** Urinary alkalinizer **Dose:** *Adults.* 10–30 mL in 1–3 oz H₂O pc & hs. *Peds.* 5–15 mL in 1–3 oz H₂O pc & hs; best after meals **W/P:** [C, +] **CI:** Al-based antacids; severe renal impair or Na-restricted diets **Disp:** 15- or 30-mL unit dose: 16 (473 mL) or 4 (118 mL) fl oz **SE:** Tetany, metabolic alkalosis, ↑ K⁺, GI upset; avoid use of multiple 50-mL amps; can cause ↑ Na⁺/hyperosmolality **Notes:** 1 mL = 1 mEq Na & 1 mEq bicarbonate

Sodium Oxybate (Xyrem) [C-III]

BOX: Known drug of abuse even at recommended doses; confusion, depression, resp depression may occur **Uses:** *Narcolepsy-associated cataplexy* **Acts:** Inhibitory neurotransmitter **Dose:** *Adults & Peds > 16 y.* 2.25 g PO qhs, 2nd dose 2.5–4 h later; may ↑ 9 g/d max **W/P:** [B, ?/–] **CI:** Succinic semialdehyde dehydrogenase deficiency; potentiates EtOH **Disp:** 500 mg/mL (180-mL) PO soln **SE:** Confusion, depression, ↓ diminished level of consciousness, incontinence, sig ↓ Sxs, resp depression, psychological Sxs **Notes:** May lead to dependence; synonym for γ-hydroxybutyrate (GHB), abused as a "date rape drug"; controlled distribution (prescriber & pt registration); must be administered when pt in bed

Sodium Phosphate (Visicol)

Uses: *Bowel prep prior to colonoscopy*, short-term constipation **Acts:** Hyperosmotic laxative **Dose:** 3 Tabs PO w/ at least 8 oz clear liq q15min (20 tabs total night before procedure); 3–5 h before colonoscopy, repeat) **W/P:** [C, ?] Renal impair, electrolyte disturbances **CI:** Megacolon, bowel obst, CHF, ascites, unstable angina, gastric retention, bowel perforation, colitis, hypomotility **Disp:** Tabs 0.398, 1.102 g **SE:** ↑ QT, ↑ PO₄³⁻, ↓ K⁺, Na¹⁺, D, flatulence, cramps, Abd bloating/pain

Sodium Polystyrene Sulfonate (Kayexalate) Uses: *Rx of ↑ K+* Acts: Na+/K+ ion-exchange resin Dose: *Adults.* 15–60 g PO or 30–60 g PR q6h based on serum K+. *Peds.* 1 g/kg/dose PO or PR q6h based on serum K+ (given w/ agent, e.g., sorbitol, to promote movement through the bowel) W/P: [C, M] CI: ↑ Na+ Disp: Powder; susp 15 g/60 mL sorbitol SE: ↑ Na+, ↓ K+, Na retention, GI upset, fecal impaction Notes: Enema acts more quickly than PO; PO most effective, onset action > 2 h

Solifenacin (Vesicare) Uses: *OAB* Acts: Antimuscarinic, ↓ detrusor contractions Dose: 5 mg PO daily, 10 mg/d max; ↓ w/ renal/hepatic impair W/P: [C, ?/–] BOO or GI obst, ulcerative colitis, MyG, renal/hepatic impair, QT prolongation risk CI: NAG, urinary/gastric retention Disp: Tabs 5, 10 mg SE: Constipation, xerostomia, dyspepsia, blurred vision, drowsiness Notes: CYP3A4 substrate; azole antifungals ↑ levels; recent concern over cognitive effects

Somatropin (Serostim) Uses: *HIV-assoc wasting/cachexia* Acts: Anabolic peptide hormone Dose: 0.1 mg/kg SQ hs W/P: [B, ?] CI: Active neoplasm; acute critical illness post-op; benzyl alcohol sens; hypersens Disp: Powder for Inj SE: Arthralgia, edema, ↑ blood glucose

Sorafenib (Nexavar) Uses: *Advanced RCC*, metastatic liver CA Acts: Kinase inhib Dose: *Adults.* 400 mg PO bid on empty stomach W/P: [D, –] w/ Irinotecan, doxorubicin, warfarin; avoid conception (male/female) Disp: Tabs 200 mg SE: Hand–foot synd; Tx-emergent hypertension; bleeding, ↑ INR, cardiac infarction/ischemia; ↑ pancreatic enzymes, hypophosphatemia, lymphopenia, anemia, fatigue, alopecia, pruritus, D, GI upset, HA, neuropathy Notes: Monitor BP 1st 6 wk; may require ↓ dose (daily or q other day); impaired metabolism w/Asian descent; may effect wound healing, D/C before major surgery

Sorbitol (Generic) Uses: *Constipation* Acts: Laxative Dose: 30–60 mL PO of a 20–70% soln PRN W/P: [B, +] CI: Anuria Disp: Liq 70% SE: Edema, electrolyte loss, lactic acidosis, GI upset, xerostomia Notes: Vehicle for many liq formulations (e.g., zinc, Kayexalate)

Sotalol (Betapace) BOX: To minimize risk of induced arrhythmia, pts initiated/reinitiated on *Betapace AF* should be placed for a minimum of 3 d (on their maint) in a facility that can provide cardiac resuscitation, cont ECG monitoring, & calculations of CrCl. *Betapace* should not be substituted for *Betapace AF* because of labeling Uses: *Ventricular arrhythmias, AF* Acts: β-Adrenergic-blocking agent Dose: *Adults. CrCl > 60 mL/min:* 80 mg PO bid, may ↑ to 240–320 mg/d. CrCl 30–60 mL/min: 80 mg q24h. CrCl 10–30 mL/min: Dose 80 mg q36–48h. *ECC 2010. SVT and ventricular arrhythmias:* 1–1.5 mg/kg IV over 5 min. *Peds Neonates.* 9 mg/m² tid. *1–19 mo:* 20.4 mg/m² tid. *20–23 mo:* 29.1 mg/m² tid. *≥2 y:* 30 mg/m² tid; to max dose of 90 mg/m² tid; ↓ w/ renal impair W/P: [B (1st tri) (D if 2nd or 3rd tri), +] CI: Asthma, COPD, ↓ HR, ↑ prolonged QT interval, 2nd-/3rd-degree heart block w/o pacemaker, cardiogenic shock, uncontrolled CHF Disp: Tabs 80, 120, 160, 240 mg SE: ↓ HR, CP, palpitations, fatigue, dizziness, weakness, dyspnea

Sotalol (Betapace AF) **BOX:** See sotalol (*Betapace*) **Uses:** *Maintain sinus rhythm for symptomatic AF/A flutter* **Acts:** β-Adrenergic-blocking agent **Dose:** *Adults. CrCl > 60 mL/min:* 80 mg PO q12h, max 320 mg/d. *CrCl 40–60 mL/min:* 80 mg PO q24h; ↑ to 120 mg during hospitalization; monitor QT interval 2–4 h after each dose, dose reduction or D/C if QT interval ≥ 500 msec. *Peds Neonates.* 40 mg/m² tid. *1–19 mo:* 20 mg/m² tid. *20–23 mo:* 29.1 mg/m² tid. *≥ 2 y:* 30 mg/m² tid; can double all doses as max daily dose; allow ~36 h between changes **W/P:** [B (1st tri; D if 2nd or 3rd tri), +] when converting from other antiarrhythmic **CI:** Asthma, ↓ HR, ↑ QT interval, 2nd/3rd-degree heart block w/o pacemaker, cardiogenic shock, uncontrolled CHF, CrCl < 40 mL/min **Disp:** Tabs 80, 120, 160 mg **SE:** ↓ HR, CP, palpitations, fatigue, dizziness, weakness, dyspnea **Notes:** Follow renal Fxn & QT interval; Betapace should not be substituted for Betapace AF because of differences in labeling

Spinosad (Natroba) **Uses:** *Head lice* **Acts:** Neuronal excitation of lice, w/ paralysis & death **Dose:** Cover dry scalp with suspension, then apply to dry hair; rinse off in 10 min **W/P:** [B, ?/–] **CI:** < 6 mo **Disp:** 0.9% topical susp **SE:** Scalp/ocular erythema **Notes:** Shake well before use; use w/ overall lice management program; in benzyl alcohol, serious Rxns in neonates, in breast milk, pump and discard milk for 8 h after use

Spironolactone (Aldactone) **BOX:** Tumorogenic in anmial studies; avoid unnecessary use **Uses:** *Hyperaldosteronism, HTN, class III/IV CHF, ascites from cirrhosis* **Acts:** Aldosterone antagonist; K⁺-sparing diuretic **Dose:** *Adults. CHF* (NYHA class III–IV) 12.5–25 mg/d (w/ ACE and loop diuretic); *HTN* 25–50 mg/d; *Ascites:* 100–400 mg q A.M with 40–160 mg of furosemide, start w 100 mg/40 mg, wait at least 3 d before ↑ dose *Peds.* 1–3.3 mg/kg/24 h PO ÷ bid-qid. *Neonates:* 0.5–1 mg/kg dose q8h; take w/ food **W/P:** [D, +] **CI:** ↑ K⁺, acute renal failure, anuria **Disp:** Tabs 25, 50, 100 mg **SE:** ↑ K⁺ & gynecomastia, arrhythmia, sexual dysfunction, confusion, dizziness, D/N/V, abnormal menstruation

Starch, Topical, Rectal (Tucks Suppositories [OTC]) **Uses:** *Temporary relief of anorectal disorders (itching, etc)* **Acts:** Topical protectant **Dose:** *Adults & Peds ≥12 y.* Cleanse, rinse and dry, insert 1 sup rectally 6×/d × 7 d max. **W/P:** [?, ?] **CI:** None **Disp:** Supp SE: D/C w/ or if rectal bleeding occurs or if condition worsens or does not improve w/in 7 d

Stavudine (Zerit) **BOX:** Lactic acidosis & severe hepatomegaly w/ steatosis & pancreatitis reported **Uses:** *HIV in combo w/ other antiretrovirals* **Acts:** Reverse transcriptase inhib **Dose:** *Adults > 60 kg:* 40 mg bid. *< 60 kg:* 30 mg bid. *Peds Birth–13 d.* 0.5 mg/kg q12h. *> 14 d & < 30 kg:* 1 mg/kg q12h. *≥30 kg:* Adult dose; ↓ w/ renal Insuff **W/P:** [C, +] **CI:** Allergy **Disp:** Caps 15, 20, 30, 40 mg; soln 1 mg/mL **SE:** Peripheral neuropathy, HA, chills, fever, malaise, rash, GI upset, anemias, lactic acidosis, ↑ LFTs, pancreatitis **Notes:** Take w/ plenty of H_2O

Steroids, Systemic (See Table 2, p 283) The following relates only to the commonly used systemic glucocorticoids **Uses:** *Endocrine disorders (adrenal insuff), *rheumatoid disorders, collagen–vascular Dzs, derm Dzs, allergic states, cerebral edema*, nephritis, nephrotic synd, immunosuppression for transplantation, ↑ Ca^{2+}, malignancies (breast, lymphomas), pre-op (pt who has been on steroids in past year, known hypoadrenalism, pre-op for adrenalectomy); Inj into joints/tissue **Acts:** Glucocorticoid **Dose:** Varies w/ use & institutional protocols.

- *Adrenal Insuff, acute: Adults.* Hydrocortisone: 100 mg IV; then 300 mg/d ÷ q6h; convert to 50 mg PO q8h × 6 doses, taper to 30–50 mg/d ÷ bid. *Peds. Hydrocortisone:* 1–2 mg/kg IV, then 150–250 mg/d ÷ tid.
- *Adrenal Insuff, chronic (physiologic replacement):* May need mineralocorticoid supl such as Florinef. *Adults. Hydrocortisone:* 20 mg PO q A.M., 10 mg PO q P.M.; *cortisone:* 0.5–0.75 mg/kg/d ÷ bid; *cortisone:* 0.25–0.35 mg/kg/d IM; *dexamethasone:* 0.03–0.15 mg/kg/d or 0.6–0.75 mg/m^2/d ÷ q6–12h PO, IM, IV. *Peds. Hydrocortisone:* 0.5–0.75 mg/kg/d PO tid; *hydrocortisone succinate:* 0.25–0.35 mg/kg/d IM.
- *Asthma, acute: Adults. Methylprednisolone* 60 mg PO/IV q6h or *dexamethasone* 12 mg IV q6h. *Peds. Prednisolone* 1–2 mg/kg/d or *prednisone* 1–2 mg/kg/d ÷ daily-bid for up to 5 d; *methylprednisolone* 2–4 mg/kg/d IV ÷ tid; *dexamethasone* 0.1–0.3 mg/kg/d ÷ q6h.
- *Congenital adrenal hyperplasia: Peds.* Initial *hydrocortisone* 30–36 mg/m^2/d PO ÷ 1/3 dose q A.M., 2/3 dose q P.M.; maint 20–25 mg/m^2/d ÷ bid.
- *Extubation/airway edema: Adults. Dexamethasone:* 0.5–1 mg/kg/d IM/IV ÷ q6h (start 24 h prior to extubation; continue × 4 more doses). *Peds. Dexamethasone:* 0.1–0.3 mg/kg/d ÷ q6h × 3–5 d (start 48–72 h before extubation)
- *Immunosuppressive/anti-inflammatory: Adults & Older Peds. Hydrocortisone:* 15–240 mg PO, IM, IV q12h; *methylprednisolone:* 4–48 mg/d PO, taper to lowest effective dose; *methylprednisolone Na succinate:* 10–80 mg/d IM. *Adults. Prednisone or prednisolone:* 5–60 mg/d PO ÷ daily-qid. *Infants & Younger Children. Hydrocortisone:* 2.5–10 mg/kg/d PO ÷ q6–8h; 1–5 mg/kg/d IM/IV ÷ bid.
- *Nephrotic synd: Peds. Prednisolone or prednisone:* 2 mg/kg/d PO tid-qid until urine is protein-free for 5 d, use up to 28 d; for persistent proteinuria, 4 mg/kg/dose PO q other day max 120 mg/d for an additional 28 d; maint 2 mg/kg/dose q other day for 28 d; taper over 4–6 wk (max 80 mg/d).
- *Septic shock (controversial): Adults. Hydrocortisone:* 500 mg–1 g IM/IV q2–6h. *Peds. Hydrocortisone:* 50 mg/kg IM/IV, repeat q4–24 h PRN.
- *Status asthmaticus: Adults & Peds. Hydrocortisone:* 1–2 mg/kg/dose IV q6h; then ↓ by 0.5–1 mg/kg q6h.
- *Rheumatic Dz: Adults. Intra-articular: Hydrocortisone acetate:* 25–37.5 mg large joint, 10–25 mg small joint *Methylprednisolone acetate:* 20–80 mg large joint, 4–10 mg small joint. *Intrabursal: Hydrocortisone acetate:* 25–37.5 mg. *Intra-ganglial: Hydrocortisone acetate:* 25–37.5 mg. *Tendon sheath: Hydrocortisone acetate:* 5–12.5 mg.

- *Perioperative steroid coverage: Hydrocortisone:* 100 mg IV night before surgery, 1 h pre-op, intraoperative, & 4, 8, & 12 h post-op; post-op day No. 1 100 mg IV q6h; post-op day No. 2 100 mg IV q8h; post-op day No. 3 100 mg IV q12h; post-op day No. 4 50 mg IV q12h; post-op day No. 5 25 mg IV q12h; resume prior PO dosing if chronic use or D/C if only perioperative coverage required.
- *Cerebral edema: Dexamethasone:* 10 mg IV; then 4 mg IV q4–6h

W/P: [C, ?/−] **CI:** Active varicella Infxn, serious Infxn except TB, fungal infxns **Disp:** Table 2, p 301 **SE:** ↑ Appetite, hyperglycemia, ↓ K+, osteoporosis, nervousness, insomnia, "steroid psychosis," adrenal suppression **Notes:** Hydrocortisone succinate for systemic, acetate for intraarticular; never abruptly D/C steroids, taper dose; also used for bacterial and TB meningitis

Steroids, Topical (See Table 3, p 284) **Uses:** *Steroid-responsive dermatoses (seborrheic/atopic dermatitis, neurodermatitis, anogenital pruritus, psoriasis)* **Action:** Glucocorticoid; ↓ capillary permeability, stabilizes lysosomes to control inflammation; controls protein synthesis; ↓ migration of leukocytes, fibroblasts **Dose:** Use lowest potency produce for shortest period for effect (see Table 3, p 284) **W/P:** [C, +] Do not use occlusive dressings; high potency topical products not for rosacea, perioral dermatitis; not for use on face, groin, axillae; none for use in a diapered area. **CI:** Component hypersens **Disp:** See Table 3, p 284 **SE:** Skin atrophy w/ chronic use; chronic administration or application over large area may cause adrenal suppression or hyperglycemia

Streptokinase (Streptase, Kabikinase) **Uses:** *Coronary artery thrombosis, acute massive PE, DVT, & some occluded vascular grafts* **Acts:** Activates plasminogen to plasmin that degrades fibrin **Dose:** *Adults.* *PE:* Load 250,000 units peripheral IV over 30 min, then 100,000 units/h IV for 24–72 h. *Coronary artery thrombosis:* 1.5 mill units IV over 60 min. *DVT or arterial embolism:* Load as w/ PE, then 100,000 units/h for 72 h; *ECC 2010. AMI:* 1.5 mill units over 1 h. *Peds.* 3500–4000 units/kg over 30 min, then 1000–1500 units/h. *Occluded catheter (controversial):* 10,000–25,000 units in NS to final vol of catheter (leave in for 1 h, aspirate & flush w/ NS) **W/P:** [C, +] **CI:** Streptococcal Infxn or streptokinase in last 6 mo, active bleeding, CVA, TIA, spinal surgery/trauma in last month, vascular anomalies, severe hepatic/renal Dz, endocarditis, pericarditis, severe uncontrolled HTN **Disp:** Powder for Inj 250,000, 750,000, 1,500,000 units **SE:** Bleeding, ↓ BP, fever, bruising, rash, GI upset, hemorrhage, anaphylaxis **Notes:** If Inf inadequate to keep clotting time 2–5× control, see PI for adjustments; antibodies remain 3–6 mo following dose

Streptomycin **BOX:** Neuro/oto/renal tox possible; neuromuscular blockage w/ resp paralysis possible **Uses:** *TB combo Rx therapy* streptococcal or enterococcal endocarditis **Acts:** Aminoglycoside; ↓ protein synth **Dose:** *Adults.* *Endocarditis:* 1 g q12h 1–2 wk, then 500 mg q12h 1–4 wk; *TB:* 15 mg/kg/d (up to 1 g), directly observed therapy (DOT) 2× wk 20–30 mg/kg/dose (max 1.5 g), DOT 3× wk 25–30 mg/kg/dose (max 1 g). *Peds.* 15 mg/kg/d; DOT 2× wk 20–40 mg/kg/

dose (max 1 g); DOT 3× wk 25–30 mg/kg/dose (max 1 g); ↓ w/ renal Insuff, either IM or IV over 30–60 min **W/P:** [D, +] **CI:** PRG **Disp:** Inj 400 mg/mL (1-g vial) **SE:** ↑ Incidence of vestibular & auditory tox, ↑ neurotox risk in pts w/ impaired renal fxn **Notes:** Monitor levels: *Peak:* 20–30 mcg/mL; *Trough:* < 5 mcg/mL; *Toxic peak:* > 50 mcg/mL, *Trough:* > 10 mcg/mL; IV over 30–60 min

Streptozocin (Zanosar) **Uses:** *Pancreatic islet cell tumors* & carcinoid tumors **Acts:** DNA–DNA (intrastrand) cross-linking; DNA, RNA, & protein synth inhib **Dose:** Per protocol; ↓ in renal failure **W/P:** w/ Renal failure [D, ?/–] **CI:** w/ Rotavirus vaccine, PRG **Disp:** Inj 1 g **SE:** N/V/D, duodenal ulcers, depression, ↓ BM rare (20%) & mild; nephrotox (proteinuria & azotemia dose related), hypophosphatemia dose limiting; hypo-/hyperglycemia; Inj site Rxns **Notes:** Monitor Cr

Succimer (Chemet) **Uses:** *Lead poisoning (levels > 45 mcg/mL)* **Acts:** Heavy metal-chelating agent **Dose:** *Adults & Peds.* 10 mg/kg/dose q8h × 5 d, then 10 mg/kg/dose q12h for 14 d; ↓ in renal Insuff **W/P:** [C, ?] **CI:** Allergy **Disp:** Caps 100 mg **SE:** Rash, fever, GI upset, hemorrhoids, metallic taste, drowsiness, ↑ LFTs **Notes:** Monitor lead levels, maintain hydration, may open caps

Succinylcholine (Anectine, Quelicin, Sucostrin, Others) **BOX:** Risk of cardiac arrest from hyperkalemic rhabdomyolysis **Uses:** *Adjunct to general anesthesia, facilitates ET intubation; induce skeletal muscle relaxation during surgery or mechanical ventilation* **Acts:** Depolarizing neuromuscular blocker; rapid onset, short duration (3–5 min) **Dose:** *Adults.* Rapid sequence intubation 1–2 mg/kg IV over 10–30 s or 2–4 mg/kg IM (*ECC 2005*). *Peds.* 1–2 mg/kg/dose IV, then by 0.3–0.6 mg/kg/dose q5min; ↓ w/ severe renal/hepatic impair **W/P:** See Box [C, M] **CI:** w/ Malignant hyperthermia risk, myopathy, recent major burn, multiple trauma, extensive skeletal muscle denervation, NAG, pseudocholinesterase deficiency **Disp:** Inj 20, 50, 100 mg/mL **SE:** Fasciculations, ↑ IOP, ICP, intragastric pressure, salivation, myoglobinuria, malignant hyperthermia, resp depression, prolonged apnea; multiple drugs potentiate CV effects (arrhythmias, ↓ BP, brady/tachycardia) **Notes:** May be given IV push/Inf/IM deltoid; hyperkalemic rhabdomyolysis in children w/ undiagnosed myopathy such as Duchenne muscular dystrophy

Sucralfate (Carafate) **Uses:** *Duodenal ulcers*, gastric ulcers, stomatitis, GERD, preventing stress ulcers, esophagitis **Acts:** Forms ulcer-adherent complex that protects against acid, pepsin, & bile acid **Dose:** *Adults.* 1 g PO qid, 1 h prior to meals & hs. *Peds.* 40–80 mg/kg/d ÷ q6h; continue 4–8 wk unless healing demonstrated by x-ray or endoscopy; separate from other drugs by 2 h; take on empty stomach ac **W/P:** [B, +] **CI:** Component allergy **Disp:** Tabs 1 g; susp 1 g/10 mL **SE:** Constipation; D, dizziness, xerostomia **Notes:** Al may accumulate in renal failure

Sulfacetamide (Bleph-10, Cetamide, Sodium Sulamyd) **Uses:** *Conjunctival infxns* **Acts:** Sulfonamide antibiotic **Dose:** 10% oint apply qid & hs; soln for keratitis apply q2–3h based on severity **W/P:** [C, M] **CI:** Sulfonamide sensitivity; age < 2 mo **Disp:** Oint 10%; soln 10, 15, 30%; topical cream 10%; foam, gel, lotion, pad all 10% **SE:** Irritation, burning, blurred vision, brow ache, SJS, photosens

Sulfacetamide & Prednisolone (Blephamide, Others) Uses: *Steroid-responsive inflammatory ocular conditions w/ Infxn or a risk of Infxn* Acts: Antibiotic & anti-inflammatory Dose: *Adults & Peds > 2 y.* Apply oint lower conjunctival sac daily-qid; soln 1–3 gtt 2–3 h while awake W/P: [C, ?/–] Sulfonamide sensitivity; age < 2 mo Disp: *Oint:* sulfacetamide 10%/prednisolone 0.5%, sulfacetamide 10%/prednisolone 0.2%, sulfacetamide 10%/prednisolone 0.25%. *Susp:* sulfacetamide 10%/prednisolone 0.25%, sulfacetamide 10%/prednisolone 0.5%, sulfacetamide 10%/prednisolone 0.2% SE: Irritation, burning, blurred vision, brow ache, SJS, photosens Notes: OK ophthal susp use as otic agent

Sulfasalazine (Azulfidine, Azulfidine EN) Uses: *Ulcerative colitis, RA, juvenile RA*, active Crohn Dz, ankylosing spondylitis, psoriasis Acts: Sulfonamide; actions unclear Dose: *Adults. Ulcerative colitis:* Initial, 1 g PO tid-qid; ↑ to a max of 8 g/d in 3–4 ÷ doses; maint 500 mg PO qid. *RA:* (EC tab) 0.5–1 g/d, ↑ weekly to maint 2 g ÷ bid. *Peds. Ulcerative colitis:* Initial: 40–60 mg/kg/24 h PO ÷ q4–6h; maint: 20–30 mg/kg/24 h PO ÷ q6h. *RA > 6 y:* 30–50 mg/kg/d in 2 doses, start w/ 1/4–1/3 maint dose, ↑ weekly until dose reached at 1 mo, 2 g/d max; ↓ w/ renal Insuff W/P: [B (D if near term), M] CI: Sulfonamide or salicylate sensitivity, porphyria, GI or GU obst; avoid in hepatic impair Disp: Tabs 500 mg; EC DR tabs 500 mg SE: GI upset; discolors urine; dizziness, HA, photosens, oligospermia, anemias, SJS Notes: May cause yellow-orange skin/contact lens discoloration; avoid sunlight exposure

Sulfinpyrazone Uses: *Acute & chronic gout* Acts: ↓ Renal tubular absorption of uric acid Dose: 100–200 mg PO bid for 1 wk, ↑ PRN to maint of 200–400 mg bid; max 800 mg/d; take w/ food or antacids, & plenty of fluids; avoid salicylates W/P: [C (D if near term), ?/–] CI: Renal impair, avoid salicylates; peptic ulcer; blood dyscrasias, near-term PRG, allergy Disp: Tabs 100 mg; caps 200 mg SE: N/V, stomach pain, urolithiasis, leukopenia Notes: Take w/ plenty of H_2O

Sulindac (Clinoril) BOX: May ↑ risk of CV events & GI bleeding; do not use for post CABG pain control Uses: *Arthritis & pain* Acts: NSAID; ↓ prostaglandins Dose: 150–200 mg bid, 400 mg/d max; w/ food W/P: [B (D if 3rd tri or near term), ?/–] CI: NSAID or ASA sensitivity, w/ ketorolac, ulcer, GI bleeding, post-op pain in coronary artery bypass graft Disp: Tabs 150, 200 mg SE: Dizziness, rash, GI upset, pruritus, edema, ↓ renal blood flow, renal failure (? fewer renal effects than other NSAIDs), peptic ulcer, GI bleeding

Sumatriptan (Alsuma, Imitrex Injection, Imitrex Nasal Spray, Imitrex Oral) Uses: *Rx acute migraine and cluster HA* Acts: Vascular serotonin receptor agonist Dose: *Adults.* SQ: 6 mg SQ as a single-dose PRN; repeat PRN in 1 h to a max of 12 mg/24 h. PO: 25–100 mg, repeat in 2 h, PRN, 200 mg/d max. *Nasal spray:* 1 spray into 1 nostril, repeat in 2 h to 40 mg/ 24 h max. *Peds. Nasal spray: 6–9 y:* 5–20 mg. *10–17 y:* 5–20 mg, up to 40 mg/d W/P: [C, M] CI: IV use, angina, ischemic heart dz, CV syndromes, uncontrolled HTN, severe hepatic impair, ergot use, MAOI use w/in 14 d, hemiplegic or basilar migraine **Disp:** *Imitrex Oral:* OD tabs 25, 50, 100 mg; *Imitrex Injection:* 6, 8, 12 mg/mL;, ODTs 25, 50, 100 mg; *Imitrex Nasal Spray:* 5, 10, 20 mg/spray; *Alsuma Auto-Injector:* 6 mg/0.5 mL **SE:** Pain & bruising at Inj site; dizziness, hot flashes, paresthesias, CP, weakness, numbness, coronary vasospasm, HTN

Sumatriptan & Naproxen Sodium (Treximet) **BOX:** ↑ Risk of serious CV (MI, stroke) serious GI events (bleeding, ulceration, perforation) of the stomach or intestines **Uses:** *Prevent migraines* **Acts:** Anti-inflammatory NSAID w/ 5-HT₁ receptor agonist, constricts CNS vessels **Dose:** *Adults.* 1 tab PO; repeat PRN after 2 h; max 2 tabs/24 h, w/ or w/o food **W/P:** [C, –] **CI:** CV Dz, severe hepatic impair, severe ↑ BP **Disp:** Tab naproxen/sumatriptan 500 mg/85 mg **SE:** Dizziness, somnolence, paresthesia, N, dyspepsia, dry mouth, chest/neck/throat/jaw pain, tightness, pressure **Notes:** Do not split/crush/chew

Sumatriptan Needleless System (Sumavel DosePro) **Uses:** *Rx acute migraine and cluster HA* **Acts:** Vascular serotonin receptor agonist **Dose:** *Adults.* SQ: 6 mg SQ as a single-dose PRN; repeat PRN in 1 h to a max of 12 mg/24h; administer in abdomen/thigh. **W/P:** [C, M] **CI:** See Sumatriptan **Disp:** Needle-free SQ injector 6 mg/0.5 mL **SE:** Injection site Rxn, tingling, warm/hot/burning sensation, feeling of heaviness/pressure/tightness/numbness, feeling strange, lightheadedness, flushing, tightness in chest, discomfort in nasal cavity/sinuses/jaw, dizziness/vertigo, drowsiness/sedation, HA

Sunitinib (Sutent) **Uses:** *Advanced GI stromal tumor (GIST) refractory/intolerant of imatinib; advanced RCC; well-differentiated pancreatic neuroendocrine tumors unresecable, locally advanced, metastatic* **Acts:** Multi-TKI **Dose:** *Adults.* 50 mg PO daily × 4 wk, followed by 2 wk holiday = 1 cycle; ↓ to 37.5 mg w/ CYP3A4 inhib (Table 10, p 301), to ↑ 87.5 mg w/ CYP3A4 inducers **CI:** w/ Atazanavir **W/P:** [D, –] Multiple interactions require dose modification (e.g., St. John's wort) **Disp:** Caps 12.5, 25, 50 mg **SE:** ↓ WBC & plt, bleeding, ↑ BP, ↓ ejection fraction, ↑ QT interval, pancreatitis, DVT, Szs, adrenal insufficiency, N/V/D, skin discoloration, oral ulcers, taste perversion, hypothyroidism **Notes:** Monitor left ventricular ejection fraction, ECG, CBC/plts, chemistries (K⁺/Mg²⁺/phosphate), TFT & LFTs periodically; ↓ dose in 12.5-mg increments if not tolerated

Tacrine (Cognex) **Uses:** *Mild–mod Alzheimer dementia* **Acts:** Cholinesterase inhib **Dose:** 10–40 mg PO qid to 160 mg/d; separate doses from food **W/P:** [C, ?] **CI:** Previous tacrine-induced jaundice **Disp:** Caps 10, 20, 30, 40 mg **SE:** ↑ LFTs, HA, dizziness, GI upset, flushing, confusion, ataxia, myalgia, ↓ HR **Notes:** Serum conc > 20 ng/mL have more SE; monitor LFTs

Tacrolimus [FK506] (Prograf, Protopic) **BOX:** ↑ Risk of Infxn and lymphoma **Uses:** *Prevent organ rejection*, eczema **Acts:** Macrolide immunosuppressant **Dose:** *Adults.* IV: 0.05–0.1 mg/kg/d cont Inf. PO: 0.1–0.2 mg/kg/d ÷ 2 doses. *Peds.* IV: 0.03–0.05 mg/kg/d as cont Inf. PO: 0.15–0.2 mg/kg/d PO ÷ q 12 h. *Adults & Peds. Eczema:* Apply bid, continue 1 wk after clearing; take on empty stomach; ↓

w/ hepatic/renal impair **W/P:** [C, –] w/ Cyclosporine; avoid topical if < 2 y of age; Neuro & nephrotox, increased risk opportunistic infections **CI:** Component allergy, castor oil allergy w/ IV form **Disp:** Caps 0.5, 1, 5 mg; Inj 5 mg/mL; oint 0.03, 0.1% **SE:** HTN, edema, HA, insomnia, fever, pruritus, ↓/↑ K^+, hyperglycemia, GI upset, anemia, leukocytosis, tremors, paresthesias, pleural effusion, Szs, lymphoma, posterior reversible encephalopathy syndrome (PRES), BK nephropathy, PML **Notes:** Monitor levels; *Trough:* 5–20 ng/mL based on indication and time since transplant; reports of ↑ CA risk; topical use for short-term/2nd-line

Tadalafil (Cialis) **Uses:** *ED BPH* **Acts:** PDE5 inhib, ↑ cyclic guanosine monophosphate & NO levels; relaxes smooth muscles, dilates cavernosal arteries **Dose:** *Adults. PRN:* 10 mg PO before sexual activity (5–20 mg max based on response) 1 dose/24 h. *Daily dosing:* 2.5 mg q day, may ↑ to 5 mg q day *BPH;* 5 mg PO q day; w/o regard to meals; ↓ w/ renal/hepatic Insuff **W/P:** [B, –] w/ α-Blockers (except tamsulosin); use w/ CYP3A4 inhib (Table 10, p 301) (e.g., ritonavir, ketoconazole, itraconazole) 2.5 mg/daily dose or 5 mg PRN dose; CrCl < 30 mL/min/hemodialysis/ severe hepatic impair do not use daily dosing **CI:** Nitrates, severe hepatic impair **Disp:** Tabs 2.5, 5-, 10-, 20-mg **SE:** HA, flushing, dyspepsia, back/limb pain, myalgia, nasal congestion, urticaria, SJS, dermatitis, visual field defect, NIAON, sudden ↓/loss of hearing, tinnitus **Notes:** Longest acting of class (36 h); daily dosing may ↑ drug interactions; excessive EtOH may ↑ orthostasis; transient global amnesia reports

Tadalafil (Adcirca) **Uses:** *Pulmonary artery hypertension* **Acts:** PDE5 inhib, ↑ cyclic guanosine monophosphate & NO levels; relaxes pulm artery smooth muscles **Dose:** 40 mg 1 × d w/o regard to meals; ↓ w/ renal/hepatic insuff **W/P:** [B, –] w/ CV Dz, impaired autonomic control of BP, aortic stenosis α-blockers (except tamsulosin); use w/ CYP3A4 inhib/inducers (e.g., ritonavir, ketoconazole); monitor for sudden ↓/ loss of hearing or vision (NAION), tinnitus, priapism **CI:** w/ Nitrates, component hypersens **Disp:** Tabs 20 mg **SE:** HA **Notes:** See Tadalafil (*Cialis*) for ED

Talc (Sterile Talc Powder) **Uses:** *↓ Recurrence of malignant pleural effusions (pleurodesis)* **Acts:** Sclerosing agent **Dose:** Mix slurry: 50 mL NS w/ 5-g vial, mix, distribute 25 mL into two 60-mL syringes, vol to 50 mL/syringe w/ NS. Infuse each into chest tube, flush w/ 25 mL NS. Keep tube clamped; have pt change positions q15min for 2 h, unclamp tube **W/P:** [X, –] **CI:** Planned further surgery on site **Disp:** 5-g powder **SE:** Pain, Infxn **Notes:** May add 10–20 mL 1% lidocaine/ syringe; must have chest tube placed, monitor closely while tube clamped (tension pneumothorax); not antineoplastic

Tamoxifen (Generic) **BOX:** CA of the uterus, stroke, and blood clots can occur **Uses:** *Breast CA [postmenopausal, estrogen receptor(+)], ↓ risk of breast CA in high-risk, met male breast CA*, ductal carcinoma in situ, mastalgia, pancreatic CA, gynecomastia, ovulation induction **Acts:** Nonsteroidal antiestrogen; mixed agonist–antagonist effect **Dose:** 20–40 mg/d; doses > 20 ÷ bid. *Prevention:* 20 mg PO/d × 5 y **W/P:** [D, –] w/ ↓ WBC, ↓ plts, hyperlipidemia **CI:** PRG, undiagnosed vag bleeding, Hx thromboembolism **Disp:** Tabs 10, 20 mg; oral soln

10 mg/5 mL **SE:** Uterine malignancy & thrombosis events seen in breast CA prevention trials; menopausal Sxs (hot flashes, N/V) in premenopausal pts; vag bleeding & menstrual irregularities; skin rash, pruritus vulvae, dizziness, HA, peripheral edema; acute flare of bone metastasis pain & ↑ Ca^{2+}; retinopathy reported (high dose) **Notes:** ↑ Risk of PRG in premenopausal women (induces ovulation); brand Nolvadex suspended in US

Tamsulosin (Flomax, Generic) **Uses:** *BPH* **Acts:** Antagonist of prostatic α-receptors **Dose:** 0.4 mg/d, may ↑ to 0.8 mg PO daily **W/P:** [B, ?] **CI:** Female gender **Disp:** Caps 0.4 mg **SE:** HA, dizziness, syncope, somnolence, ↓ libido, GI upset, retrograde ejaculation, rhinitis, rash, angioedema, IFIS **Notes:** Not for use as antihypertensive; do not open/crush/chew; approved for use w/ dutasteride for BPH

Tapentadol (Nucynta) [C-II] **Uses:** *Mod/severe acute pain* **Acts:** Mu-opioid agonist and norepinephrine reuptake inhib **Dose:** 50–100 mg PO q 4–6 h PRN (max 600 mg/d); w/ mod hepatic impair: 50 mg q8h PRN (max 3 doses/24 h) **W/P:** [C, −] Hx of seizures, CNS depression; ↑ ICP, severe renal impair, biliary tract Dz; elderly, serotonin synd w/ concomitant serotonergic agents **CI:** ↓ pulm fxn, use w/ or w/in 14 d of MAOI **Disp:** Tabs 50, 75, 100 mg **SE:** N/V, dizziness, somnolence, headache **Notes:** Taper dose w/ D/C

Tazarotene (Tazorac, Avage) **Uses:** *Facial acne vulgaris; stable plaque psoriasis up to 20% BSA* **Acts:** Keratolytic **Dose:** *Adults & Peds > 12 y. Acne:* Cleanse face, dry, apply thin film qhs lesions. *Psoriasis:* Apply qhs **W/P:** [X, ?/−] **CI:** Retinoid sensitivity **Disp:** Gel 0.05, 0.1%; cream 0.05, 0.1% **SE:** Burning, erythema, irritation, rash, photosens, desquamation, bleeding, skin discoloration **Notes:** D/C w/ excessive pruritus, burning, skin redness, or peeling until Sxs resolve

Telavancin (Vibativ) **BOX:** Fetal risk; must have pregnancy test prior to use in childbearing age **Uses:** *Complicated skin/skin structure infxns d/t susceptible Gram-positive bacteria* **Action:** lipoglycopeptide antibacterial; **Spectrum:** Good gram(+) aerobic and anaerobic include MRSA,MSSA some VRE; poor gram(−) **Dose:** 10 mg/kg IV q24h; 7.5 mg/kg q24h w/CrCl 30–50 mL/min; 10 mg/kg q48h w/CrCl 10–30 mL/min **W/P:** [C, ?] Nephrotoxicity, C. difficile-associated disease, ↑ QTc, interferes w/coag tests **CI:** Pregnancy **Disp:** Inj 250, 750 mg **SE:** Taste disturbance, N, V, foamy urine **Notes:** ↓ Efficacy w/ mod—severe renal impair

Telbivudine (Tyzeka) **BOX:** May cause lactic acidosis and severe hepatomegaly w/ steatosis when used alone or w/ antiretrovirals; D/C of the drug may lead to exacerbations of hep B; monitor LFTs **Uses:** *Rx chronic hep B* **Acts:** Nucleoside RT inhib **Dose:** *CrCl > 50 mL/min:* 600 mg PO daily; *CrCl 30–49 mL/min:* 600 mg q 48 h; *CrCl < 30 mL/min:* 600 mg q 72 h; *ESRD:* 600 mg q96h; dose after hemodialysis **W/P:** [B, ?/−]; may cause myopathy; follow closely w/ other myopathy causing drugs **Disp:** Tabs 600 mg **SE:** Fatigue, Abd pain, N/V/D, HA, URI, nasopharyngitis, ↑ LFTs/creatine phosphokinase, myalgia/myopathy, flu-like Sxs, dizziness, insomnia, dyspepsia **Notes:** Use w/ PEG-interferon may ↑ peripheral neuropathy risk

Telithromycin (Ketek) BOX: CI in myasthenia MyG **Uses:** *Mild–mod CAP* **Acts:** Unique macrolide, blocks ↓ protein synth; bactericidal. *Spectrum: S. aureus, S. pneumoniae, H. influenzae, M. catarrhalis, C. pneumoniae, M. pneumoniae* **Dose:** *CAP:* 800 mg (2 tabs) PO daily × 7–10 d **W/P:** [C, M] Pseudomembranous colitis, ↑ QTc interval, visual disturbances, hepatic dysfunction; dosing in renal impair unknown **CI:** Macrolide allergy, w/ pimozide, w/ MyG **Disp:** Tabs 300, 400 mg **SE:** N/V/D, dizziness, blurred vision **Notes:** A CYP450 inhib; multiple drug interactions; hold statins d/t ↑ risk of myopathy

Telmisartan (Micardis) BOX: Use of renin-angiotensin agents in PRG can cause fetal injury and death, D/C immediately when PRG detected **Uses:** *HTN, CHF* **Acts:** Angiotensin II receptor antagonist **Dose:** 40–80 mg/d **W/P:** [C (1st tri; D 2nd & 3rd tri), ?/–] **CI:** Angiotensin II receptor antagonist sensitivity **Disp:** Tabs 20, 40, 80 mg **SE:** Edema, GI upset, HA, angioedema, renal impair, orthostatic ↓ BP

Telmisartan and Amlodipine (Twynsta) BOX: Use of renin-angiotensin agents in PRG can cause fetal injury and death, D/C immediately when PRG detected **Uses:** *Hypertension* **Acts:** CCB; relaxes coronary vascular smooth muscle & angiotensin II receptor antagonist **Dose:** Telmisartan/amlodipine; max 80/10 mg PO/d; ↑ dose after 2 wk **W/P:** [C 1st tri; D 2nd, 3rd; ?/–] **CI:** PRG **Disp:** Tabs mg telmisartan/mg amlodipine 40/5; 40/10; 80/5; 80/10 **SE:** HA, edema, dizziness, N, ↓ BP **Notes:** Titrate w/ hepatic/renal impair; avoid w/ ACE/other ARBs; correct hypovolemia before; w/ CHF monitor; w/ CAD, CCBs may cause ACS

Temazepam (Restoril) [C-IV] Uses: *Insomnia*, anxiety, depression, panic attacks **Acts:** Benzodiazepine **Dose:** 15–30 mg PO hs PRN; ↓ in elderly **W/P:** [X, ?/–] Potentiates CNS depressive effects of opioids, barbs, EtOH, antihistamines, MAOIs, TCAs **CI:** NAG **Disp:** Caps 7.5, 15, 22.5, 30 mg **SE:** Confusion, dizziness, drowsiness, hangover **Notes:** Abrupt D/C after > 10 d use may cause withdrawal

Temozolomide (Temodar) Uses: *Glioblastoma multiforme (GBM), refractory anaplastic astrocytoma* **Acts:** Alkylating agent **Dose:** *GBM, new:* 75 mg/m² PO/IV/d × 42 days w/ RT, maint 150 mg/m²/d days 1–5 of 28 day cycle × 6 cycles; may ↑ to 200 mg/m²/day × 5 days every 28 days in cycle 2; *Refractory astrocytoma:* 150 mg/m² PO/IV/day × 5 days per 28-day cycle; Adjust dose based on ANC and plt count (per PI and local protocols). **W/P:** [D, ?/–] w/ Severe renal/hepatic impair, myelosuppression (monitor ANC & plt), myelodysplastic synd, secondary malignancies, PCP pneumonia (PCP prophylaxis required) **CI:** Hypersens to components or dacarbazine **Disp:** Caps 5, 20, 100, 140, 180, & 250 mg; Powder for Inj 100 mg **SE:** N/V/D, fatigue, HA, asthenia, seizure, hemiparesis, fever, dizziness, coordination abnormality, alopecia, rash, constipation, anorexia, amnesia, insomnia, viral Infxn, ↓ WBC, plt **Notes:** Infuse over 90 min; swallow caps whole; if caps open avoid inhalation and contact w/ skin/mucous membranes

Temsirolimus (Torisel) Uses: *Advanced RCC* **Acts:** Multikinase inhib, ↓ mTOR (mammalian target of rapamycin), ↓ hypoxic-induced factors, ↓ VEGF **Dose:** 25 mg IV 30–60 min 1×/wk. Hold w/ ANC < 1000 cells/mcL, plt < 75,000 cells/mcL, or NCI grade 3 tox. Resume when tox grade 2 or less, restart w/ dose ↓ 5 mg/wk not < 15 mg/wk. w/ CYP3A4 Inhib: ↓ 12.5 mg/wk. w/ CYP3A4 Inducers ↑ 50 mg/wk **W/P:** [D, –] Avoid live vaccines, ✓ wound healing, avoid periop **CI:** None **Disp:** Inj 25 mg/mL w/ 250 mL diluent **SE:** Rash, asthenia, mucositis, N, bowel perforation, anorexia, edema, ↑ lipids, ↑ glucose, ↑ triglycerides, ↑ LFTs, ↑ Cr, ↑ WBC, ↓ HCT, ↓ plt, ↓ PO$_4$ **Notes:** Premedicate w/ antihistamine; ✓ lipids, CBC, plt, Cr, glucose; w/ sunitinib dose-limiting tox likely; females use w/ contraception

Tenecteplase (TNKase) Uses: *Restore perfusion & ↓ mortality w/ AMI* **Acts:** Thrombolytic; TPA **Dose:** 30–50 mg; see table below **W/P:** [C, ?], ↑ Bleeding w/ NSAIDs, ticlopidine, clopidogrel, GPIIb/IIIa antagonists **CI:** Bleeding, CVA, CNS neoplasm, uncontrolled ↑ BP, major surgery (intracranial, intraspinal) or trauma w/in 2 mo **Disp:** Inj 50 mg, reconstitute w/ 10 mL sterile H$_2$O only **SE:** Bleeding, allergy **Notes:** Do not shake w/ reconstitution; start ASA ASAP, IV heparin ASAP w/ aPTT 50–70 s

Tenecteplase Dosing (From one vial of reconstituted TNKase)

Weight (kg)	TNKase (mg)	TNKase Volume (mL)
< 60	30	6
60–69	35	7
70–79	40	8
80–89	45	9
≥90	50	10

Tenofovir (Viread) **BOX:** Lactic acidosis & severe hepatomegaly w/ steatosis, including fatal cases, have been reported w/ the use of nucleoside analogs alone or in combo w/ other antiretrovirals. Not OK w/ chronic hep; effects in pts co infected w/ hep B & HIV unknown Uses: *HIV Infxn* **Acts:** Nucleotide RT inhib **Dose:** 300 mg PO daily w/ or w/o meal; CrCl ≥50 mL/min Δ q24h, CrCl 30–49 mL/min q48H, CrCl 10–29 mL/min 2×/wk **W/P:** [B, ?/–] Didanosine (separate administration times), lopinavir, ritonavir w/ known risk factors for liver Dz **CI:** Hypersens **Disp:** Tabs 300 mg **SE:** GI upset, metabolic synd, hepatotox; separate didanosine doses by 2 h **Notes:** Combo product w/ emtricitabine is Truvada

Tenofovir/Emtricitabine (Truvada) **BOX:** Lactic acidosis & severe hepatomegaly w/ steatosis, including fatal cases, have been reported w/ the use of nucleoside analogs alone or in combo w/ other antiretrovirals. Not OK w/ chronic hep; effects in pts coinfected w/ hep B & HIV unknown Uses: *HIV Infxn* **Acts:** Dual nucleotide RT inhib **Dose:** 300 mg PO daily w/ or w/o a meal; adjust w/ renal impair **W/P:** [B, ?/–] w/ Known risk factors for liver Dz **CI:** CrCl < 30 mL/min; **Disp:** Tabs 200 mg emtricitabine/300 mg tenofovir **SE:** GI upset, rash, metabolic synd, hepatotox

Terazosin (Hytrin) Uses: *BPH & HTN* Acts: α_1-Blocker (blood vessel & bladder neck/prostate) Dose: Initial, 1 mg PO hs; ↑ 20 mg/d max; may ↓ w/ diuretic or other BP medicine W/P: [C, ?] w/ β-Blocker, CCB, ACE inhib; use w/ phosphodiesterase-5 (PDE5) inhib (e.g., sildenafil) can cause ↓ BP CI: α-Antagonist sensitivity Disp: Tabs 1, 2, 5, 10 mg; caps 1, 2, 5, 10 mg SE: ↓ BP, & syncope following 1st dose or w/ PDE5 inhib; dizziness, weakness, nasal congestion, peripheral edema, palpitations, GI upset Notes: Caution w/ 1st dose syncope; if for HTN, combine w/ thiazide diuretic

Terbinafine (Lamisil, Lamisil AT, Others [OTC]) Uses: *Onychomycosis, athlete's foot, jock itch, ringworm*, cutaneous candidiasis, pityriasis versicolor Acts: ↓ Squalene epoxidase resulting in fungal death Dose: *PO:* 250 mg/d PO for 6–12 wk. *Topical:* Apply to area tinea pedis bid, tinea cruris & corporus q day-bid, tinea versicolor soln bid; ↓ PO in renal/hepatic impair W/P: [B, –] PO ↑ effects of drug metabolism by CYP2D6, w/ liver/renal impair CI: CrCl < 50 mL/min, WBC < 1000/mm³, severe liver Dz Disp: Tabs 250 mg; *Lamisil AT* [OTC] cream, gel, soln 1% SE: HA, dizziness, rash, pruritus, alopecia, GI upset, taste perversion, neutropenia, retinal damage, SJS, ↑ LFTs Notes: Effect may take months d/t need for new nail growth; topical not for nails; do not use occlusive dressings; PO follow CBC/LFTs

Terbutaline (Brethine) Uses: *Reversible bronchospasm (asthma, COPD); inhibit labor* Acts: Sympathomimetic; tocolytic Dose: *Adults. Bronchodilator:* 2.5–5 mg PO qid or 0.25 mg SQ; repeat in 15 min PRN; max 0.5 mg in 4 h. *Metered-dose inhaler:* 2 inh q4–6h. *Premature labor:* Acutely 2.5–10 mg/min/IV, gradually ↑ as tolerated q10–20min; maint 2.5–5 mg PO q4–6h until term. *Peds. PO:* 0.05–0.15 mg/kg/dose PO tid; max 5 mg/24h; ↓ in renal failure W/P: [B, +] ↑ Tox w/ MAOIs, TCAs; DM, HTN, hyperthyroidism, CV Dz, convulsive disorders, ↓ K⁺ Disp: Tabs 2.5, 5 mg; Inj 1 mg/mL; metered-dose inhaler SE: HTN, hyperthyroidism, β_1-adrenergic effects w/ high dose, nervousness, trembling, tachycardia, HTN, dizziness

Terconazole (Terazol 7) Uses: *Vag fungal Infxns* Acts: Topical triazole antifungal Dose: 1 applicator-full or 1 supp intravag hs × 3–7 d W/P: [C, ?] CI: Component allergy Disp: Vag cream 0.4, 0.8%, vag supp 80 mg SE: Vulvar/ vag burning Notes: Insert high into vagina

Teriparatide (Forteo) BOX: ↑ Osteosarcoma risk in animals, use only where potential benefits outweigh risks Uses: *Severe/refractory osteoporosis* Acts: PTH (recombinant) Dose: 20 mcg SQ daily in thigh or Abd W/P: [C, ?/–]; caution in urolithiasis CI: w/ Paget Dz, prior radiation, bone metastases, ↑ Ca²⁺; Disp: 3-mL Prefilled device (discard after 28 d) SE: Orthostatic ↓ BP on administration, N/D, ↑ Ca²⁺; leg cramps Notes: 2 y max use

Tesamorelin (Egrifta) Uses: *↓ Excess abd fat in HIV-infected patients w/ lipodystrophy* Acts: Binds/stimulates growth hormone-releasing factor receptors Dose: 2 mg SQ/d; W/P: [X; HIV-infected mothers should not breast feed] CI: Hypothalamic-pituitary axis disorders; head radiation/trauma; malignancy; PRG; child w/

open epiphyses **Disp:** Vial 1 mg **SE:** Arthralgias, Inj site Rxn, edema, myalgia, ↑ glucose , N, V **Notes:** ✓ Gluc, ? ↑ mortality w/ acute critical illness; ↑ IGF

Testosterone (AndroGel 1%, AndroGel 1.62% Androderm, Axiron, Fortesta, Striant, Testim, Testopel) [C-III] **BOX:** Virilization reported in children exposed to topical testosterone products. Children to avoid contact w/ unwashed or unclothed application sites **Uses:** *Male hypogonadism (congenital/ acquired)* **Acts:** Testosterone replacement; ↑ lean body mass, libido **Dose:** All daily applications *AndroGel 1%:* 50 mg (4 pumps); *AndroGel 1.62%:* (40.5 mg (2 pumps); apply to clean skin on upper body only. *Androderm:* Two 2.5-mg or one 5-mg patch daily. *Axiron:* 60 mg (1 pump = 30 mg each axilla) qAM. *Fortesta:* 40 mg (4 pumps) on clean, dry thighs; adjust form 1-7 pumps based on blood test 2 h after (days 14 and 35). *Striant:* 30-mg Buccal tabs bid. *Testim:* One 5-g gel tube. *Testopel:* 150–450 mg (2–6 pellets) SQ implant q3–6mo (implant 2 75-mg pellets for each 25 mg testosterone required weekly; eg: For 75 mg/wk, implant 450 mg (6 pellets). **W/P:** [X, –] may cause polycythemia, worsening of BPH Sx **CI:** PCa, male breast CA, pregnant or breast-feeding women **Disp:** *AndroGel 1%:* 12.5 mg/pump; *AndroGel 1.62%:* 20.25 mg/pump; *Androderm:* 2.5-, 5-mg patches; *Axiron:* Metered-dose pump 30 mg/pump; *Fortesta:* Metered-dose gel pump 10 mg/pump; *Striant:* 30-mg buccal tab. *Testopel:* 75 mg/implant **SE:** Site Rxns, acne, edema, wgt gain, gynecomastia, HTN, ↑ sleep apnea, prostate enlargement, ↑ PSA **Notes:** IM testosterone enanthate (*Delatestryl; Testro-L.A.*) & cypionate (*Depo-Testosterone*) dose q14–28d w/ variable serum levels; PO agents (methyltestosterone & oxandrolone) associated w/ hepatic tumors; transdermal/mucosal forms preferred; wash hands immediately after topical applications *AndroGel* formulations not equivalent; ✓ levels and adjust PRN (300–1,000 ng/dL testosterone range)

Tetanus Immune Globulin **Uses:** Prophylaxis *passive tetanus immunization* (suspected contaminated wound w/ unknown immunization status, see Table 7, p 297), or Tx of tetanus **Acts:** Passive immunization **Dose:** *Adults & Peds. Prophylaxis:* 250–500 units IM (< 7 y 4 unit/kg) 500 units if Tx delayed; *Tx:* children 500–3,000 units, adults 3,000–6,000 units **W/P:** [C, ?] **CI:** Thimerosal sensitivity **Disp:** Inj 250-unit vial/syringe **SE:** Pain, tenderness, erythema at site; fever, angioedema, anaphylaxis **Notes:** May begin active immunization series at different Inj site if required

Tetanus Toxoid (TT) **Uses:** *Tetanus prophylaxis* **Acts:** Active immunization **Dose:** Based on previous immunization, Table 7, p 297 **W/P:** [C, ?/–] **CI:** Chloramphenicol use, neurologic Sxs w/ previous use, active Infxn w/ routine primary immunization **Disp:** Inj tetanus toxoid fluid, 5 Lf units/0.5 mL; tetanus toxoid adsorbed, 5 units/0.5 mL **SE:** Inj site erythema, induration, sterile abscess; arthralgias, fever, malaise, neurologic disturbances **Notes:** DTaP rather than TT or Td all adults 19–64 y who have not previously received one dose of DTaP (protection adult pertussis); also use DT or Td instead of TT to maintain diphtheria immunity; if IM, use only preservative-free Inj; Do not confuse Td (for adults) w/ DT (for children)

Tetrabenazine (Xenazine) BOX: ↑ Risk of depression, suicide w/ Huntington Dz Uses: *Rx chorea in Huntington Dz* Acts: Monoamine depleter Dose: 25–100 mg/d ÷ doses; 12.5 mg PO/d × 1 wk, ↑ to 12.5 mg bid, may ↑ to 12.5 mg tid after 1 wk; if > 50 mg needed, ✓ for CYP2D6 gene; if poor metabolizer, 25 mg max; 50 mg/d max; extensive/indeterminate metabolizer 37.5 mg dose max, 100 mg/d max W/P: [C, ?/–] 1/2 dose w/ strong CYP2D6 inhib (paroxetine, fluoxetine); wait 20 d after reserpine D/C before use CI: Suicidality, untreated or inadequately treated depression; hepatic impair; w/ MOAI or reserpine Disp: Tabs 12.5, 25 mg SE: Sedation, insomnia, depression, anxiety, irritability, akathisia, Parkinsonism, balance difficulties, neuroleptic malignant syndrome, fatigue, N, V, dysphagia, ↑ QT

Tetracycline (Achromycin V, Sumycin) Uses: *Broad-spectrum antibiotic* Acts: Bacteriostatic; ↓ protein synth. *Spectrum:* Gram(+): *Staphylococcus, Streptococcus.* Gram(–): *H. pylori.* Atypicals: *Chlamydia, Rickettsia, & Mycoplasma* Dose: *Adults.* 250–500 mg PO bid-qid. *Peds > 8 y.* 25–50 mg/kg/24 h PO q6–12h; ↓ w/ renal/hepatic impair, w/o food preferred W/P: [D, +] CI: PRG, antacids, w/ dairy products, children < 8 y Disp: Caps 100, 250, 500 mg; tabs 250, 500 mg; PO susp 250 mg/5 mL SE: Photosens, GI upset, renal failure, pseudotumor cerebri, hepatic impair Notes: Can stain tooth enamel & depress bone formation in children

Thalidomide (Thalomid) BOX: Restricted use; use associated w/ severe birth defects and ↑ risk of venous thromboembolism Uses: *Erythema nodosum leprosum (ENL)*, GVHD, aphthous ulceration in HIV(+) Acts: ↓ Neutrophil chemotaxis, ↓ monocyte phagocytosis Dose: *GVHD:* 100–1600 mg PO daily. *Stomatitis:* 200 mg bid for 5 d, then 200 mg daily up to 8 wk. *Erythema nodosum leprosum:* 100–300 mg PO qhs W/P: [X, –] May ↑ HIV viral load; Hx Szs CI: PRG; sexually active males not using latex condoms, or females not using 2 forms of contraception Disp: 50-, 100-, 200-mg caps SE: Dizziness, drowsiness, rash, fever, orthostasis, SJS, peripheral neuropathy, Szs Notes: MD must register w/ STEPS risk-management program; informed consent necessary; immediately D/C if rash develops

Theophylline (Theo24, Theochron) Uses: *Asthma, bronchospasm* Acts: Relaxes smooth muscle of the bronchi & pulm blood vessels Dose: *Adults.* 900 mg PO ÷ q6h; SR products may be ÷ q8–12h (maint). *Peds.* 16–22 mg/kg/24 h PO ÷ q6h; SR products may be ÷ q8–12h (maint); ↓ in hepatic failure W/P: [C, +] Multiple interactions (e.g., caffeine, smoking, carbamazepine, barbiturates, β-blockers, ciprofloxacin, E-mycin, INH, loop diuretics) CI: Arrhythmia, hyperthyroidism, uncontrolled Szs Disp: Elixir 80 mg/15 mL; soln 80 mg/15 mL; syrup 80, 150 mg/15 mL; caps 100, 200, 250 mg; tabs 100, 125, 200, 250, 300 mg; SR caps 100, 125, 200, 250, 260, 300 mg; SR tabs 100, 200, 300, 400, 450, 600 mg SE: N/V, tachycardia, Szs, nervousness, arrhythmias Notes: IV Levels: Sample 12–24 h after Inf started; *Therapeutic:* 5–15 mcg/mL; *Toxic:* > 20 mcg/mL. PO Levels: *Trough:* just before next dose; *Therapeutic:* 5–15 mcg/mL

Thiamine [Vitamin B$_1$] Uses: *Thiamine deficiency (beriberi), alcoholic neuritis, Wernicke encephalopathy* Acts: Dietary supl Dose: **Adults.** *Deficiency:* 100 mg/d IM for 2 wk, then 5–10 mg/d PO for 1 mo. *Wernicke encephalopathy:* 100 mg IV single dose, then 100 mg IM for 2 wk. **Peds.** 10–25 mg/d IM for 2 wk, then 5–10 mg/24 h PO for 1 mo W/P: [A (C if does exceed RDA), +] CI: Component allergy Disp: Tabs 5, 10, 25, 50, 100, 250, 500 mg; Inj 100, 200 mg/mL SE: Angioedema, paresthesias, rash, anaphylaxis w/ rapid IV Notes: IV use associated w/ anaphylactic Rxn; give IV slowly

Thiethylperazine (Torecan) Uses: *N/V* Acts: Antidopaminergic antiemetic Dose: 10 mg PO, PR, or IM daily-tid; ↓ in hepatic failure W/P: [X, ?] CI: Phenothiazine & sulfite sensitivity, PRG Disp: Tabs 10 mg; supp 10 mg; Inj 5 mg/mL SE: EPS, xerostomia, drowsiness, orthostatic ↓ BP, tachycardia, confusion

6-Thioguanine [6-TG] (Tabloid) Uses: *AML, ALL, CML* Acts: Purine-based antimetabolite (substitutes for natural purines interfering w/ nucleotide synth) Dose: 2–3 mg/kg/d; ↓ in severe renal/hepatic impair W/P: [D, −] CI: Resistance to mercaptopurine Disp: Tabs 40 mg SE: ↓ BM (leucopenia/thrombocytopenia), N/V/D, anorexia, stomatitis, rash, hyperuricemia, rare hepatotox

Thiopental Sodium (Pentothal) [C-III] Uses: *Induce anesthesia, short procedure anesthesia; Sz control after anesthesia, neurosurg pts w/ ↑ ICP & adequate ventilation, narcoanalysis* Acts: Ultrashort-acting barbiturate (hypnotic & anesthetic) Dose: **Adults.** *Anesthesia, slow-induction:* 50–75 mg IV q20–40s, then 25–50 mg IV PRN pt moves. *Anesthesia, rapid-induction:* 3–4 mg/kg IV ÷ in 2–4 doses *Anesthesia, maint:* 0.2–0.4% IV, adj to effect. *Szs post-anesthesia:* 75–125 mg IV, may ↑ to 250 mg over 10 min. *Narcoanalysis w/ ↑ ICP:* 1.5–3.5 mg/kg IV PRN. *Narcoanalysis:* 100 mg/min IV, D/C when pt confused counting backwards from 100; 0.2% in D5W at 50 mL/min max; 25–75 mg IV over 60 s to assess tolerance W/P: [C, +/−] Levels as low as 1 mg/dL may be lethal CI: Hypersens, porphyria, poor IV access Disp: Inj SE: ↓ Resp, myocardial depression, ↓ BP, hangover, laryngospasm Notes: Slow Inj ↓ risk of OD & resp depression; do not use conc < 2% in SWFI

Thioridazine (Mellaril) BOX: Dose-related QT prolongation Uses: *Schizophrenia*, psychosis Acts: Phenothiazine antipsychotic Dose: **Adults.** Initial, 50–100 mg PO tid; maint 200–800 mg/24 h PO in 2–4 ÷ doses. **Peds >2 y.** 0.5–3 mg/kg/24 h PO in 2–3 ÷ doses W/P: [C, ?] Phenothiazines, QTc-prolonging agents, AI CI: Phenothiazine sensitivity Disp: Tabs 10, 15, 25, 50, 100, 150, 200 mg; PO conc 30, 100 mg/mL SE: Low incidence of EPS; ventricular arrhythmias; ↓ BP, dizziness, drowsiness, neuroleptic malignant synd, Szs, skin discoloration, photosens, constipation, sexual dysfunction, blood dyscrasias, pigmentary retinopathy, hepatic impair Notes: Avoid EtOH, dilute PO conc in 2–4 oz liq

Thiothixene (Navane) BOX: Not for dementia-related psychosis; increased mortality risk in elderly on antipsychotics Uses: *Psychosis* Acts: ? may Antagonize dopamine receptors Dose: **Adults & Peds > 12 y.** *Mild–mod psychosis:* 2 mg

PO tid, up to 20–30 mg/d. *Severe psychosis:* 5 mg PO bid; ↑ to max of 60 mg/24 h PRN. *IM use:* 16–20 mg/24 h ÷ bid-qid; max 30 mg/d. *Peds < 12 y.* 0.25 mg/kg/24 h PO ÷ q6–12h **W/P:** [C, ?] Avoid w/ ↑ QT interval or meds that can ↑ QT **CI:** Phenothiazine sensitivity **Disp:** Caps 1, 2, 5, 10, 20 mg; PO conc 5 mg/mL; Inj 10 mg/mL **SE:** Drowsiness, EPS most common; ↓ BP, dizziness, drowsiness, neuroleptic malignant synd, Szs, skin discoloration, photosens, constipation, sexual dysfunction, leukopenia, neutropenia and agranulocytosis, pigmented retinopathy, hepatic impair **Notes:** Dilute PO conc immediately before use

Tiagabine (Gabitril) Uses: *Adjunct in partial Szs*, bipolar disorder **Acts:** Antiepileptic, enhances activity of GABA **Dose:** *Adults & Peds ≥12 y.* Initial 4 mg PO, ↑ by 4 mg during 2nd wk; ↑ PRN by 4–8 mg/d based on response, 56 mg/d max; take w/ food **W/P:** [C, M] May ↑ suicidal risk **CI:** Component allergy **Disp:** Tabs 2, 4, 12, 16, 20 mg **SE:** Dizziness, HA, somnolence, memory impair, tremors **Notes:** Use gradual withdrawal; used in combo w/ other anticonvulsants

Ticagrelor (Brilinta) BOX: ↑ Bleeding risk; can be fatal; daily aspirin > 100 mg may ↓ effectiveness; do not start w/ active bleeding, Hx intracranial bleed, planned CABG; if hypotensive and recent procedure, suspect bleeding; manage any bleed w/o D/C of ticagrelor Uses: *↓ CV death and heart attack in ACS* **Acts:** Oral anti-platelet; reversibly binding ADP receptor antagonist inhibitor **Dose:** Initial 180 mg PO w/ ASA 325 mg, then 90 mg bid w/ ASA 75–100 mg/day **W/P:** [D, –] w/mod hepatic impair; w/strong CYP3A inhibitors or CYP3A inducers **CI:** Hx intracranial bleed, active pathologic bleeding, severe hepatic impair **Disp:** Tabs 90 mg **SE:** Bleeding, SOB **Notes:** REMS; D/C 5 days pre-op

Ticarcillin/Potassium Clavulanate (Timentin) Uses: *Infxns of the skin, bone, resp & urinary tract, Abd, sepsis* **Acts:** Carboxy-PCN; bactericidal; ↓ cell wall synth; clavulanic acid blocks β-lactamase. *Spectrum:* Good gram(+), not MRSA; good gram(–) & anaerobes **Dose:** *Adults.* 3.1 g IV q4–6h max 24 g ticarcillin component/d. *Peds.* 200–300 mg/kg/d IV ÷ q4–6h; ↓ in renal failure **W/P:** [B, +/–] PCN sensitivity **Disp:** Inj ticarcillin/clavulanate acid 3.1 g/0.1 g vial **SE:** Hemolytic anemia, false(+) proteinuria **Notes:** Often used in combo w/ aminoglycosides; penetrates CNS w/ meningeal irritation

Ticlopidine (Ticlid) BOX: Neutropenia/agranulocytosis, TTP, aplastic anemia reported Uses: *↓ Risk of thrombotic stroke*, protect grafts status post-coronary artery bypass graft, diabetic microangiopathy, ischemic heart Dz, DVT prophylaxis, graft prophylaxis after renal transplant **Acts:** Plt aggregation inhibitor **Dose:** 250 mg PO bid w/ food **W/P:** [B, ?/–], ↑ Tox of ASA, anticoagulation, NSAIDs, theophylline; do not use w/ clopidogrel (↓ effect) **CI:** Bleeding, hepatic impair, neutropenia, ↓ plt **Disp:** Tabs 250 mg **SE:** Bleeding, GI upset, rash, ↑ LFTs **Notes:** ✓ CBC 1st 3 mo

Tigecycline (Tygacil) Uses: *Rx complicated skin & soft-tissue Infxns, & complicated intra-Abd Infxns* **Acts:** New class: related to tetracycline; *Spectrum:*

Broad gram(+), gram(−), anaerobic, some mycobacterial; *E. coli, E. faecalis* (van-comycin-susceptible isolates), *S. aureus* (methicillin-susceptible/resistant), *Streptococcus* (agalactiae, anginosus grp, pyogenes), *Citrobacter freundii, Enterobacter cloacae, B. fragilis* group, *C. perfringens, Peptostreptococcus* **Dose:**100 mg, then 50 mg q12h IV over 30–60 min **W/P:** [D, ?] Hepatic impair, monotherapy w/ intestinal perforation, not OK in peds, w/ tetracycline allergy **CI:** Component sensitivity **Disp:** Inj 50 mg vial **SE:** N/V, Inj site Rxn

Timolol (Blocadren)   BOX: Exacerbation of ischemic heart Dz w/ abrupt D/C **Uses:** *HTN & MI* **Acts:** β-Adrenergic receptor blocker, β₁, β₂ **Dose:** *HTN:* 10–20 mg bid, up to 60 mg/d. *MI:* 10 mg bid **W/P:** [C (1st tri; D if 2nd or 3rd tri), +] **CI:** CHF, cardiogenic shock, ↓ HR, heart block, COPD, asthma **Disp:** Tabs 5, 10, 20 mg **SE:** Sexual dysfunction, arrhythmia, dizziness, fatigue, CHF

Timolol, Ophthalmic (Timoptic) **Uses:** *Glaucoma* **Acts:** β-Blocker **Dose:** 0.25% 1 gt bid; ↓ to daily when controlled; use 0.5% if needed; 1-gtt/d gel **W/P:** [C (1st tri; D 2nd or 3rd), ?/+] **Disp:** Soln 0.25/0.5%; Timoptic XE (0.25, 0.5%) gel-forming soln **SE:** Local irritation

Tinidazole (Tindamax) Off-label use discouraged (animal carcinogenicity w/ other drugs in class) **Uses:** *Adults/children > 3 y:* *Trichomoniasis & giardiasis; intestinal amebiasis or amebic liver abscess* **Acts:** Antiprotozoal nitroimidazole; *Spectrum: Trichomonas vaginalis, Giardia duodenalis, Entamoeba histolytica* **Dose: Adults.** *Trichomoniasis:* 2 g PO; Rx partner. *Giardiasis:* 2 g PO. *Amebiasis:* 2 g PO daily × 3 d. *Amebic liver abscess:* 2 g PO daily × 3–5 d. *Peds. Trichomoniasis:* 50 mg/kg PO, 2 g/d max. *Giardiasis:* 50 mg/kg PO, 2 g max. *Amebiasis:* 50 mg/kg PO daily × 3 d, 2 g/d max. *Amebic liver abscess:* 50 mg/kg PO daily × 3–5 d, 2 g/d max; take w/ food **W/P:** [C, D in 1st tri, −] May be cross-resistant w/ metronidazole; Sz/peripheral neuropathy may require D/C; w/ CNS/hepatic impair **CI:** Metronidazole allergy, 1st tri PRG, w/ EtOH use **Disp:** Tabs 250, 500 **SE:** CNS disturbances; blood dyscrasias, taste disturbances, N/V, darkens urine **Notes:** D/C EtOH during & 3 d after Rx; potentiates warfarin & Li; clearance ↓ w/ other drugs; crush & disperse in cherry syrup for peds; removed by HD

Tinzaparin (Innohep)   BOX: Risk of spinal/epidural hematomas development w/ spinal anesthesia or lumbar puncture **Uses:** *Rx of DVT w/ or w/o PE* **Acts:** LMW heparin **Dose:** 175 units/kg SQ daily at least 6 d until warfarin dose stabilized **W/P:** [B, ?] Pork allergy, active bleeding, mild–mod renal impair, morbid obesity **CI:** Allergy to sulfites, heparin, benzyl alcohol; HIT **Disp:** Inj 20,000 units/mL **SE:** Bleeding, bruising, ↓ plts, Inj site pain, ↑ LFTs **Notes:** Monitor via anti-Xa levels; no effect on bleeding time, plt Fxn, PT, aPTT

Tioconazole (Vagistat) **Uses:** *Vag fungal Infxns* **Acts:** Topical antifungal **Dose:** 1 Applicator-full Intravag hs (single dose) **W/P:** [C, ?] **CI:** Component allergy **Disp:** Vag oint 6.5% **SE:** Local burning, itching, soreness, polyuria **Notes:** Insert high into vagina; may damage condom or diaphragm

Tiotropium (Spiriva) **Uses:** Bronchospasm w/ COPD, bronchitis, emphysema **Acts:** Synthetic anticholinergic like atropine **Dose:** 1 Caps/d inhaled using HandiHaler, *do not* use w/ spacer **W/P:** [C, ?/–] BPH, NAG, MyG, renal impair **CI:** Acute bronchospasm **Disp:** Inh caps 18 mcg **SE:** URI, xerostomia **Notes:** Monitor FEV1 or peak flow

Tirofiban (Aggrastat) **Uses:** *Acute coronary synd* **Acts:** Glycoprotein IIB/IIIa inhib **Dose:** Initial 0.4 mcg/kg/min for 30 min, followed by 0.1 mcg/kg/min 12–24h; use in combo w/ heparin; *ECC 2010. ACS or PCI:* 0.4 mcg/kg/min IV for 30 min, then 0.1 mcg/kg/min for 18–24 h post PCI; ↓ in renal Insuff **W/P:** [B, ?/–] **CI:** Bleeding, intracranial neoplasm, vascular malformation, stroke/surgery/trauma w/in last 30 d, severe HTN **Disp:** Inj 50, 250 mcg/mL **SE:** Bleeding, ↓ HR, coronary dissection, pelvic pain, rash

Tizanidine (Zanaflex) **Uses:** *Rx spasticity* **Acts:** α_2-adrenergic agonist **Dose:** *Adults.* 4 mg q6–8h, ↑ 2–4 mg PRN max 12 mg/dose or 36 mg/d; ↓ w/ CrCl < 25 mL/min. *Peds.* Not rec. **W/P:** [C, ?/–] Do not use w/ potent CYP1A2 inhib or other α_2-adrenergic agonists **CI:** w/ Fluvoxamine, ciprofloxacin; hypersens **Disp:** Caps 2, 4, 6 mg; Tabs 2, 4 mg **SE:** ↓ BP, ↓ HR, somnolence, hepatotox **Notes:** ✓ LFT and BP; do not abruptly D/C, taper dose; take consistently w/ or w/o food

Tobramycin (Nebcin) **Uses:** *Serious gram(–) Infxns* **Acts:** Aminoglycoside; ↓ protein synth. *Spectrum:* Gram(–) bacteria (including *Pseudomonas*) **Dose:** *Adults.* Conventional dosing: 1–2.5 mg/kg/dose IV q8–12h. *Once-daily dosing:* 5–7 mg/kg/dose q24h. *Peds.* 2.5 mg/kg/dose IV q8h; ↓ w/ renal Insuff **W/P:** [C, M] **CI:** Aminoglycoside sensitivity **Disp:** Inj 10, 40 mg/mL **SE:** Nephro/ototox **Notes:** Follow CrCl & levels. Levels: *Peak:* 30 min after Inf; *Trough:* < 0.5 h before next dose; *Therapeutic Conventional: Peak:* 5–10 mcg/mL, *Trough:* < 2 mcg/mL

Tobramycin Ophthalmic (AKTob, Tobrex) **Uses:** *Ocular bacterial Infxns* **Acts:** Aminoglycoside **Dose:** 1–2 gtt q4h; oint bid–tid; if severe, use oint q3–4h, or 2 gtt q30–60 min, then less frequently **W/P:** [C, M] **CI:** Aminoglycoside sensitivity **Disp:** Oint & soln tobramycin 0.3% **SE:** Ocular irritation

Tobramycin & Dexamethasone Ophthalmic (TobraDex) **Uses:** *Ocular bacterial Infxns associated w/ sig inflammation* **Acts:** Antibiotic w/ antiinflammatory **Dose:** 0.3% Oint apply q3–8h or soln 0.3% apply 1–2 gtt q1–4h **W/P:** [C, M] **CI:** Aminoglycoside sensitivity **Disp:** Oint & susp 2.5, 5, & 10 mL tobramycin 0.3% & dexamethasone 0.1% **SE:** Local irritation/edema **Notes:** Use under ophthalmologist's direction

Tocilizumab (Actemra) **BOX:** May cause serious Infxn (TB, bacterial, invasive fungal, viral, opportunistic); w/ serious infection stop tocilizumab until Infxn controlled **Uses:** *Mod–severe RA, SJIA* **Acts:** IL-6 receptor inhib **Dose:** RA 4–8 mg/kg; SJIA if < 30 kg 12 mg/kg; if > 30 kg 8 mg/kg **W/P:** [C, ?/–] **CI:** ANC > 2000/mm³, plt ct < 100,000, AST/ALT > 1.5 ULN; serious infection; high risk bowel perforation **Disp:** Inj **SE:** URI, nasopharyngitis, HA, HTN, ↑ ALT, ↑ AST, ↑ LDL, ↓ ANC **Notes:** Do not give live vaccines; ✓ CBC/plt counts, LFTs, lipids;

PPD, if + treat before starting, w/ prior Hx retreat unless adequate Tx confirmed, monitor for TB, even if –PPD; ↓ mRNA expression of several CYP450 isoenzymes (CYP3A4)

Tolazamide (Tolinase) Uses: *Type 2 DM* Acts: Sulfonylurea; ↑ pancreatic insulin release; ↑ peripheral insulin sensitivity; ↓ hepatic glucose output Dose: 100–500 mg/d (no benefit > 1 g/d) W/P: [C, +/–] Elderly, hepatic or renal impair Disp: Tabs 100, 250, 500 mg SE: HA, dizziness, GI upset, rash, hyperglycemia, photosens, blood dyscrasias

Tolazoline (Priscoline) Uses: *Peripheral vasospastic disorders, persistent pulm hypertension of newborn* Acts: Competitively blocks α-adrenergic receptors Dose: Adults. 10–50 mg IM/IV/SQ qid. Neonates. 1–2 mg/kg IV over 10–15 min, then 1–2 mg/kg/h (adjust w/ ↓ renal Fxn) W/P: [C, ?] Avoid alcohol, w/ CAD, renal impair, CVA, PUD, ↓ BP CI: CAD Disp: Inj 25 mg/mL SE: ↓ BP, peripheral vasodilation, tachycardia, arrhythmias, GI upset & bleeding, blood dyscrasias, renal failure

Tolbutamide (Orinase) Uses: *Type 2 DM* Acts: Sulfonylurea; ↑ pancreatic insulin release; ↑ peripheral insulin sensitivity; ↓ hepatic glucose output Dose: 500–1000 mg bid; 3 g/d max; ↓ in hepatic failure W/P: [C, +] CI: Sulfonylurea sensitivity Disp: Tabs 250, 500 mg SE: HA, dizziness, GI upset, rash, photosens, blood dyscrasias, hypoglycemia, heartburn

Tolcapone (Tasmar) BOX: Cases of fulminant liver failure resulting in death have occurred Uses: *Adjunct to carbidopa/levodopa in Parkinson Dz* Acts: Catechol-O-methyltransferase inhib slows levodopa metabolism Dose: 100 mg PO tid w/ 1st daily levodopa/carbidopa dose, then dose 6 & 12 h later; ↓ /w/ renal Insuff W/P: [C, ?] CI: Hepatic impair; w/ nonselective MAOI Disp: Tabs 100, 200 mg SE: Constipation, xerostomia, vivid dreams, hallucinations, anorexia, N/D, orthostasis, liver failure, rhabdomyolysis Notes: Do not abruptly D/C or ↓ dose; monitor LFTs

Tolmetin (Tolectin) BOX: May ↑ risk of CV events & GI bleeding Uses: *Arthritis & pain* Acts: NSAID; ↓ prostaglandins Dose: 200–600 mg PO tid; 2000 mg/d max W/P: [C (D in 3rd tri or near term), +] CI: NSAID or ASA sensitivity; use for pain post-coronary artery bypass graft Disp: Tabs 200, 600 mg; caps 400 mg SE: Dizziness, rash, GI upset, edema, GI bleeding, renal failure

Tolnaftate (Tinactin) [OTC] Uses: *Tinea pedis, cruris, corporis, manus, versicolor* Acts: Topical antifungal Dose: Apply to area bid for 2–4 wk W/P: [C, ?] CI: Nail & scalp infxns Disp: OTC 1% liq; gel; powder; topical cream; ointment, powder, spray soln SE: Local irritation Notes: Avoid ocular contact, Infxn should improve in 7–10 d

Tolterodine (Detrol, Detrol LA) Uses: *OAB (frequency, urgency, incontinence)* Acts: Anticholinergic Dose: Detrol: 1–2 mg PO bid; Detrol LA: 2–4 mg/d W/P: [C, ?/–] w/ CYP2D6 & 3A3/4 inhib (Table 10, p 301) CI: Urinary retention, gastric retention, or uncontrolled NAG Disp: Tabs 1, 2 mg; Detrol LA tabs 2, 4 mg SE: Xerostomia, blurred vision, headache, constipation Notes: LA form may see "intact" pill in stool

Tolvaptan (Samsca) BOX: Hospital use only w/ close monitoring of Na⁺ Uses: *Hypervolemic or euvolemic ↓ Na⁺* Acts: Vasopressin V₂-receptor antagonist Dose: *Adults.* 15 mg PO daily; after ≥ 24 h, may ↑ to 30 mg × 1 daily; max 60 mg × daily; titrate at 24-h intervals to Na⁺ goal W/P: [C, –] Monitor Na⁺, volume, neurologic status; GI bleed risk w/ cirrhosis, avoid w/ CYP3A inducers and moderate inhib, ↓ dose w/ P-gp inhib, ↑ K⁺ CI: Hypovolemic hyponatremia; urgent need to raise Na⁺; in pts incapable of sensing/reacting to thirst; anuria; w/ strong CYP3A inhib Disp: Tabs 15, 30 mg SE: N, xerostomia, pollakiuria, polyuria, thirst, weakness, constipation, hyperglycemia Notes: Monitor K⁺

Topiramate (Topamax) Uses: *Adjunctive Rx for complex partial Szs & tonic-clonic Szs*, bipolar disorder, neuropathic pain, migraine prophylaxis Acts: Anticonvulsant Dose: *Adults:* neuropathic pain,. *Seizures:* Total dose 400 mg/d; see PI for 8-wk titration schedule. *Migraine prophylaxis:* titrate 100 m/d total. *Peds 2–16 y. Initial:* 1–3 mg/kg/d PO qhs; titrate per insert to 5–9 mg/kg/d; ↓ w/ renal impair W/P: [C, ?/–] CI: Component allergy Disp: Tabs 25, 50, 100, 200 mg; caps sprinkles 15, 25, 50 mg SE: Wgt loss, memory impair, metabolic acidosis, kidney stones, fatigue, dizziness, psychomotor slowing, paresthesias, GI upset, tremor, nystagmus, acute glaucoma requiring D/C Notes: Metabolic acidosis responsive to ↓ dose or D/C; D/C w/ taper

Topotecan (Hycamtin) BOX: Chemotherapy precautions, for use by physicians familiar w/ chemotherapeutic agents, BM suppression possible Uses: *Ovarian CA (cisplatin-refractory), cervical CA, NSCLC*, sarcoma, ped NSCLC Acts: Topoisomerase I inhib; ↓ DNA synth Dose: 1.5 mg/m²/d as a 1-h IV Inf × 5 d, repeat q3wk; ↓ w/ renal impair W/P: [D, –] CI: PRG, breast-feeding Disp: Inj 4-mg vials SE: ↓ BM, N/V/D, drug fever, skin rash, interstitial lung disease

Torsemide (Demadex) Uses: *Edema, HTN, CHF, & hepatic cirrhosis* Acts: Loop diuretic; ↓ reabsorption of Na⁺ & Cl⁻ in ascending loop of Henle & distal tubule Dose: 5–20 mg/d PO or IV; 200 mg/d max W/P: [B, ?] CI: Sulfonylurea sensitivity Disp: Tabs 5, 10, 20, 100 mg; Inj 10 mg/mL SE: Orthostatic ↓ BP, HA, dizziness, photosens, electrolyte imbalance, blurred vision, renal impair Notes: 10–20 mg torsemide = 40 mg furosemide = 1 mg bumetanide

Tramadol (Rybix ODT, Ryzolt ER, Ultram, Ultram ER) Uses: *Mod-severe pain* Acts: Centrally acting synthetic opioid analgesic Dose: *Adults.* 50–100 mg PO q4–6h PRN, start 25 mg PO q A.M., ↑ q3d to 25 mg PO qid; ↑ 50 mg q3d, 400 mg/d max (300 mg if > 75 y); ER 100–300 mg PO daily; Rybix ODT individualize ↑ 50 mg/day q3d to 200 mg/d or 50 mg qid; after titration 50–100 mg q4–6 PRN, 400 mg/day max. *Peds.* (ER form not rec) 0.5–1 mg/kg PO q4–6h PRN; ↓ w/ renal Insuff W/P: [C, ?/–] Suicide risk in addiction prone, w/tranquilizers or antidepressants CI: Opioid dependency; w/ MAOIs; sensitivity to codeine Disp: Tabs 50 mg; ER 100, 200, 300 mg; Rybix ODT 50 mg SE: Dizziness, HA, somnolence, GI upset, resp depression, anaphylaxis Notes: ↓ Sz threshold; tolerance/dependence may develop; abuse potential d/t mu-opioid agonist activity; Avoid EtOH; do not cut, chew ODT tabs

Tramadol/Acetaminophen (Ultracet) Uses: *Short-term Rx acute pain (< 5 d)* Acts: Centrally acting analgesic; nonnarcotic analgesic Dose: 2 tabs PO q4–6h PRN; 8 tabs/d max. *Elderly/renal impair:* Lowest possible dose; 2 tabs q12h max if CrCl < 30 mL/min W/P: [C, –] Szs, hepatic/renal impair, suicide risk in addiction prone; w/tranquilizers or antidepressants CI: Acute intoxication Disp: Tab 37.5 mg tramadol/325 mg APAP SE: SSRIs, TCAs, opioids, MAOIs ↑ risk of Szs; dizziness, somnolence, tremor, HA, N/V/D, constipation, xerostomia, liver tox, rash, pruritus, ↑ sweating, physical dependence Notes: Avoid EtOH; abuse potential mu-opioid agonist activity (tramadol); see acetaminophen note, p 34

Trandolapril (Mavik) BOX: Use in PRG in 2nd/3rd tri can result in fetal death Uses: *HTN*, heart failure, LVD, post-AMI Acts: ACE inhib Dose: *HTN:* 1–4 mg/d. *Heart failure/LVD:* Start 1 mg/d, titrate to 4 mg/d; ↓ w/ severe renal/hepatic impair W/P: [D, +] ACE inhib sensitivity, angioedema w/ ACE inhib Disp: Tabs 1, 2, 4 mg SE: ↓ BP, ↓ HR, dizziness, ↑ K⁺, GI upset, renal impair, cough, angioedema Notes: African Americans minimum dose is 2 mg vs. 1 mg in caucasians

Tranexamic Acid (Lysteda) Uses: *↓ Cyclic heavy menstrual bleeding* Acts: ↓ Dissolution of hemostatic fibrin by plasmin Dose: 2 tabs tid (3900 mg/d) 5 d max during monthly menstruation; ↓ w/ renal impair (see label) W/P: [B, +/–] ↑ thrombosis risk; w/ subarachnoid hemorrhage CI: Component sensitivity; active or ↑ thrombosis risk Disp: Tabs 650 mg SE: HA, sinus and nasal symptoms, abd pain, back/musculoskeletal/joint pain, cramps, migraine, anemia, fatigue, retinal/ocular occlusion; allergic Rxns

Tranylcypromine (Parnate) BOX: Antidepressants ↑ risk of suicidal thinking and behavior in children and adolescents w/ major depressive and other psychiatric disorders Uses: *Depression* Acts: MAOI Dose: 30 mg/d PO ÷ doses, may ↑ 10 mg/d over 1–3 wk to max 60 mg/d W/P: [C, +/–] minimize foods w/ tyramine CI: CV Dz, cerebrovascular defects, Pheo, w/ MAOIs, TCAs, SSRIs, SNRIs, sympathomimetics, bupropion, meperidine, dextromethorphan, buspirone Disp: Tabs 10 mg SE: Orthostatic hypotension, ↑ HR, sex dysfunction, xerostomia Notes: False(+) amphetamine drug test

Trastuzumab (Herceptin) BOX: Can cause cardiomyopathy and ventricular dysfunction; Inf Rxns and pulm tox reported Uses: *Met breast CA that over express the HER2/neu protein*, breast CA adjuvant, w/ doxorubicin, cyclophosphamide, and paclitaxel if pt HER2/neu(+) Acts: MoAb; binds human epidermal growth factor receptor 2 protein (HER2) mediates cellular cytotoxicity Dose: Per protocol, typical 2 mg/kg/IV/wk W/P: [B, ?] CV dysfunction, allergy/Inf Rxns Disp: Live vaccines Disp: Inj 21 mg/mL SE: Anemia, cardiomyopathy, nephrotic synd, pneumonitis Notes: Inf-related Rxns minimized w/ acetaminophen, diphenhydramine, & meperidine

Trazodone (Desyrel, Oleptro) BOX: Closely monitor for worsening depression or emergence of suicidality, particularly in pts < 24 y. Oleptro not approved in peds Uses: *Depression*, hypnotic, augment other antidepressants Acts: Antidepressant; ↓ reuptake of serotonin & norepinephrine Dose: *Adults & Adolescents. Desyrel:*

50–150 mg PO daily–qid; max 600 mg/d. *Sleep:* 50 mg PO, qhs, PRN. **Adults.** *Oleptro:* Start 150 mg PO qd, may ↑ by 75 mg q3d, max 375 mg/d; take qhs on empty stomach **W/P:** [C, ?/–] Serotonin/neuroleptic malignant syndromes reported; ↑ QTc; may activate manic states; syncope reported; may ↑ bleeding risk; avoid w/in 14 d of MAOI **CI:** Component allergy **Disp:** *Desyrel:* Tabs 50, 100, 150, 300 mg; *Oleptro:* Scored tabs 150, 300 mg **SE:** Dizziness, HA, sedation, N, xerostomia, syncope, confusion, tremor, hep, EPS **Notes:** Takes 1–2 wk for Sx improvement; may interact w/ CYP3A4 inhib to ↑ trazodone concentrations, carbamazepine ↓ trazodone concentrations

Treprostinil (Remodulin, Tyvaso)   Uses: *NYHA class II–IV pulm arterial HTN* Acts: Vasodilation, ↓ plt aggregation Dose: *Remodulin* 0.625–1.25 ng/kg/min cont Inf/SQ (preferred), titrate to effect; Tyvaso: Initial: 18 mcg (3 inhal) q4h 4 times/day; if not tolerated, ↓ to 1–2 inhalations, then ↑ to 3 inhal; Maint: ↑ additional 3 inhal 1–2 wk intervals; 54 mcg (or 9 inhal) 4 ×/day max W/P: [B, ?/–] CI: Component allergy Disp: *Remodulin* Inj 1, 2.5, 5, 10 mg/mL; *Tyvaso:* 0.6 mg/mL (2.9 mL) ~6 mcg/inhal SE: Additive effects w/ anticoagulants, antihypertensives; Inf site Rxns; D, N, HA, ↓ BP Notes: Initiate in monitored setting; do not D/C or ↓ dose abruptly

Tretinoin, Topical [Retinoic Acid] (Avita, Retin-A, Renova, Retin-A Micro)   Uses: *Acne vulgaris, sun-damaged skin, wrinkles* (photo aging), some skin CAs Acts: Exfoliant retinoic acid derivative Dose: *Adults & Peds > 12 y.* Apply daily hs (w/ irritation, ↓ frequency). *Photoaging:* Start w/ 0.025%, ↑ to 0.1% over several mo (apply only q3d if on neck area; dark skin may require bid use) W/P: [C, ?] CI: Retinoid sensitivity Disp: Cream 0.02, 0.025, 0.05, 0.1%; gel 0.01, 0.025, micro formulation gel 0.1, 0.04%; liq 0.05% SE: Avoid sunlight; edema; skin dryness, erythema, scaling, changes in pigmentation, stinging, photosens

Triamcinolone (Azmacort)   Uses: *Chronic asthma* Actions: Topical steroid Dose: 2 Inh tid-qid or 4 Inh bid W/P: [C, ?] CI: Component allergy Disp: Aerosol, metered inhaler 100-mcg spray SE: Cough, oral candidiasis Notes: Instruct pts to rinse mouth after use; not for acute asthma; contains ozone-depleting CFCs; will be gradually removed from US market

Triamcinolone & Nystatin (Mycolog-II)   Uses: *Cutaneous candidiasis* Acts: Antifungal & anti-inflammatory Dose: Apply lightly to area bid; max 25 mg/d W/P: [C, ?] CI: Varicella; systemic fungal infxns Disp: Cream & oint 15, 30, 60, 120 mg SE: Local irritation, hypertrichosis, pigmentation changes Notes: For short-term use (< 7 d)

Triamterene (Dyrenium)   Uses: *Edema associated w/ CHF, cirrhosis* Acts: K+-sparing diuretic Dose: *Adults.* 100–300 mg/24 h PO ÷ daily-bid. *Peds. HTN:* 2–4 mg/kg/d in 1–2 ÷ doses; ↓ w/ renal/hepatic impair W/P: [B (manufacturer; D ed. opinion), ?/–] CI: ↑ K+, renal impair; caution w/ other K+-sparing diuretics Disp: Caps 50, 100 mg SE: ↓ K+, blood dyscrasias, liver damage, other Rxns

Triazolam (Halcion) [C-IV]   Uses: *Short-term management of insomnia* Acts: Benzodiazepine Dose: 0.125–0.25 mg/d PO hs PRN; ↓ in elderly W/P: [X, ?/–] CI: NAG; cirrhosis; concurrent fosamprenavir, ritonavir, nelfinavir, itraconazole, ketoconazole, nefazodone **Disp:** Tabs 0.125, 0.25 mg **SE:** Tachycardia, CP, drowsiness, fatigue, memory impair, GI upset **Notes:** Additive CNS depression w/ EtOH & other CNS depressants, avoid abrupt D/C, do not prescribe > 1 mo supply

Triethanolamine (Cerumenex) [OTC] **Uses:** *Cerumen (ear wax) removal* **Acts:** Ceruminolytic agent **Dose:** Fill ear canal & insert cotton plug; irrigate w/ H_2O after 15 min; repeat PRN **W/P:** [C, ?] **CI:** Perforated tympanic membrane, otitis media **Disp:** Soln 6, 12 mL **SE:** Local dermatitis, pain, erythema, pruritus

Triethylenethiophosphoramide (Thiotepa, Thioplex, Tespa, TSPA)
Uses: *Hodgkin Dz & NHLs; leukemia; breast, ovarian CAs, preparative regimens for allogeneic & ABMT w/ high doses, intravesical for bladder CA* **Acts:** Polyfunctional alkylating agent **Dose:** 0.5 mg/kg q1–4wk, 6 mg/m² IM or IV × 4 d q2–4wk, 15–35 mg/m² by cont IV Inf over 48 h; 60 mg into the bladder & retained 2 h q1–4wk; 900–125 mg/m² in ABMT regimens (highest dose w/o ABMT is 180 mg/m²); 1–10 mg/m² (typically 15 mg) IT 1 or 2×/wk; 0.8 mg/kg in 1–2 L of soln may be instilled intraperitoneally; ↓ in renal failure **W/P:** [D, –] **CI:** Component allergy **Disp:** Inj 15, 30 mg **SE:** ↓ BM, N/V, dizziness, HA, allergy, paresthesias, alopecia **Notes:** Intravesical use in bladder CA infrequent today

Trifluoperazine (Stelazine) **Uses:** *Psychotic disorders* **Acts:** Phenothiazine; blocks postsynaptic CNS dopaminergic receptors **Dose:** *Adults.* 2–10 mg PO bid. *Peds 6–12 y.* 1 mg PO daily-bid initial, gradually ↑ to 15 mg/d; ↓ in elderly/debilitated pts **W/P:** [C, ?/–] **CI:** Hx blood dyscrasias; phenothiazine sensitivity **Disp:** Tabs 1, 2, 5, 10 mg; PO conc 10 mg/mL; Inj 2 mg/mL **SE:** Orthostatic ↓ BP, EPS, dizziness, neuroleptic malignant synd, skin discoloration, lowered Sz threshold, photosens, blood dyscrasias **Notes:** PO conc must be diluted to 60 mL or more prior to administration; requires several wk for onset of effects

Trifluridine Ophthalmic (Viroptic) **Uses:** *Herpes simplex keratitis & conjunctivitis* **Acts:** Antiviral **Dose:** 1 gtt q2h, max 9 gtt/d; ↓ to 1 gtt q4h after healing begins; Rx up to 21 d **W/P:** [C, M] **CI:** Component allergy **Disp:** Soln 1% **SE:** Local burning, stinging

Trihexyphenidyl (Artane) **Uses:** *Parkinson Dz* **Acts:** Blocks excess acetylcholine at cerebral synapses **Dose:** 2–5 mg PO daily-qid **W/P:** [C, +] **CI:** NAG, GI obst, MyG, BOO **Disp:** Tabs 2, 5 mg; elixir 2 mg/5 mL **SE:** Dry skin, constipation, xerostomia, photosens, tachycardia, arrhythmias

Trimethobenzamide (Tigan) **Uses:** *N/V* **Acts:** ↓ Medullary chemoreceptor trigger zone **Dose:** *Adults.* 300 mg PO or 200 mg IM tid-qid PRN. *Peds.* 20 mg/kg/24 h PO in 3–4 ÷ doses **W/P:** [C, ?] **CI:** Benzocaine sensitivity **Disp:** Caps 300 mg; Inj 100 mg/mL **SE:** Drowsiness, ↓ BP, dizziness; hepatic impair, blood dyscrasias, Szs, parkinsonian-like synd **Notes:** In the presence of viral infxns, may mask emesis or mimic CNS effects of Reye synd

Trimethoprim (Primsol, Proloprim, Trimpex) **Uses:** *UTI d/t susceptible gram(+) & gram(–) organisms; Rx PCP w/ dapsone* suppression of UTI **Acts:** ↓ Dihydrofolate reductase. *Spectrum:* Many gram(+) & (–) except *Bacteroides,*

Branhamella, Brucella, Chlamydia, Clostridium, Mycobacterium, Mycoplasma, Nocardia, Neisseria, Pseudomonas, & *Treponema* **Dose: Adults.** 100 mg PO bid or 200 mg PO q day; PCP 5 mg/kg tid × 21 d w/ dapsone. **Peds.** 4 mg/kg/d in 2 ÷ doses; ↓ w/ renal failure **W/P:** [C, +] **CI:** Megaloblastic anemia d/t folate deficiency **Disp:** Tabs 100 mg; PO soln 50 mg/5 mL **SE:** Rash, pruritus, megaloblastic anemia, hepatic impair, blood dyscrasias **Notes:** Take w/ plenty of H2O

Trimethoprim (TMP)–Sulfamethoxazole (SMX) [Co-Trimoxazole, TMP-SMX] (Bactrim, Septra) Uses: *UTI Rx & prophylaxis, otitis media, sinusitis, bronchitis, prevent PCP pneumonia (w/CD4 count < 200 cells/mm^3)* **Acts:** SMX ↓ synth of dihydrofolic acid, TMP ↓ dihydrofolate reductase to impair protein synth. *Spectrum:* Includes *Shigella*, PCP, & *Nocardia* Infxns, *Mycoplasma, Enterobacter* sp, *Staphylococcus, Streptococcus,* & more **Dose: Adults.** 1 DS tab PO bid or 5–20 mg/kg/24 h (based on TMP) IV in 3–4 ÷ doses. *PCP:* 15–20 mg/kg/d IV or PO (TMP) in 4 ÷ doses. *Nocardia:* 10–15 mg/kg/d IV or PO (TMP) in 4 ÷ doses. PCP prophylaxis: 1 reg tab daily or DS tab 3 × wk *UTI prophylaxis:* 1 PO daily. **Peds.** 8–10 mg/kg/24 h (TMP) PO ÷ into 2 doses or 3–4 doses IV; do not use in newborns; ↓ in renal failure; maintain hydration **W/P:** [B (D if near term), +] **CI:** Sulfonamide sensitivity, porphyria, megaloblastic anemia w/ folate deficiency, sig hepatic impair **Disp:** Regular tabs 80 mg TMP/400 mg SMX; DS tabs 160 mg TMP/800 mg SMX; PO susp 40 mg TMP/200 mg SMX/5 mL; Inj 80 mg TMP/400 mg SMX/5 mL **SE:** Allergic skin Rxns, photosens, GI upset, SJS, blood dyscrasias, hep **Notes:** Synergistic combo, interacts w/ warfarin

Trimetrexate (NeuTrexin) **BOX:** Must be used w/ leucovorin to avoid tox Uses: *Mod–severe PCP* **Acts:** ↓ Dihydrofolate reductase **Dose:** 45 mg/m^2 IV q24h for 21 d; administer w/ leucovorin 20 mg/m^2 IV q6h for 24 d; ↓ in hepatic impair **W/P:** [D, ?/–] **CI:** MTX sensitivity **Disp:** Inj 25, 200 mg/vial **SE:** Sz, fever, rash, GI upset, anemias, ↑ LFTs, peripheral neuropathy, renal impair **Notes:** Use cytotoxic cautions; Inf over 60 min

Triptorelin (Trelstar 3.75, Trelstar 11.25, Trelstar 22.5) Uses: *Palliation of advanced PCa* **Acts:** LHRH analog; ↓ GNRH w/ cont dosing; transient ↑ in LH, FSH, testosterone, & estradiol 7–10 d after 1st dose; w/ chronic use (usually 2–4 wk), sustained ↓ LH & FSH w/ ↓ testicular & ovarian steroidogenesis similar to surgical castration **Dose:** 3.75 mg IM q4wk; or 11.25 mg IM q12wk or 22.5 mg q24wk **W/P:** [X, N/A] **CI:** Not indicated in females **Disp:** Inj Depot 3.75 mg; 11.25 mg; 22.5 mg **SE:** Dizziness, emotional lability, fatigue, HA, insomnia, HTN, D, V, ED, retention, UTI, pruritus, anemia, Inj site pain, musculoskeletal pain, osteoporosis, allergic Rxns **Notes:** Only 6 month formulation, ✓ periodic testosterone levels

Trospium (Sanctura, Sanctura XR) Uses: *OAB w/ Sx of urge incontinence, urgency, frequency* **Acts:** Muscarinic antagonist, ↓ bladder smooth muscle tone **Dose:** 20 mg tab PO bid; 60 mg ER caps PO q day A.M., 1 h ac or on empty stomach. ↓ w/ CrCl < 30 mL/min and elderly **W/P:** [C, +/–] w/ EtOH use, in hot environments, ulcerative colitis, MyG, renal/hepatic impair **CI:** Urinary/gastric retention, NAG **Disp:** Tab 20 mg; caps ER 60 mg **SE:** Dry mouth, constipation, HA, rash

Ulipristal Acetate (Ella) **Uses:** *Emergency contraceptive for PRG prevention (unprotected sex/contraceptive failure)* **Acts:** Progesterone agonist/antagonist, delays ovulation **Dose:** 1 tab PO ASAP w/in 5 d of unprotected sex or contraceptive failure **W/P:** [X, –] CYP3A4 inducers ↓ effect **CI:** PRG **Disp:** Tab 30 mg **SE:** HA, N, abd, dysmenorrhea **Notes:** NOT for routine contraception; fertility after use unchanged, maintain routine contraception; use any day of menstrual cycle

Urokinase (Abbokinase) **Uses:** *PE, DVT, restore patency to IV catheters* **Acts:** Converts plasminogen to plasmin; causes clot lysis **Dose:** *Adults & Peds. Systemic effect:* 4400 units/kg IV over 10 min, then 4400–6000 units/kg/h for 12 h. *Restore catheter patency:* Inject 5000 units into catheter & aspirate up to 2 doses **W/P:** [B, +] **CI:** Do not use w/in 10 d of surgery, delivery, or organ biopsy; bleeding, CVA, vascular malformation **Disp:** Powder for Inj, 250,000-unit vial **SE:** Bleeding, ↓ BP, dyspnea, bronchospasm, anaphylaxis, cholesterol embolism **Notes:** aPTT should be < 2× nl before use and before starting anticoagulants after

Ustekinumab (Stelara) **Uses:** *Moderate-to-severe plaque psoriasis* **Action:** Human IL-12 and -23 antagonist **Dose:** Wgt < 100 kg, 45 mg SQ initial and 4 wks later, then 45 mg q 12 wks. Wgt > 100 kg, 90 mg SQ initially and 4 wks later, then 90 mg q 12 wks. **W/P:** [B/?] **Disp:** Prefilled syringe and single dose vial 45 mg/0.5 mL, 90 mg/1 mL **SE:** Nasopharyngitis, URI, HA, fatigue **Notes:** Do not use with live vaccines

Valacyclovir (Valtrex) **Uses:** *Herpes zoster; genital herpes; herpes labialis* **Acts:** Prodrug of acyclovir; ↓ viral DNA replication. *Spectrum:* Herpes simplex I & II **Dose:** *Zoster:* 1 g PO tid × 7 d. *Genital herpes(initial episode):* 1 g bid × 7–10 d, *(recurrent)* 500 mg PO bid × 3 d or 1 g PO q day × 5 d. *Herpes prophylaxis:* 500–1000 mg/d. *Herpes labialis:* 2 g PO q12h × 1 d ↓ w/ renal failure **W/P:** [B, +] ↑ CNS effects in elderly **Disp:** Caplets 500, 1000 mg **SE:** HA, GI upset, dizziness, pruritus, photophobia

Valganciclovir (Valcyte) **BOX:** Granulocytopenia, anemia, and thrombocytopenia reported. Carcinogenic, teratogenic, and may cause aspermatogenesis **Uses:** *CMV retinitis and CMV prophylaxis in solid-organ transplantation* **Acts:** Ganciclovir prodrug; ↓ viral DNA synth **Dose:** *CMV Retinitis induction:* 900 mg PO bid w/ food × 21 d, then 900 mg PO daily; *CMV prevention:* 900 mg PO q day × 100 d posttransplant, ↓ w/ renal dysfunction **W/P:** [C, ?/–] Use w/ imipenem/ cilastatin, nephrotoxic drugs **CI:** Allergy to acyclovir, ganciclovir, valganciclovir; ANC < 500 cells/mcL; plt < 25,000 cells/mcL; Hgb < 8 g/dL **Disp:** Tabs 450 mg **SE:** BM suppression, headache, GI upset **Notes:** Monitor CBC & Cr

Valproic Acid (Depakene, Depakote, Stavzor) **BOX:** Fatal hepatic failure (usually during 1st 6 mo of Tx, peds < 2 y high risk, monitor LFTs at baseline and frequent intervals), teratogenic effects, and life-threatening pancreatitis reported **Uses:** *Rx epilepsy, mania; prophylaxis of migraines*, Alzheimer behavior disorder **Acts:** Anticonvulsant; ↑ availability of GABA **Dose:** *Adults & Peds.*

Szs: 30–60 mg/kg/24 h PO ÷ tid (after initiation of 10–15 mg/kg/24 h). *Mania:* 750 mg in 3 ÷ doses, ↑ 60 mg/kg/d max. *Migraines:* 250 mg bid, ↑ 1000 mg/d max; ↓ w/ renal impair **CI:** [D, +] Multiple drug interactions **CI:** Severe hepatic impair, urea cycle disorder **Disp:** Caps 250 mg; caps w/ coated particles 125 mg; tabs DR 125, 250, 500 mg; tabs ER 250, 500 mg; Caps DR (Stavzor) 125, 250,500 mg; syrup 250 mg/5 mL; Inj 100 mg/mL **SE:** Somnolence, dizziness, GI upset, diplopia, ataxia, rash, thrombocytopenia↓ plt, hep, pancreatitis, ↑ bleeding times, alopecia, ↑ wgt ↑, hyperammonemic encephalopathy in pts w/ urea cycle disorders; if taken during pregnancy may cause lower IQ tests in children **Notes:** Monitor LFTs & levels: *Trough:* Just before next dose; *Therapeutic: Peak:* 50–100 mcg/mL; *Toxic Trough:* > 100 mcg/mL. *Half-life:* 5–20 h; phenobarbital & phenytoin may alter levels

Valsartan (Diovan) BOX: Use during 2nd/3rd tri of PRG can cause fetal harm **Uses:** HTN, CHF, DN **Acts:** Angiotensin II receptor antagonist **Dose:** 80–160 mg/d, max 320 mg/d **W/P:** [D, ?/–] w/ K⁺-sparing diuretics or K⁺ supls **CI:** Severe hepatic impair, biliary cirrhosis/obst, primary hyperaldosteronism, bilateral RAS **Disp:** Tabs 40, 80, 160, 320 mg **SE:** ↓ BP, dizziness, HA, viral Infxn, fatigue, Abd pain, D, arthralgia, fatigue, back pain, hyperkalemia, cough, ↑ Cr

Vancomycin (Vancocin, Vancoled) **Uses:** *Serious MRSA Infxns; enterococcal Infxns; PO Rx of *S. aureus* and *C. difficile* pseudomembranous colitis* **Acts:** ↓ Cell wall synth. *Spectrum:* Gram(+) bacteria & some anaerobes (including MRSA, *Staphylococcus, Enterococcus, Streptococcus* sp, *C. difficile*) **Dose:** *Adults.* 1 g IV q12h or 15–20 mg/kg/dose; *C. difficile:* 125–500 mg PO q6h × 7–10 d. *Peds.* 40–60 mg/kg/d IV in ÷ doses q6–12 h; *C. difficile:* 40–60 mg/kg/d PO × 7–10 d. *Neonates.* 10–15 mg/kg/dose q12h; ↓ w/ renal Insuff **W/P:** [C, M] **CI:** Component allergy; avoid in Hx hearing loss **Disp:** Caps 125, 250 mg; powder 250 mg/5 mL, 500 mg/6 mL for PO soln; powder for Inj 500 mg, 1000 mg, 10 g/vial **SE:** Oto-/nephrotoxic, GI upset (PO); **Notes:** Not absorbed PO, effect in gut only; give IV slowly (over 1–3 h) to prevent "red-man synd" (flushing of head/neck/upper torso); IV product used PO for colitis. *Levels: Peak:* 1 h after Inf; *Trough:* < 0.5 h before next dose; *Therapeutic: Peak:* 20–40 mcg/mL; *Trough:* 10–20 mcg/mL; *Toxic Peak:* > 50 mcg/mL; *Trough:* > 20 mcg/mL. *1/2:* 6–8 h

Vardenafil (Levitra, Staxyn) **Uses:** *ED* **Acts:** PDE5 inhib, increases cyclic guanosine monophosphate (cGMP) and NO levels; relaxes smooth muscles, dilates cavernosal arteries **Dose:** *Levitra* 10 mg PO 60 min before sexual activity; titrate; max × 1 = 20 mg; 2.5 mg w/ CYP3A4 inhib (Table 10, p 301); *Staxyn* (10 mg ODT) 60 min before sex **W/P:** [B, –] w/ CV, hepatic, or renal Dz or if sex activity not advisable; potentiate the hypotensive effects of nitrates, alpha-blockers, and antihypertensives **CI:** w/ Nitrates, **Disp:** *Levitra* Tabs 2.5, 5, 10, 20 mg tabs; *Staxyn* 10 mg ODT (contains phenylalanine) **SE:** ↑ QT interval ↓ BP, HA, dyspepsia, priapism, flushing, rhinitis, sinusitis, flu synd, sudden ↓/loss of hearing, tinnitus, NIAON. **Notes:** Concomitant α-blockers may cause ↓ BP; transient global amnesia reports; place Staxyn on tongue to disintegrate w/o liquids; ODT not equal to oral pill; gets higher levels

Varenicline (Chantix) **BOX:** Serious neuropsychiatric events (depression, suicidal ideation/attempt) reported. **Uses:** *Smoking cessation* **Acts:** Nicotine receptor partial agonist **Dose:** *Adults.* 0.5 mg PO daily × 3 d, 0.5 mg bid × 4 d, then 1 mg PO bid for 12 wk total; after meal w/ glass of water **W/P:** [C, ?/–] ↓ Dose w/ renal impair, may increase risk of CV events in pts w/ CV disease **Disp:** Tabs 0.5, 1 mg **SE:** Serious psychological disturbances, N, V, insomnia, flatulence, unusual dreams **Notes:** Slowly ↑ dose to ↓ N; initiate 1 wk before desired smoking cessation date; monitor for changes in behavior

Varicella Immune Globulin (VarZIG) (Investigational, call (800)843-7477]) **Uses:** Post-exposure prophylaxis for persons w/o immunity, exposure likely to result in Infxn (household contact, > 5 min) and ↑ risk for severe Dz (immunosuppression, PRG) **Acts:** Passive immunization **Dose:** 125 units/10 kg up to 625 units IV (over 3–5 min) or IM (deltoid or proximal thigh); give w/in 4–5 days (best < 72 h) of exposure **W/P:** [?, –] Indicated for PRG women exposed to varicella **CI:** IgA deficiency **Disp:** Inj, 125-mg unit vials **SE:** Inj site Rxn, dizziness, fever, HA, N; ARF, thrombosis rare **Notes:** Wait 5 mo before varicella vaccination after varicella immune globulin; may ↓ vaccine effectiveness; observe for varicella for 28 d; if VariZIG admin not possible w/in 96 hours of exposure consider admin of IGIV (400 mg/kg)

Varicella Virus Vaccine (Varivax) **Uses:** *Prevent varicella (chickenpox)* **Acts:** Active immunization w/ live attenuated virus **Dose:** *Adults & Peds (> 12 mo).* 0.5 mL SQ, repeat 4–8 wk **W/P:** [C, M] **CI:** Immunosuppression; PRG, fever, untreated TB, neomycin-anaphylactoid Rxn; **Disp:** Powder for Inj **SE:** Varicella rash, generalized or at Inj site, arthralgias/myalgias, fatigue, fever, HA, irritability, GI upset **Notes:** OK for all children & adults who have not had chickenpox; avoid PRG for 3 mo after; do not give w/in 3 mo of immunoglobulin (IgG) and no IgG w/in 2 mo of vaccination; avoid ASA for 6 wk; avoid high-risk people for 6 wk after vaccination

Vasopressin [Antidiuretic Hormone, ADH] (Pitressin) **Uses:** *DI; Rx post-op Abd distention*; adjunct Rx of GI bleeding & esophageal varices; asystole, PEA, pulseless VT & VF, adjunct systemic vasopressor (IV drip) **Acts:** Posterior pituitary hormone, potent GI, and peripheral vasoconstrictor **Dose:** *Adults & Peds. DI:* 2.5–10 units SQ or IM tid-qid. *GI hemorrhage:* 0.2–0.4 units/min; ↓ in cirrhosis; caution in vascular Dz. *VT/VF:* 40 units IV push × 1. *Vasopressor:* 0.01–0.04 units/min. *Peds. ECC 2010. Cardiac arrest:* 0.4–1 unit/kg IV/IO bolus; max dose 40 units; *Hypotension:* 0.2–2 mill units/kg/min cont inf **W/P:** [B, +] w/ Vascular Dz **CI:** Allergy **Disp:** Inj 20 units/mL **SE:** HTN, arrhythmias, fever, vertigo, GI upset, tremor **Notes:** Addition of vasopressor to concurrent norepinephrine or epi infusions

Vecuronium (Norcuron) **BOX:** To be administered only by appropriately trained individuals **Uses:** *Skeletal muscle relaxation* **Acts:** Nondepolarizing neuromuscular blocker; onset 2–3 min **Dose: *Adults & Peds.*** 0.1–0.2 mg/kg IV bolus (also rapid intubation *(ECC 2005)*; maint 0.010–0.015 mg/kg after 25–40 min; additional doses q12–15 min PRN; ↓ w/in severe renal/hepatic impair **W/P:** [C, ?] Drug interactions cause ↑ effect (e.g., aminoglycosides, tetracycline, succinylcholine) **Disp:** Powder for Inj 10, 20 mg **SE:** ↓ HR, ↓ BP, itching, rash, tachycardia, CV collapse **Notes:** Fewer cardiac effects than succinylcholine

Venlafaxine (Effexor, Effexor XR)   **BOX:** Monitor for worsening depression or emergence of suicidality, particularly in ped pts **Uses:** *Depression, generalized anxiety*, social anxiety disorder; panic disorder*, OCD, chronic fatigue synd, ADHD, autism **Acts:** Potentiation of CNS neurotransmitter activity **Dose:** 75–225 mg/d ÷ into 2–3 equal doses (IR) or q day (ER); 375 mg IR or 225 mg ER max/d ↓ w/ renal/hepatic impair **W/P:** [C, ?/–] **CI:** MAOIs **Disp:** Tabs IR 25, 37.5, 50, 75, 100 mg; ER caps 37.5, 75, 150 mg **SE:** HTN, ↑ HR, HA, somnolence, GI upset, sexual dysfunction; actuates mania or Szs **Notes:** Avoid EtOH

Verapamil (Calan, Covera HS, Isoptin, Verelan)   **Uses:** *Angina, HTN, PSVT, AF, atrial flutter*, migraine prophylaxis, hypertrophic cardiomyopathy, bipolar Dz **Acts:** CCB **Dose: *Adults. Arrhythmias:*** 2nd line for PSVT w/ narrow QRS complex & adequate BP 2.5–5 mg IV over 1–2 min; repeat 5–10 mg in 15–30 min PRN (30 mg max). *Angina:* 80–120 mg PO tid, ↑ 480 mg/24 h max. *HTN:* 80–180 mg PO tid or SR tabs 120–240 mg PO daily to 240 mg bid; *ECC 2010.* Reentry SVT w/ narrow QRS: 2.5–5 mg IV over 2 min (slower in older pts); repeat 5–10 mg, in 15–30 min, PRN max of 20 mg; or 5 mg bolus q15min (max 30 mg). *Peds < 1 y.* 0.1–0.2 mg/kg IV over 2 min (may repeat in 30 min). *1–16 y:* 0.1–0.3 mg/kg IV over 2 min (may repeat in 30 min); 5 mg max. *PO: 1–5 y:* 4–8 mg/kg/d in 3 ÷ doses. > *5 y:* 80 mg q6–8h; ↓ in renal/hepatic impair **W/P:** [C, +] Amiodarone/β-blockers/flecainide can cause ↓ HR; statins, midazolam, tacrolimus, theophylline levels may be ↑; use w/clonidine may cause severe ↓ HR w/ elderly pts **CI:** Conduction disorders, cardiogenic shock; β-blocker/thiazide combo, dofetilide, pimozide, ranolazine **Disp:** *Calan SR:* Caps 120, 180, 240 mg; *Verelan SR:* Caps 120, 180, 240, 360 mg *Verelan PM:* caps (ER) 100, 200, 300 mg; *Calan:* Tabs 40, 80, 120 mg; *Covera HS* tabs ER/controlled release 180, 240 mg; *Isoptin SR* 24-h 120, 180, 240 mg; Inj 2.5 mg/mL **SE:** Gingival hyperplasia, constipation, ↓ BP, bronchospasm, HR or conduction disturbances; ↓ BP and bradyarrhythmias taken w/ telithromycin

Vigabatrin (Sabril)   **BOX:** Vision loss reported **Uses:** *Refractory complex partial Sz disorder, infantile spasms* **Action:** ↓ Gamma-aminobutyric acid transaminase (GABA-T) to ↑ levels of brain GABA **Dose: *Adults.*** Initially 500 mg 2×/d, then ↑ daily dose by 500 mg at weekly intervals based on response and tolerability; **Peds.** *Seizures:* 10–15 kg: 0.5–1 g/day divided 2×/d; 16–30 kg: 1–1.5 g/day divided 2×/d; 31–50 kg: 1.5–3 g/day divided 2×/d; > 50 kg: 2–3 g/day divided 2×/d; *Infantile spasms:* Initially 50 mg/kg/day twice daily, ↑ 150 mg/kg/day max **W/P:** [C, +/–] ↓ dose by 25% w/ CrCl 50–80 mL/min, ↓ dose 50% w/ CrCl 30–50 mL/min, ↓ dose 75% w/ CrCl 10–30 mL/min; MRI signal changes reported in some infants **Disp:** Tabs 500 mg, powder/oral soln 500 mg/packet **SE:** vision loss/blurring, anemia, peripheral neuropathy, fatigue, somnolence, nystagmus, tremor, memory impairment, ↑ wgt, arthralgia, abnormal coordination, confusion **Notes:** ↓ Phenytoin levels reported; taper slowly to avoid withdrawal Szs; restricted distribution

Vilazodone (Viibryd) **BOX:** ↑ Suicide risk in children/adolescents/young adults on antidepressants for major depressive disorder (MDD) and other psych disorders **Uses:** *MDD* **Acts:** SSRI and 5HT1A receptor partial agonist **Dose:** 40 mg/d; start 10 mg PO/d × 7 d, then 20 mg/d × 7 d, then 40 mg/d; ↓ to 20 mg w/ CYP3A4 inhib **W/P:** [C, ?/–] **CI:** MOAI, < 14 d between D/C MAOI and start **Disp:** Tabs 10, 20, 40 mg **SE:** Serotonin syndrome, neuroleptic malignant syndrome, N/V/D, dry mouth, dizziness, insomnia, restlessness, abnormal dreams, sexual dysfunction **Notes:** NOT approved for peds; w/ D/C, ↓ dose gradually

Vinblastine (Velban, Velbe) **BOX:** Chemotherapeutic agent; handle w/ caution **Uses:** *Hodgkin Dz & NHLs, mycosis fungoides, CAs (testis, renal cell, breast, NSCLC), AIDS-related Kaposi sarcoma*, choriocarcinoma, histiocytosis **Acts:** ↓ Microtubule assembly **Dose:** 0.1–0.5 mg/kg/wk (4–20 mg/m²); ↓ in hepatic failure **W/P:** [D, ?] **CI:** Intrathecal IT use **Disp:** Inj 1 mg/mL in 10 mg vial **SE:** ↓ BM (especially leukopenia), N/V, constipation, neurotox, alopecia, rash, myalgia, tumor pain

Vincristine (Oncovin, Vincasar PFS) **BOX:** Chemotherapeutic agent; handle w/ caution; fatal if administered intrathecally **Uses:** *ALL, breast & small-cell lung CA, sarcoma (e.g., Ewing tumor, rhabdomyosarcoma), Wilms tumor, Hodgkin Dz & NHLs, neuroblastoma, multiple myeloma* **Acts:** Promotes disassembly of mitotic spindle, causing metaphase arrest **Dose:** 0.4–1.4 mg/m² (single doses 2 mg/max); ↓ in hepatic failure **W/P:** [D, ?] **CI:** Intrathecal IT use **Disp:** Inj 1 mg/mL, 5 mg vial **SE:** Neurotox commonly dose limiting, jaw pain (trigeminal neuralgia), fever, fatigue, anorexia, constipation & paralytic ileus, bladder atony; no sig ↓ BM w/ standard doses; tissue necrosis w/ extrav

Vinorelbine (Navelbine) **BOX:** Chemotherapeutic agent; handle w/ caution **Uses:** *Breast CA & NSCLC* (alone or w/ cisplatin) **Acts:** ↓ Polymerization of microtubules, impairing mitotic spindle formation; semisynthetic vinca alkaloid **Dose:** 30 mg/m²/wk; ↓ in hepatic failure **W/P:** [D, ?] **CI:** Intrathecal IT use, granulocytopenia (< 1000/mm³) **Disp:** Inj 10 mg **SE:** ↓ BM (leukopenia), mild GI, neurotox (6–29%); constipation/paresthesias (rare); tissue damage from extrav

Vitamin B₁ See Thiamine (p 257)
Vitamin B₆ See Pyridoxine (p 228)
Vitamin B₁₂ See Cyanocobalamin (p 88)
Vitamin K See Phytonadione (p 220)
Vitamin, Multi See Multivitamins (Table 12, p 304)

Voriconazole (VFEND) Uses: *Invasive aspergillosis, candidemia, serious fungal infxns* Acts: ↓ Ergosterol synth. *Spectrum: Candida, Aspergillus, Scedosporium, Fusarium* sp Dose: *Adults & Peds > 12 y.* IV: 6 mg/kg q12h × 2, then 4 mg/kg bid; may ↓ to 3 mg/kg/dose. PO: < 40 kg: 100 mg q12h, up to 150 mg; > 40 kg: 200 mg q12h, up to 300 mg; ↓ w/ mild–mod hepatic impair; IV w/ renal CYP3A4 substrates (Table 10, p 301); do not use w/ clopidogrel (↓ effect) Disp: Tabs 50, 200 mg; susp 200 mg/5 mL; 200 mg Inj SE: Visual changes, fever, rash, GI upset, ↑ LFTs Notes: ✓ for multiple drug interactions (e.g., ↑ dose w/ phenytoin)

Vorinostat (Zolinza) Uses: *Rx cutaneous manifestations in cutaneous T-cell lymphoma* Acts: Histone deacetylase inhib Dose: 400 mg PO daily w/ food; if intolerant ↓ 300 mg PO d × 5 consecutive days each wk W/P: [D, ?/–] w/ Warfarin (↑ INR) Disp: Caps 100 mg SE: N/V/D, dehydration, fatigue, anorexia, dysgeusia, DVT, PE, ↓ plt, anemia, hyperglycemia, QTc prolongation, Notes: Monitor CBC, lytes (K, Mg, Ca), glucose, & SCr q2wk × 2 mo then monthly; baseline & periodic ECGs; drink 2 L fluid/d

Warfarin (Coumadin) BOX: Can cause major or fatal bleeding Uses: *Prophylaxis & Rx of PE & DVT, AF w/ embolization*, other post-op indications Acts: ↓ Vit K-dependent clotting factors in this order: VII-IX-X-II Dose: *Adults.* Titrate, INR 2.0–3.0 for most; mechanical valves INR is 2.5–3.5. *American College of Chest Physicians guidelines:* 5 mg initial, may use 7.5–10 mg; ↓ if pt elderly or w/other bleeding risk factors; maint 2–10 mg/d PO, follow daily INR initial to adjust dosage (Table 8, p 299). *Peds.* 0.05–0.34 mg/kg/24 h PO or IV; follow PT/INR to adjust dosage; monitor vit K intake; ↓ w/ hepatic impair/elderly W/P: [X, +] CI: Severe hepatic/renal Dz, bleeding, peptic ulcer, PRG Disp: Tabs 1, 2, 2.5, 3, 4, 5, 6, 7.5, 10 mg; Inj SE: Bleeding d/t over-anticoagulation or injury & therapeutic INR; bleeding, alopecia, skin necrosis, purple toe synd Notes: Monitor vit K intake (↓ effect); INR preferred test; to rapidly correct over-anticoagulation: vit K, fresh-frozen plasma, or both; highly teratogenic. Caution pt on taking w/ other meds, especially ASA. *Common warfarin interactions: Potentiated by:* APAP, EtOH (w/ liver Dz), amiodarone, cimetidine, ciprofloxacin, cotrimoxazole, erythromycin, fluconazole, flu vaccine, isoniazid, itraconazole, metronidazole, omeprazole, phenytoin, propranolol, quinidine, tetracycline. *Inhibited by:* barbiturates, carbamazepine, chlordiazepoxide, cholestyramine, dicloxacillin, nafcillin, rifampin, sucralfate, high–vit K foods. Consider genotyping for VKORC1 & CYP2C9

Witch Hazel (Tucks Pads, Others [OTC]) Uses: After bowel movement cleansing to decrease local irritation or relieve hemorrhoids; after anorectal surgery, episiotomy, vag hygiene Acts: Astringent; shrinks blood vessels locally Dose: Apply PRN W/P: [?, ?] External use only CI: None Supplied: Presoaked pads SE: Mild itching or burning

Zafirlukast (Accolate) Uses: *Adjunctive Rx of asthma* Acts: Selective & competitive inhib of leukotrienes Dose: *Adults & Peds > 12 y.* 20 mg bid. *Peds 5–11 y.* 10 mg PO bid (empty stomach) W/P: [B, –] Interacts w/ warfarin, ↑ INR

CI: Component allergy **Disp:** Tabs 10, 20 mg **SE:** Hepatic dysfunction, usually reversible on D/C; HA, dizziness, GI upset; Churg-Strauss synd, neuropsych events (agitation, restlessness, suicidal ideation) **Notes:** Not for acute asthma

Zaleplon (Sonata) [C-IV] **Uses:** *Insomnia* **Acts:** A nonbenzodiazepine sedative/hypnotic, a pyrazolopyrimidine **Dose:** 5–20 mg hs PRN; not w/ high-fat meal; ↓ w/ renal/hepatic Insuff, elderly **W/P:** [C, ?/–] w/ Mental/psychological conditions **CI:** Component allergy **Disp:** Caps 5, 10 mg **SE:** HA, edema, amnesia, somnolence, photosens **Notes:** Take immediately before desired onset

Zanamivir (Relenza) **Uses:** *Influenza A & B w/ Sxs < 2 d; prophylaxis for influenza* **Acts:** ↓ Viral neuraminidase **Dose:** *Adults & Peds > 7 y.* 2 Inh (10 mg) bid × 10 d, initiate w/in 48 h of Sxs. *Prophylaxis household:* 10 mg q day × 10 d. *Adults & Peds > 12 y. Prophylaxis Community:* 10 mg q day × 28 d **W/P:** [C, M] Not OK for pt w/ airway Dz **CI:** Pulm Dz **Disp:** Powder for Inh 5 mg **SE:** Bronchospasm, HA, GI upset, allergic Rxn, abnormal behavior, ear, nose, throat Sx **Notes:** Uses a Disk-haler for administration; dose same time each day; 2009 H1N1 strains susceptible

Ziconotide (Prialt) **BOX:** Psychological, cognitive, neurologic impair may develop over several wk; monitor frequently; may necessitate D/C **Uses:** *IT Rx of severe, refractory, chronic pain* **Acts:** N-type CCB in spinal cord **Dose:** 2.4 mcg/d IT at 0.1 mcg/h; may ↑ 2.4 mcg/d 2–3×/wk to max 19.2 mcg/d (0.8 mcg/h) by day 21 **W/P:** [C, ?/–] w/ Neuro-psych impair **CI:** Psychosis **Disp:** Inj 25, 100 mcg/mL **SE:** Dizziness, N/V, confusion, psych disturbances, abnormal vision, meningitis; may require dosage adjustment **Notes:** May D/C abruptly; uses specific pumps; do not ↑ more frequently than 2–3×/wk

Zidovudine (Retrovir) **BOX:** Neutropenia, anemia, lactic acidosis, myopathy & hepatomegaly w/ steatosis **Uses:** *HIV Infxn, prevent maternal HIV transmission* **Acts:** ↓ RT **Dose:** *Adults.* 200 mg PO TID or 300 mg PO bid or 1 mg/dose IV q4h. *PRG:* 100 mg PO 5×/d until labor; during labor 2 mg/kg IV over 1 h then 1 mg/kg/h until cord clamped. *Peds 4 wk–18 y.* 160 mg/m²/dose TID or see table below; in renal failure **W/P:** [C, ?/–] w/ganciclovir, interferon alfa,ribavirin; may alter many other meds (see PI) **CI:** Allergy **Disp:** Caps 100 mg; tabs 300 mg; syrup 50 mg/5 mL; Inj 10 mg/mL **SE:** Hematologic tox, HA, fever, rash, GI upset, malaise, myopathy, fat redistribution **Notes:** w/severe anemia/neutropenia dosage interruption may be needed

Recommended Pediatric Dosage of Retrovir

Body Weight (kg)	Total Daily Dose	Dosage Regimen and Dose	
		bid	tid
4 to < 9	24 mg/kg/day	12 mg/kg	8 mg/kg
≥9 to < 30	18 mg/kg/day	9 mg/kg	6 mg/kg
≥30	600 mg/day	300 mg	200 mg

Zidovudine & Lamivudine (Combivir)   BOX: Neutropenia, anemia, lactic acidosis, myopathy & hepatomegaly w/ steatosis **Uses:** *HIV Infxn* **Acts:** Combo of RT inhib **Dose:** *Adults & Peds > 12 y.* 1 tab PO bid; ↓ in renal failure **W/P:** [C, ?/–] **CI:** Component allergy **Disp:** Tab zidovudine 300 mg/lamivudine 150 mg **SE:** Hematologic tox, HA, fever, rash, GI upset, malaise, pancreatitis **Notes:** Combo product ↓ daily pill burden

Zileuton (Zyflo, Zyflo CR)   **Uses:** *Chronic Rx asthma* **Acts:** Leuko-triene inhib (↓ 5-lipoxygenase) **Dose:** *Adults & Peds > 12 y.* 600 mg PO qid; CR 1200 mg bid w/in 1 h of A.M./P.M. meal **W/P:** [C, ?/–] **CI:** Hepatic impair **Disp:** Tabs 600 mg; CR tabs 600 mg **SE:** Hepatic damage, HA, GI upset, leukopenia, neuropsych events (agitation, restlessness, suicidal ideation) **Notes:** Monitor LFTs q mo × 3, then q2–3mo; take regularly; not for acute asthma; do not chew/crush CR

Ziprasidone (Geodon)   BOX: ↑ Mortality in elderly w/ dementia-related psychosis **Uses:** *Schizophrenia, acute agitation* **Acts:** Atypical antipsychotic **Dose:** 20 mg PO bid, may ↑ in 2-d intervals up to 80 mg bid; agitation 10–20 mg IM PRN up to 40 mg/d; separate 10 mg doses by 2 h & 20 mg doses by 4 h (w/ food) **W/P:** [C, –] w/ ↓ Mg²⁺, ↓ K⁺ **CI:** QT prolongation, recent MI, uncompensated heart failure, meds that ↑ QT interval **Disp:** Caps 20, 40, 60, 80 mg; susp 10 mg/mL; Inj 20 mg/mL **SE:** ↓ HR; rash, somnolence, resp disorder, EPS, wt gain, orthostatic ↓ BP **Notes:** ✓ Lytes

Zoledronic Acid (Zometa, Reclast)   **Uses:** *↑ Ca²⁺ of malignancy (HCM), ↓ skeletal-related events in CAP, multiple myeloma, & metastatic bone lesions (Zometa)*; *prevent/Rx of postmenopausal osteoporosis, Paget Dz, ↑ bone mass in men w/ osteoporosis, steroid induced osteoporosis (Reclast)* **Acts:** Bisphosphonate; ↓ osteoclastic bone resorption **Dose:** *Zometa HCM:* 4 mg IV over ≥15 min; may retreat in 7 d w/ adequate renal Fxn. *Zometa bone lesions/myeloma:* 4 mg IV over > 15 min, repeat q3–4wk PRN; extend w/ ↑ Cr. *Reclast Rx osteoporosis:* 5 mg IV annually. *Reclast:* prevent postmenopausal osteoporosis 5 mg IV q2y. *Paget's:* 5 mg IV X 1. **W/P:** [C, ?/–] w/ Diuretics, aminoglycosides; ASA-sensitive asthmatics; avoid invasive dental procedures **CI:** Bisphosphonate allergy; urticaria, angioedema, w/ dental procedures, CrCl < 35 **Disp:** Vial 4 mg, 5 mg **SE:** All ↑ w/ renal dysfunction: fever, flu-like synd, GI upset, insomnia, anemia; electrolyte abnormalities, bone, joint, muscle pain, AF, osteonecrosis of jaw, atyp femur Fx **Notes:** Requires vigorous prehydration; do not exceed rec doses/Inf duration to ↓ renal dysfunction; follow Cr; effect prolonged w/ Cr ↑; avoid oral surgery; dental exam recommended prior to Rx; ↓ dose w/ renal dysfunction; give Ca²⁺ and vit D supls; may ↑ atypical subtrochanteric femur fractures

Zolmitriptan (Zomig, Zomig XMT, Zomig Nasal)   **Uses:** *Acute Rx migraine* **Acts:** Selective serotonin agonist; causes vasoconstriction **Dose:** Initial 2.5 mg PO, may repeat after 2 h, 10 mg max in 24 h; nasal 5 mg; if HA returns, repeat after 2 h, 10 mg max 24 h **W/P:** [C, ?/–] **CI:** Ischemic heart Dz, Prinzmetal angina, uncontrolled HTN, accessory conduction pathway disorders, ergots,

MAOIs **Disp:** Tabs 2.5, 5 mg; rapid tabs (XMT) 2.5, 5 mg; nasal 5 mg, **SE:** Dizziness, hot flashes, paresthesias, chest tightness, myalgia, diaphoresis

Zolpidem (Ambien IR, Ambien CR, Edluar, ZolpiMist) [C-IV]

Uses: *Short-term Tx of insomnia; *Ambien and Edluar* w/ difficulty of sleep onset; *Ambien CR* w/difficulty of sleep onset and/or sleep maint* **Acts:** Hypnotic agent **Dose:** *Adults. Ambien:* 5–10 mg or 12.5 mg *CR* PO qhs; *Edluar:* 10 mg SL q hs; *Zolpimist:* 10 mg spray qhs; ↓ dose in elderly, debilitated, & hepatic impair (5 mg or 6.25 mg CR) **W/P:** [C, −] may cause anaphylaxis, angioedema, abnormal thinking, CNS depression, withdrawal; evaluate for other comorbid conditions **CI:** None **Disp:** *Ambien IR:* Tabs 5, 10 mg; *Ambien CR* 6.25, 12.5 mg; *Edluar:* SL tabs 5, 10 mg; *Zolpimist:* oral soln 5 mg/spray (60 actuations/unit) **SE:** Drowsiness, dizziness, D, drugged feeling, HA, dry mouth, depression **Notes:** Take tabs on empty stomach; be able to sleep 7–8 hrs; *Zolpimist:* Prime w/ 5 sprays initially, and w/ 1 spray if not used in 14 days; store upright.

Zonisamide (Zonegran)

BOX: ↑ Risk of suicidal thoughts or behavior **Uses:** *Adjunct Rx complex partial Szs* **Acts:** Anticonvulsant **Dose:** Initial 100 mg/d PO; may ↑ to 400 mg/d **W/P:** [C, −] ↑ tox w/ CYP3A4 inhib; ↓ levels w/ carbamazepine, phenytoin, phenobarbital, valproic acid **CI:** Allergy to sulfonamides; oligohidrosis & hypothermia in peds **Disp:** Caps 25, 50, 100 mg **SE:** Metabolic acidosis, dizziness, drowsiness, confusion, ataxia, memory impair, paresthesias, psychosis, nystagmus, diplopia, tremor, anemia, leukopenia; GI upset, nephrolithiasis (? d/t metabolic acidosis), SJS; monitor for ↓ sweating & ↑ body temperature **Notes:** Swallow caps whole

Zoster Vaccine, Live (Zostavax)

Uses: *Prevent varicella zoster in adults > 60 y* **Acts:** Active immunization (live attenuated varicella) virus **Dose:** *Adults.* 0.65 mL SQ × 1 **CI:** Gelatin, neomycin anaphylaxis; fever, untreated TB, immunosuppression **W/P:** [C, ?/−] **Disp:** Single dose vial **SE:** Inj site Rxn, HA **Notes:** May be used if previous Hx of zoster; do not use in place of Varicella Virus Vaccine in children; contact precautions not necessary; antivirals and immune globulins may ↓ effectiveness

NATURAL AND HERBAL AGENTS

The following is a guide to some common herbal products. These may be sold separately or in combo with other products. According to the FDA, "Manufacturers of dietary supplements can make claims about how their products affect the structure or function of the body, but they may not claim to prevent, treat, cure, mitigate, or diagnose a disease without prior FDA approval." The table on p 280 summarizes some of the common dangerous aspects of natural and herbal agents.

Black Cohosh Uses: Sx of menopause (e.g., hot flashes), PMS, hypercholesterolemia, peripheral arterial Dz; has anti-inflammatory & sedative effects **Efficacy:** May have short-term benefit on menopausal Sx **Dose:** 20–40 mg bid **W/P:** May further ↓ lipids &/or BP w/ prescription meds **CI:** PRG (miscarriage, prematurity reports); lactation **SE:** w/ OD, N/V, dizziness, nervous system & visual changes, ↓ HR, & (possibly) Szs, liver damage/failure

Chamomile Uses: Antispasmodic, sedative, anti-inflammatory, astringent, antibacterial. **Dose:** 10–15 g PO daily (3 g dried flower heads tid-qid between meals; can steep in 250 mL hot H_2O) **W/P:** w/ Allergy to chrysanthemums, ragweed, asters (family *Compositae*) **SE:** Contact dermatitis; allergy, anaphylaxis **Interactions:** w/ Anticoagulants, additive w/ sedatives (benzodiazepines); delayed ↓ gastric absorption of meds if taken together (↓ GI motility)

Cranberry (*Vaccinium macrocarpon*) Uses: Prevention & Rx UTI. **Efficacy:** Possibly effective **Dose:** 300–400 mg bid in 6-oz. juice qid; tincture 1/2–1 tsp up to 3×/d, tea 2–3 tsps of dried flowers/cup; creams apply topically 2–3×/d PO **W/P:** May ↑ kidney stones in some susceptible individuals, V **SE:** None known **Interactions:** May potentiate warfarin

Dong Quai (*Angelica polymorpha, sinensis*) Uses: Uterine stimulant; anemia, menstrual cramps, irregular menses, & menopausal Sx; anti-inflammatory, vasodilator, CNS stimulant, immunosuppressant, analgesic, antiasthmatic **Efficacy:** Possibly effective for menopausal Sx **Dose:** 3–15 g daily, 9–12 g PO tab bid. **W/P:** Avoid in PRG & lactation **SE:** D, photosens, skin CA **Interactions:** Anticoagulants (↑ INR w/ warfarin)

Echinacea (*Echinacea purpurea*) Uses: Immune system stimulant; prevention/Rx URI of colds, flu; supportive care in chronic Infxns of the resp/lower urinary tract **Efficacy:** Not established; may ↓ severity & duration of URI **Dose:** Caps 500 mg, 6–9 mL expressed juice or 2–5 g dried root PO **W/P:** Do not use w/ progressive systemic or immune Dzs (e.g., TB, collagen–vascular disorders, MS); may interfere w/ immunosuppressive Rx, not OK w/ PRG; do not use > 8 consecutive wk; possible immunosuppression; 3 different commercial forms **SE:** N; rash **Interactions:** Anabolic steroids, amiodarone, MTX, corticosteroids, cyclosporine

Ephedra/Ma Huang **Uses:** Stimulant, aid in wgt loss, bronchial dilation. **Dose:** Not OK d/t reported deaths (> 100 mg/d can be life-threatening); US sales banned by FDA in 2004; bitter orange w/ similar properties has replaced this compound in most wgt-loss supls **W/P:** Adverse cardiac events, strokes, death **SE:** Nervousness, HA, insomnia, palpitations, V, hyperglycemia **Interactions:** Digoxin, antihypertensives, antidepressants, diabetic meds

Evening Primrose Oil **Uses:** PMS, diabetic neuropathy, ADHD **Efficacy:** Possibly for PMS, not for menopausal Sx **Dose:** 2–4 g/d PO **SE:** Indigestion, N, soft stools, HA **Interactions:** ↑ Phenobarbital metabolism, ↓ Sz threshold

Fish Oil Supplements (Omega-3 Polyunsaturated Fatty Acid)
Uses: CAD, hypercholesterolemia, hypertriglyceridemia, type 2 DM, arthritis **Efficacy:** No definitive data on ↓ cardiac risk in general population; may ↓ lipids and help w/ secondary MI prevention **Dose:** One FDA approved (see Lovaza, p 205); OTC 1500–3000 mg/d; AHA rec: 1 g/d **W/P:** Mercury contamination possible, some studies suggest ↑ cardiac events **SE:** ↑ Bleeding risk, dyspepsia, belching, aftertaste **Interactions:** Anticoagulants

Feverfew (Tanacetum parthenium) **Uses:** Prevent/Rx migraine; fever; menstrual disorders; arthritis; toothache; insect bites **Efficacy:** Weak for migraine prevention **Dose:** 125 mg PO of dried leaf (standardized to 0.2% of parthenolide) PO **W/P:** Do not use in PRG **SE:** Oral ulcers, gastric disturbance, swollen lips, Abd pain; long-term SE unknown **Interactions:** ASA, warfarin

Garlic (Allium sativum) **Uses:** Antioxidant; hyperlipidemia; HTN; anti-infective (antibacterial, antifungal); tick repellant (oral) **Efficacy:** ↓ Cholesterol by 4–6%; soln ↓ BP; possible ↑ GI/CAP risk **Dose:** 2–5 g, fresh garlic; 0.4–1.2 g of dried powder; 2–5 mg oil; 300–1000 mg extract or other formulations to 2–5 mg of allicin daily, 400–1200 mg powder (2–5 mg allicin) PO **W/P:** Do not use in PRG (abortifacient); D/C 7 d pre-op **SE:** ↑ Insulin/lipid/alcohol levels, anemia, oral burning sensation, N/V/D **Interactions:** Warfarin & ASA (↓ plt aggregation), additive w/ DM agents (↑ hypoglycemia), CYP 3A4 inducer (may ↑ cyclosporine, HIV antivirals, oral contraceptives)

Ginger (Zingiber officinale) **Uses:** Prevent motion sickness; N/V d/t anesthesia **Efficacy:** Benefit in ↓ N/V w/ motion or PRG; weak for post-op or chemotherapy **Dose:** 1–4 g rhizome or 0.5–2 g powder PO daily **W/P:** Pt w/ gallstones; excessive dose (↑ depression, & may interfere w/ cardiac Fxn or anticoagulants) **SE:** Heartburn **Interactions:** Excessive consumption may interfere w/ cardiac, DM, or anticoagulant meds (↓ plt aggregation)

Ginkgo Biloba **Uses:** Memory deficits, dementia, anxiety, improvement Sx peripheral vascular Dz, vertigo, tinnitus, asthma/bronchospasm, antioxidant, premenstrual Sx (especially breast tenderness), impotence, SSRI-induced sexual dysfunction **Dose:** 60–80 mg standardized dry extract PO bid-tid **Efficacy:** Small cognition benefit w/ dementia; no other demonstrated benefit in healthy adults **W/P:** ↑ Bleeding risk (antagonism of plt-activating factor), concerning w/ anti-platlet agents (D/C 3 d pre-op); reports of ↑ Sz risk **SE:** GI upset, HA, dizziness, heart palpitations, rash **Interactions:** ASA, salicylates, warfarin

Ginseng **Uses:** "Energy booster" general; also for pt undergoing chemotherapy, stress reduction, enhance brain activity & physical endurance (adaptogenic), anti-oxidant, aid to control type 2 DM; Panax ginseng being studied for ED **Efficacy:** Not established **Dose:** 1–2 g of root or 100–300 mg of extract (7% ginsenosides) PO tid **W/P:** w/ Cardiac Dz, DM, ↓ BP, HTN, mania, schizophrenia, w/ corticosteroids; avoid in PRG; D/C 7 d pre-op (bleeding risk) **SE:** Controversial "ginseng abuse synd" w/ high dose (nervousness, excitation, HA, insomnia); palpitations, vag bleeding, breast nodules, hypoglycemia **Interactions:** Warfarin, antidepressants, & caffeine (↑ stimulant effect), DM meds (↑ hypoglycemia)

Glucosamine Sulfate (Chitosamine) and Chondroitin Sulfate **Uses:** Osteoarthritis (glucosamine: rate-limiting step in glycosaminoglycan synth), ↑ cartilage rebuilding; *Chondroitin:* biological polymer, flexible matrix between protein filaments in cartilage; draws fluids/nutrients into joint, "shock absorption") **Efficacy:** Controversial **Dose:** Glucosamine 500 PO tid, chondroitin 400 mg PO tid **W/P:** Many forms come from shellfish, so avoid if have shellfish allergy **SE:** ↑ Insulin resistance in DM; concentrated in cartilage, theoretically unlikely to cause toxic/teratogenic effects **Interactions:** *Glucosamine:* None. *Chondroitin:* Monitor anticoagulant Rx

Kava Kava (Kava Kava Root Extract, *Piper methysticum*) **Uses:** Anxiety, stress, restlessness, insomnia **Efficacy:** Possible mild anxiolytic **Dose:** Standardized extract (70% kavalactones) 100 mg PO bid-tid **W/P:** Hepatotox risk, banned in Europe/Canada. Not OK in PRG, lactation. D/C 24 h pre-op (may ↑ sedative effect of anesthetics) **SE:** Mild GI disturbances; rare allergic skin/rash Rxns, may ↑ cholesterol; ↑ LFTs/jaundice; vision changes, red eyes, puffy face, muscle weakness **Interactions:** Avoid w/ sedatives, alcohol, stimulants, barbiturates (may potentiate CNS effect)

Melatonin **Uses:** Insomnia, jet lag, antioxidant, immunostimulant **Efficacy:** Sedation most pronounced w/ elderly pts w/ ↓ endogenous melatonin levels; some evidence for jet lag **Dose:** 1–3 mg 20 min before HS (w/ CR 2 before hs) **W/P:** Use synthetic rather than animal pineal gland, "heavy head," HA, depression, daytime sedation, dizziness **Interactions:** β-Blockers, steroids, NSAIDs, benzodiazepines

Milk Thistle (*Silybum marianum*) **Uses:** Prevent/Rx liver damage (e.g., from alcohol, toxins, cirrhosis, chronic hep); preventive w/ chronic toxin exposure (painters, chemical workers, etc) **Efficacy:** Use before exposure more effective than use after damage has occurred **Dose:** 80–200 mg PO tid **SE:** GI intolerance **Interactions:** None

Red Yeast Rice **Uses:** Hyperlipidemia **Efficacy:** HMG-CoA reductase activity, naturally occurring lovastatin; ↓ LDL, ↓ triglycerides, ↑ HDL; ↓ secondary CAD events **Dose:** 1,200–1,800 mg bid **W/P:** CI w/PRG, lactation; do not use w/ liver Dz, recent surgery, serious infection; may contain a mycotoxin, citrinin, can cause renal failure **Disp:** Caps 600–1,200 mg **SE:** N, V, abd pain, hepatitis, myopathy, rhabdomyolysis **Interactions:** Possible interactions many drugs, avoid w/ CYP3A4 inhibitors or EtOH **Notes:** Use only in adults; generic lovastatin cheaper

Resveratrol **Uses:** Cardioprotective, prevent aging; ? antioxidant **Efficacy:** Limited human research **W/P:** Avoid w/ Hx of estrogen responsive CA or w/ CYP3A4 metabolized drugs **Disp:** Caps, tabs 20–500 mg, skins of red grapes, plums, blueberries, cranberries, red wine **SE:** D/N, anorexia, insomnia, anxiety, jt pain, antiplatelet aggregation **Interactions:** Avoid w/ other antiplatelet drugs or anticoagulants; CYP3A4 inhibitor

Saw Palmetto (*Serenoa repens*) **Uses:** Rx BPH, hair tonic, PCa prevention (weak 5α-reductase inhib like finasteride, dutasteride) **Efficacy:** Small, no sig benefit for prostatic Sx **Dose:** 320 mg daily **W/P:** Possible hormonal effects, avoid in PRG, w/ women of childbearing years **SE:** Mild GI upset, mild HA, D w/ large amounts **Interactions:** ↑ Iron absorption; ↑ estrogen replacement effects

St. John's Wort (*Hypericum perforatum*) **Uses:** Mild–mod depression, anxiety, gastritis, insomnia, vitiligo; anti-inflammatory; immune stimulant/anti-HIV/antiviral **Efficacy:** Variable; benefit w/ mild–mod depression in several trials, but not always seen in clinical practice **Dose:** 2–4 g of herb or 0.2–1 mg of total hypericin (standardized extract) daily. *Common preparations:* 300 mg PO tid (0.3% hypericin) **W/P:** Excess doses may potentiate MAOI, cause allergic Rxn, not OK in PRG **SE:** Photosens, xerostomia, dizziness, constipation, confusion, fluctuating mood w/ chronic use **Interactions:** CYP 3A enzyme inducer; do not use w/ Rx antidepressants(especially MAOI); ↓ cyclosporine efficacy (may cause rejection), digoxin (may ↑ CHF), protease inhib, theophylline, OCP; potency varies between products/batches

Valerian (*Valeriana officinalis*) **Uses:** Anxiolytic, sedative, restlessness, dysmenorrhea **Efficacy:** Probably effective sedative (reduces sleep latency) **Dose:** 2–3 g in extract PO daily-bid added to 2/3 cup boiling H_2O, tincture 15–20 drops in H_2O, oral 400–900 mg hs (combined w/ OTC sleep product Alluna) **W/P:** Hepatotoxicity with long-term use **SE:** Sedation, hangover effect, HA, cardiac disturbances, GI upset **Interactions:** Caution w/ other sedating agents (e.g., alcohol, or prescription sedatives); may cause drowsiness w/ impaired Fxn

Yohimbine (*Pausinystalia yohimbe*) Yocon, Yohimex **Uses:** Improve sexual vigor, Rx ED **Efficacy:** Variable **Dose:** 1 tab = 5.4 mg PO tid (use w/ physician supervision) **W/P:** Do not use w/ renal/hepatic Dz; may exacerbate schizophrenia/mania (if pt predisposed). α_2-Adrenergic antagonist (↓ BP, Abd distress, weakness w/ high doses), OD can be fatal; salivation, dilated pupils, arrhythmias **SE:** Anxiety, tremors, dizziness, ↑ BP, ↑ HR **Interactions:** Do not use w/ antidepressants (e.g., MAOIs or similar agents)

(Adapted from Haist SA and Robbins JB: *Internal Medicine on Call*, 4th ed., 2005 McGraw-Hill; and the FDA @ http://dietarysupplements.nlm.nih.gov/dietary/index.jsp (Accessed July 2011)).

Unsafe Herbs With Known Toxicity

Agent	Toxicities
Aconite	Salivation, N/V, blurred vision, cardiac arrhythmias
Aristolochic acid	Nephrotox
Calamus	Possible carcinogenicity
Chaparral	Hepatotox, possible carcinogenicity, nephrotox
"Chinese herbal mixtures"	May contain ma huang or other dangerous herbs
Coltsfoot	Hepatotox, possibly carcinogenic
Comfrey	Hepatotox, carcinogenic
Ephedra/Ma huang	Adverse cardiac events, stroke, Sz
Juniper	High allergy potential, D, Sz, nephrotox
Kava kava	Hepatotox
Licorice	Chronic daily amounts (> 30 g/mo) can result in increased K^+, Na/fluid retention w/HTN, myoglobinuria, hyporeflexia
Life root	Hepatotox, liver CA
Ma huang/ephedra	Adverse cardiac events, stroke, Sz
Pokeweed	GI cramping, N/D/V, labored breathing, increased BP, Sz
Sassafras	V, stupor, hallucinations, dermatitis, abortion, hypothermia, liver CA
Usnic acid	Hepatotox
Yohimbine	Hypotension, Abd distress, CNS stimulation (mania/& psychosis in predisposed individuals)

Source: Haist SA, Robbins JB. *Internal Medicine On Call.* 4th ed. New York, NY: McGraw-Hill; 2005.

Tables

TABLE 1
Local Anesthetic Comparison Chart for Commonly Used Injectable Agents

Agent	Proprietary Names	Onset	Duration	Maximum Dose	
				mg/kg	Volume in 70-kg Adult[a]
Bupivacaine	Marcaine	7–30 min	5–7 h	3	70 mL of 0.25% solution
Lidocaine	Xylocaine, Anestacon	5–30 min	2 h	4	28 mL of 1% solution
Lidocaine with epinephrine (1:200,000)		5–30 min	2–3 h	7	50 mL of 1% solution
Mepivacaine	Carbocaine	5–30 min	2–3 h	7	50 mL of 1% solution
Procaine	Novocaine	Rapid	30 min–1 h	10–15	70–105 mL of 1% solution

[a] To calculate the maximum dose if not a 70-kg adult, use the fact that a 1% solution has 10 mg/mL drug.

282

TABLE 2
Comparison of Systemic Steroids (See also page 244)

Drug	Relative Equivalent Dose (mg)	Relative Mineralo-corticoid Activity	Duration (h)	Route
Betamethasone	0.75	0	36–72	PO, IM
Cortisone (Cortone)	25	2	8–12	PO, IM
Dexamethasone (Decadron)	0.75	0	36–72	PO, IV
Hydrocortisone (Solu-Cortef, Hydrocortone)	20	2	8–12	PO, IM, IV
Methylprednisolone acetate (Depo-Medrol)	4	0	36–72	PO, IM, IV
Methylprednisolone succinate (Solu-Medrol)	4	0	8–12	PO, IM, IV
Prednisone (Deltasone)	5	1	12–36	PO
Prednisolone (Delta-Cortef)	5	1	12–36	PO, IM, IV

TABLE 3
Topical Steroid Preparations (See also page 246)

Agent	Common Trade Names	Potency	Apply
Alclometasone dipropionate	Aclovate, cream, oint 0.05%	Low	bid/tid
Amcinonide	Cyclocort, cream, lotion, oint 0.1%	High	bid/tid
Betamethasone			
Betamethasone valerate	Valisone cream, lotion 0.01%	Low	q day/bid
Betamethasone valerate	Valisone cream 0.01, 0.1%, oint, lotion 0.1%	Intermediate	q day/bid
Betamethasone dipropionate	Diprosone cream 0.05%	High	q day/bid
Betamethasone dipropionate	Diprosone aerosol 0.1%	Ultrahigh	q day/bid
Betamethasone dipropionate, augmented	Diprolene oint, gel 0.05%	Ultrahigh	q day/bid
Clobetasol propionate	Temovate cream, gel, oint, scalp, soln 0.05%	Ultrahigh	bid (2 wk max)
Clocortolone pivalate	Cloderm cream 0.1%	Intermediate	q day–qid
Desonide	DesOwen, cream, oint, lotion 0.05%	Low	bid–qid
Desoximetasone			
Desoximetasone 0.05%	Topicort LP cream, gel 0.05%	Intermediate	q day–qid
Desoximetasone 0.25%	Topicort cream, oint	High	q day–bid
Dexamethasone base	Aeroseb-Dex aerosol 0.01%	Low	bid–qid
	Decadron cream 0.1%	Ultrahigh	bid/qid
Diflorasone diacetate	Psorcon cream, oint 0.05%		
Fluocinolone			
Fluocinolone acetonide 0.01%	Synalar cream, soln 0.01%	Low	bid/tid
Fluocinolone acetonide 0.025%	Synalar oint, cream 0.025%	Intermediate	bid/tid

284

Fluocinolone acetonide 0.2%	Synalar-HP cream 0.2%	High	bid/tid
Fluocinonide 0.05%	Lidex, anhydrous cream, gel, oint, soln 0.05%	High	bid/tid
Flurandrenolide	Lidex-E aqueous cream 0.05%		bid/tid
	Cordran cream, oint 0.025% cream, lotion, oint 0.05% tape, 4 mcg/cm²	Intermediate Intermediate Intermediate	bid/tid bid/tid q day
Fluticasone propionate	Cutivate cream 0.05%, oint 0.005%	Intermediate	bid
Halobetasol	Ultravate cream, oint 0.05%	Very high	bid
Halcinonide	Halog cream 0.025%, emollient base 0.1% cream, oint, soln 0.1%	High	q day/tid
Hydrocortisone Hydrocortisone	Cortizone, Caldecort, Hycort, Hytone, etc—aerosol 1%, cream 0.5, 1, 2.5%, gel 0.5%, oint 0.5, 1, 2.5%, lotion 0.5, 1, 2.5%, paste 0.5% soln 1%	Low	tid/qid
Hydrocortisone acetate	Corticaine cream, oint 0.5, 1%	Low	tid/qid
Hydrocortisone butyrate	Locoid oint, soln 0.1%	Intermediate	bid/tid
Hydrocortisone valerate	Westcort cream, oint 0.2%	Intermediate	bid/tid

(Continued)

TABLE 3 (continued)
Topical Steroid Preparations (See also page 246)

Agent	Common Trade Names	Potency	Apply
Mometasone furoate	Elocon 0.1% cream, oint, lotion	Intermediate	q day
Prednicarbate	Dermatop 0.1% cream	Intermediate	bid
Triamcinolone			
Triamcinolone acetonide 0.025%	Aristocort, Kenalog cream, oint, lotion 0.025%	Low	tid/qid
Triamcinolone acetonide 0.1%	Aristocort, Kenalog cream, oint, lotion 0.1%	Intermediate	tid/qid
Triamcinolone acetonide 0.5%	Aerosol 0.2-mg/2-sec spray Aristocort, Kenalog cream, oint 0.5%	High	tid/qid

TABLE 4
Comparison of Insulins (See also page 153)

Type of Insulin	Onset (h)	Peak (h)	Duration (h)
Ultra Rapid			
Apidra (glulisine)	<0.25	0.5–1.5	3–4
Humalog (lispro)	<0.25	0.5–1.5	3–4
NovoLog (aspart)	<0.25	0.5–1.5	3–4
Rapid (regular insulin)			
Humulin R, Novolin R	0.5–1	2–3	4–6
Intermediate			
Humulin N, Novolin L	1–4	6–10	10–16
Prolonged			
Lantus (insulin glargine)	1–4	No peak	24
Levemir (insulin detemir)	1–4	No peak	24
Combination Insulins			
Humalog Mix 75/25 (lispro protamine/ lispro)	<0.25	Dual	Up to 10–6
Humalog Mix 50/50 (lispro protamine/ lispro)	<0.25	Dual	Up to 10–16
NovoLog Mix 70/30 (aspart protamine/ aspart)	<0.25	Dual	Up to 10–16
Humulin 70/30, Novolin 70/30 (NPH/regular)	0.5–1	Dual	Up to 10–16

Note: Do not confuse Humalog, NovoLog, Humalog Mix, and NovoLog Mix with each other or with other agents as serious medication errors can result.

TABLE 5
Oral Contraceptives (See also page 206)

[Note: 21 = 21 Active pills; 24 = 24 Active pills; Standard for most products is 28 [unless specified] = 21 Active pills + 7 Placebo[a]]

Drug (Manufacturer)	Estrogen (mcg)	Progestin (mg)	Content of Additional Pills (d = days)
Monophasics			
Alesse 21, 28 (Wyeth)	Ethinyl estradiol (20)	Levonorgestrel (0.1)	
Apri (Barr)	Ethinyl estradiol (30)	Desogestrel (0.15)	
Aviane (Barr)	Ethinyl estradiol (20)	Levonorgestrel (0.1)	
Balziva (Barr)	Ethinyl estradiol (35)	Norethindrone (0.4)	
Beyaz (Bayer) f(super)	Ethinyl estradiol (20)	Drospirenone (3.0)	0.451 mg levomefolate in all including 7 placebo
Brevicon (Watson)	Ethinyl estradiol (35)	Norethindrone (0.5)	
Cryselle (Barr)	Ethinyl estradiol (30)	Norgestrel (0.3)	
Demulen 1/35 21, 28 (Pfizer)	Ethinyl estradiol (35)	Ethynodiol diacetate (1)	
Demulen 1/50 21, 28 (Pfizer)	Ethinyl estradiol (50)	Ethynodiol diacetate (1)	
Desogen (Organon)	Ethinyl estradiol (30)	Desogestrel (0.15)	
Emoquette (Qualitest/Endo)	Ethinyl estradiol (30)	Desogestrel (0.15)	
Femcon Fe (Warner-Chilcott)	Ethinyl estradiol (35)	Norethindrone (0.4)	75 mg Fe × 7 d
Junel Fe 1/20, 21, 28 (Barr)	Ethinyl estradiol (20)	Norethindrone acetate (1)	75 mg Fe × 7 d
Junel Fe 1.5/30, 28 (Barr)	Ethinyl estradiol (30)	Norethindrone acetate (1.5)	75 mg Fe × 7 d
Kariva (Barr)	Ethinyl estradiol (20, 0, 10)	Desogestrel (0.15)	2 inert; 2 ethinyl estradiol (10)
Kelnor 1/35 (Barr)	Ethinyl estradiol (35)	Ethynodiol Diacetate (1)	
Lessina (Barr)	Ethinyl estradiol (20)	Levonorgestrel (0.1)	

288

Brand	Estrogen	Progestin	Notes
Levlen 21, 28 (Bayer)	Ethinyl estradiol [30]	Levonorgestrel [0.15]	
Levlite (Bayer)	Ethinyl estradiol [20]	Levonorgestrel [0.1]	
Levora (Watson)	Ethinyl estradiol [30]	Levonorgestrel [0.15]	
Loestrin 24 Fe (Warner-Chilcott)	Ethinyl estradiol [20]	Norethindrone (1)	75 mg Fe × 4 d
Loestrin Fe 1.5/30 21, 28 (Warner-Chilcott)	Ethinyl estradiol [30]	Norethindrone acetate (1.5)	75 mg Fe × 7 d in 28 d
Loestrin Fe 1/20 21, 28 (Warner-Chilcott)	Ethinyl estradiol [20]	Norethindrone acetate (1)	75 mg Fe × 7 d in 28 d
Loestrin 1/20 21 (Warner-Chilcott)	Ethinyl estradiol [20]	Norethindrone acetate (1)	
Loestrin 1.5/30 21 (Warner-Chilcott)	Ethinyl estradiol [30]	Norethindrone acetate (1.5)	
Lo/Ovral 21, 28 (Wyeth)	Ethinyl estradiol [30]	Norgestrel [0.3]	
Low-Ogestrel (Watson)	Ethinyl estradiol [30]	Norgestrel [0.3]	
Lutera (Watson)	Ethinyl estradiol [20]	Levonorgestrel [0.1]	
Microgestin 1/20 21, 28 (Watson)	Ethinyl estradiol [20]	Norethindrone acetate (1)	
Microgestin 1.5/30 21, 28 (Watson)	Ethinyl estradiol [30]	Norethindrone acetate (1.5)	
Microgestin Fe 1/20 21, 28 (Watson)	Ethinyl estradiol [20]	Norethindrone acetate (1)	75 mg Fe × 7 d in 28 d
Microgestin Fe 1.5/30 21, 28 (Watson)	Ethinyl estradiol [30]	Norethindrone acetate (1.5)	75 mg Fe × 7 d in 28 d
Mircette (Organon)	Ethinyl estradiol [20, 0, 10]	Desogestrel (0.15)	2 inert; 2 ethinyl estradiol (10)
Modicon (Ortho-McNeil)	Ethinyl estradiol [35]	Norethindrone (0.5)	
MonoNessa (Watson)	Ethinyl estradiol [35]	Norgestimate (0.25)	
Necon 0.5/35 (Watson)	Mestranol [35]	Norethindrone (0.5)	
Necon 1/50 (Watson)	Mestranol [50]	Norethindrone (1)	

(Continued)

TABLE 5 (continued)
Oral Contraceptives (See also page 206)

[Note: 21 = 21 Active pills; 24 = 24 Active pills; Standard for most products is 28 [unless specified] = 21 Active pills + 7 Placebo^q]

Drug (Manufacturer)	Estrogen (mcg)	Progestin (mg)	Content of Additional Pills (d = days)
Monophasics			
Necon 1/35 (Watson)	Ethinyl estradiol (35)	Norethindrone (0.5)	
Necon 1/35 (Watson)	Ethinyl estradiol (35)	Norethindrone (1)	
Nordette 21, 28 (King)	Ethinyl estradiol (30)	Levonorgestrel (0.15)	
Norinyl 1/35 (Watson)	Ethinyl estradiol (35)	Norethindrone (1)	
Norinyl 1/50 (Watson)	Mestranol (50)	Norethindrone (1)	
Nortrel 0.5/35 (Barr)	Ethinyl estradiol (35)	Norethindrone (0.5)	
Nortrel 1/35 21, 28 (Barr)	Ethinyl estradiol (35)	Norethindrone (1)	
Ocella (Barr)	Ethinyl estradiol (30)	Drospirenone (3)	
Ogestrel 0.5/50 (Watson)	Ethinyl estradiol (50)	Norgestrel (0.5)	
Ortho-Cept (Ortho-McNeil)	Ethinyl estradiol (30)	Desogestrel (0.15)	
Ortho-Cyclen (Ortho-McNeil)	Ethinyl estradiol (35)	Norgestimate (0.25)	
Ortho-Novum 1/35 (Ortho-McNeil)	Ethinyl estradiol (35)	Norethindrone (1)	
Ortho-Novum 1/50 2 (Ortho-McNeil)	Mestranol (50)	Norethindrone (1)	
Ovcon 35 21, 28 (Warner-Chilcott)	Ethinyl estradiol (35)	Norethindrone (0.4)	
Ovcon 35 FE (Warner-Chilcott)	Ethinyl estradiol (35)	Norethindrone (0.4)	75 mg Fe × 7 d in 28 d
Ovcon 50 (Warner-Chilcott)	Ethinyl estradiol (50)	Norethindrone (1)	
Ovral 21, 28 (Wyeth-Ayerst)	Ethinyl estradiol (50)	Norgestrel (0.5)	

Drug	Estrogen (mg)	Progestin (mcg)	Content of Additional Pills
Portia (Barr)	Ethinyl estradiol (30)	Levonorgestrel (0.15)	
Reclipsen (Watson)	Ethinyl estradiol (30)	Desogestrel (0.15)	
Safyral (Bayer) f(super)	Ethinyl estradiol (30)	Drospirenone (3.0)	0.451 mg levomefolate in all including 7 placebo
Solia (Prasco)	Ethinyl estradiol (30)	Desogestrel (0.15)	
Sprintec (Barr)	Ethinyl estradiol (35)	Norgestimate (0.25)	
Sronyx (Watson)	Ethinyl estradiol (20)	Levonorgestrel (0.1)	
Yasmin (Bayer)[e] (generics Ocella, Syeda, Zarah)	Ethinyl estradiol (30)	Drospirenone (3.0)	
Yaz (Bayer) 28 day[b,d,e] (generics Gianvi, Loryna)	Ethinyl estradiol (20)	Drospirenone (3.0)	4 inert in 28 d
Zenchent (Watson)	Ethinyl estradiol (35)	Ethynodiol diacetate (0.4)	
Zovia 1/35 (Watson)	Ethinyl estradiol (35)	Ethynodiol diacetate (1)	

Multiphasics

Drug	Estrogen (mg)	Progestin (mcg)	Content of Additional Pills
Aranelle (Barr)	Ethinyl estradiol (35)	Norethindrone (0.5, 1, 0.5)	
Cesia (Prasco)	Ethinyl estradiol (25)	Desogestrel (0.1, 0.125, 0.15)	
Cyclessa (Organon)	Ethinyl estradiol (25)	Desogestrel (0.1, 0.125, 0.15)	
Enpresse (Barr)	Ethinyl estradiol (30, 40, 30)	Levonorgestrel (0.05, 0.075, 0.125)	
Estrostep (Warner-Chilcott)[b]	Ethinyl estradiol (20, 30, 35)	Norethindrone acetate (1)	
Estrostep Fe (Warner-Chilcott)[b]	Ethinyl estradiol (20, 30, 35)	Norethindrone acetate (1)	75 mg Fe × 7 d in 28 d

(Continued)

TABLE 5 (continued)

Oral Contraceptives (See also page 206)

(Note: 21 = 21 Active pills; 24 = 24 Active pills; Standard for most products is 28 [unless specified] = 21 Active pills + 7 Placebo[q])

Drug	Estrogen (mg)	Progestin (mcg)	Content of Additional Pills
Generess Fe (Watson) (Note: Chewable tablets)	Ethinyl estradiol (25)	Norethindrone acetate (0.8)	75 mg Fe × 4 d
Leena (Watson)	Ethinyl estradiol (35)	Norethindrone (0.5, 1, 0.5)	
Lessina (Watson)	Ethinyl estradiol (20)	Levonorgestrel (0.1)	
Lutera (Watson)	Ethinyl estradiol (20)	Levonorgestrel (0.1)	
Natazia (Bayer) (see footnote g)			
Necon 10/11 21, 28 (Watson)	Ethinyl estradiol (35)	Norethindrone (0.5, 1)	
Necon 7/7/7 (Watson)	Ethinyl estradiol (35)	Norethindrone (0.5, 0.75, 1)	
Nortrel 7/7/7 (Barr)	Ethinyl estradiol (35)	Norethindrone (0.5, 0.75, 1)	
Orsythia (Qualitest)	Ethinyl estradiol (20)	Levonorgestrel (0.1)	
Ortho-Novum 10/11 (Ortho-McNeil)	Ethinyl estradiol (35)	Norethindrone (0.5, 1)	
Ortho-Novum 7/7/7 21 [Ortho-McNeil]	Ethinyl estradiol (35, 35, 35)	Norethindrone (0.5, 0.75, 1)	
Ortho Tri-Cyclen 21, 28 [Ortho-McNeil]	Ethinyl estradiol (25)	Norgestimate (0.18, 0.215, 0.25)	
Ortho Tri-Cyclen Lo 21, 28 (Ortho-McNeil)	Ethinyl estradiol (35, 35, 35)	Norgestimate (0.18, 0.215, 0.25)	
Previfem (Teva)	Ethinyl estradiol (35)	Norgestimate (0.25)	
Tilia Fe (Watson)	Ethinyl estradiol (20, 30, 35)	Norethindrone (1)	75 mg Fe × 7 d in 28 d

Multiphasics

292

Drug	Estrogen (mg)	Progestin (mcg)	Content of Additional Pills
Tri-Legest (Barr)	Ethinyl estradiol (20, 30, 35)	Norethindrone (1)	
Tri-Legest Fe (Barr)	Ethinyl estradiol (20, 30, 35)	Norethindrone (1)	75 mg Fe × 7 d in 28 d
Tri-Levlen (Bayer)	Ethinyl estradiol (30, 40, 30)	Levonorgestrel (0.05, 0.075, 0.125)	
Tri-Nessa (Watson)	Ethinyl estradiol (35)	Norgestimate (0.18, 0.215, 0.25)	
Tri-Norinyl 21, 28 (Watson)	Ethinyl estradiol (35, 35, 35)	Norethindrone (0.5, 1, 0.5)	
Tri-Previfem (Teva)	Ethinyl estradiol (35)	Norgestimate (0.18, 0.215, 0.25)	

Oral Contraceptives (See also page 206)

(Note: 21 = 21 Active pills; 24 = 24 Active pills; Standard for most products is 28 [unless specified] = 21 Active pills + 7 Placebo²) Fe = iron supplement

Drug	Estrogen (mg)	Progestin (mcg)	Content of Additional Pills

Multiphasics

Drug	Estrogen (mg)	Progestin (mcg)	Content of Additional Pills
Tri-Sprintec (Barr)	Ethinyl estradiol (35)	Norgestimate (0.18, 0.215, 0.25)	
Triphasil 21, 28 (Wyeth)	Ethinyl estradiol (30, 40, 30)	Levonorgestrel (0.05, 0.075, 0.125)	
Trivora 28 (Watson)	Ethinyl estradiol (30, 40, 30)	Levonorgestrel (0.05, 0.075, 0.125)	
Velivet (Barr)	Ethinyl estradiol (25)	Desogestrel (0.1, 0.125, 0.15)	

Drug	Estrogen (mg)	Progestin (mcg)	Content of Additional Pills

Progestin Only (aka "mini-pills")

Drug	Estrogen (mg)	Progestin (mcg)	Content of Additional Pills
Camila (Barr)	None	Norethindrone (0.35)	
Errin (Barr)	None	Norethindrone (0.35)	

(Continued)

TABLE 5 (continued)
Oral Contraceptives (See also page 206)

(Note: 21 = 21 Active pills; 24 = 24 Active pills; Standard for most products is 28 [unless specified] = 21 Active pills + 7 Placebo[a])

Drug	Estrogen (mg)	Progestin (mcg)	Content of Additional Pills

Progestin Only (aka "mini-pills")

Drug	Estrogen (mg)	Progestin (mcg)	Content of Additional Pills
Jolivette 28 (Watson)	None	Norethindrone (0.35)	
Micronor (Ortho-McNeil)	None	Norethindrone (0.35)	
Nor-QD (Watson)	None	Norethindrone (0.35)	
Nora-BE (Ortho-McNeil)	None	Norethindrone (0.35)	

Extended-Cycle Combination (aka COCP [combined oral contraceptive pills])

Drug	Estrogen (mg)	Progestin (mcg)	Content of Additional Pills
Jolessa (Barr) 91-d pack	Ethinyl estradiol (30)	Levonorgestrel (0.15)	7 inert
Lybrel (Wyeth) 28-d pack[c]	Ethinyl estradiol (20)	Levonorgestrel (0.09)	None
Quasense (Watson)	Ethinyl estradiol (30)	Levonorgestrel (0.15)	7 inert

294

| Seasonique (Duramed) 91-d pack | Ethinyl estradiol (30) | Levonorgestrel (0.15) | 7 (10 mcg ethinyl estradiol) |
| Seasonale (Duramed) 91-d pack | Ethinyl estradiol (30) | Levonorgestrel (0.15) | 7 inert |

Source: The Medical Letter, Volume 49 (Issue 1266) 2007, manufacturers insert and web sites as of August 29, 2009.

[a] The designations 21 and 28 refer to number of days in regimen available.

[b] Also approved for acne.

[c] First FDA-approved pill for 365 d dosing.

[d] Approved for premenstrual dysphoric disorder (PMDD) in women who use contraception for birth control.

[e] Avoid in patients with hyperkalemia risk.

[f] Raises folate levels to help decrease neural tube defect risk with eventual pregnancy.

[g] First "four phasic" OCP. Varies doses of estrogen (estradiol valerate) with progestin (dienogest) throughout cycle with 2 inert pills at end of cycle.

TABLE 6
Oral Potassium Supplements

Brand Name	Salt	Form	mEq Potassium/ Dosing Unit
Glu-K	Gluconate	Tablet	2 mEq/tablet
Kaon elixir	Gluconate	Liquid	20 mEq/15 mL
Kaon-Cl 10	KCl	Tablet, SR	10 mEq/tablet
Kaon-Cl 20%	KCl	Liquid	40 mEq/15 mL
K-Dur 20	KCl	Tablet, SR	20 mEq/tablet
KayCiel	KCl	Liquid	20 mEq/15 mL
K-Lor	KCl	Powder	20 mEq/packet
K-lyte/Cl	KCl/bicarbonate	Effervescent tablet	25 mEq/tablet
Klorvess	KCl/bicarbonate	Effervescent tablet	20 mEq/tablet
Klotrix	KCl	Tablet, SR	10 mEq/tablet
K-Lyte	Bicarbonate/ citrate	Effervescent tablet	25 mEq/tablet
Klor-Con/EF	Bicarbonate/ citrate	Effervescent tablet	25 mEq/tablet
K-Tab	KCl	Tablet, SR	10 mEq/tablet
Micro-K	KCl	Capsule, SR	8 mEq/capsule
Potassium Chloride 10%	KCl	Liquid	20 mEq/15 mL
Potassium Chloride 20%	KCl	Liquid	40 mEq/15 mL
Slow-K	KCl	Tablet, SR	8 mEq/tablet
Tri-K	Acetate/ bicarbonate and citrate	Liquid	45 mEq/15 mL
Twin-K	Citrate/gluconate	Liquid	20 mEq/5 mL

SR = sustained release.

Note: Alcohol and sugar content vary between preparations.

TABLE 7
Tetanus Prophylaxis (See also page 255)

History of Absorbed Tetanus Toxoid Immunization	Clean, Minor Wounds		All Other Wounds[a]	
	Td[b]	TIG[c]	Td[d]	TIG[c]
Unknown or <3 doses	Yes	No	Yes	Yes
=3 doses	No[e]	No	No[f]	No

[a] Such as, but not limited to, wounds contaminated with dirt, feces, soil, saliva, etc; puncture wounds; avulsions; and wounds resulting from missiles, crushing, burns, and frostbite.

[b] Td = tetanus-diphtheria toxoid (adult type), 0.5 mL IM.
- For children <7 y, DPT (DT, if pertussis vaccine is contraindicated) is preferred to tetanus toxoid alone.
- For persons >7 y, Td is preferred to tetanus toxoid alone.
- DT = diphtheria-tetanus toxoid (pediatric), used for those who cannot receive pertussis.

[c] TIG = tetanus immune globulin, 250 units IM.

[d] If only 3 doses of fluid toxoid have been received, then a fourth dose of toxoid, preferably an adsorbed toxoid, should be given.

[e] Yes, if >10 y since last dose.

[f] Yes, if >5 y since last dose.

Source: Guidelines from the Centers for Disease Control and Prevention and reported in *MMWR* (*MMWR*, December 1, 2006; 55(RR-15):1-48).

TABLE 8
Oral Anticoagulant Standards of Practice (See also warfarin page 272)

Thromboembolic Disorder	INR	Duration
Deep Venous Thrombosis & Pulmonary Embolism		
Treatment of single episode		
Transient risk factor	2–3	3 mo
Idiopathic[a]	2–3	long-term
Recurrent systemic embolism	2–3	long-term
Prevention of Systemic Embolism		
Atrial fibrillation (AF)[b]	2–3	long-term
AF: cardioversion	2–3	3 wk prior; 4 wk post sinus rhythm
Mitral valvular heart dx[c]	2–3	long-term
Cardiomyopathy (usually ASA)[d]	2–3	long-term
Acute Myocardial Infarction		
High risk[e]	2–3 + low-dose aspirin	long-term
All other infarcts (usually ASA)[f]		

TABLE 8
Oral Anticoagulant Standards of Practice (See also warfarin page 272) (continued)

Thromboembolic Disorder	INR	Duration
Prosthetic Valves		
Bioprosthetic heart valves		
Mitral position	2–3	3 mo
Aortic position[g]	2–3	3 mo
Bileaflet mechanical valves in aortic position[h]	2–3	long-term
Other mechanical prosthetic valves[i]	2.5–3.5	long-term

[a] 3 mo if mod or high risk of bleeding or distal DVT; if low risk of bleeding, then long-term for proximal DVT/PE.

[b] Paroxysmal AF or ≥2 risk factors (age >75, hx, BP, DM, mod-severe LV dysfunction or CHF), then warfarin; 1 risk factor warfarin or 75–325 mg ASA; 0 risk factors ASA.

[c] Mitral valve Dz: rheumatic if hx systemic embolism, or AF or LA thrombus or LA >55 mm; MVP: only if AF, systemic embolism or TIAs on ASA; mitral valve calcification: warfarin if AF or recurrent embolism on ASA; aortic valve w/ calcification: warfarin not recommended.

[d] In adults only ASA; only indication for anticoagulation cardiomyopathy in children, to begin no later than their activation on transplant list.

[e] High risk = large anterior MI, significant CHF, intracardiac thrombus visible on TE, AF, and hx of a thromboembolic event.

[f] If meticulous INR monitoring and highly skilled dose titration are expected and widely accessible, then INR 3.5 (3.0–4.0) w/o ASA or 2.5 (2.0–3.0) w ASA long-term (4 years).

[g] Usually ASA 50–100 mg; warfarin if hx embolism, LA thrombus, AF, low EF, hypercoagulable state, 3 mo, or until thrombus resolves.

[h] Target INR 2.5–3.5 if AF, large anterior MI, LA enlargement, hypercoagulable state, or low EF.

[i] Add ASA 50–100 mg if high risk (AF, hypercoagulable state, low EF, or hx of ASCVD).

Source: Antithrombotic and thrombolytic therapy: American College of Chest Physicians Evidence-Based Clinical Practice Guidelines (8th Edition). *Chest.* 2008;133(6 suppl):110S–112S.

TABLE 9
Antiarrhythmics: Vaughn Williams Classification

Class I: Sodium Channel Blockade

A. **Class Ia:** Lengthens duration of action potential ($\uparrow$ the refractory period in atrial and ventricular muscle, in SA and AV conduction systems, and Purkinje fibers)
 1. Amiodarone (also classes II, III, IV)
 2. Disopyramide (Norpace)
 3. Imipramine (MAO inhibitor)
 4. Procainamide (Pronestyl)
 5. Quinidine
B. **Class Ib:** No effect on action potential
 1. Lidocaine (Xylocaine)
 2. Mexiletine (Mexitil)
 3. Phenytoin (Dilantin)
 4. Tocainide (Tonocard)
C. **Class Ic:** Greater sodium current depression (blocks the fast inward Na$^+$ current in heart muscle and Purkinje fibers, and slows the rate of $\uparrow$ of phase 0 of the action potential)
 1. Flecainide (Tambocor)
 2. Propafenone

Class II: β-Blocker

D. Amiodarone (also classes Ia, III, IV)
E. Esmolol (Brevibloc)
F. Sotalol (also class III)

Class III: Prolong Refractory Period via Action Potential

G. Amiodarone (also classes Ia, II, IV)
H. Sotalol

Class IV: Calcium Channel Blocker

I. Amiodarone (also classes Ia, II, III)
J. Diltiazem (Cardizem)
K. Verapamil (Calan)

TABLE 10
Cytochrome P-450 Isoenzymes and Common Drugs
They Metabolize, Inhibit, and Induce[a]

CYP1A2

Substrates:	Acetaminophen, caffeine, cyclobenzaprine, clozapine, imipramine, mexiletine, naproxen, theophylline, propranolol
Inhibitors:	Cimetidine, most fluoroquinolone antibiotics, fluvoxamine, verapamil
Inducers:	Tobacco smoking, charcoal-broiled foods, cruciferous vegetables, omeprazole

CYP2C9

Substrates:	Most NSAIDs (including COX-2), glipizide, irbesartan, losartan, phenytoin, warfarin
Inhibitors:	Amiodarone, fluconazole, ketoconazole, metronidazole
Inducers:	Barbiturates, rifampin

CYP2C19

Substrates:	Diazepam, amitriptyline, lansoprazole, omeprazole, phenytoin, pantoprazole, rabeprazole, clopidogrel
Inhibitors:	Omeprazole, lansoprazole, isoniazid, ketoconazole, fluoxetine, fluvoxamine
Inducers:	Barbiturates, rifampin

CYP2D6

Substrates:	**Antidepressants:** Most tricyclic antidepressants, clomipramine, fluoxetine, paroxetine, venlafaxine **Antipsychotics:** Aripiprazole, clozapine, haloperidol, risperidone, thioridazine **Beta blockers:** Carvedilol, metoprolol, propranolol, timolol **Opioids:** Codeine, hydrocodone, oxycodone, propoxyphene, tramadol **Others:** Amphetamine, dextromethorphan, duloxetine, encainide, flecainide, mexiletine, ondansetron, propafenone, selegiline, tamoxifen
Inhibitors:	Amiodarone, bupropion, cimetidine, clomipramine, doxepin, duloxetine, fluoxetine, haloperidol, methadone, paroxetine, quinidine, ritonavir
Inducers:	Unknown

(Continued)

TABLE 10
Cytochrome P-450 Isoenzymes and Common Drugs
They Metabolize, Inhibit, and Induce[a] (continued)

	CYP3A

Substrates:
Anticholinergics: Darifenacin, oxybutynin, solifenacin, tolterodine
Benzodiazepines: Alprazolam, diazepam, midazolam, triazolam
Ca channel blockers: Amlodipine, diltiazem, felodipine, nimodipine, nifedipine, nisoldipine, verapamil
Chemotherapy: Cyclophosphamide, erlotinib, ifosfamide, paclitaxel, tamoxifen, vinblastine, vincristine
HIV protease inhibitors: Amprenavir, atazanavir, indinavir, nelfinavir, ritonavir, saquinavir
HMG-CoA reductase inhibitors: Atorvastatin, lovastatin, simvastatin
Immunosuppressive agents: Cyclosporine, tacrolimus
Macrolide-type antibiotics: Clarithromycin, erythromycin, telithromycin, troleandomycin
Opioids: Alfentanil, cocaine, fentanyl, methadone, sufentanil
Steroids: Budesonide, cortisol, $17\text{-}\beta\text{-estradiol}$, progesterone
Others: Acetaminophen, amiodarone, carbamazepine, delavirdine, efavirenz, nevirapine, quinidine, repaglinide, sildenafil, tadalafil, trazodone, vardenafil

Inhibitors:
Amiodarone, amprenavir, aprepitant, atazanavir, ciprofloxacin, cisapride, clarithromycin, diltiazem, erythromycin, fluconazole, fluvoxamine, grapefruit juice (in high ingestion), indinavir, itraconazole, ketoconazole, nefazodone, nelfinavir, norfloxacin, ritonavir, saquinavir, telithromycin, troleandomycin, verapamil, voriconazole

Inducers:
Carbamazepine, efavirenz, glucocorticoids, modafinil, nevirapine, phenytoin, phenobarbital, rifabutin, rifapentine, rifampin, St. John's wort

---

[a] Increased or decreased (primarily hepatic cytochrome P-450) metabolism of medications may influence the effectiveness of drugs or result in significant drug-drug interactions. Understanding the common cytochrome P-450 isoforms (e.g., CYP2C9, CYP2D9, CYP2C19, CYP3A4) and common drugs that are metabolized by (aka "substrates"), inhibit, or induce activity of the isoform helps minimize significant drug interactions. CYP3A is involved in the metabolism of >50% of drugs metabolized by the liver.

Source: Katzung B (ed): Basic and Clinical Pharmacology, 11th ed. McGraw-Hill, New York, 2009; The Medical Letter, Volume 47, July 4, 2004; N Engl J Med 2005:352:2211-21.

TABLE 11
SSRIs/SNRIs/Triptans and Serotonin Syndrome

A life-threatening condition, when selective serotonin reuptake inhibitors (SSRIs) and 5-hydroxytryptamine receptor agonists (triptans) are used together. However, many other drugs have been implicated (see below). Signs and symptoms of serotonin syndrome include the following:

Restlessness, coma, N/V/D, hallucinations, loss of coordination, overactive reflexes, ↑ HR/temperature, rapid changes in BP, increased body temperature

Class	Drugs
Antidepressants	MAOIs, TCAs, SSRIs, SNRIs, mirtazapine, venlafaxine
CNS stimulants	Amphetamines, phentermine, methylphenidate, sibutramine
5-HT$_1$ agonists	Triptans
Illicit drugs	Cocaine, methylenedioxymethamphetamine (ecstasy), lysergic acid diethylamide (LSD)
Opioids	Tramadol, pethidine, oxycodone, morphine, meperidine
Others	Buspirone, chlorpheniramine, dextromethorphan, linezolid, lithium, selegiline, tryptophan, St. John's wort

Management includes removal of the precipitating drugs and supportive care. To control agitation, serotonin antagonists (cyproheptadine or methysergide) can be used. When symptoms are mild, discontinuation of the medication or medications and the control of agitation with benzodiazepines may be needed. Critically ill patients may require sedation and mechanical ventilation as well as control of hyperthermia. (Boyer EW, Shanon M. The serotonin syndrome. *N Engl J Med.* 2005;352(11):1112–1120.)

MOAI = monoamine oxidase inhibitor.
TCA = tricyclic antidepressant.
SNRI = serotonin-norepinephrine reuptake inhibitors.

TABLE 12
Multivitamins, Oral OTC

Composition of Selected Multivitamins and Multivitamins with Mineral and Trace Element Supplements. Listings Show Vitamin Content (Part 1) and Then the Mineral Trace Element and Other Components (Part 2) of Popular US Brands. Values Listed Are a Percentage of Daily Value.

Part 1. Vitamins

	Fat Soluble				Water Soluble								
	A	D	E	K	C	B$_1$	B$_2$	B$_3$	B$_6$	Folate	B$_{12}$	Biotin	B$_5$
Centrum[a]	70	100	100	31	150	100	100	100	100	125	100	10	100
Centrum Performance[a]	70	100	200	31	200	300	300	200	300	100	300	17	100
Centrum Silver[a]	50	125	167	38	150	100	100	100	150	125	417	10	100
Nature Made Multi Complete	50	250	167	100	300	100	100	100	100	100	100	10	100
Nature Made Multi Daily	60	100	100	0	100	100	100	100	100	100	100	0	100
Nature Made Multi Max	60	100	500	50	500	3333	2941	250	2500	100	833	17	500
Nature Made Multi 50+	60	100	200	13	200	200	200	100	200	100	417	10	100
One-A-Day 50 Plus	50	100	110	25	200	300	200	100	300	100	417	10	150
One-A-Day Essential	60	100	100	0	100	100	100	100	100	100	100	0	100

304

One-A-Day Maximum[b]	50	100	100	31	100	150	200	200	100	100	100	10	100
Therapeutic Vitamin	100	100	100	0	150	200	200	200	100	100	150	10	100
Theragran-M Advanced High Protein	100	200	100	35	150	200	200	300	100	100	200	10	100
Theragran-M Premier High Potency	70	200	100	31	200	267	235	200	125	100	150	10	100
Theragran-M Premier 50 Plus High Potency	70	200	100	13	125	200	176	300	125	100	500	12	150
Therapeutic Vitamin + Minerals[b]	100	200	100	0	200	100	100	100	100	100	100	10	100
Unicap M	100	100	100	0	100	100	100	100	100	100	100	0	100
Unicap Sr.	100	50	100	NA	100	80	82	80	110	100	50	0	100
Unicap T	100	100	100	0	833	667	588	500	300	100	300	0	250

(Continued)

TABLE 12 (continued)
Multivitamins, Oral OTC

Part 2. Minerals, trace elements, and other components

	Minerals						Trace Elements						Other
	Ca	P	Mg	Fe	Zn	I	Se	K	Mn	Cu	Cr	Mo	
Centrum[a]	20	11	25	100	73	100	79	2	115	45	29	60	Lutein, lycopene
Centrum Performance[a]	10	5	10	100	73	100	100	2	200	45	100	100	Gingko, ginseng
Centrum Silver[a]	22	11	13	0	73	100	79	2	115	45	38	60	Lutein, lycopene
Nature Made Multi Complete	16	NA	25	100	100	100	35	NA	200	100	100	100	
Nature Made Multi Daily	45	0	0	100	100	0	0	0	0	0	0	0	
Nature Made Multi Max	10	4	6	50	100	100	100	1	100	100	100	0	Lutein
Nature Made Multi 50+	20	5	25	0	100	100	71	2	100	100	100	33	Lutein
One-A-Day 50 Plus	12	0	25	0	150	100	150	1	200	100	150	120	Lutein
One-A-Day Essential	5	0	0	100	0	100	0	0	0	0	0	0	
One-A-Day Maximum	16	11	25	100	100	100	29	2	175	100	54	213	
Therapeutic Vitamin[b]	0	0	0	0	0	0	0	0	0	0	0	0	

Theragran-M Advanced High Potency	4	3	25	50	100	100	100	1	100	100	42	100	
Theragran-M Premier High Potency	17	11	25	100	100	100	286	2	100	175	100	107	Lutein, lycopene, coenzyme Q10
Theragran-M Premier 50 Plus High Potency	20	5	25	0	113	100	286	2	100	100	21	100	Lutein, coenzyme Q10
Therapeutic Vitamin + Minerals[b]	4	3	10	50	100	50	36	<1	100	100	42	100	
Unicap M	6	5	0	100	100	100	0	<1	50	100	0	0	
Unicap Sr.	10	8	8	56	100	100	0	<1	50	100	0	0	
Unicap T	0	0	0	100	100	100	14	<1	50	100	0	0	

Common multivitamins available without a prescription are listed. Most chain drug stores have generic versions of many of the multivitamin supplements listed above; thus, specific generic brands are not listed. Many specialty vitamin combinations are available, but not included in this list (examples are B vitamins plus C, supplements for a specific condition or organ, pediatric and infant formulations, and prenatal vitamins). Values are listed as percentages of the Daily Value (also known as %DV) based on Recommended Dietary Allowances of vitamins and minerals based on Dietary Reference Intakes (Food and Nutrition Board, Institute of Medicine, National Academy of Science). Additional information may be available for many other supplements from the NIH Dietary Supplements Labels Database http://dietarysupplements.nlm.nih.gov/dietary

[a] New formulation October 2007.

[b] Formulations may vary. Consult with pharmacy for current product.

[c] Common generic brands (when other than the store name itself) are: Osco Drug Central-Vite (Albertson's); Spectravite (CVS); Kirkland Signature Daily Multivitamin (Costco); Whole Source, PharmAssure (Rite Aid); Central-Vite (Safeway); Member's Mark (Sam's Club); Vitasmart (Kmart); Century (Target); A thru Z Select, Super Aytinal, Ultra Choice (Walgreens); Equate Complete or Spring Valley Sentury-Vite (Wal-Mart).

Vitamins: B_1 = thiamine; B_2 = riboflavin; B_3 = niacin; B_5 = pantothenic acid; B_6 = pyridoxine; B_{12} = cyanocobalamin. Elements: Ca = calcium; Cr = chromium; Cu = copper; Fe = iron; I = iodine; K = potassium; Mg = magnesium; Mn = manganese; Mo = molybdenum; P = phosphorus; Se = selenium; Zn = zinc; 0 = not applicable or not available.

Index

Page numbers followed by *t* indicate tables.

Generic (Trade)	Adult Dose (continued)
Magnesium sulfate	**VF/pulseless VT arrest with torsade de pointes:** 1–2 g IV push (2–4 mL 50% solution) in 10 mL D5W. If pulse present, then 1–2 g in 50–100 mL D5W over 5–60 min.
Metoprolol	**AMI:** 5 mg slow IV q5min, total 15 mg; then 50 mg PO, titrate to effect.
Morphine	**STEMI:** 2–4 mg slow IV (over 1–5 min), then give 2–8 mg IV q5–15min as needed. **NSTEMI:** 1–5 mg slow IV if Sxs unrelieved by nitrates or recur; use w/ caution; can be reversed with 0.4–2mg IV naloxone.
Nitroglycerin	IV bolus: 12.5–25 mcg (if no spray or SL dose given); Inf: Start 10 mcg/min, ↑ by 10 mcg/min q3–5min until desired effect; ceiling dose typically 200 mcg/min. SL: 0.3–0.4 mg; repeat q5min. Aerosol spray: Spray 0.5–1 s at 5-min intervals.
Nitroprusside	0.1 mcg/kg/min start, titrate (max dose 5–10 mcg/kg/min).
Procainamide	**Stable monomorphic VT, refractory reentry SVT, stable wide-complex tachycardia, AFib w/ WPW:** 20 mg/min IV until one of these: arrhythmia stopped, hypotension, QRS widens >50%, total 17 mg/kg; then maintenance infusion of 1–4 mg/min.
Propranolol (Inderal)	**SVT:** 0.5 to 1 mg IV given over 1 min; repeat PRN up to 0.1 mg/kg.
Reteplase, recombinant (Retavase)	10 Units IV bolus over 2 min; 30 min later, 10 units IV bolus over 2 min w/NS flush before and after each dose.
Sodium bicarbonate	**Cardiac Arrest w/ good ventilation, hyperkalemia, OD of TCAs, ASA, cocaine, diphenhydramine:** 1 mEq/kg IV bolus; repeat 1/2 dose q10min PRN. If rapidly available, use ABG to guide therapy (ABG results unreliable in cardiac arrest).
Sotalol (Betapace)	**SVT and ventricular arrhythmias:** 1–1.5 mg/kg IV over 5 min.
Streptokinase	**AMI:** 1.5 million units over 1 h.
Tirofiban (Aggrastat)	**ACS or PCI:** 0.4 mcg/kg/min IV for 30 min, then 0.1 mcg/kg/min for 18–24 h post PCI.
Verapamil	**Reentry SVT w/ narrow QRS:** 2.5–5 mg IV over 2 min (slower in older pts); repeat 5–10 mg, in 15–30 min PRN max of 20 mg; or 5 mg bolus q15min (max 30 mg).

ABG: arterial blood gas, QRS: electrocardiogram complex

Based on data from 2010 American Heart Association Guidelines for Cardiopulmonary Resuscitation and Emergency Cardiovascular Care. *Circulation.* 2010;122(18 suppl 3):S639. Available online at: http://circ.ahajournals.org/content/vol122/18_suppl_3/.

Generic (Trade)	Adult Dose
Clopidogrel	ACS: 300–600 mg PO loading dose, then 75 mg/d PO; full effect takes several days.
Diltiazem (Cardizem)	Acute rate control: 0.25 mg/kg (15–20 mg) over 2 min; 0.35 mg/kg (20–25 mg) over 2 min; maint inf 5–15 mg/h.
Dobutamine (Dobutrex)	2–20 mcg/kg/min.
Dopamine	2–20 mcg/kg/min: titrate to HR not >10% of baseline.
Epinephrine	ACS: 0.1–0.5 mcg/kg/min, titrate, ET 2–2.5 mg in 20 mL NS. Profound bradycardia/ hypotension: 2–10 mcg/min (1 mg in 250 mL D5W) IV/IO push, repeat q3–5 min (0.2 mg/kg max) if 1 mg dose fails. Inf: 0.1–0.5 mcg/kg/min, titrate. ET 2–2.5 mg in 20 mL NS. Profound bradycardia/ hypotension: 2–10 mcg/min (1 mg in 250 mL D5W). Allergic Rxn: 0.3–0.5 mg (0.3–0.5 mL of 1:1000 soln) SQ. Anaphylaxis: 0.3–0.5 (3–5 mL of 1:1000 soln) IV.
Eptifibatide (Integrilin)	ACS: 180 mcg/kg/min IV bolus over 1–2 min, then 2 mcg/kg/min, then repeat bolus in 10 min; continue infusion 18–24 h post PCI.
Esmolol (Brevibloc)	0.5 mg/kg (500 mcg/kg) over 1 min, then 0.05 mg/kg/min (50 mcg/kg/min) inf; if inadequate response after 5 min, repeat 0.5 mg/kg bolus, then titrate inf up to 0.2 mg/kg/ min (200 mcg/kg/min); maximum 0.3 mg/kg/min (300 mcg/kg/min).
Glucagon	β-Blocker or CCB overdose: 3–10 mg slow IV over 3–5 min; follow with inf of 3–5 mg/h; Hypoglycemia: 1 mg IV, IM, or SQ.
Heparin (unfractionated)	STEMI: Bolus 60 units/kg (max 4000 units); then 12 units/kg/h (max 1000 units/h) round to nearest 50 units; keep aPTT 1.5–2 X control 48 h or until angiography.
Ibutilide	SVT (AFib and AFlutter): ≥60 kg, 1 mg (10 mL) over 10 min, a second dose may be used: <60 kg 0.01 mg/kg over 10 min.
Labetalol (Trandate)	10 mg IV over 1–2 min; repeat or double dose q10min (150 mg max); or initial bolus, then 2–8 mg/min.
Lidocaine	Cardiac arrest from VF/VT refractory, VF: Initial: 1–1.5 mg/kg IV/IO, additional 0.5–0.75 mg/kg IV push, repeat in 5–10 min, max total 3 mg/kg, ET: 2–4 mg/kg as last resort. Reperfusing stable VT, wide complex tachycardia or ectopy: Doses of 0.3–0.75 mg/kg to 1–1.5 mg/kg may be used initially; repeat 0.5–0.75 mg/kg q5–10min; max dose 3 mg/kg.

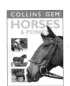

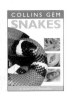

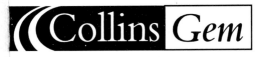

Collins Gem

FAMILY & PARTY GAMES

Trevor Bounford and
The Diagram Group

HarperCollins*Publishers*

HarperCollins*Publishers*
Westerhill Road, Bishopbriggs, Glasgow G64 2QT

A Diagram book first created by Diagram Visual Information
Limited of 195 Kentish Town Road, London NW5 2JU

Additional photography: Andrew Pearce ARPS

First published 2001

Reprint 10 9 8 7 6 5 4 3 2 1 0

© Diagram Visual Information Limited 2001

ISBN 0 00 712270-5

Printed in Italy by Amadeus S.p.A.

Introduction

An essential ingredient for any family get-together, or party, is a good selection of games to play. With a little thought and planning, games can help to provide amusement for all concerned, and provide a welcome break during the proceedings.

Collins Gem Family & Party Games is a fascinating, highly illustrated guide to almost 150 games and activities, most of which can be played by children over the age of five, and by adults of any age. Each game details the minimum age group, the optimum number of players, the aim of the game, any preparation required, and the various stages in the game itself. With each activity there are step-by-step instructions and clear, accurate diagrams showing techniques and methods that are easy to follow. The games are arranged under specific categories, such as action, musical, racing, dice or spoken word games, and include old favourites such as Hide and Seek, Pin the Tail on the Donkey, and Tongue-twisters, as well as newer activities such as Aggression, Botticelli and Telegrams. Additionally, to make finding the right game easy, this book includes indexes of games by appropriate age and games defined by a certain number of players, plus sections on organising games and useful equipment.

Collins Gem Family & Party Games is an attractive companion volume to *Gem Card Games*.

Contents

Action Games

Ball Games

Blindfold Games

Contest Games

Musical Games

Fivestones and Jacks

Pen and Paper Games

Games by Age

◐ Games particularly suitable for a party.

Games for age 5–10

Games for age 7+

Games for age 8+

Games for age 9+

Games for age 10+

Games by Players

Games for 2 players

Games for groups of players

Games for teams of players

Advice for Giving a Party

At the best parties everything seems to be spontaneous and fun. Invariably, such parties have been carefully planned and prepared.

As a general rule, the younger the party-goers, the less planning you have to do. Very young children up to five years old don't need much more than a few simple games to keep them happy. Five to 10-year-olds are more demanding and will expect a variety of games and activities. For the over-10s you will need to choose games and activities imaginatively. Young people are often self-conscious and easily embarrassed.

Choose the games you want to play well in advance, and make sure that you have the equipment you need for each game. It is important to select a good mix of games, bearing in mind the ages and characters of your guests. Try to avoid playing too many active games one after the other – mix active games with quiet games or quizzes to give the guests a chance to recuperate.

Prepare more games than you think you will need, and have a good supply of prizes. If you are planning some outdoor games, remember to prepare extra indoor games in case the weather is against you. Many games, such as Musical Bumps, need to have someone in charge to control the music and settle disputes. And games involving rough and tumble may need supervision to stop them getting out of hand.

HANDY RULES

- Give clear instructions to everyone before each game.
- Don't let any one game go on too long.
- Have plenty of space if players need to move about.
- Consolation prizes for losers are often a good idea.
- Boisterous games are best played before any meal.

Useful Equipment

The equipment required is specified at the beginning of each game. Some of the games require specific equipment, such as dice, spellicans or tiddlywinks, but most of the other things you will need can be found around the house. Each category of game uses similar equipment, but in general the following will be handy.

- A scarf to serve as a blindfold.
- Pencils (one for each player with a few in reserve) and plenty of paper.
- Wrapping paper, blank postcards.
- A cassette player or musical instruments.
- A selection of different-sized balls.
- String and rope.
- Plenty of balloons are essential for any children's party, and some of the games make use of them.

Action Games

MY LITTLE BIRD
Age 3+

Players
Group

This game is
played in countries
all over the world.
Other names for it
include Flying High and
Birds Fly.

PLAY

- One player is the leader
  and the others stand in a
  row in front of him.
  Alternatively, everyone sits
  around a table.

- The leader starts by saying 'My little bird is
  lively, is lively,' and then goes on to name
  something followed by the word 'fly' – for
  example, he might say 'eggs fly.'

- If whatever he names can fly – for example, cockatoos –
  the players raise their arms and wave them about. If it
  cannot fly – as with eggs – the players should remain still.

- A player who makes a mistake is out. The last player left
  in the game wins.

DEAD LIONS

Age 3+   **Players** Group

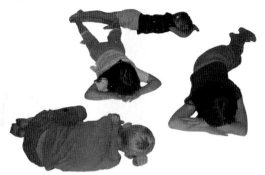

Aim
The player staying still the longest is the winning dead lion.

Preparation
The organiser gets all the players to lie motionless on the ground or floor.

Play
- The organiser disqualifies every player who moves until only one dead lion is left lying. This last player is the winner. All disqualified players try to make the others move without actually touching them.

CHARADES

Age 7+

Players Teams

Charades is probably the best-known and most popular of all games involving acting.

AIM

For one team to guess a word with several syllables, or the title of a book or film, that are acted out in mime by another team.

EQUIPMENT

Some dressing-up clothes will add to the fun but are not absolutely necessary.

Book   **Film**

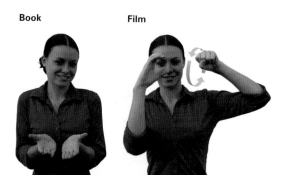

PREPARATION

It is probably a good idea to prepare some good subjects beforehand if children are involved. Good examples include words such as Bandage, Carpet, Earring and Knapsack, or film and book titles.

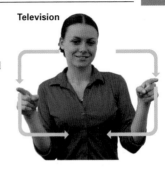

Television

PLAY

• The first team chooses its title or word and indicates the type of subject using one of the set mimes shown here.

Play/theatre

Song/musical

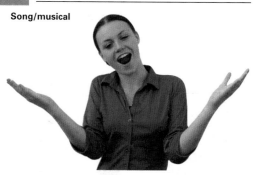

The team then indicates how many words and syllables the title contains by holding up fingers. It then acts out each word or syllable separately, or the whole word or title together. There are several ways of giving clues, such as indicating a short word, the word 'the', the word of the title sounds like the one being mimed.

- The second team tries to guess what the word or title is.

- The game is played in turn by the teams, with the team with most correct guesses the winner.

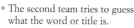

Sounds like

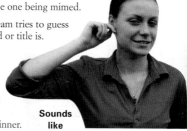

Number of words

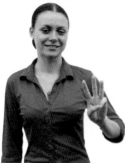

Number of syllables

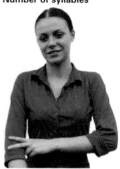

Small word

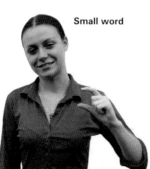

'The'

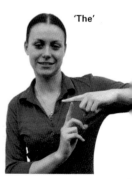

HIDE AND SEEK

Age 7+   **Players** Group

One of the best-loved and most enduring of all children's games.

Aim

To get 'home' without being touched.

Play

- One player is made 'seeker' and covers his or her eyes and counts to 40 while the others go and hide.

- The seeker then has to try to find players and touch them.

- The players must try to reach home without being touched – better still, without being seen by the seeker. The players who are caught are out.

- The last player to be caught is the winner and can take the place of the seeker.

HUNT THE THIMBLE

Age 5+   **Players** Group

This very popular game is usually played with a thimble, but any other small object will do just as well.

Play

- All the players but one leave the room while the player left behind hides the thimble somewhere in the room or on his or her person. He then calls the other players back into the room to look for it.

- The game is won by the first player to find the thimble and take it to the player who hid it. The finder then has a turn at hiding the thimble.

TREASURE HUNT
Age 5+   Players Group

PREPARATION

Considerable preparation is required because the host has to write a story about buried treasure. The story should not be too long and should contain a number of clues as to where the treasure can be found. For example, a reference in the story to the beach could be a clue to a sandpit in the garden. The 'treasure' may be any item and may be hidden indoors or out.

PLAY

- Players are given a copy of the story, or the host reads it out to them. The players then set off to search for the treasure. They must not talk to each other during the hunt. A time limit of, say, 15 minutes should be allowed.

- The winner is the first player to find the treasure, which may double as a prize.

IN THE MANNER OF THE WORD
Age 9+
Players Group

This is an amusing acting game in which players attempt to guess adverbs.

PLAY

• One player chooses an adverb, such as rapidly, quietly or amusingly. The other players in turn then ask him to carry out some action 'in the manner of the word'. For example, a player might say; 'Eat in the manner of the word,' 'Walk in the manner of the word,' or 'Laugh in the manner of the word.'

• The player who chooses the adverb must do as the other players ask, and the other players may make guesses as soon as acting begins.

• The first player to guess an adverb correctly scores one point. If no one guesses the word after each of the players has asked for an action, the player who chose the adverb receives one point.

• The game is won by the player with most points after each of the players has had a turn at choosing the adverb.

MATCHING PAIRS

Age 5–10

Players Group

EQUIPMENT
A number of everyday articles are needed and some wrapping paper.

PREPARATION
The host thinks of a 'pair' of items for each of the guests. Examples might include: salt and pepper, knife and fork, sock and shoe, a pair of gloves, a cup and saucer, a King and Queen (from a set of playing cards). The host wraps up one part of each 'pair' and hides the other somewhere in the room.

PLAY
- Players are given a part of their 'pair'.
- They have to look for what they think is likely to be the other, which has been hidden by the host.
- Every player who matches his pair within ten minutes or so is a winner.

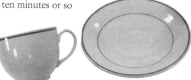

SARDINES

Age 7+   **Players Group**

This is a type of Hide and Seek (see page 26) usually
played in the dark. The more rooms that can be played in
the more exciting the game becomes.

AIM
To find and join the 'sardine'.

PLAY
- One player is chosen as 'sardine' to go and hide
  (preferably somewhere big enough for most of the
  others to squeeze in, too) while all the others cover their
  eyes and count to 30.

- The seekers then go off individually to find the sardine.

- When a seeker locates the sardine, he or she joins the
  sardine in the hiding place. Eventually the hiding place
  is full of hiders, while fewer and fewer seekers remain.

- There are no winners in this game. The last player to
  find the hiding place becomes the next sardine.

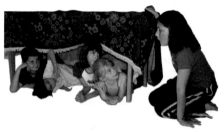

SIMON SAYS
Age 3+
Players Group

This is an old party
game that remains a
great favourite.

PLAY
- One player is the
  leader and the others
  spread around the
  room in front of him
  or her.

- The leader orders the
  others to make various
  actions – such as touching their
  toes or raising their arms. Whether
  or not they must obey the orders
  depends on how the orders are given.

- If the leader begins the order with the
  words 'Simon says,' the players must obey. If he
  does not begin with these words, they must not make
  the action. If a player makes a mistake, he or she is out
  of the game. The leader can encourage mistakes by
  giving rapid orders; by developing a rhythm with a
  repeated pattern of movements and then breaking it; or
  by making the actions himself for the others to follow.

- The last person left in the game is the winner and
  becomes the next leader.

TRIANGULAR TUG-OF-WAR

Age 10+   **Players** Group

EQUIPMENT
A 2–3 m (6–9 ft) length of rope (or cord) and three handkerchiefs are required.

PREPARATION
Tie the ends of the rope together. If indoors, make sure you have a large area clear of furniture. Get three players to stand outside the rope and hold it with one hand behind them to form a triangle. Place a handkerchief on the ground in front of each player.

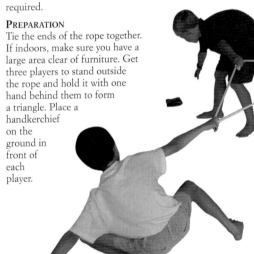

PLAY

- The players have to hold on to the rope behind them and pick up the handkerchief in front of them. Each should be aware of his opponents though, and pull the rope to make sure they don't get to their handkerchiefs first.

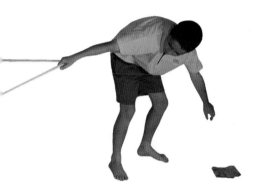

- The player who manages to pick up his handkerchief first, while holding on to the rope, wins.

WHAT'S THE TIME, MR WOLF?
Age 5+

Players Group

PREPARATION
One player chooses to be or is
chosen as Mr Wolf.

PLAY
- Mr Wolf stands with his
  back to the others, who
  advance one step at a
  time towards him
  from a reasonable
  distance. At each
  step, one member
  of the advancing
  group shouts,
  'What's the time,
  Mr Wolf?'

- The time is given by
  him, and the group
  takes another step
  forward.

- At a moment of his
  own choosing Mr
  Wolf will, instead,
  shout the reply, 'Dinner Time!'
  He then turns rapidly and chases the others.
  The player who's caught becomes Mr Wolf.

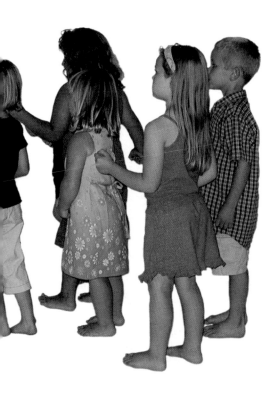

Ball Games

BROKEN BOTTLES
Age 10+
Players Group

EQUIPMENT
A soft ball is needed.

PLAY
- Players form a circle and throw the ball to each other, catching with both hands.

- When a player drops or misses the ball, he or she pays a penalty. The first penalty is to use only the right hand. The second is to use only the left. The third is to have one knee on the floor, but use both hands, the fourth, to be on both knees. The fifth, to be on both knees and use only the right

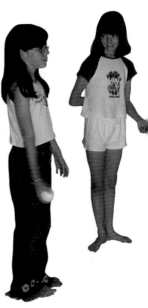

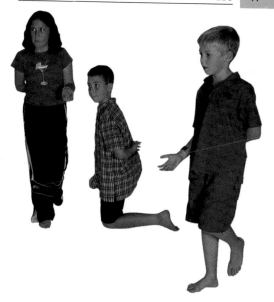

hand, and lastly, sixth, to be on both knees and to use only the left hand. After that, the player drops out.

- The player who survives longest wins.

BUCKET BALL

Age 3+   **Players Group**

AIM

To get the ball into the bucket.

PLAY

- A plastic household bucket is weighed down with a large stone or brick.

- Players stand around it and take turns to throw a ball into it. Young players can stand fairly close, older ones further back. For players who are good at it, a smaller ball can be used since this makes the game more of a challenge.

- The player who gets the ball into the bucket most often wins.

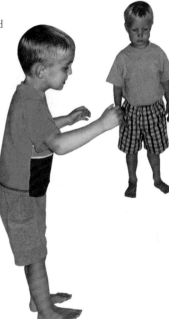

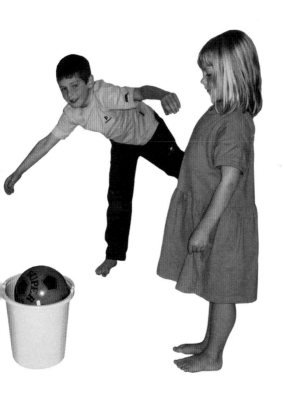

CIRCLE BALL

Age 5–10   **Players** Group

This game is best played on a hard surface. It is a fast and energetic game played only for enjoyment.

Aim

Players bounce a ball to each other in turn.

Play

- A circle about 1 m (3 ft) across is drawn, and players form a circle around it, standing several metres back.

- A ball is thrown from player to player in order, and must bounce inside the drawn circle. Players must catch it before it bounces again.

FRENCH CRICKET

Age 10+ **Players** Group

EQUIPMENT
A tennis ball and tennis racket or cricket bat are needed.

PLAY

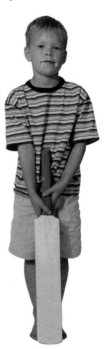

- Each player takes a turn at holding the racket or bat.

- Another player then tries to get him or her out by bowling and hitting his or her legs below the knees. The batter, meanwhile, protects the legs with the bat or racket and tries to hit the ball. Each time a player hits the ball, he or she scores a point and has another turn.

- If the batter hits the ball, he or she can face the way the ball will be coming from next. If not, he or she has to stay in the same position, making it difficult to protect the legs if the ball is coming from behind.

- The ball must be bowled from where it lands.

- A player who is hit below the knees is out.

GUARD THE GATE

Age 5-10   **Players** Group

AIM
To roll a ball through the 'gate' formed by the space between players.

PLAY
- Players form a circle, each being one arm's length away from the next. The gate is the space to his or her right.

- The ball (a tennis ball would be suitable, or a larger ball for younger players) is rolled by hand by the players, each trying to send it through any of the spaces between players – the gates. At the same time the players must guard their own gates to stop the ball going through. Players who let the ball through their gates drop out.

- The player who succeeds in defending his or her gate the longest wins.

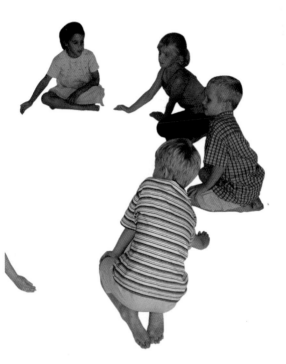

HOT POTATO

Age 5–10   **Players Group**

Aim

For the players to keep the ball away from the player in
the middle.

Play

- The players form a circle and one is chosen to stand in
  the centre.

- The ball is thrown from player
  to player, and the one in
  the middle tries
  to intercept. He
  or she may win

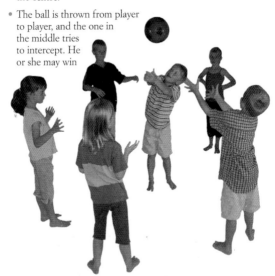

the ball by touching it at any time, even if one of the other players is holding it, or it falls outside the circle. Whoever makes the mistake that allows the player in the middle to touch the ball takes his or her place.

- The game goes on until all the players have a turn in the middle. The one who holds out longest may be declared the winner.

WALL GAME

Age 5+   **Players Group**

AIM
To throw and catch a ball quickly.

PLAY
- Each player is given a number. They stand near the wall in no particular order.
- The first player starts the game by throwing the ball against the wall, at the same time calling the number of one of the other players.
- That player has to try to catch the ball after the first bounce.
- If the player succeeds, he or she throws the ball and calls another number.
- If he or she fails, the first player throws again and calls a different number.
- The game can be scored, with points given for every successful catch. The highest score within a time limit wins.

Blindfold Games

BLIND MAN'S BLUFF

Age 7+   **Players Group**

AIM

A blindfolded player tries to catch and identify another
player.

PLAY

- A blind person is chosen and blindfolded. He or she is
  turned around three times in the centre of the room and
  then left alone.

- The other players dance around, taunting the
  blindfolded person and dodging out of his or her way to
  avoid capture.

- When the blindfolded person catches someone, he or
  she has two or three guesses at the name of the prisoner.
  If he guesses correctly, the prisoner becomes the new
  blind man. If wrong, he continues to be the blind man
  and tries to catch another player.

BLIND JUDGEMENT

Age 7+   **Players Group**

PLAY

- One player is blindfolded and placed on a 'seat of
  judgement'.

- Another player then stands quietly in front of him, and

the player in the judgement seat gives a brief description of whoever he thinks might be standing in front of him.

- If the other players think that the 'blind judgement' was reasonably accurate, the player in front of the blindfolded player becomes the new blind man.

- If his judgement was inaccurate, the original blind man must pass judgement on another player.

THIEVES

Age 7+   **Players Group**

AIM

A blindfolded player tries to catch players stealing from him or her.

PLAY

- One player is blindfolded and given a rolled paper or other soft implement to hold in his or her hand.

- The blindfolded player sits in the middle of a circle made by the other players, and a pile of treasure – necklaces, brooches, bracelets, etc. – is placed in front of him or her.

- Players in the circle quietly take it in turns to steal a piece of treasure. If the blindfolded person hears a thief, he or she strikes at him or her with the newspaper and calls 'thief, thief.'

- If he or she touches a thief, the thief must return empty-handed to his or her place to await the next turn.

- The thief who collects most treasure wins the game.

BLIND MAN'S TREASURE HUNT

Age 7+   **Players** Group

EQUIPMENT

Parcels of different sizes and shapes, at least one for each player, plus several extra to allow choice for all players, and a blindfold, are needed.

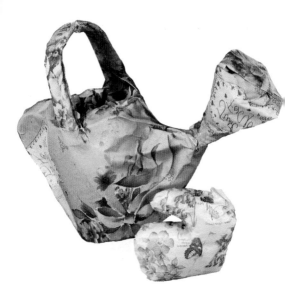

PREPARATION

All the players must be sent out of the room. The parcels are then placed on a table in the middle of the room.

PLAY

- Bring in the guests one by one, blindfolded.

- Lead them up to the table and tell them they may choose one present, but must not open it until everyone has chosen.

- Everyone 'wins' something in this game. The fun lies in the opening of the presents, and guessing what they are from their shape and sound.

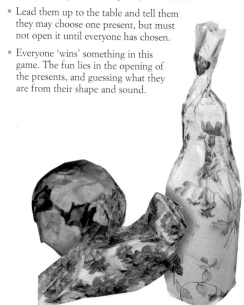

PIN THE TAIL ON THE DONKEY

Age 5+   **Players Group**

AIM

Blindfolded players try to pin a tail in the correct position on a drawing of a tail-less donkey.

PREPARATION

The organiser draws a large picture of a donkey without a tail and fastens it onto a pinboard propped upright. He also makes a donkey's tail out of cardboard or wool and sticks a large pin through the body end.

PLAY

- Each player in turn is blindfolded and turned around so that he is in front of and facing the donkey. He is then given the tail and attempts to pin it on the correct part of the donkey.

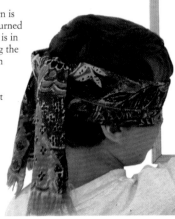

- The organiser marks the position of each player's attempt.

- The player who pins nearest the correct place is the winner.

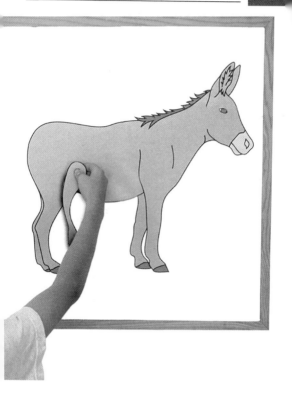

SQUEAK-PIGGY-SQUEAK

Age 7+   **Players Group**

AIM

A blindfolded player attempts to identify another player by getting him to squeak.

PLAY

- One player is blindfolded, given a cushion, and turned around three times in the centre of the room. The others sit down around the room.

- The blindfolded person must then place his or her cushion on another player's lap and sit on it, and then call 'squeak-piggy-squeak'. The person he or she is sitting on squeaks like a pig.

- If the blindfolded person recognises the person, they change places. Once the new person is blindfolded, the players all change seats before he or she tries to sit on a player's lap.

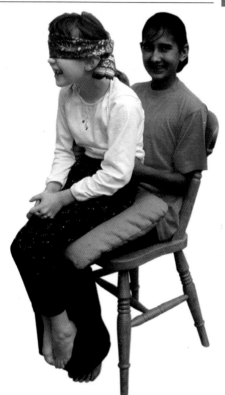

Contest Games

AGGRESSION

Age 9+   **Players 2**

AIM
Players fight imaginary battles and try to occupy the maximum amount of territory.

EQUIPMENT
Each player must have a crayon of a different colour.

PLAYING AREA
A large sheet of paper is used. One player begins by drawing the boundaries of an imaginary country; the other player then draws the outline of another imaginary country. Any agreed number of countries may be drawn (20 is an average number), and they can be any shape or size. When the agreed number of countries has been drawn, each is clearly marked with a different letter of the alphabet.

ARMIES
Each player is allotted 100 armies. Taking turns, each chooses a country (who drew the boundary has no bearing on the choice) that he or she intends to occupy and writes within it how many armies he or she is allocating to it. (Once a country has been occupied, no player may add further armies to it.) This procedure continues until all the countries have been occupied or until each player has allocated all his or her armies.

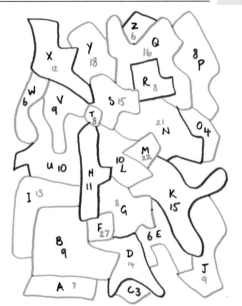

Green: used 100 armies, won 6 countries.
Blue: used 100 armies, won 9 countries.
Red: used 91 armies, won 11 countries

PLAY

- The player who chose the first country has the opening move.

- The player's aim is to retain more occupied countries than his or her opponent; to achieve this, he or she 'attacks' enemy armies in adjacent countries. The player announces which of his or her territories will attack which neighbour. (Adjacent countries are defined as those with a common boundary.)

- A player may attack with armies from more than one country, provided they are all in countries that have a common border with the country under attack. If the number of armies located in the attacking country or countries is greater than those located in the defending country, the defending army is conquered; its armies are crossed off and can take no further part in the game. (The armies used to conquer a country may be reused.)

- Players take it in turns to conquer countries until one or both of them cannot mount any further attacks.

- At the end of the game the players total the number of countries each of them retains.

- The winner is the player with the highest number of unconquered countries – he or she need not necessarily be the player who made the greatest number of conquests.

APPLE BOBBING

Age 5+   **Players Group**

EQUIPMENT

A large bowl, lots of apples, newspapers (in case of spillage) and a towel are needed.

PREPARATION

Fill the bowl with water, place it on newspapers and put a number of apples into the water.

PLAY

- Players take turns in trying to retrieve an apple from the bowl, using only their mouths.

- There are no real winners, since everybody should end up with an apple. Perhaps a small prize could be given to the player who gets his or her apple in the shortest time.

APPLE ON A STRING

Age 7+   **Players Group**

This game is an old favourite for Hallowe'en. Players try, without using their hands, to eat apples suspended from strings.

PLAY

- A piece of string is hung across the room, well above head height. An apple (or doughnut) per person is suspended from it, also on a string.

- The players try to eat their apples or doughnuts without using their hands.

- The first player to eat the apple down to its core, or to finish eating the doughnut, is the winner.

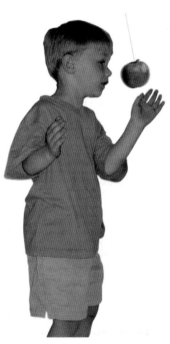

ARM WRESTLING

Age 7+   **Players 2**

PLAY

- Two players sit facing each other at either side of a table. Resting their right elbows on the table so that the elbows touch and with crooked arms, they clasp each other's right hands. (Both players may use their left arms if they prefer.)

- On the signal to begin, each player tries to force his opponent's right hand back until it touches the table. Elbows must be kept firmly on the table.

- The winner is the first to succeed.

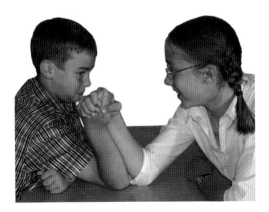

BATTLESHIPS

Age 10+   **Players 2**

AIM

The objective is to destroy an opponent's entire fleet by a series of 'hits'.

PLAY

- The players should sit so that they cannot see each other's papers. Each of them draws two identical playing areas, 10 squares by 10 squares in size. In order to identify each square, the playing areas have numbers down one side and letters across the top (thus the top left-hand square is A1; the bottom left-hand square is A10, etc.).

- Each player marks one playing area his or her 'home fleet' and the other playing area the 'enemy fleet'. Players have their own fleet of ships that they may position anywhere within their home fleet area. A fleet comprises:

  a) one battleship, four squares long;

  b) two cruisers, each three squares long;

  c) three destroyers, each two squares long; and

  d) four submarines, each one square only.

a   **b**

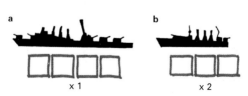

x 1   x 2

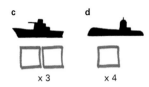

- Players 'position' their ships by outlining the appropriate number of squares. The squares representing each ship must be in a row or column (see page 66). There must also be at least one vacant square between ships. Players take turns.

- In each turn, a player may attempt three hits: he or she calls out the names of any three squares, marking them on the enemy fleet area as he or she does so.

- The player's opponent must then consult his or her own home fleet area to see whether any of these squares are occupied.

- If they are, he or she must state how many and the category of ship hit. In order to sink a ship, every one of its component squares must receive a hit.

- The game continues with both players marking the state of their own and the enemy's fleet – this may be done by shading or outlining squares, or in some other manner (see page 67). There is no limit to the number of hits each player may attempt.

- The winner is the player who first destroys his or her opponent's fleet.

Battleships: Player 1's positions

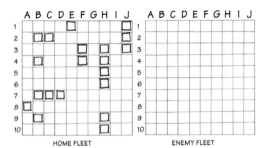

HOME FLEET   ENEMY FLEET

Battleships: Player 2's positions

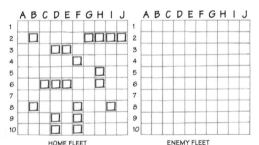

HOME FLEET   ENEMY FLEET

Game in progress: Player 1

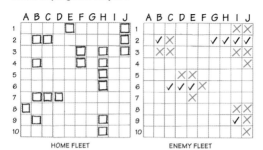

HOME FLEET

ENEMY FLEET

Game in progress: Player 2

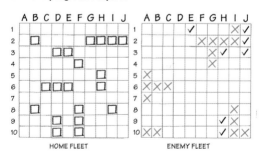

HOME FLEET

ENEMY FLEET

BOXES

Age 5+   **Players 2**

Aim

Players try to draw and initial as many boxes as they can.

Play

- Any number of dots is drawn on a piece of paper in rows. About ten rows by ten is a good number.

- Players take turns. In each turn they may draw a horizontal or vertical line to join up any two dots that are next to each other.

- Whenever a player completes a box, he or she initials it and may then draw another line that does not complete a box.

- As soon as there are no more dots to be joined – all the boxes having been completed – the game ends.

Example of grid

Game in progress

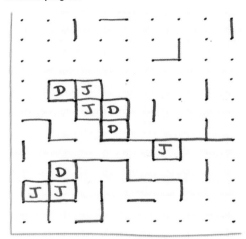

WINNING

The player with the highest number of initialled boxes is the winner.

VARIATION

Another way of playing is to try to form as few boxes as possible – the players join up as many dots as they can before being forced to complete a box. The winner is the player with the lowest number of initialled boxes.

CRYSTALS

Age 10+   **Players 2**

In this sophisticated pattern-visualising game, each player tries to form symmetrical shapes known as 'crystals'.

AIM

Each player attempts to 'grow' crystals on a piece of paper with the aim of filling more squares than his or her opponent.

EQUIPMENT

All that is needed is a large sheet of squared (graph) paper and a differently coloured crayon for each player.

PREPARATION

A grid of 20 rows of 20 squares each would form a suitable area. A player does not score points for the number of crystals he or she grows, but for the number of squares covered by the crystals he or she claims.

A crystal is made up of 'atoms', each of which occupies a single square. Atoms added by either of the players until the crystal is completed.

In growing crystals, players must observe certain rules of symmetry that determine whether or not a crystal is legitimate. The symmetry of a crystal can be determined by visualising four axes through its centre: horizontal, vertical and two diagonal axes. Once the axes have been 'drawn', it should theoretically be possible to fold the crystal along each of the four axes to produce corresponding 'mirror' halves that, when folded, exactly overlay each other (i.e. are the same shape and size).

Crystals: rules for building

✔ = legitimate crystals   ✘ = not legitimate

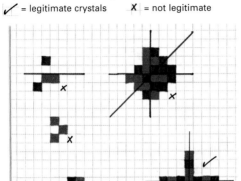

In addition to the rules of symmetry, players must observe the following:

a) a legitimate crystal may be formed from four or more atoms drawn by one player only;

b) the atoms forming a crystal must be joined along their sides – they may not be connected only by their corners;

c) a crystal may not contain any empty atoms (i.e. holes).

PLAY

- Players decide on their playing order, and each one in turn shades in any one square of his or her choice.

- In the first few turns, players rarely try to grow crystals. Instead, they place single atoms around the playing area in order to establish potential crystal sites.

- As play progresses, players will see which atoms are best placed for growing crystals and add to them as appropriate.

- When a player thinks he or she has grown a crystal, he or she declares it, and rings the area that it covers. A player with a winning advantage will try to retain the lead by either blocking his or her opponents' attempts at growing crystals, or by growing several small crystals that – although not high scoring – restrict the playing area. Play ends when no blank squares are left or when the players agree that no more crystals can be formed.

- Players work out which of the crystals are legitimate (ticked in the game opposite), and count the number of squares each covers. Any crystal that does not demonstrate symmetry around each of the four axes is not legitimate and does not score.

- The number of squares in the legitimate crystals that each player has grown are added up, and the player with most squares wins the game.

Crystals: examples

✓ = legitimate crystals ✗ = not legitimate

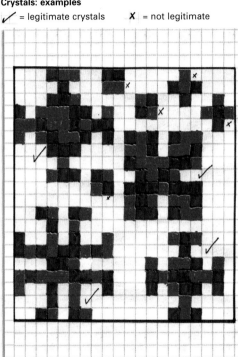

MURDER IN THE DARK

Age 10+   **Players Group**

EQUIPMENT
Envelopes, paper and a pen.

PREPARATION
One person must hand out sealed envelopes to the players.
Only two of them have anything written on the piece of
paper inside. On one is written 'You are the murderer.'
The other says 'You
are the detective.'

PLAY
- The players open
  their envelopes,
  and the player
  who has been
  chosen to play the
  'detective' lets
  everyone know of
  this. (The others
  must keep quiet
  about the contents
  of their envelopes,
  of course.)

- When all the
  players are ready,
  the detective turns
  out the lights for
  one minute.

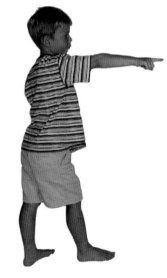

- During this time, the players mill about in the dark and the 'murderer' commits the crime by *very gently* squeezing someone's neck.

- The moment the victim feels the murderer's hands, he or she must scream loudly and fall to the floor.

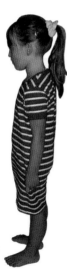

- Meanwhile, the 'murderer' must try to get as far away from the scene of the crime as possible in order to appear innocent.

- A few seconds after the scream, the detective puts the lights back on, noting the positions of all the players.

- The detective asks the players questions about the 'murder'. They must all answer truthfully, except the murderer, who may lie as much as he or she likes.

- When the detective thinks he or she has deduced the identity of the murderer, he officially accuses someone.

- If the detective is correct, the murderer must confess. But if he is wrong (and he only gets one guess), the murderer wins and the mystery remains unsolved.

NOUGHTS AND CROSSES

Age 5+   Players 2

AIM
To place three adjoining marks on a grid.

PLAY
- Two vertical lines are drawn with two horizontal lines crossing them, forming nine spaces. Players decide which of them is to draw noughts (circles) and which of them crosses.

- Taking turns, players make their mark in any vacant space.

- The winner is the player who manages to get three of his or her marks in a row (horizontally, vertically or diagonally). He or she then draws a line through his or her winning row and the game comes to an end. If neither player succeeds in forming a row, the game is considered drawn. As the player who draws first has a better chance of winning, players usually swop their starting order after each game.

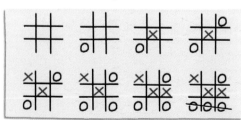

THREE-DIMENSIONAL NOUGHTS AND CROSSES

Age 10+   Players 2

Based on the standard game, the three-dimensional version offers a lengthier and more challenging alternative. It can be bought as a game but can equally well be played with pencil and paper.

Three-dimensional noughts and crosses

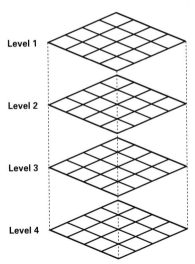

Level 1

Level 2

Level 3

Level 4

Aim

Players aim to complete a line of their marks in any of the three dimensions.

Play

- The cube may be represented diagrammatically by 64 squares – as shown overleaf. For actual play, each 'layer' of the cube is drawn out individually.

- Play then proceeds as in Noughts and Crosses.

- The winner is the first player to get four of his or her marks in a row (illustrations overleaf show winning rows).

Horizontal win

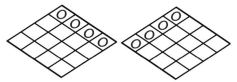

From side to side on the same level

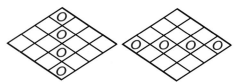

From corner to corner on the same level

Vertical win

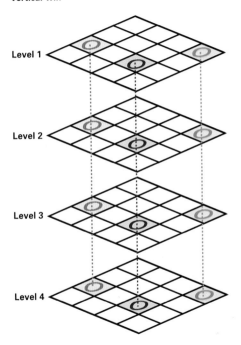

Level 1

Level 2

Level 3

Level 4

Vertical diagonal win

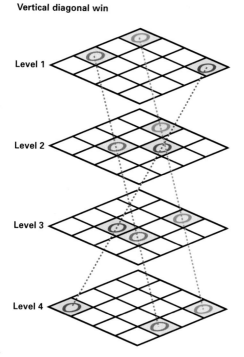

SCISSORS, PAPER, STONE
Age 10+   Players 2

This ancient game, also known as Hic, Haec, Hoc and by many other names, is played all over the world. Three objects (scissors, a piece of paper and a stone) are indicated by different positions of the hand:

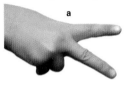

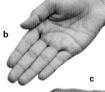

a) two fingers making a V shape represent scissors;

b) an open hand represents a piece of paper; and

c) a clenched fist represents a stone.

AIM
To guess correctly and to win the maximum number of rounds.

PLAY
- Two players hide one hand behind their backs and adopt one of the three positions.
- One player calls 'One, two, three' (or 'Hic, haec, hoc') and as the third number or word is called the players show their hands.

- The winner of a round is decided with reference to the following statements: scissors can cut paper; paper may be wrapped around a stone; and a stone can blunt the scissors. Thus, if one player chooses scissors and the other player paper, the player who chooses scissors wins the round. If both players decide on the same object, the round is a draw. Players usually play a predetermined number of rounds.

- The winner is the player who wins the largest number of rounds.

Scissors cut paper

Paper wraps stone

Stone blunts scissors

SHAPING UP

Age 10+   **Players 2**

EQUIPMENT

In advance, prepare the shapes shown here from card.
There should be one whole set per player. Note that each
shape comprises five squares.

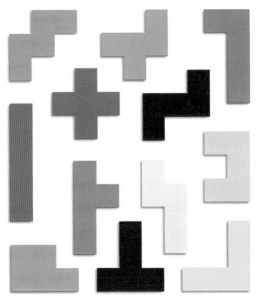

PLAY

- Players are asked to make up different shapes and are given a time limit, perhaps 4 or 5 minutes, for each. Examples might include a rectangle that is 5 by 12 squares, 3 by 20 squares, and so on.

- Each square used scores one point. For example, a rectangle of 5 by 12 squares would score 60 points.

- After, say, six test challenges, the player with the most points is declared the winner.

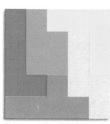

25 points

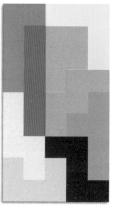

45 points

60 points

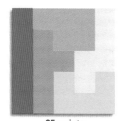

25 points

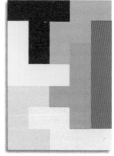

35 points

SPROUTS

Age 5–10 **Players 2**

Sprouts has certain similarities with Boxes, but needs rather more ingenuity to win!

Aim

The players try to be the last to complete a 'sprout' within the allowed moves.

Play

- About six or so dots are drawn – well spaced out – on a sheet of paper (more may be drawn for a longer game).

- Taking turns, each player draws a line joining any two dots or joining a dot to itself.

- This player then draws a dot anywhere along the line he or she has just made, and his or her turn ends. When drawing a line, the following rules must be observed:

  a) no line may cross itself;

  b) no line may cross a line that has already been drawn;

  c) no line may be drawn through a dot;

  d) a dot may have no more than three lines leaving it.

- The last person able to draw a legitimate line is the winner.

Sprouts: foul lines

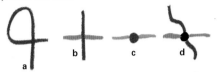

Sprouts: a sample game

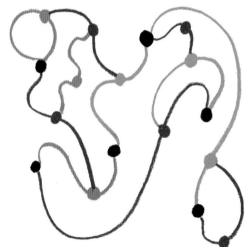

Musical Games

HERE WE GO ROUND THE MULBERRY BUSH

Age 3+ **Players** Group

PLAY

- The players form a circle and hold hands.

- During the first verse, they dance round in a circle.

- For each of the subsequent verses they perform the actions described and then join hands again for the chorus.

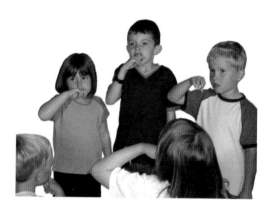

Chorus

Here we go round the mulberry bush, the mulberry bush,
the mulberry bush,
Here we go round the mulberry bush,
On a cold and frosty morning.

1

This is the way we wash our face, wash our face, wash our face,
This is the way we wash our face
On a cold and frosty morning.

2

This is the way we brush our teeth, brush our teeth,
brush our teeth,
This is the way we brush our teeth,
On a cold and frosty morning.

3

This is the way we comb our hair, comb our hair, comb our hair,
This is the way we comb our hair,
On a cold and frosty morning.

4

This is the way we walk to school, walk to school, walk to school,
This is the way we walk to school,
On a cold and frosty morning.

5

This is the way we run home from school, run home from school,
run home from school,
This is the way we run home from school,
On a cold and frosty morning.

LONDON BRIDGE

Age 3+   **Players** Group

PREPARATION

Two players are chosen to be the bridge. Each chooses to be either silver or gold.

PLAY

- The bridge is formed by the two players joining hands.

- The rest dance in a circle, passing under the bridge. On the word 'lady' the arms of the bridge come down and catch one of the dancers.

- They ask, 'What will you pay me, silver or gold?' Depending on the answer, the captured player stands

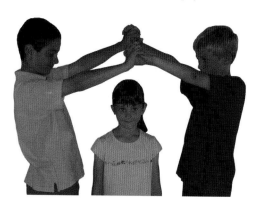

behind one side of the bridge and the game goes on until all the dancers are caught. Often, the game ends with the two lines of players having a tug-of-war.

London Bridge is falling down, falling down, falling down,
London Bridge is falling down,
My fair lady.

Build it up with sticks and stones, sticks and stones, sticks and
stones,
Build it up with sticks and stones,
My fair lady.

Sticks and stones will fall away, fall away, fall away,
Sticks and stones will fall away,
My fair lady.

Build it up with iron bars, iron bars, iron bars,
Build it up with iron bars,
My fair lady.

Irons bars will bend and break, bend and break, bend and break,
Iron bars will bend and break,
My fair lady.

Build it up with pins and nails, pins and nails, pins and nails,
Build it up with pins and nails,
My fair lady.

Pins and nails will rust and break, rust and break, rust and break,
Pins and nails will rust and break,
My fair lady.

OLD MACDONALD HAD A FARM

Age 3+   **Players** Group

PLAY

- The players form a circle, standing or sitting.

- As each verse is sung, they imitate the animal sounds, and repeat all the other noises of the previous verses, so that as the game proceeds it becomes very raucous and exciting. The game can be extended for several more verses to include, for instance, cats, pigs, frogs, horses, and so on.

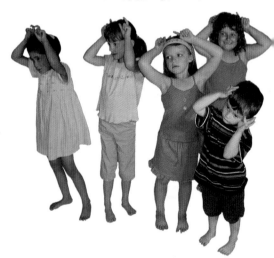

Old MacDonald had a farm, ee-aye-ee-aye-o,
And on that farm he had some cows, ee-aye-ee-aye-o,
With a Moo-moo here, a Moo-moo there,
Here a Moo, there a Moo, everywhere a Moo-moo,
Old MacDonald had a farm, ee-aye-ee-aye-o.

Old MacDonald had a farm, ee-aye-ee-aye-o,
And on that farm he had some ducks, ee-aye-ee-aye-o,
With a Quack-quack here, a Quack-quack there,
Here a Quack, there a Quack, everywhere a Quack-quack,
With a Moo-moo here, a Moo-moo there,
Here a Moo, there a Moo, everywhere a Moo-moo,
Old MacDonald had a farm, ee-aye-ee-aye-o.

Old MacDonald had a farm, ee-aye-ee-aye-o,
And on that farm he had some sheep, ee-aye-ee-aye-o,
With a Baa-baa here, a Baa-baa there,
Here a Baa, there a Baa, everywhere a Baa-baa,
With a Quack-quack here, a Quack-quack there,
Here a Quack, there a Quack, everywhere a Quack-quack,
With a Moo-moo here, a Moo-moo there,
Here a Moo, there a Moo, everywhere a Moo-moo,
Old MacDonald had a farm, ee-aye-ee-aye-o.

Old MacDonald had a farm, ee-aye-ee-aye-o,
And on that farm he had some dogs, ee-aye-ee-aye-o,
With a Woof-woof here, a Woof-woof there,
Here a Woof, there a Woof, everywhere a Woof-woof,
With a Baa-baa here, a Baa-baa there,
Here a Baa, there a Baa, everywhere a Baa-baa,
With a Quack-quack here, a Quack-quack there,
Here a Quack, there a Quack, everywhere a Quack-quack,
With a Moo-moo here, a Moo-moo there,
Here a Moo, there a Moo, everywhere a Moo-moo,
Old MacDonald had a farm, ee-aye-ee-aye-o.

THE FARMER'S IN THE DELL

Age 3+   **Players Group**

PLAY

- The players form a circle and hold hands, with one player in the centre, who is the farmer.

- As they sing, the players walk or dance around the farmer. At the end of the first verse, the farmer picks one of the others to be his wife, and the chosen one joins him in the circle.

- At the end of the second verse, the wife chooses a child, and so on for each verse.

- When patting the cheese, make sure the children are gentle.

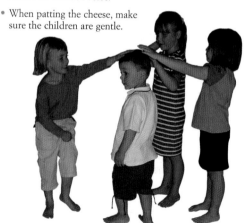

The farmer's in the dell, the farmer's in the dell,
Heigh-ho, merry-o,
The farmer's in the dell.

The farmer wants a wife, the farmer wants a wife,
Heigh-ho, merry-o,
The farmer wants a wife.

The wife wants a child, the wife wants a child,
Heigh-ho, merry-o,
The wife wants a child.

The child wants a nurse, the child wants a nurse,
Heigh-ho, merry-o,
The child wants a nurse.

The nurse wants a dog, the nurse wants a dog,
Heigh-ho, merry-o,
The nurse wants a dog.

The dog wants a cat, the dog wants a cat,
Heigh-ho, merry-o,
The dog wants a cat.

The cat wants a rat, the cat wants a rat,
Heigh-ho, merry-o,
The cat wants a rat.

The rat wants a cheese, the rat wants a cheese,
Heigh-ho, merry-o,
The rat wants a cheese,

We all pat the cheese, we all pat the cheese,
Heigh-ho, merry-o,
we all pat the cheese.

THE WHEELS ON THE BUS

Age 3+   **Players Group**

PLAY

- The players stand in a circle and perform the actions described in the verses.

- For the first verse, they roll their hands over each other, for the second they make engine noises, for the third they make bell-pulling actions, for the fourth they cry like babies, for the fifth they stand and sit down. Extra verses and actions can be added.

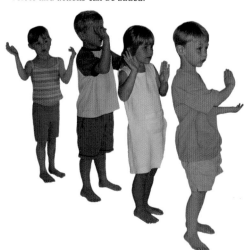

The wheels on the bus go round and round,
Round and round, round and round,
The wheels on the bus go round and round,
All day long.

The engine on the bus goes Brrrmm-Brrrmm-Brrrmm!
Brrrmm-Brrrmm-Brrrmm!, Brrrmm-Brrrmm-Brrrmm!
The engine on the bus goes Brrrmm-Brrrmm-Brrrmm!
All day long.

The bell on the bus goes Ding! Ding! Ding!
Ding! Ding! Ding!, Ding! Ding! Ding!
The bell on the bus goes Ding! Ding! Ding!
All day long.

The baby on the bus goes Wahh! Wahh! Wahh!
Wahh! Wahh! Wahh!, Wahh! Wahh! Wahh!
The baby on the bus goes Wahh! Wahh! Wahh!
All day long.

The people on the bus stand up, sit down,
Stand up, sit down, stand up, sit down,
The people on the bus stand up, sit down,
All day long.

THIS OLD MAN

Age 3+   **Players Group**

PLAY

• The players form a circle, standing or sitting.

• As they sing the first line of each verse, the players hold up the appropriate number of fingers, and hold up, point to or mime the thing named, for the second line they slap their knees in time to the rhythm, and for the last line they can roll about on the floor if space allows, or rotate their hands around in front of their bodies.

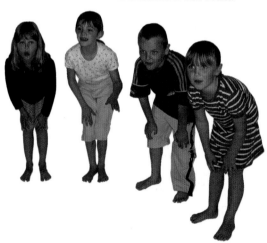

This old man, he played one, he played nick-nack on my thumb
    With a nick-nack paddy-whack give the dog a bone,
        This old man came rolling home.

This old man, he played two, he played nick-nack on my shoe,
    With a nick-nack paddy-whack give the dog a bone,
        This old man came rolling home.

This old man, he played three, he played nick-nack on my knee
    With a nick-nack paddy-whack give the dog a bone,
        This old man came rolling home.

This old man, he played four, he played nick-nack on my floor
    With a nick-nack paddy-whack give the dog a bone,
        This old man came rolling home.

This old man, he played five, he played nick-nack on a bee hive
    With a nick-nack paddy-whack give the dog a bone,
        This old man came rolling home.

This old man, he played six, he played nick-nack with some sticks
    With a nick-nack paddy-whack give the dog a bone,
        This old man came rolling home.

This old man, he played seven, he played nick-nack up in heaven
    With a nick-nack paddy-whack give the dog a bone,
        This old man came rolling home.

This old man, he played eight, he played nick-nack on my gate
    With a nick-nack paddy-whack give the dog a bone,
        This old man came rolling home.

This old man, he played nine, he played nick-nack on the line
    With a nick-nack paddy-whack give the dog a bone,
        This old man came rolling home.

This old man, he played ten, he played nick-nack on my hen
    With a nick-nack paddy-whack give the dog a bone,
        This old man came rolling home.

MUSICAL PATTERNS
Age 5+   **Players Teams**

EQUIPMENT
A cassette player, or a musical instrument such as a piano, is needed to provide the music.

PREPARATION
The players are arranged into teams of equal numbers.

PLAY
- The music starts and the players march, or dance, around the room as they wish.

- The host calls out a shape and stops the music, whereupon the players rush to find their team-mates and form the shape. The host should start with easy shapes, such as a circle and a square, and progress to more complicated ones, such as letters of the alphabet. Some suggestions are given on these pages.

- One point may be awarded in each round for the team with the best shape. The team that scores the highest number of points wins.

MUSICAL CHAIRS
Age 5+   **Players Group**

EQUIPMENT
Chairs and something to play music on.

PREPARATION
Chairs are placed around the room in a large circle. There should be one chair fewer than the number of players.

PLAY
- The players stand in the circle and, when the music starts, all dance around.

- When the music stops, each player tries to sit on a seat. The player left without a seat is eliminated.

- One chair is then removed from the circle and the music is restarted.

- The last person to stay in the game is the winner.

MUSICAL BUMPS

Age 5+   Players Group

This is like Musical Chairs, except that it is played without the chairs.

EQUIPMENT
Something to play music on.

PLAY
- When the music stops, players sit down on the floor. The last person to sit down is out.

- The last person to stay in the game is the winner.

MUSICAL ISLANDS
Age 3+

Players Group

EQUIPMENT
A small carpet and
something to play
music on.

PLAY
- The music starts
  and the players
  walk around in
  a circle. A small
  carpet is placed
  in the path of
  the circle.
  Players must
  step on it when
  they pass round
  the circle.

- When the music
  stops, the player
  who is standing on
  the carpet drops
  out. If no player is
  standing on the
  carpet at that
  moment, no one
  drops out.

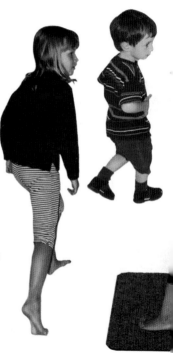

- The game continues until there is only one player remaining. That player is the winner.

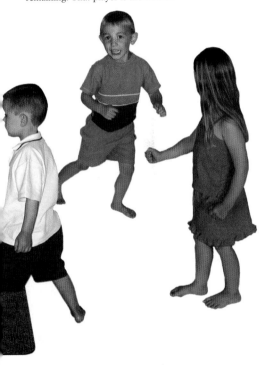

MUSICAL NUMBERS

Age 5+ **Players Group**

EQUIPMENT

Something to play music on.

PLAY

- The players march, walk or dance around the room as the music plays. From time to time, the host stops the music and calls out a number. If the number is three, the players must arrange themselves into groups of three. If he calls out four, then they must form groups of four.

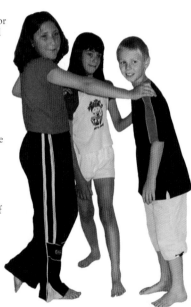

- Any players finding themselves not part of a group drop out of the game.

- The game ends when there are only three or four players remaining, too few with which to continue the game.

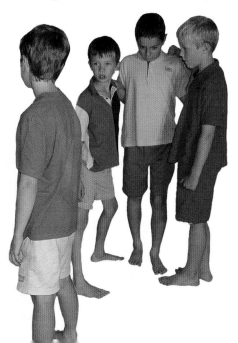

MUSICAL STATUES

Age 3+

Players Group

This game is an enjoyable 'quiet' alternative to Musical Chairs.

EQUIPMENT
Something to play music on.

PLAY

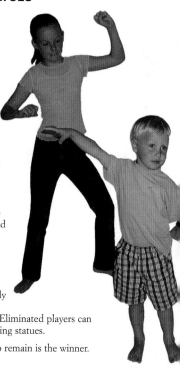

- Players dance around the room to music. When the music stops, the players immediately stop dancing and stand as still as statues.

- Any player seen moving is out.

- The music is started again fairly quickly, and the game continues. Eliminated players can help to spot moving statues.

- The last player to remain is the winner.

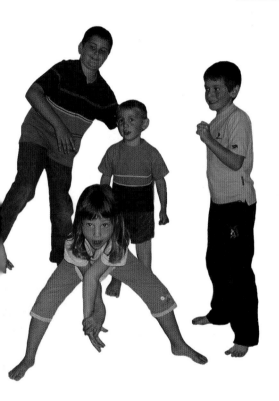

PASS THE PARCEL

Age 5+   **Players Group**

PREPARATION

A small present is wrapped in layer after layer of paper. Each layer should be secured with thread, glue, or a rubber band. Music – to be started and stopped by someone not taking part in the game – is also needed.

PLAY

- Players sit in a circle and one of them holds the parcel. When the music starts, players pass the parcel around the circle to the right.

- When the music stops, whoever is holding the parcel unwraps one layer of wrapping. The music is then restarted and the parcel passed on again.

- The game continues in this way until someone takes off the final wrapping and so wins the present.

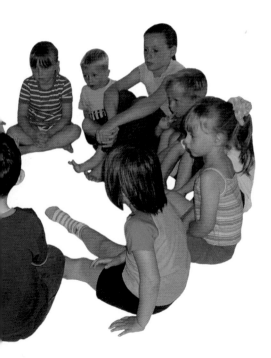

Picture Games

BUTTERFLIES

Age 5+   **Players 2**

EQUIPMENT
You will need about six tubes of brightly coloured oil paints, scissors, and a piece of paper for each player. This game can be quite messy.

PREPARATION
Fold each piece of paper in two.

PLAY
- Get those taking part to squeeze blobs of three different colours of paint on one half of their piece of paper (**a**). They should try to put some blobs near to the crease.

- Each player should then fold the paper together, and open it out (**b**). The result should resemble a butterfly, which could be cut out.

- The results are judged and a prize awarded to the creator of the best 'butterfly'.

a

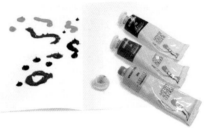

b

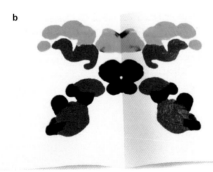

LIGHTS OUT!

Age 10+ **Players** Group

EQUIPMENT

A pencil and a piece of paper are needed for each player.
A non-playing judge is also needed.

PLAY

- Make sure the players are sitting comfortably and then turn out the lights.

- Ask them to draw a lake.

- When they have all finished and expect you to turn the light back on, ask them to draw a boat on the lake.

- When this has been done to the best of their ability, ask them to draw a house on the shore.

- Again, wait until they have finished and then ask them to draw a man in the boat, a tree by the house, a fisherman by the shore, some clouds in the sky, and so on until the picture has a number of elements.

- At this point turn the lights back on.

- The winner will be whoever is judged to have created the most recognisable scene.

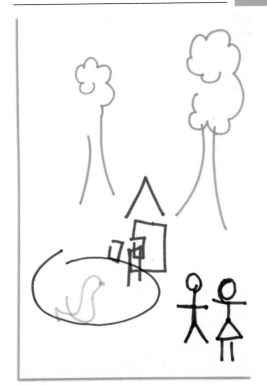

PICTURE CONSEQUENCES

Age 5+   **Players Group**

AIM

Players cooperate to produce a funny picture.

PLAY

- The players draw parts of an animal or a person dressed in funny clothing, according to choice. They start with the head, then fold the paper so only the neck is showing.

- Each person passes the paper to his or her neighbour, who draws the next section, and so on.

- After drawing the feet, players may write down the name of the person whom they want the figure to represent!

- There is no winner, the game is played for fun.

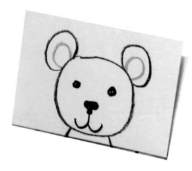

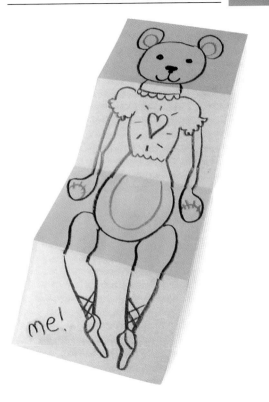

SQUIGGLES

Age 5–10   **Players** Group

Aim

The players make drawings, using squiggles as their
starting point.

Play

• Each player scribbles very quickly on his or her piece of
  paper – the more abstract the squiggle, the better.

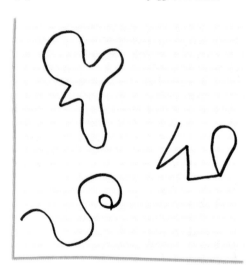

- Players then exchange papers and set themselves a time limit of, for example, two minutes, in which they must use every bit of the squiggle to make a picture. Ingenuity is more important than artistic ability – the challenge is to use your squiggle inventively!

- There are no winners, the game is just for the fun of it.

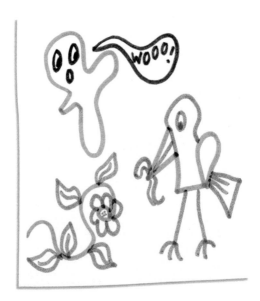

Racing Games

ASSAULT COURSE

Age 5+   **Players Teams**

EQUIPMENT

Lots of obstacles and varied items are needed for the course – dressing-up clothes, sacks, balls, balloons, apples, potatoes and spoons, for example.

PREPARATION

The objects are laid out in advance by the host along a course. Starting and finishing lines should be marked with string or chalk. Examples of suitable obstacles include a long jump, a potato and spoon dash, a box to be leapt over, a rope for six skips, a sack for jumping in to the next obstacle, and an old shirt to put on.

PLAY

- The host first explains what has to be done at each point along the course. The object is for each team to complete the course.

- On the word 'Go!' the first member of each team runs the course and must cope with every obstacle in turn, as instructed.

- Once he or she has completed the course and reaches the finishing line, the next team member can start.

- The team with all its members at the finishing line first wins.

BALLOON RACE

Age 5+   **Players** Teams

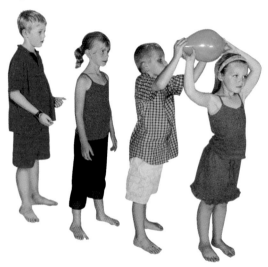

EQUIPMENT
Two balloons.

PREPARATION
Separate the players into two teams of equal numbers.

PLAY

- The teams form two lines, which stand side by side. The balloon is given to the front player in each team, who passes it backwards over his or her head to the next player.

- The balloon is passed backwards along the line to the last player, who runs to the front of the line and then passes the balloon through his or her feet to the player behind.

- This alternating process continues until the teams revert to the positions they were in at the beginning of the game.

- The first team to reach its original position wins.

EGG-CUP RACE

Age 10+   **Players Teams**

EQUIPMENT

Two egg cups and a table-tennis ball are needed for each team. The egg cups should not be so large that a table-tennis ball, when placed in one, cannot be blown out.

PREPARATION

Players are separated into two teams. They sit on opposite sides of a table.

PLAY

- After 'Go!' the first player in each team takes the egg cups and puts the table-tennis ball in the first egg-cup. The idea is to blow the ball into the next egg cup, which can be as close as the players wish to the first one.

- When this is achieved, table-tennis ball and egg cups are passed on to the next member of the team, who has to do the same.

- The first team in which everyone has managed to blow the table-tennis ball into the second egg cup is the winner.

GOING AWAY
Age 5+ **Players Teams**

EQUIPMENT
Two suitcases packed with old clothes. One will be full of female clothes and objects; the other full of male clothes and items.

PREPARATION
The players are arranged into two equal teams – one of males and one of females. The teams stand as far away from the suitcases as possible.

PLAY
- When they are told to start, the first player from each team hops to the suitcase containing male items if the player is female – or a case containing female items if the player is male.

- The players put on the clothes and, if there is any make-up, or wigs or toiletries, they should attempt to utilise these in some way. Each then picks up the suitcase and hops back to the starting line. Once there, they remove the clothes and replace them in the cases.

- They now hop back to the end of the room with the cases, drop them and run back to the start. The next player performs the same routine.

- The first team to complete the course wins.

HOOP RACE
Age 5+   Players Teams

EQUIPMENT
Two hoops. Alternatively, two rings made from string can be used.

PREPARATION
Players are divided into two teams of equal numbers.

PLAY
- The teams stand in two lines.

- When they are given the word 'Go!', the first player takes the hoop, passes it over his or her head and steps through it, before passing it on to the player behind.

- This goes on down the line.

- When the last person in the line has stepped through the hoop, he or she runs with it to the front of the line and the game continues.

- The winning team is the first that has its players back in their original positions.

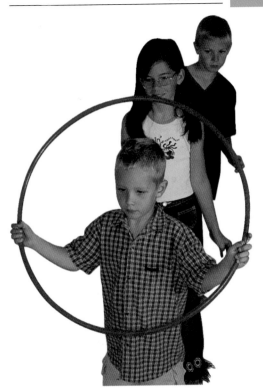

HURRY, WAITER!

Age 5+ **Players** Teams

Aim

Players try to keep a table-tennis ball balanced on a plate while weaving in and out of a line of their team-mates.

Play

- Players divide into teams and stand in a line behind their leaders. Each leader is given a table-tennis ball on a plate.

- At the word 'Go!' he weaves in and out between the players in his team as quickly as he can without dropping the ball.

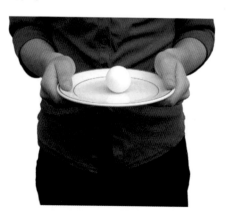

- When he reaches the end of the line, he runs straight to the head of the line again and hands the plate and ball to the next player, saying 'Here is your breakfast, Sir (or Madam)' as he does so.

- This procedure is repeated, with each player beginning at the head of the line and returning to his place as soon as he has handed the 'breakfast' to the next player in turn.

- If a player drops the ball, he must go back to the head of the line and start again. The first team to finish wins the game.

PIGGY-BACK RACE

Age 7+   **Players** Teams

This is another race in which pairs of players try to be the first to run a course.

PLAY

- Players form pairs and line up at one end of the room. One player from each pair gets on the other's back to be carried.

- At the word 'Go!' the pairs race to the other end of the room, where they must change places so that the carrier becomes the carried.

- They must then race back to the original end of the room. If a player touches the floor while he is being carried, that pair must start again.

PASSING THE ORANGE

Age 5+

Players Teams

Aim
Seated players try to pass an
orange down the line using
their chins, or (in an
alternative version) by
using their feet!

Play
- Players divide into
  teams and stand in a line
  beside their leaders.
  Each leader is given
  an orange which is
  tucked between
  chin and chest.
  On the word

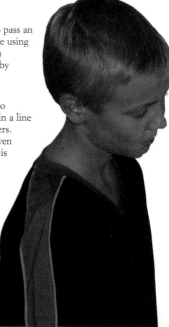

'Go!' he passes the orange to the next player – neither player may use his hands. (Alternatively, the players sit side-by-side in a line on the floor and the leader, legs together, cradles the orange on his feet. He then passes it to the feet of the next player.

- Using either one of these ways, the orange is passed from player to player. If the orange drops on the floor, or if a player uses his hands, the orange is returned to the leader to start again.

- The first team to pass the orange down the line wins.

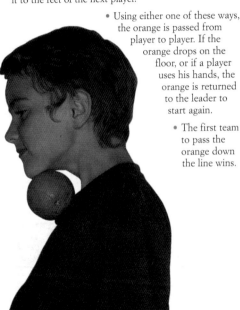

POTATO RACE

Age 5+ **Players Group**

Equipment
Five potatoes, two plates and one spoon are needed for each player.

Preparation
For each player, place a spoon on a plate at the starting line. Place another plate, holding five potatoes, on a line a few metres away.

Play
- On the word 'Go!' each player has to pick up a spoon, run to the plate containing the potatoes and – using only the spoon – scoop up the first potato. Each now runs back to the starting line and deposits the potato on the plate there.

- This procedure continues until all five potatoes have been successfully carried to the plate at the starting line.

- Players must only use one hand to carry the spoon. If a potato drops onto the ground, it must be scooped up again into the spoon.

- The winner is the first player to transport all their potatoes from one plate to the other.

THREE-LEGGED RACE

Age 5+   **Players** Group

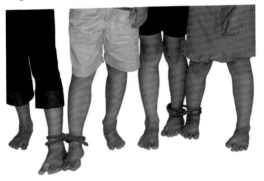

AIM

Pairs of players try to be the first to run from one end of the room to the other.

EQUIPMENT

A scarf is needed to tie together the legs of the players in each pair.

PLAY

- Players form pairs and line up at one end of the room. The scarves are used to tie the right leg of one of the players in the pair to the left leg of his or her partner. At the word 'Go!' pairs race to the other end of the room.

TORTOISE RACE
Age 5+

Players Group

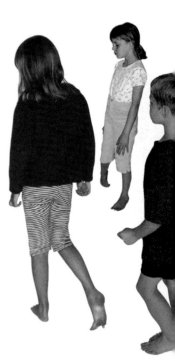

AIM
Each player tries to
be the last to finish.

PLAY
- Players line up
  along one side of
  the room. At the
  word 'Go!' they
  each start to move
  across the room as
  slowly as possible.
  They must head
  straight for the
  opposite wall.

- A player is
  disqualified if he
  or she stops
  moving or changes
  direction.

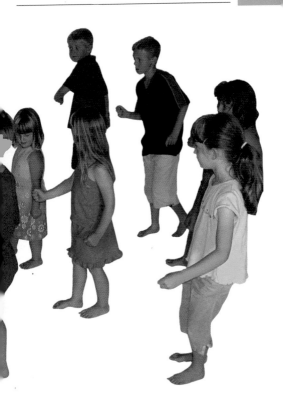

WOOL TANGLES

Age 5+   Players Teams

AIM

Teams of four players try to be first to untangle balls of yarn wrapped around chairs.

PREPARATION

A chair and four differently coloured balls of yarn are needed for each team.

PLAY

• Players form into teams of four. Each team is given four balls of yarn and a chair.

• Teams are then allowed about one minute in which to tangle their yarn around their chairs. They are not allowed to lift up their chairs or to make deliberate knots in the yarn.

• At the end of the time limit, the organiser calls 'Stop!' and teams must move around to a different chair.

• At the word 'Go!' teams start to disentangle the yarn from their new chair. Each player winds one of the balls of yarn. Players are not allowed to pick up the chair or deliberately break the yarn.

• The game is won by the first team to untangle the yarn into four separate balls.

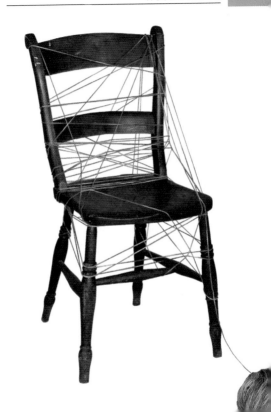

Dice Games

Dice games were played in ancient times and remain universally popular.

DICE
A standard modern die is a regular cube, with the six sides numbered with dots from 1 to 6. Any two opposing sides add up to 7.

ODDS
With one true die, each face has an equal chance of landing face up. With two dice thrown together, some scores are more likely than others because there are more ways in which they can be made.

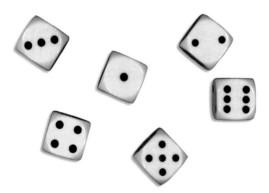

BEETLE

Age 8+   **Players 2**

EQUIPMENT

1) One die, either an ordinary one or a special 'beetle die' marked B (body), H (head), L (legs), E (eye), F (feeler) and T (tail);

2) a simple drawing of a beetle as a guide, showing its various parts and (when an ordinary die is used) their corresponding numbers (1=B; 2=H; 3=L; 4=E; 5=F; 6=T);

3) a pencil and a piece of paper for each player.

AIM

Each player, by throwing the die, tries to complete his drawing of the beetle.

PLAY

- Each player throws the die once only in each round. Each player must begin by throwing a B (or a 1); this permits the player to draw the body.

- When this has been drawn, he or she can throw for other parts of the beetle that can be joined to the body. An H or a 2 must be thrown to link the head to the body before the feelers (F or 5) and eyes (E or 4) can be added.

- Each eye or feeler requires its own throw. A throw of L or 3 permits the player to add three legs to one side of the body.

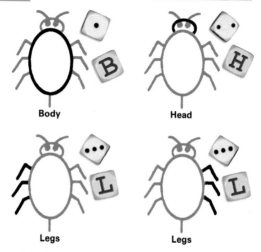

Body

Head

Legs

Legs

- A further throw of L or 3 is necessary for the other three legs. Sometimes it is agreed that a player may continue to throw during a turn for as long as he or she throws parts of the body that can be used.

- The first to complete his or her beetle scores 13 points and is the winner. The 13 points represent the total of each part of the beetle (body, head, tail, two feelers, two eyes and six legs).

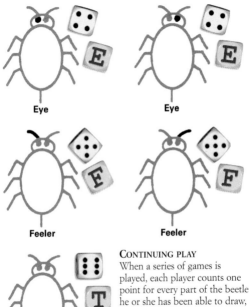

Eye

Eye

Feeler

Feeler

Tail

CONTINUING PLAY

When a series of games is played, each player counts one point for every part of the beetle he or she has been able to draw, and cumulative scores are carried from round to round. The winner is the player with the highest score at the end of the series or the first to reach a previously agreed total score.

CENTENNIAL
Age 10+   Players 2

Also known as Martinetti or Ohio.

Equipment
l) Three dice;

2) a long board or piece of paper marked with a row of boxes numbered 1 to 12;

3) a distinctive counter or some other object for each player.

Aim
Each player tries to be the first to move his or her counter, in accordance with throws of the dice, from 1 to 12 and back.

Play
• A preliminary round determines who will take the first turn (the player with the highest score).

• Each player on a turn throws all three dice at once.

• Turns pass clockwise around the table. In order to place his or her counter in the first box, a player must throw a 1. He or she can try then for a 2, a 3, and so on, box by box up to 12 and back again. He or she can make any number with one or more dice. For example, a 3 can be scored with one 3, a 1 and a 2, or with three 1s. It is possible to move through more than one box on a single throw. For example, a throw of 1, 2, 3 would not only take him or her through the first three boxes, but on through the fourth (1 + 3 = 4), to the fifth (2 + 3 = 5)

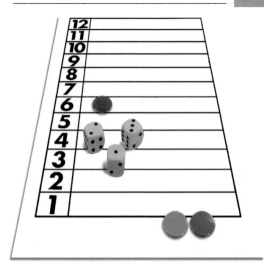

and finally the sixth (1 + 2 + 3 = 6). Other players' throws must be watched constantly. If a player throws a number he or she needs but overlooks and does not use it, that number may be claimed by any other player, who must do this as soon as the dice are passed and must be able to use it at once.

- The first player to get to 12 and back wins.

CHICAGO

Age 8+   **Players 2**

EQUIPMENT
Two dice are used.

AIM
To score each of 11 combinations in turn.

PLAY
- The game is based on the 11 possible combinations of the two dice – 2, 3, 4, 5, 6, 7, 8, 9, 10, 11 and 12 – and so consists of 11 rounds.

- Each player in turn rolls the dice once in each round. During the first round, he or she will try to make a total of 2, during the second, a total of 3, and so on, up to 12. Each time the player is successful, that number of points is added to his or her score. For example, if he or she is shooting for 5 and throws a total of 5, the player gains 5 points. If he or she fails to make the desired number, he or she scores nothing on that throw.

- The player with the highest score after the 11 rounds is the winner.

	Player 1	Player 2
Round 1	= 0	= 2

	Player 1	Player 2
Round 2	= 0	= 0
Round 3	= 4	= 0
Round 4	= 0	= 5
Round 5	= 6	= 6
Round 6	= 0	= 0
Round 7	= 0	= 0
Round 8	= 9	= 0
Round 9	= 10	= 0
Round 10	= 0	= 11
Round 11	= 0	= 12
TOTAL	29	36

CHEERIO
Age 10+   **Players 2**

EQUIPMENT

1) Five dice;

2) a dice cup;

3) a sheet of paper showing the various combinations and a scoring column for each player.

AIM

Each player tries to score the maximum possible for each of the 11 scoring combinations. Games are often played as a series, the player who wins the most games in the series being the overall winner. Alternatively, the scores in each game can be carried forward to the next game until a player has reached a previously agreed cumulative total. If two or more players exceed the total, the player with the highest score wins. Ties are settled by an extra game.

PLAY

• Each player in turn rolls all five dice.

• Having rolled the dice once, he or she may pick up all or any of them and roll once more in an attempt to improve the score. He or she does not have to try for combinations in any particular order, and does not have to declare the combination until he or she has finished rolling. This gives the player considerable freedom of choice. For example, if he or she has rolled 6, 6, 2, 3, 3 he or she might call 'Sixes' (score 12). But if he or she wanted to keep Sixes for a later turn, when he or she might roll more than two of them, the player could call a different combination even if this would give him or her a lower score or no score. A player cannot call the same combination more than once in a game.

- The player with the highest total score wins the game.

COMBINATIONS

Ones Scores one point for each die showing one spot (max. score five points – score here = 3 points).

Twos Scores two for each two-spot die (max. 10 – score here = 4 points).

Threes Scores three for each three-spot die (max. 15 – score here = 9 points).

Fours Scores four for each four-spot die (max. 20 – score here = 12 points).

Fives Scores five for each five-spot die (max. 25 – score here = 15 points).

Sixes Scores six for each six-spot die (max. 30 – score here = 18 points).

Little straight A show of 1, 2, 3, 4, 5 scores 20.

Big straight A show of 2, 3, 4, 5, 6 scores 25.

Full house Three of a kind plus two of a kind scores according to the numbers shown on the dice (6, 6, 6, 5, 5 scores the maximum 28 points – score here = 16 points).

Big hand The total spot value of the dice (6, 6, 6, 6, 6 scores the maximum 30 points – score here = 28 points).

Cheerio Five of a kind in any value, 1 to 6. Always scores 50 points.

Cheerio score sheet

	Jason	Debbie	Katie	Paul
1s	3		3	2
2s		8	4	
3s	3	9		
4s	16			12
5s		20		
6s				24
Little straight				
Big straight			25	
Full house	22		16	
Big hand				30
Cheerio		50		

DROP DEAD

Age 8+   **Players 2+**

EQUIPMENT

l) Five dice;

2) paper on which to record players' scores.

AIM

Players aim to make the highest total score.

PLAY

- At his or her turn, each player begins by rolling the five dice. Each time he or she makes a throw that does not contain a 2 or a 5, he or she scores the total spot value of that throw and is entitled to another throw with all five dice.

- Whenever a player makes a throw containing a 2 or a 5, nothing is scored for that throw and any die or dice that showed a 2 or a 5 must be excluded from any further throws. A player's turn continues until his or her last remaining die shows a 2 or a 5 – at which point he or she 'drops dead' and play passes to the next player.

- The player who gains the highest score wins. The total score in the example shown here is 42 points.

Example of play

throw 1

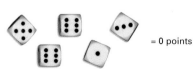

= 0 points

throw 2

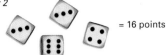 = 16 points

throw 3

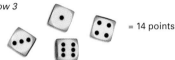 = 14 points

throw 4

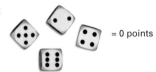 = 0 points

throw 5

= 9 points

throw 6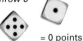

= 0 points

throw 7
= 3 points

throw 8
= 0 points

total score = 42

FIFTY

Age 8+

Players 2

EQUIPMENT
Two dice.

PLAY
- Each player in turn rolls the two dice, but scores only when identical numbers are thrown (two 1s, two 2s, and so on). All these doubles, except two 6s and two 3s, score five points. A double 6 scores 25 points; and a double 3 wipes out the player's total score and he or she has to start again.

- The winner is the first player to reach the score of 50 points.

 two 1s
= 5 points

 two 2s
= 5 points

 two 3s
= wipe score

 two 4s
= 5 points

 two 5s
= 5 points

 two 6s
= 25 points

GENERAL

Age 10+   **Players** 2

AIM

Each player or partnership aims to win by scoring a 'big general' (see Five of a kind, page 150) or by scoring most points for the 10 general combinations. As in Cheerio, each combination may be scored only once in a game.

EQUIPMENT

1) Five dice;

2) a score sheet showing combinations and players' names.

ORDER OF PLAY

Determined by a preliminary round in which each player rolls the dice once. The player with the lowest spot score shoots first, the player with the next lowest score second, and so on.

PLAY

- A game normally consists of 10 turns ('frames') per player, but ends immediately if any player rolls a 'big general'. Players take it in turn to roll each frame.

- Each player may roll the dice once, twice, or three times during each frame. If, on the first throw, the player fails to make a combination that he or she wishes to score, he or she may pick up all or any of the dice for a second roll. But the value of any combination he or she now rolls is diminished, and a 'big general' now becomes a 'small general'.

- After the second roll the player may again, if he or she wishes, pick up all or any of the dice for a third roll.

- After the third roll, he or she must state which combination he or she is scoring.

- Play then passes to the next player.

- If the game runs its full course of 10 frames, the player with the highest score wins.

ACES WILD

'Aces' (1s) may be counted as 2 or as 6 if one or both of these are needed to complete a Straight – but not as any other number or for any other purpose.

COMBINATIONS

Numbers 1 to 6 Score their spot values.

Straight Either 1, 2, 3, 4, 5 or 2, 3, 4, 5, 6 scores 25 points if made on the first throw, but only 20 points if made on the second or third throws. Only one straight is scored.

Full house Three of a kind and two of a kind score 35 points on the first throw but only 30 points on the second or third throws.

Four of a kind Scores 45 points on the first throw, but only 40 points on the second or third throws.

Five of a kind If made on the first throw it ranks as the 'big general' and immediately wins the game. Made on the second or third throws it is a 'small general' and scores 60 points.

Player 1

frame 1

throw 1

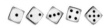

throw 2

= straight = 20 points

frame 2

throw 1

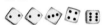

throw 2

= full house = 30 points

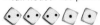

Player 2

throw 1

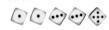

throw 2

= straight = 20 points

throw 1

throw 2

throw 3

= fours = 12 points

Player 1

Player 2

frame 3

throw 1

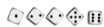

throw 1

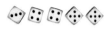

throw 2

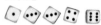

throw 2

throw 3

throw 3

= 3s = 6 points

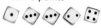

= full house = 30 points

	Player 1	Player 2
1s		
2s		
3s	6	
4s		12
5s		
6s		
Straight	20	20
Full house	30	30
Four of a kind		
Five of a kind		

DOUBLE CAMEROON

Age 10+   **Players 2**

This game is like General, but with important differences.

EQUIPMENT
Ten dice.

PLAY
- After a player has rolled the dice for the third time in each turn, he or she divides them into two groups of five, and then allots the score of each group to one of the 10 combinations in the game. So in the course of a game, each player has five turns.

COMBINATIONS
Numbers 1 to 6 Score their spot values.

Full house Scores its spot value.

Little Cameroon 1, 2, 3, 4, 5 scores 21 points.

Big Cameroon 2, 3, 4, 5, 6 scores 30 points.

Five of a kind Scores 50 points.

NB: Unlike in General, a score does not decrease if the combination is made on a second or third throw.

GOING TO BOSTON

Age 8+   Players 2

Also known as Newmarket or Yankee Grab.

EQUIPMENT
Three dice.

AIM
Players try to win as many of an agreed number of rounds as they can.

PLAY
- Each player in turn rolls the three dice together.

- After the first roll, the player leaves the dice showing the highest number on the table then rolls the other two again. Of these, the die with the highest number is also left on the table and the remaining die is rolled again.

- This completes the player's throw: the total of the three dice is his or her score.

- When all players have thrown, the player with the highest score wins the round. Ties are settled by further rolling.

- The player who wins the most rounds is the winner. Alternatively, each player can contribute counters to a pool that is won at the end of each game.

VARIATION
A variation known as Multiplication is played like Going to Boston, but with one important difference. When each player has completed a turn, his or her score is the sum of

the spot values of the first two dice retained, multiplied by that of the third. For example, if the player's first throw is 5, the second throw 4, and the final throw 6, the score will be 54: (5 + 4) x 6.

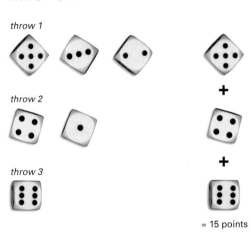

throw 1

throw 2

throw 3

+

+

= 15 points

multiplication

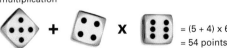

= (5 + 4) x 6
= 54 points

HEARTS

Age 10+

Players 2

AIM

Players try to score more than their opponents over an agreed series of rounds, or a single round, or to be the first to reach an agreed total.

EQUIPMENT

Six dice. Special dice marked with the letters H, E, A, R, T, S instead of numbers are sometimes used, but the game is now more commonly played with ordinary dice.

PLAY

- A preliminary round decides the first shooter (the player with the highest score).

- Each player in turn rolls the six dice once and calculates his or her score according to the following ratings:

  1 (H) = 5 points;
  1, 2 (HE) = 10 points;
  1, 2, 3 (HEA) = 15 points;
  1, 2, 3, 4 (HEAR) = 20 points;
  1, 2, 3, 4, 5 (HEART) = 25 points;
  1, 2, 3, 4, 5, 6 (HEARTS) = 35 points.

  If any numbers are missing from the sequence, the player can score only up to the missing number: i.e, 1, 2, 3, 5, 5, 6 will only score 15 points; 2, 3, 4, 4, 5, 6 will score nothing at all. If a double (two dice of the same spot value) or a treble appears in the throw, only one of the numbers or letters counts. But if three 1s (or Hs) are thrown, the player's whole score is wiped out and he or she has to start again.

- The player with the highest score wins.

Player 1 *round 1*

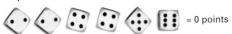 = 0 points

Player 2 *round 1*

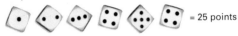 = 25 points

Player 1 *round 2*

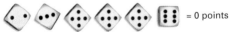 = 0 points

Player 2 *round 2*

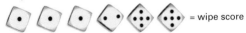 = wipe score

Player 1 *round 3*

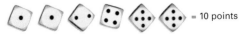 = 10 points

Player 2 *round 3*

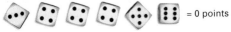 = 0 points

PIG

Age 8+   **Players 2**

AIM

Using one die, players try to reach an agreed total score (usually 100) before the other players.

ORDER OF PLAY

This is determined by a preliminary round. Each player throws the die once and the player with the lowest score becomes first shooter. The next lowest scoring player shoots second, and so on. The order of play is important because the first and last shooters have natural advantages.

PLAY

- The first shooter begins. Like the other players, he or she may roll the die as many times as he or she wishes.

- The score is totalled throw by throw until he or she elects to end his or her turn.

- He or she passes the die to the next player, memorising his or her score so far.

- But if a player throws a 1, he or she loses the entire score he or she has made on that turn, and the die passes to the next player.

- Play passes from player to player until someone reaches the total score agreed.

Given a little luck, the first shooter is the player most likely to win. But his or her advantage can be counteracted by other players continuing until they have had the same number of turns. The last shooter still has the advantage of knowing the scores made by all his or her opponents. Provided a player does not roll a 1, he or she can continue throwing until all those scores are beaten. The fairest way of playing the game is to organise it as a series, with each player in turn becoming first shooter.

- The winner is the first player to reach the previously agreed total score.

Player 1	Player 2	Player 3	Player 4

Player 3 — out

Player 2 — stops, scores 21

Player 4 — stops, scores 23

Player 1 — out

ROUND THE CLOCK

Age 8+   **Players** 2

AIM

Players try to throw 1 to 12 in the correct sequence.

EQUIPMENT

Two dice.

PLAY

- Players throw both dice once in each turn. From 1 to 6, a player can score with either one of the two dice or with both of them – e.g. a throw of 3 and 1 can be counted as 3, 1 or 4. It is also possible at this stage to score twice on one throw, e.g. if a player needs 2 and throws a 2 and a 3 he or she can count both of these numbers. From 7 to 12, however, a player will obviously always need the combined spot values of both dice to score. The table shows the combinations possible.

- The winner is the first to complete the correct sequence.

2			
3			
4			

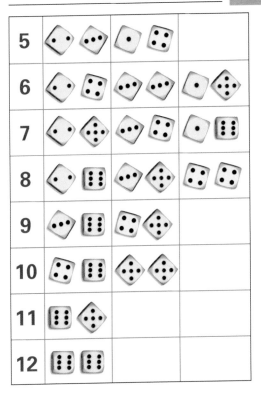

SHUT THE BOX

Age 8+   Players 2

AIM
Players aim to cover as many of the numbers as possible, in accordance with the throws of the dice.

EQUIPMENT
1) Two dice;

2) a board or sheet of paper with nine drawn boxes numbered 1 to 9;

3) nine counters used to cover the boxes in play.

PLAY
- The player taking the first turn throws the two dice and then decides which two boxes he or she will cover. Any two boxes that have the same total as the throw may be covered – e.g. a throw of 5 and 3 (total 8) would allow the player to cover 5 and 3, 4 and 4 or 6 and 2.

 a

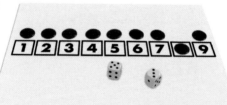

- The same player then throws the two dice again and tries to cover another two boxes. He or she is not allowed to use combinations involving numbers that he has already covered. In the example, with the 8 covered (**a**) and two sixes thrown, only 9 and 3 or 7 and 5 could be covered (**b**).

- A player's turn continues until he or she is unable to make use of a combination from his or her latest throw. (Note that as the two dice must be used for every throw a player with only the 1 uncovered cannot continue.) All the uncovered numbers are then added up and become the player's penalty score.

- Play then passes to the next player.

- The winner is the player with the lowest penalty score from uncovered boxes.

b

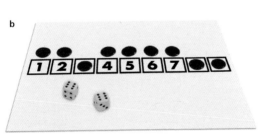

TWENTY-ONE

Age 10+   **Players 2**

EQUIPMENT
One die, paper, pencil and a box of matches (or several counters).

PLAY
- Each player is given an equal number of matches (or counters). They all contribute one to the 'bank'. One player is chosen to start off.

- The player rolls the die as many times as he or she likes, trying to get as close to a total of 21 as possible. At any stage, the player can 'stick', and the total is recorded. For example, if a player has scored 19 after a few throws, the chances are that the next throw will take the score to over 21, so the player may decide to 'stick' with what he or she has got.

- The other players then make their attempts to score 21. Any player throwing a number that takes the total over 21 goes 'bust'.

- At the end of each round, the player with the highest total, not exceeding 21, takes all the matches in the bank. Players who score the same amount can either share the winnings or have a play-off to decide who takes them.

- After a few rounds, unlucky – or unskilful – players may run out of matches. They must then drop out of the game.

- The game can continue for a fixed period of time, after which the player with the highest number of matches will be the winner. Alternatively, the first player to amass a certain number of matches may be declared the winner.

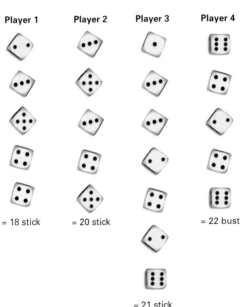

| Player 1 | Player 2 | Player 3 | Player 4 |

= 18 stick   = 20 stick   = 22 bust

= 21 stick

Fivestones and Jacks

Age 8+　　　　**Players 2**

Fivestones is an old game, known
in different places by different
names such as Knucklebones
(because it used to be played
with the knucklebones of
sheep) and Chuckies.

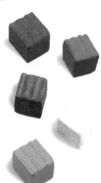

Aim

To complete a sequence of
small games, chiefly using
only one hand. If played with
other players, the aim is to
complete the sequence
ahead of the others.

ONES

Play

• All the fivestones are held in the palm of one hand.

• They are thrown upwards; while they are in the air the
hand is turned over and the player tries to catch the
fivestones on the back of the hand. If successful, he or
she moves on to the next game of Twos. If the player
catches only some of the stones, he or she puts all but
one on the floor, throws the remaining one in the air and
tries to pick the rest up one by one with the throwing
hand before catching the one in the air with the same
hand. The stones can be transferred to the free hand.

TWOS

PLAY

- Four of the fivestones are scattered on the floor.

- The remaining one is thrown in the air and the player tries to pick up two of the four with the throwing hand in time to catch the one in the air with the same hand.

- If successful, he or she throws again to pick up the remaining pair. Beginners are allowed to use their throw to nudge the scattered fivestones closer together. Experts must pick them up where they lie.

THREES

PLAY

- Four fivestones are scattered on the floor.

- The remaining one is thrown, and the player picks up one from the ground.

- He or she throws again and picks up the remaining three, all with the throwing hand.

FOURS

PLAY

- Played like Twos and Threes, but all four scattered fivestones must be picked up at once.

PECKS

PLAY

- The four fivestones are scattered, and must be picked up one by one.

- The stones picked up cannot be transferred to the free hand and must be kept in the throwing hand.

BUSHELS

PLAY

- The fivestones are thrown up (**1**) and caught on the back of the hand (**2**), thrown again and caught in the palm.

- Any not caught are then picked up one by one (**3**), but none of the stones may be transferred to the free hand.

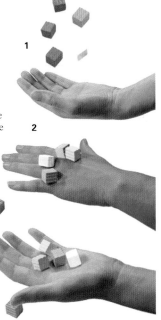

CLAWS

PLAY

- The fivestones are thrown and caught on the back of the hand.

- If all are caught they are thrown again and caught in the palm.

- If some are dropped, the caught ones are kept on the back of the hand, and the others are picked up between the fingers or finger and thumb.

- Then the stones on the back of the hand are thrown and caught in the palm, and the stones between the fingers manoeuvred into the palm. If the stones on the back of the hand fall at any stage, the player must begin again.

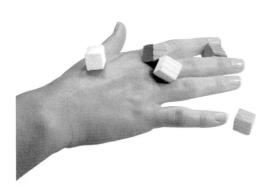

ONES UNDER THE ARCH

PLAY

- The free hand forms an arch with the thumb and forefinger. The stones are scattered and one picked up to throw.

- As the stone is thrown, one of the scattered stones is knocked through the arch with the throwing hand before the stone in the air is caught.

- This is repeated until all the stones are through the arch. Beginners can take a throw to manoeuvre the stone before knocking it through the arch.

TWOS UNDER THE ARCH

PLAY

- The game proceeds as Ones Under the Arch, but the scattered stones must be pushed through the arch two at a time. As before, beginners may take a throw to manoeuvre the scattered stones before knocking them through.

THREES UNDER THE ARCH

PLAY

- As before, but three stones must be pushed through in one throw, and then the remaining one.

FOURS UNDER THE ARCH

PLAY

- As before, but all four stones must be knocked through the arch in one throw.

STABLES

PLAY

- The game is played in a way similar to Under the Arches games, but instead of an arch, the free hand forms a series of 'stables' between the fingers.

- One stone should be knocked into each stable. As before, beginners can take throws to manoeuvre the stones first.

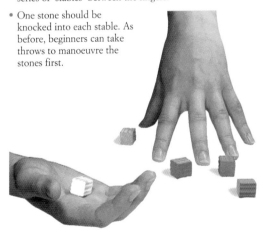

TOAD-IN-THE-HOLE

PLAY

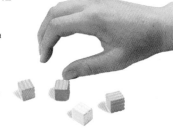

- The game is a bit like Under the Arch, but instead of an arch, the free hand forms a 'cave' in the way shown.

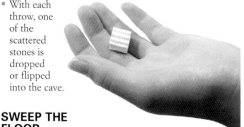

- With each throw, one of the scattered stones is dropped or flipped into the cave.

SWEEP THE FLOOR

PLAY

- This is a sequence of actions, accompanied by spoken words. The stones, except for one throwing stone, are scattered.

- First, the stone is thrown and the throwing hand wipes the table as the player says, 'Sweep the floor!'

- Second, one of the scattered stones is moved as the player says, 'Move the chair!'

- Third, the 'chair' is picked up and the player says 'Pick it up!'

- Last, the chair is put back on the table or ground again, 'Put it down!'

- In the second round, all these actions are repeated, but the table receives two wipes, and two chairs are moved, picked up and put down.

- In the third round everything is done in threes, and in threes, and in the fourth, by fours.

Players who make any mistakes return to the beginning of that round.

SNAKE IN THE GRASS

PLAY

- Four of the fivestones are placed in a line a few inches apart.

- The remaining stone is thrown, and the first of the four in a row is moved as far as possible in and out of the others until it is brought back to where it started. Players can take as many throws as they like, but obviously the fewer the better.

BIG BEN

PLAY

- A tower is built of four of the fivestones.

- The remaining stone is thrown and the topmost stone from the tower is removed and placed in the non-throwing hand. If the tower topples, it must be rebuilt and the game started again.

- The game continues until the tower has been dismantled.

- When the last stone is picked up, the throwing stone should be caught in the non-throwing hand, so that all the stones are together in that hand.

- The game can also be played in reverse, the four stones held in the non-throwing hand, and each stone placed on top of the next in throws.

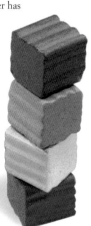

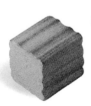

JACKS

Nearly all of the games for fivestones can also be played with jacks and a rubber ball. There are five jacks. Only the ball is thrown, and is allowed one bounce before being caught.

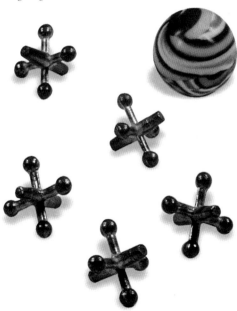

Spellicans

Age 5+   **Players 2**

This game, which originated in China, is also called
Spillikins. Players try their skill at removing straws or small
sticks from a pile, one at a time and without disturbing any
of their neighbours. Any number of players can take part.

EQUIPMENT

Spellicans is played with a set of about 30 thin strips of
wood or plastic. These strips, called spellicans, have
carved heads representing animals, people, etc. There is
also a carved hook for moving the strips.

START OF PLAY

The order of play is determined by the throw of a die or
some other means. The last person in the playing order
then takes all the spellicans in one hand and drops them
onto the table or floor. He must not interfere with any
spellican after it has left his hand.

PLAY

- At his or her turn, each player takes the carved hook
  and attempts to remove a spellican from the pile without
  disturbing any of the others. Once a player has started
  moving a particular spellican, he or she is not permitted
  to transfer the attack to a different spellican.

- If the player successfully removes a spellican from the
  pile, he or she keeps it and tries to remove another
  spellican from the pile. A player's turn continues until a
  spellican other than the one being attacked is disturbed.

- Play continues in this way until all the spellicans have been taken.

- Each spellican has a points value, and a game is won by the player with the highest score. Spellicans that are generally fairly easy to move have a low value, and more elaborate and difficult to move spellicans have a correspondingly higher value.

JACKSTRAWS

Age 5+   **Players 2**

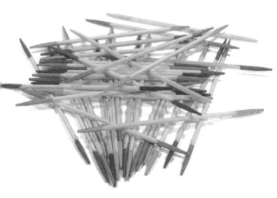

The game is similar to Spellicans. Alternative names are Jackstraws/Jerkstraws, Juggling Sticks and Pick-a-stick.

Equipment

Jackstraws is played with about 50 wood or plastic sticks or straws. These are about 15 cm (6 in) long, rounded and with pointed ends, and they are coloured according to their point value.

Play

* The rules are the same as for Spellicans except that players remove the sticks with their fingers or, in some versions of the game, may use a stick of a specified colour after they have drawn one from the pile.

LAST MATCH

Age 5–10   Players 2

Preparation

A box of about 50 matches is needed, and they should be struck first to eliminate any risk of children doing so.

Aim

To be able to pick up the last match.

Play

* Each player decides on a number between 1 and 10 – this is the maximum number of matches he may pick up in any round.

* The matches are tipped in a heap, and players pick up as many matches as they wish, within their limit.

* They continue until all the matches have been picked up.

* The player who picks up the last match wins.

SQUAYLES

Age 5-10   Players 2

PREPARATION

As with the other matchstick games, the matches should
be struck and extinguished before being used. Any
number of matches are arranged in a pattern of squares.

AIM

To be able to pick up the last match.

PLAY

- The players take turns to pick up matches. They may
take one or two at a time, provided the two are next to
each other, though they do not have to be in a straight
line.

- The winner is the player who picks up the last match.

Start of play

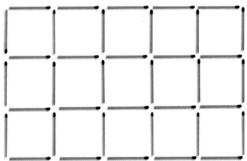

Tiddlywinks

Age 5+ **Players 2**

In the standard game of Tiddlywinks, each player attempts to put small discs or 'winks' into a cup by shooting them with a larger disc called a 'shooter'. Variations include games based on sports such as tennis and golf.

EQUIPMENT

Each player usually has a shooter and four winks. A target cup is also needed. Winks and shooters must be slightly pliable and are commonly made of bone or plastic. Winks are usually about 1.5 cm (about 0.5 in) and shooters about 2.5 cm (1 in) in diameter. Each player's winks and shooters should be of a different colour.

Target cups are made of plastic, wood, or glass and are about 4 cm (1.5 in) across and 2.5–5 cm (1–2 in) high.

shooters

PLAYING AREA

Games are played on the floor or on a table. Any shape of table may be used but a square or round one is best if there are more than two players. The table should be covered with a thick cloth or piece of felt.

winks

STANDARD TIDDLYWINKS

SHOOTING

A player shoots a wink by stroking and then pressing the edge of the shooter against the top edge of the wink and so making the wink jump into the air. A wink is shot from where it lies after the player's previous turn.

PLAY

- The cup is placed in the centre of the playing area, and each player places his or her winks in a line in front of him.

- Order of play is often decided by a preliminary shot – first shot of the game going to the player who gets his or her wink nearest the cup.

- Play is then usually clockwise around the players. Each player shoots one wink in a turn plus one extra shot each time he or she gets a wink into the cup. Any wink that is partly covered by another is out of play. A player whose wink is covered by an opponent's wink must either wait until the opponent moves his or her wink or must attempt to remove the opponent's wink by hitting it with one of his or her own winks. Any wink that stops against the side of the cup is out of play until it is knocked level onto the table by another wink. A wink that is shot off the table does not go out of play. It must be replaced on the table at the point where it went off.

- Tiddlywinks may be scored in two ways:

  a) players count the number of games they win;

  b) players score one point for each wink in the cup.

- The game is won by the first player to get all his or her tiddlywinks in the cup.

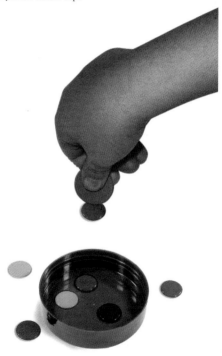

TARGET TIDDLYWINKS

This involves shooting winks at numbered targets. A typical layout is a target with concentric circles each worth a different set number of points.

PLAY

- Target Tiddlywinks is played in the same way as the standard game except that:

  a) players score a set number of points for landing their winks on different parts of the target (a wink touching two scoring areas always scores the lower number);

  b) a wink may not be shot again once it has landed on any part of the target, but may be knocked by another wink.

- The player with the highest score wins. This player has scored 50 + 10 + 5 + 5 = 70 points.

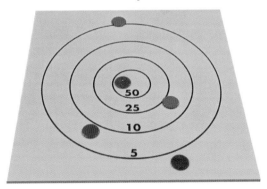

TIDDLYWINKS TENNIS

PREPARATION

The lines of a tennis court should be marked on the floor
or the tiddlywinks cloth. (Dimensions for the court should
be varied to suit the skill of the players and the height of
the net.) An improvised net can be made with folded
paper or card, or with a row of books.

PLAY

- Players shoot a wink back and forth over the net,
  gaining points whenever their opponents fail to get the
  wink over the net or shoot it so that it goes outside the
  limits of the court. The game can be played by two
  players (singles) or four players (doubles). In the
  doubles version, partners take alternate turns to shoot
  the wink from their side of the net. Rules for service can
  be modified to suit the skill of the players – e.g. extra
  shots allowed to get the wink over the net or no
  restrictions on where in the opponent's court the wink
  must land.

- A match is scored in games and sets as in ordinary
  tennis, with the first player to win three sets taking
  the match.

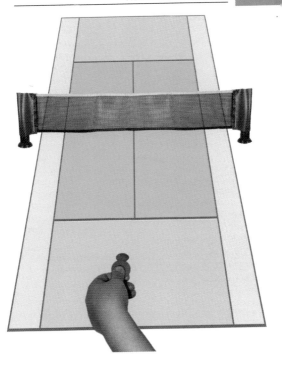

Spoken Word Games

ALL'S WELL THAT ENDS WELL
Age 10+   **Players** Group

PLAY

- Players must first choose a category – for example, food, places, animals or famous sports stars.

- The first player says a word from that category. If food is chosen, she might say 'eggs'.

- The next player then has to name a food that begins with the last letter of the previous word. So he might respond with 'salami'.

- The next player could say 'ice cream', and so on.

- Players who cannot think of a new food, who answer with a food that has already been said, or answer with a word that is not in the correct category, drop out. Players can make it difficult for one another by saying a food that ends with an awkward letter.

- The winner is the last player left in after the others have been eliminated.

EGGS
SALAMI
ICE CREAM
MERINGUE
ENDIVE
E?

ANIMAL, VEGETABLE OR MINERAL

Age 5–10   **Players** Group

Sometimes called Twenty Questions, this game is one of the oldest and most familiar word-guessing games.

AIM

Players try to guess an object thought of by one of the others.

PLAY

- One of the players thinks of an object. It may be general (e.g. 'a ship'), specific (e.g. 'the Lusitania'), or a feature (e.g. 'the bridge of the Lusitania').

- He or she then tells the others the composition of his chosen object (i.e. animal, vegetable or mineral). The three categories may be defined as follows:

  1) animal: all forms of animal life or anything of animal origin, e.g. a centipede, a tortoiseshell button;

  2) vegetable: all forms of vegetable life or anything of vegetable origin, e.g. a wooden cotton reel, a carrot;

  3) mineral: anything inorganic or of inorganic origin, e.g. glass, a car. Objects are often a combination of categories, for example, a can of beer or a leather shoe.

- The other players then ask up to 20 questions to try to guess the object. They should ask questions of a general nature rather than make random guesses, until they feel confident that they are near to knowing the object.

- As each question is put to the player, he or she must reply either 'Yes' or 'No', or 'I don't know', as appropriate.

- The first player to guess the object correctly may choose an object for a new round of play. If no one has guessed the object by the time 20 questions have been asked, the players are told what it was, and the same person may choose an object for the next round or – if two teams are playing – a person in the other team may choose.

BOTTICELLI

Age 10+   **Players Group**

AIM

Players try to guess the identity of a personality by asking questions.

PLAY

- One player chooses the name of a famous person and tells the other players the initial of the name. For example, he or she might say 'M' for Madonna.

- Taking turns, each player must think of a character whose name begins with that letter, and describe the character without naming the person he or she has in mind. If he or she thought of Mickey Mouse, he would ask, 'Are you a Walt Disney character?'

- If the first player recognises the description, he or she answers, 'No, I am not Mickey Mouse,' and another player may make a guess.

- If the first player does not recognise the description, however, the player who gave it may then ask a direct question that will give him or her and the other players a lead, such as 'Are you in the entertainment business?'

- The first player must give a truthful 'Yes' or 'No' reply. The first person to guess the personality wins the round and may choose the next character. If nobody succeeds in guessing the personality after a reasonable length of time, the first player tells them the answer and may choose again for the new round.

BUZZ
Age 10+   **Players** Group

This game should be played as briskly as possible for maximum enjoyment.

AIM
To count numbers remembering which ones to replace with the word 'Buzz'.

PLAY
- The players sit in a circle.

- One player calls out 'One', the next player 'Two', the next 'Three', and so on.

- As soon as the number five, or any multiple of five, is reached, the players must say 'Buzz'. If the number contains a five but is not a multiple of five, only part of it is replaced by buzz. (For example, 52 would be 'Buzz two'.) If a player forgets to say 'Buzz' or hesitates too long, he or she drops out.

- The last player remaining in the game is the winner.

Buzz

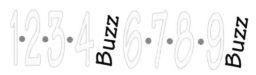

1·2·3·4·*Buzz*·6·7·8·9·*Buzz*

VARIATIONS

A variation is called Fizz. This is played exactly like Buzz, except that players say 'Fizz' for seven or multiples of seven. Another variation, Buzz-Fizz, combines the two games, so that 57, for example, becomes Buzz-Fizz.

Fizz

5·6·*Fizz*·8·9·10·11·12·13·*Fizz*

Buzz-Fizz

1·2·3·4·*Buzz*·6·*Fizz*·8·9·*Buzz*

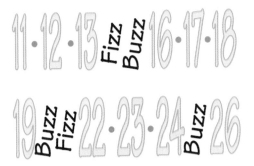

CHINESE WHISPERS

Age 5+   **Players** Group

PLAY

- Players sit in a circle on the floor or along the length of a table. Get one of them to think of a sentence. It should not be spoken out loud.

- The first player quietly whispers the sentence to the person on his or her left.

- That person then whispers the sentence to the next person in the line. The sentence should only be spoken once and never out loud. On and on it goes until the last player.

- The last person then announces the sentence in the form that it has arrived at the end of the line. The first person then announces what the original sentence was. It will probably have changed quite a lot from the original version, causing a great deal of merriment.

- There are no winners in this game: it is played just for fun.

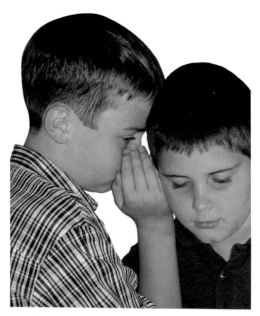

CRAZY CHEF

Age 5-10   Players Group

PREPARATION

Players form a circle, with one of them standing in the centre, who acts as the 'chef'.

PLAY

- The player in the centre must point to someone in the circle, saying – for example – 'I only like the letter M. What shall I cook for supper?'

- The player who has been pointed at now has to suggest something suitable for supper that contains that letter – for example, meat or hamburgers. Anything suggested must be edible and cooked, rather than eaten raw. If the player pointed at fails to come up with a suitable 'meal', he or she is out and leaves the circle.

- After each turn, the 'chef' asks for suggestions using another letter, but X, Y and Z are not allowed.

- 'Meals' cannot be suggested more than once. The game continues in this way until only one player is left.

- The last player left wins.

GHOSTS

Age 10+   **Players Group**

AIM

Players take it in turns to contribute a letter to an unstated word while trying to avoid completing any word.

PLAY

- The first player begins by thinking of any word (e.g. rabbit) and calls out the first letter (R).

- The next player then thinks of a word beginning with R (e.g. rescue) and calls out its second letter (E).

- Play then continues in this way until one of the players is unable to contribute a letter that does not complete a word.

- Whenever a player completes a word – and the other players notice – that player loses a 'life'. This is true even if the player completes a word by accident because they were thinking of another word.

- If a player is unable to think of a suitable word, they may try to bluff their way out of the situation by calling out a letter of an imaginary word.

- If, however, they hesitate for too long or the other players suspect that they have no particular word in mind, they may challenge the player. The challenged player must state the word and if they cannot do so lose a life. If the explanation is satisfactory, however, the challenger loses a life. Whenever a player loses a first life they becomes 'a third of a ghost'. Losing a second life makes them 'two-thirds of a ghost', and if a player loses a third life they become a whole ghost and must drop out of the game.

- The game is won by the player who manages to survive the longest.

R (abbit)
R E (scue)
R E P (lica)
R E P E (at)
R E P E A (t)
R E P E A L

I LOVE MY LOVE

Age 10+   **Players Group**

AIM

Players think of an adjective beginning with each letter of
the alphabet to complete a given statement.

PLAY

- The first player starts by saying, 'I love my love because
  he [or she] is . . .' using any adjective beginning with A.

- The next person repeats the phrase, but his or her
  adjective must begin with B, the next person's with C,
  and so on through the alphabet. Alternatively, each
  player must make a different statement as well as using
  an adjective with a different letter. Examples of suitable
  statements are: Her name is (Anna), she lives in
  (Arnhem), and I shall give her (an aardvark).

- Players may write down the chosen statements if they
  wish, but there must be no hesitation over the answers.

- Any player who hesitates or gives an incorrect answer
  drops out of the game.

- The winner is the last person left in.

VARIATION

A similar game, known as A Was An Apple Pie, involves
players thinking of a verb instead of an adjective. The first
player says: 'A was an apple pie. A ate it,' and other
players might add 'B baked it,' 'C chose it,' 'D dropped it,'
and so on.

Adjectives for playing I Love My Love

A attractive, attentive, alluring, appreciative
B bashful, beautiful, brainy, burlesque
C charming, cute, courteous, courageous
D dainty, dextrous, daring, different
E eccentric, effeminate, errant, extravagant
F fair, fun, flamboyant, forceful
G gallant, gorgeous, groovy, generous
H happy, hilarious, hearty, humble
I ingenious, illustrious, imaginative, intelligent
J jaunty, jolly, jubilant, joyful
K keen, kind, knowledgeable, kooky
L lenient, loyal, lively, lavish
M mad, mischievous, modish, mysterious
N natty, notorious, noble, nice
O obedient, optimistic, open-minded, outspoken
P polite, patient, prestigious, profound
Q quiet, qualitative, queenly, quick
R rebellious, resolute, resourceful, responsible
S silly, sagacious, sedate, skilful
T timid, thin, thoughtful, tolerant
U upstanding, understanding, unselfish, unflappable
V voracious, virtuous, vivacious, valiant
W warm, wholesome, wise, wonderful
X —
Y young, youthful, yummy
Z zany, zappy, zealous, zippy

I SPY
Age 5–10   Players Group

AIM
Each player tries to be the first to guess which visible object one of them has spied.

PLAY
- Two or more people can play, and one of them is chosen to start.

- He or she says, 'I spy, with my little eye, something beginning with . . .' and gives the first letter of an object that he or she has chosen and that is visible to all the players. (They may have to turn their heads in order to see the object, but they should not need to move about.) For example, if the player chose a vase, he or she would give the letter V or, if a two-word object was chosen, the first letter of each word (e.g. PF for picture frame). If the player chooses an object, such as a chair, of which there may be more than one in the room, the other players must guess the particular chair he or she has in mind.

- The game ends as soon as someone has spotted the object that was chosen – he or she may then spy the next object.

VARIATION
I spy may be played by very young children if colours rather than first letters are given. For example, a player may say, 'I spy, with my little eye, something red,' and the others then look for the red object that he or she has in mind.

I WENT ON A TRIP

Age 10+   Players Group

AIM
Players try to remember and repeat a growing list of items.

PLAY
- One of the players chooses an article – for example an umbrella – and says, 'I went on a trip and took my umbrella.'

- The next player repeats that sentence and adds a second item after 'umbrella'. In this way the players gradually build up a list of articles.

- Each time his or her turn comes, a player repeats the list and adds another item. Whenever a player cannot repeat the list correctly, the list is closed and the next player in the group begins a new list.

VARIATION
A variation known as City of Boston is very similar to I Went on a Trip, but players must add to a list of items for sale. Thus the first player might say 'I shall sell you a bunch of violets when you come to the City of Boston'. The other players then repeat that sentence in turn and add an item that he or she will sell.

I WENT SHOPPING

Age 10+   **Players** Group

PLAY

- The first player begins by saying something like: 'I went shopping and I bought some apples' (the first item must begin with the letter 'A').

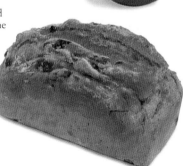

- The next player must add something beginning with 'B' to the list. For example: 'I went shopping and I bought some apples and some bread.' The whole list must be repeated in the course of each round.

- The third player might add 'carrots' to the list. If a player gets the list wrong, or cannot think of an item beginning with the next letter of the alphabet, he or she must drop out of the game.

- The winner is the last player left in the game.

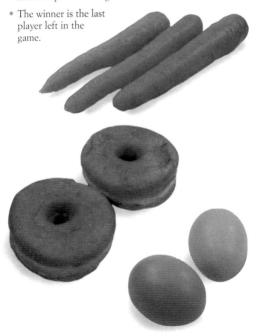

INITIAL ANSWERS

Age 10+   Players Group

AIM
To be the last remaining person in the game.

PLAY
- The players sit in a circle and one of them starts by thinking of any letter of the alphabet (e.g. S).

- He or she must then think of a three-letter word beginning with that letter and give a definition of the word; for example 'S plus two letters is a father's child'.

- The second person in the circle has to try to guess the word ('son'), and he or she then thinks of a word of four letters also beginning with S. He or she might choose 'soup' and define it as 'S plus three letters makes a tasty start to a meal' for the person sitting next to him or her to guess.

- This next person, after guessing the word correctly, must think of a five-letter word – perhaps 'snail' – defining it as 'S plus four letters carries a house on its back'.

- The game continues in this way, with each person having to think of a word beginning with the chosen letter, and each word having one letter more than the previous word. Any player who fails to think of an appropriate word, or who fails to guess a word, must drop out.

- The last person left in the game is the winner. A different letter of the alphabet should be chosen for the next round.

INITIAL LETTERS

Age 10+   Players Group

AIM
To be the last remaining person in the game.

PLAY
- The players sit in a circle.

- One of them puts a question – it may be as far-fetched as he or she likes – to the others.

- Each of them in turn must reply with a two-word answer, beginning with the initials of his or her names. Players have only five seconds in which to think of an answer. For example, if the question was, 'What is your favourite food?' Brian Richards could reply 'Boiled rice,' and Rosie Collins might say 'Roquefort cheese.' When all the players have answered, the second player asks a question. Any player who fails to answer after five seconds or who gives a wrong answer drops out of the game.

- The winner is the last person to stay in.

Question: What is your favourite food?

BRIAN RICHARDS	Boiled rice
DANIEL BENNETT	Digestive biscuits
ROSIE COLLINS	Roquefort cheese
JAMES DAY	Jam doughnuts
DANIEL BENNETT	Digestive biscuits

MY FATHER KEEPS A GROCER'S SHOP
Age 5–10   Players Group

AIM
To guess the right word.

PLAY
- The players sit in a group.

- The first one chosen begins, 'My father keeps a grocer's shop, and in it he sells . . .' Instead of saying the complete word, the player just gives the first letter. If he or she was thinking of 'Carrots', he or she would say 'C'.

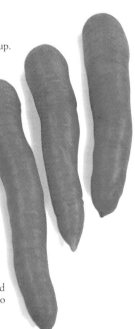

- The other players now try to guess what the word is.

- The first to guess correctly wins the round and becomes the next to think of a word.

ONE MINUTE, PLEASE

Age 10+   Players Group

AIM

To speak for one minute on a given topic.

PLAY

- One player is chosen as timekeeper and also picks topics for each player to talk about.

- When it is his or her turn to speak, a player is told his or her topic. This may be anything from a serious topic such as 'The current political situation' to something frivolous like 'Why women wear hats'. Players may choose to treat the subject in any manner they please and what they say may be utter nonsense, provided they do not deviate from the topic, hesitate unduly or repeat themselves.

- Other players may challenge the speaker if they feel he or she has broken a rule. If the timekeeper agrees, then the speaker must drop out and the next player is given a new topic.

- The winner is the player who manages to speak for an entire minute. If, however, two or more players achieve this, the others decide which of the speeches was the best, or alternatively further rounds may be played.

ONE ORANGE

Age 5–10   **Players Group**

PLAY

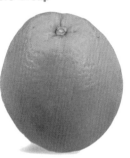

- The players are seated in a circle.

- The player chosen to lead off the game turns to the person on his or her left and says, 'One orange'.

- The phrase is repeated by each member of the circle in turn, until it returns to the player to the left of the first person.

- This player must now make up another phrase containing two items beginning with the same letter – for example, 'Two tigers'.

- This is now added to the first phrase, and both are repeated by each player in the circle until it is the turn of the last player.

- He or she will now choose a third item. After a few rounds, the phrase all the players must repeat may be something like: 'One orange, two tigers, three trains, four feathers, five fingers, six sailors, seven sausages . . .'

- When a player makes a mistake, he or she must drop out of the game. The winner is the last player remaining.

TABOO

Age 10+ **Players Group**

AIM

Players try to avoid saying a particular letter of the alphabet.

PLAY

- One player is the questioner and chooses which letter is to be 'taboo'.

- He or she then asks each of the players in turn any question he or she likes.

- Players must answer with a sensible phrase or sentence that does not contain the forbidden letter – if they do use the taboo letter, they are out.

- The last player to stay in the game wins and becomes the next questioner.

Example

F **is** TABOO

Questioner: 'Name a ball game'

Player 1 'Cricket' STAYS IN

Player 2 'Basketball' STAYS IN

Player 3 'Golf' GOES OUT

TONGUE-TWISTERS

Age 10+ **Players** Group

Equipment
A box or hat.

Preparation
The host should prepare at least ten tongue-twisters in advance and place them in a box or hat.

Play
- Each player is invited to pick out a tongue-twister from the box or hat. He or she then has to try to say it ten times in succession without stumbling or hesitating.
- Anyone who manages to say his or her tongue-twister ten times without faltering is the winner.

It can be fun compiling original tongue-twisters, perhaps based on the names or interests of one's guests.

Examples of tongue-twisters that might be used include:

Peter Piper picked a piece
of pickled pepper.

Betty bit a blue blob of
bitter blubber.

One white wren went wrong one day.

Four fraught farmers ploughing furrowed fields.

Forty throstle thrushes flit through frightful thistles.

Red lorry, yellow lorry.

The Leith police dismisseth us.

The sixth sick sheik's sixth sheep's sick.

I saw sister Susie sewing shirts for sailors.

TRAVELLER'S ALPHABET

Age 10+   **Players** Group

AIM

Players try to think up alliterative sentences.

PLAY

- The first player says, 'I am going on a journey to Amsterdam', or any other town or country beginning with A.

- The next person then asks, 'What will you do there?' The verb, adjective and noun used in the answer must all begin with A; for example, 'I shall acquire attractive antiques.'

- The second player must then give a place name and an answer using the letter B, the third player uses the letter C, and so on, around the players. Any player who cannot respond is eliminated from the game. If the players wish to make the game more taxing, they may have to give an answer that is linked with the place they have chosen. For example, a player might say, 'I am going to Greece to guzzle gorgeous grapes.' If a player gives an inappropriate answer, he or she may be challenged by another player. If the challenger cannot think of a more fitting sentence, the first player may stay in the game. Should the challenger's sentence be suitably linked, the first player is eliminated.

- The last player in the game wins.

WORD ASSOCIATION

Age 10+ **Players Group**

PLAY

• Players stand in a circle.

• The first player says the first word that enters his or her head.

• The player to the left has to respond immediately with a word that is somehow linked to the first word – for example, cup = tea = bag = paper, etc. A non-player acts as judge. Players hesitating too long before replying are eliminated. A player may be asked to explain the association between words if his or her reply does not seem to be linked to the previous word.

• The last player left in the game is the winner.

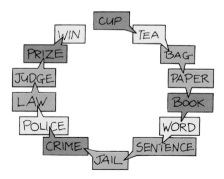

Pen and Paper Games

ACROSTICS

Age 10+   **Players 2**

AIM
Players try to build words out of a given set of letters.

PLAY
- A word of at least three letters is chosen.

- Each player writes the word in a column down the left-hand side of a sheet of paper; he or she then writes the same word, but with the letters reversed, down the right-hand side of the page.

- The player fills in the space between the two columns with the same number of words as there are letters in the keyword – and starting and ending each word with the letter at either side. For example, if the keyword is 'stem', a player's words might read: 'scream', 'trundle', 'earliest' and 'manageress'.

- The winner may be either the first person to fill in all the words, or the player with the longest or most original words.

S C R E A M

T R U N D L E

E A R L I E S T

M A N A G E R E S S

ANAGRAMS

Age 10+   **Players** Group

peilmidhun	delphinium
wodronsp	snowdrop
gamirodl	marigold
nedelarv	lavender

AIM

Players try to unscramble jumbled-up words.

PLAY

- One player prepares a list of words belonging to a particular category (e.g. flowers, cities, poets) and jumbles up the letters in each word.

- Each of the other players is given a list of the jumbled words and their category and tries to rearrange the letters back into the original words.

- The first player to rearrange all the words correctly, or the player with most correct words, after a given time, wins the game.

VARIATION

More experienced players may like to make up anagrams of their own by rearranging the letters in a word to make one or more other words. For example, 'angered' is an anagram of 'derange'.

BUILD THE TRIANGLE

Age 10+   Players Group

AIM

Players try to think of words beginning with a particular letter and of different lengths.

PLAY

- A letter of the alphabet is chosen by the host.

- Players are then asked to write it down and build a triangle of words all beginning with the chosen letter, as shown in the example below, adding one letter to each new word. If, for example, the letter chosen is A, the triangle might read as in the illustration below.

- The player with the largest triangle wins.

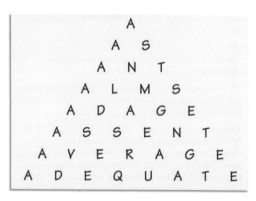

CATEGORIES

Age 10+   **Players Group**

AIM
Players try to think of words or names within particular categories beginning with particular letters.

PREPARATION
Each player is given a pencil and a piece of paper. The players decide on between six and a dozen different categories; these may be easy ones for children (e.g. girls' or boys' names, animals, colours) or more difficult for any adults who are also playing (e.g. politicians, rivers, chemicals). Each player lists the categories on his or her other paper. One of the players chooses any letter of the alphabet – preferably an 'easy' letter such as 'a' or 'd' if young children are playing. Older players can make the game more challenging by choosing difficult letters such as 'j' or 'k'. A time limit is agreed.

PLAY
- The players try to find a word beginning with the chosen letter for each of the categories.

- They write down their words next to the appropriate category, trying to think of words that none of the other players will have chosen.

- When the time is up, each player in turn reads out his or her list of words. If a player has found a word not thought of by any other player, he or she scores two points for that word. If, however, one or more of the other players has also chosen that word, each of them scores one point. If the player could not find a word at all, or if his or her choice of word did not correctly fit the category, he or she gets no points. (Disagreement about the relevance of a word to a category must be resolved by a vote among the other players.)

- The winner is the player with the highest score for his or her list of words. Any number of subsequent rounds may be played, using either the same or different categories; the chosen letter, however, must be different for each round. Players may take it in turns to choose a

	Place	Plant	Colour
P	Peru	poppy	pink
E	Eire	endive	ecru
R	Rome	reed	red
S	Seoul	soya	sepia
O	Ohio	orpine	ochre
N	New York	nemesia	navy

letter at the start of a round. Players make a note of their scores at the end of each round. The winner is the player with the highest points total at the end of the final round.

VARIATION

In a variation, known as Guggenheim, the players choose a keyword of about four to six letters, for example, 'person'. The letters of the keyword are written spaced out, and players try to find words for each of the categories beginning with each of the letters of the keyword.

Food	Wood	Name
plum	pine	Peter
egg	elm	Edward
ragout	redwood	Robin
soup	sycamore	Sally
orange	oak	Oliver
noodles	nutmeg-tree	Nicola

CROSSWORDS

Age 10+   **Players** Group

AIM

Players try to make words from letters written in a grid of squares, say five by five.

PLAY

- Each player in turn calls out any letter of the alphabet.

- As each letter is called, all players write it into any square of their choice, with the aim of forming words of two or more letters reading either across or down. Generally, abbreviations and proper nouns (names, etc.) may not be used. Once a letter has been written down, it cannot be moved to another square.

- Players continue to call out letters until all the individual squares have been filled. The number of points scored is equal to the number of letters in each word (one-letter words do not count). Thus a three-letter word scores three points. If a word fills an entire row or column, one bonus point is scored in addition to the score for that word. No ending of a word can form the beginning of another word in the same row or column. For example, if a row contains the letters 'i, f, e, n, d' a player may score four points for the word 'fend', but cannot in addition score two points for the word 'if'.

- The winning player is the one with the highest score.

Player 1

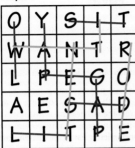

= 35 points

Player 2

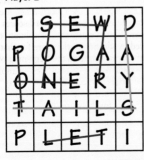

= 28 points

EMERGENCY CONSEQUENCES

Age 10+   **Players** Group

EQUIPMENT

Pencil and paper for each player.

PLAY

- Each player has to think of an 'emergency' and phrase it in the form of a question, for example: 'What would you do if your television exploded and the curtains caught fire?'

- The paper is then folded in half so the question is not visible and handed to the player on the left.

- The next player now writes down what he would do in an emergency (not knowing, of course, what the first player wrote) and the results are read out. For example, the second player might respond: 'I would boil the kettle and call a vet.'

- This game is for amusement only.

What would you do if your father fell down the stairs and broke his leg?

I would set the dog on him and call the police

FAIR AND SQUARE

Age 10+

Players Group

EQUIPMENT
Pencil and paper
for each player.

PREPARATION
Players must draw
a large square on a
piece of paper and
divide it into 25
smaller squares by
drawing four
vertical, and four
horizontal, lines
within the
outline.

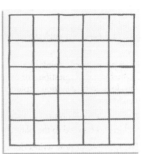

PLAY
- One player is
  chosen to start
  and calls out a
  letter of the
  alphabet. All
  the players
  must put the
  letter in one of
  their squares.

- When this is

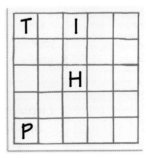

done, the next player chooses a letter and the players decide where to place it in their grids. Players may choose the same letter more than once.

- The game continues until all 25 squares are filled. The idea is to arrange your letters so that your grid contains a number of words of three or more letters. Words can run up and down. Players may, of course, choose letters to suit their own needs as their turn arises.

- Players score three points for a five-letter word, two points for a four-letter word and one point for each three-letter word.

- The winner is the person with the highest score. For example, this player's final score is 19 points, as shown opposite.

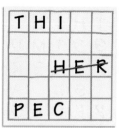

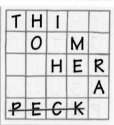

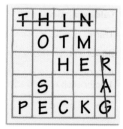

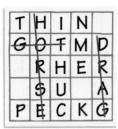

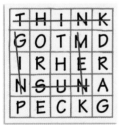

Calculating the score

THINK, HORSE: 3 points each = 6 points.

DRAG, PECK, THIN: 2 points each = 6 points.

INK, GOT, HER, SUN, GIN, MEN, RAG:
1 point each = 7 points.

Total: 19 points

FILL-INS

Age 10+   **Players Group**

Aim
Players try to guess missing letters in words.

Play
- A list of 30–40 words is prepared and kept hidden from the players.

- Each player is then given the first and last letters, the number of letters missing, and a clue for each word on the list.

- The winner is the first player to fill in all the blanks correctly. Alternatively, the players may be allowed an agreed length of time and then the winner is the player with the most correct words.

E - - - - R time for eggs (EASTER)

H - - - Y a festive plant (HOLLY)

P - - - - - C a peaceful ocean? (PACIFIC)

D - - - - - R cleaning cloth (DUSTER)

HANGMAN

Age 10+   Players 2

AIM

Players try to guess a secret word.

PLAY

- One person thinks of a word of about five or six letters.

- This player writes down the same number of dashes as there are letters in his or her word.

- The other players may then start guessing the letters in the word, calling out one letter at a time.

- If the guess is a successful one, the letter is written by the first player above the appropriate dash – if it appears more than once in a word it must be entered as often as it occurs.

- If the guess is an incorrect one, however, the first player may start to draw a hanged man – one line of the drawing representing each wrong letter. The other players must try to guess the secret word before the first player can complete the drawing of the hanged man.

- If one player guesses the word (this should become easier as the game progresses), he or she may take a turn at choosing a word. If the hanged man is completed before the word is guessed, the same player may choose another word. To make the game more difficult, longer words may be chosen. Alternatively, the player may choose a group of words making a proverb or the title of a book or film and should give the other players a clue as to the category.

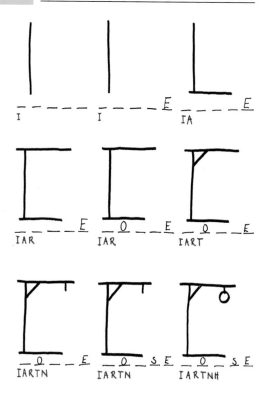

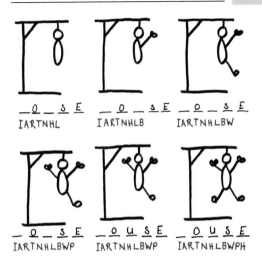

- In this game the word was 'mouse', but the hangman was completed before the word was guessed.

HEADS AND TAILS

Age 10+   **Players** Group

EQUIPMENT

A dictionary, and pencil and paper for each player.

PLAY

- Players are given 10 minutes to make a list of as many words as possible of four or more letters that begin and end with the same letter – for example, gargling, giving, noun, toot, rectangular, bomb.

- One point is given for each word, but words of six or more letters may be awarded an extra point.

- The winner is the player with the most points.

VARIATION

gargling	giving
noun	toot
rectangular	target
suspicious	grabbing
reaper	bomb
delighted	

Older participants could list words that begin and end with the same two letters – for example – church, decide, enliven, retire, tomato.

HIDDEN WORDS

Age 10+   **Players** Group

EQUIPMENT
Paper and pencil for each player.

PREPARATION
Make a list of sentences that contain, hidden in consecutive letters, the names of animals or insects – for example: 'Thomas wanted to add more sugar to his tea.' (Swan, toad) 'He knew that it would cost Richrd on keyrings alone.' (Newt, ostrich, donkey)

PLAY
- Give the players 5 or 10 minutes, depending on the number of sentences, to list all the animals they can find. There may be more than one in each sentence.

- The winner will be the player who finds the highest number of animals.

> **Thomas wanted to add more sugar to his tea.**
>
> **Transfer returned money to this slot here.**
>
> **He knew that it would cost Richard on keyrings alone.**

HOW MANY?
Age 5–10

Players Group

EQUIPMENT
Paper and pencil for each
player and some small
household items.

PREPARATION
Put the household items in
containers. Examples might
include matches, grains of
rice, buttons and peas.
Make a list of how many of
each there are in each
container.

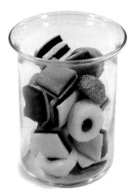

PLAY
- The containers are
  presented, one by one,
  and players write down
  how many items they
  think each contains.

- Allow players a few
  seconds to look at each
  item and then remove it
  so they cannot count the
  contents. If there are
  more than four
  competitors, the player

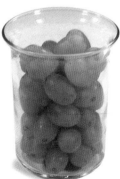

whose guess is closest to the correct total scores three points, with the next two closest scoring two and one point respectively. Bonus points could be awarded for a completely accurate guess.

• The player with the highest number of points wins.

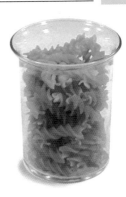

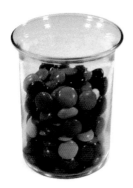

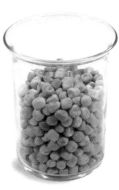

JOTTO

Age 10+   **Players Group**

EQUIPMENT

Coins, and pencil and paper for each player.

PLAY

- Players choose a partner. Each pair tosses a coin to see who will start. The first of each pair now writes down a secret five-letter word. None of the letters in that word must be repeated. Examples might include House, Chain, Water.

- The other player now tries to guess the word. He or she also chooses a five-letter word, writes it down and then shows it to the first player.

- The first player looks at the word and writes down next to it which letters in that word are in his or her own hidden word. The letters can be written in any order.

- The second player of each pair now makes another guess and writes it down underneath the first attempt.

- This word is also shown to the first player, who again writes down the letters that are correct.

- The game continues until the second player guesses the first player's word correctly.

- The second player then has a turn at thinking up a five-letter word for the first player to guess.

- The winners are the players in each pair who identify the highest number of secret words in, say, 10 minutes.

VARIATION
More challenging is for the first player to write only the number of letters in the guessed word which match those in the secret word.

HOUSE

PLACE	E
STONE	ESO
HORSE	ESOH
HOUSE	✔

CHAIN

SPACE	CA
QUACK	CA
CLAIM	CAI
CHAIR	CAIH
CHAIN	✔

NAME THEM!

Age 10+   Players Group

EQUIPMENT
Paper and pencil for each player.

PREPARATION
The host prepares a list of 20 famous people, then splits it
into 40 names. Depending on the participants, characters
may be a wide-ranging general selection or could be
related to specific activities such as sport or the film world,
etc. If a wide selection is given, then clues could be offered
such as five sports personalities, six historical figures, two
film characters, etc.

PLAY
• Players have 10 minutes to write down which surnames
  they think match up with which first names to create the
  names of 20 famous people.

• The player with the highest number of correct answers
  is the winner.

1. David	6. George
2. Robbie	7. Julia
3. Kylie	8. Zidane
4. Brad	9. Michael
5. Bill	10. Carey

11. Tony	26. Jennifer
12. Bart	27. Clinton
13. Sampras	28. Mickey
14. Owen	29. Minogue
15. Jim	30. Nelson
16. Jones	31. Roberts
17. Pitt	32. Redgrave
18. Mouse	33. ZInedine
19. Williams	34. Blair
20. Marion	35. Keating
21. Tim	36. Bush
22. Ronan	37. Mandela
23. Pete	38. Beckham
24. Aniston	39. Henman
25. Steve	40. Simpson

ODD MAN OUT

Age 10+   **Players** Group

EQUIPMENT
Paper and pencil for each player.

PREPARATION
The host prepares a number of lists, each containing one item that does not fit in with the others. The following are examples of lists with the 'odd man out' in italics:

PLAY
- Players are given a copy of the list and 10 minutes or so to write down which items are the 'odd man out'.

- The player with the highest number of correct answers is the winner.

> Thames, Severn, *Windermere*, Avon
> (the others are rivers)
>
> Zola, Proust, *Debussy*, Flaubert
> (the others were writers)
>
> Bee, scorpion, hornet, *flea*
> (the others have stings)
>
> Elizabeth, Victoria, Anne, *Belinda*
> (the others were British Queens)
>
> *New York*, Paris, Tokyo, Rome
> (the others are capital cities)
>
> Green, yellow, *pink*, blue
> (the others are colours of the rainbow)

PHOTOGRAPHIC MEMORY
Age 10+   **Players Group**

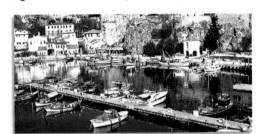

EQUIPMENT
A postcard or a picture from a magazine, and a piece of paper and a pencil for each player.

PREPARATION
Ask the guests to look at the picture for 1 minute, after which it is taken away.

PLAY
- The players should be given a piece of paper and a pencil.
- They are then asked a number of questions about the picture they have examined, testing their recall of the picture's details. The number and complexity of questions will depend on the age of the players.
- The player who answers the most questions correctly is the winner.

RIDDLEMEREE

Age 10+   **Players Group**

EQUIPMENT
Paper and pencil for each player.

PLAY
- This involves players choosing a word – an item in the room or a place name – and writing a 'riddlemeree', or riddle, giving clues to the letters in the word. Allow players about 10 minutes. The following is an example:.

  My first is in apple but not in orange,

  My second is in kitten but not in cat,

  My third is in tea but not in coffee,

  My fourth is in green but not in red,

  My fifth is in potato and also in carrot.

  Answer: 'Piano'.

- Winners are any players who write a riddle that is not solved and any player who works one out.

C   My first is in castle and also in cottage

A   My second is in barter but not in borrow

K   My third is in stake but not in stage

E   My fourth is in tree but not in twig

SCAFFOLD

Age 10+   **Players Group**

EQUIPMENT

A dictionary, and paper and pencil for each player.

PLAY

- Players are given three letters (at least one of which should be a vowel), and 10 minutes to write down words that contain all three letters. Words must be of four letters or more. Plurals are not allowed.

  For example, if the letters are A, M, T, the list of words may include: TEAM, MATE, MEAT, MATADOR, TRAMP, TOMATO, MATCH, ATTEMPT, MATTER . . .

- The player with the highest number of correct words will be the winner.

paste poster sprite step

speed spider escape response

separate precious

persistence pest spice

spare whisper

trespasser desperation sleep

EPS

SPELLING BEE

Age 7+   **Players Group**

AIM

To spell as many words as possible correctly, so gaining the maximum number of points.

PREPARATION

One person is chosen as leader, and the other players sit facing him or her. The leader may be given a previously prepared list of words or may make one up. It is a good idea to have a dictionary to hand in case of disputes.

PLAY

- The leader then reads out the first word on the list and the first player tries to spell it.

- The player is allowed 10 seconds in which to make an attempt at the correct spelling. If he or she succeeds, one point is scored and the next word is read out for the next player. If the player makes a mistake, the leader reads out the correct spelling. The player does not score for that word, and the next word is read out for the next player. (Alternatively, the player is eliminated from the game for an incorrect answer.) Play continues around the group of players until all the words on the list have been spelled.

- The winner is the player with the most points at the end of the game.

BACKWARDS SPELLING BEE

Age 7+   Players Group

In Backwards Spelling Bee, a more difficult version of the game, players must spell their words backwards. Scoring is the same as in the standard game.

VARIATION

For Right or Wrong Spelling Bee, the players should form two teams, and line up opposite each other.

PLAY

- The leader calls out a word to each player in turn, alternating between teams.

- Each time a player spells a word, the player standing opposite him must call out 'Right' or 'Wrong'.

- If he calls a correctly spelled word wrong or a misspelled word right, he is eliminated from the game and must leave the line. (Players may move around once their numbers have been depleted, so that there is a caller for each player in the other team.)

- If the caller makes a correct call, he gets the next word to spell.

- The last team to retain any players wins.

Street	TEERTS	✔
London	NODNOL	✔
Forward	DARWROF	✗

SURPRISE SENTENCES
Age 7+   Players Teams

AIM
Each team tries to write a sentence, with each player in the team writing one word of it.

PREPARATION
For each team, a large sheet of paper is attached to a wall or to a board propped upright.

PLAY
* Each team lines up opposite its sheet of paper and the leader is given a pencil.

* At the word 'Go!' the leader runs up to his or her team's paper and writes any word he or she likes and then runs back to the team, hands the pencil to the next player and goes to the end of the team.

* As soon as the next player gets the pencil, he or she goes to the paper and adds a second word either in front of, or behind, the leader's word.

* Play continues in this way with each player adding one word. The words should be chosen and put together so that they can be part of a grammatically correct sentence.

* Each player, except the last, must avoid completing the sentence. The last player should be able to complete the sentence by adding just one word and he or she also puts in the punctuation.

- Players may not confer and choose a sentence before writing their words.

- The first team to construct a sentence with one word from each player wins the game.

SWARMING ANTS

Age 10+

Players Group

EQUIPMENT
Pencil and paper for
each player.

PREPARATION
On a piece of paper,
write down the phrases
listed on the right: ('A
shining ant', 'A floating
ant', etc.).

PLAY
- The players have to
write down a word
ending in -ant that
relates to the clue.
Some examples are
shown.

- The player with the
highest number of
correct answers is the
winner.

A shining ant
brilliant

A floating ant
buoyant

A sweet-smelling ant
fragrant

A green ant
verdant

A singing ant
chant

A plentiful ant
abundant

A waiting ant
attendant

A non-stop ant
constant

A sloping ant
slant

A graceful ant
elegant

A tell-tale ant
informant

TANGLED SENTENCES
Age 5-10   Players Group

AIM
To scramble up sentences in a way that makes it hard to guess what they are meant to be.

PLAY
- Players write down a sentence, which might be a popular saying, a line from a pop song or poem, or a newspaper headline. However, instead of writing it down properly, they write it with the words scrambled in such a way as to make a strange or funny sentence, such as 'Make never wrongs a two right' from 'Two wrongs never make a right'. The sentences being scrambled might be quite simple, if the players are young, or quite complicated for older children.

- Really, this is a game played just for the fun of it, but the winner might be the player whose tangled sentence is the most difficult to unscramble.

chickens hatch before your count don't they
(DON'T COUNT YOUR CHICKENS BEFORE THEY HATCH)

feather a flock of birds together
(BIRDS OF A FEATHER FLOCK TOGETHER)

a wall sat Humpty on Dumpty
(HUMPTY DUMPTY SAT ON A WALL)

TELEGRAMS

Age 10+   **Players** Group

AIM

Players make up a message from a list of letters or a given word.

PLAY

- Players are given or make up a list of 15 letters and must use each of them – in the order given – as the initial letter of a word in a 15-word telegram. (Alternatively, the players are given or select a word of about 10–15 letters, e.g. blackberries – the first word must begin with 'b', the second with 'l', and so on.) The telegram may include one or two place names and may – if the player wishes – have the name of the 'sender' as the last word. Stops (or periods) may be used for punctuation.

- The winner is the first player to complete his or her telegram, or, if a time limit has been set, the player whose telegram is judged to be the best at the end of the time set.

TELEGRAM

tell Ellen let everyone go running after Mummy

ELEPHANT

extra long ears, particularly hares, are neatly tapered

TRANSFORMATION

Age 10+   **Players Group**

AIM

Players try to 'transform' one word into another through a series of intermediate stages.

PLAY

- Two words with the same number of letters are chosen.

- Each player writes down the two words.

- He or she then tries to change the first word into the second word by altering only one letter at a time and each time forming a new word. For example, 'dog' could be changed to 'cat' in four words as below.

- It is easiest to begin with three- or four-letter words until the players are quite practised — when five- or even six-letter words may be tried.

- The winner is the player who completes the changes using the fewest number of words.

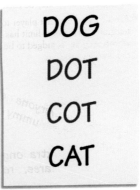

DOG
DOT
COT
CAT

WHAT'S NEXT?

Age 10+   **Players Group**

EQUIPMENT
Paper and pencil for each player.

PREPARATION
The host prepares a number of 'progressions' in advance. These can be numerical or alphabetical. Examples are:

What is the next number in this sequence? 5 6 8 11... (Answer: 15).

What is the next letter in this sequence? A E I M... (Answer: Q).

In the first example, you add one to five to make six, then add two to six to make eight, and add three to eight to make eleven. To continue the sequence, therefore, you must add four to eleven to make fifteen. Likewise, in the second example, there are three letters missing between each entry in the sequence.

PLAY
• The players are allowed 3 minutes or so to work out what letter or number comes next in each progression.

• The winner is the player with the most correct answers.

Answers to sequences on right are:
128; IR; 28; T; 32; J; 85; 34; 4,294,967,296.

1 2 4 8 16 32 64 ....

MN LO KP JQ ....

1 2 3 4 6 9 13 19 ....

Z B X D V F ....

31 28 31 30 31 ....

J F M A M J ....

5 9 13 21 33 53 ....

1 1 2 3 5 8 13 21 ....

2 4 16 256 65,536 ....

WHO IS IT?

Age 10+

Players Group

EQUIPMENT
Paper and pencil for each player, a good pile of
photographs of famous people cut out from newspapers
and magazines, and some card.

PREPARATION
The host should have cut out part of each photograph so
that it shows the eyes only. Each should then be stuck onto
the card. Each picture should now be labelled with a
number or letter, and a note, kept by the organiser, of the
celebrity whose eyes feature in each picture. Each player
should also get a list of the celebrities.

PLAYING
• The 'eyes' are passed around the table, and everyone has
  to write down the name of the personality to whom they
  belong.

• The winner is the participant making the most correct
  guesses.

WORD SQUARE

Age 10+   **Players Group**

EQUIPMENT
Pencil and paper for each player.

PREPARATION
Write, in large capital letters and, as shown below, the words 'WORLD' and 'EARTH' on each piece of paper, and give one to every player. Other combinations can be used, but make sure both words are of the same length so that the Word Square can be completed.

PLAYING
- The players have to think of words comprising five letters that can fit in between, as in the example below.

- The first player creating a Word Square is the winner.

W	r	i	t	E
O	p	e	r	A
R	o	v	e	R
L	i	g	h	T
D	i	t	c	H

WORD-MAKING

Age 10+   **Players Group**

EQUIPMENT
A dictionary, and pencil and paper for each player.

PREPARATION
Think of a long word and give each player a pencil and a sheet of paper.

PLAYING
- Players are given a long word, which they write down on the top of their sheet of paper.

- They have 10 minutes to make as many new words of at least three letters from the word they have been given. For example, if they are given HELICOPTER, they might make a list containing: TOP, CLIP, TRIPE, HOTEL, REPEL, CHOIR and POLICE.

- The player who writes down the most new words (no plurals or proper names are allowed) will be the winner. Five- or six-letter words may count double.

PHOTOGRAPHY

ANDREW	LEANNE
rat	graph
hot	hot
pat	got
pay	pot
tray	pay
harp	trap
part	tray
root	rot
hoop	gap
troop	party
graph	pray
rap	goat
hat	happy
hog	

Index

COLLINS GEM
1950s
a mine of information

COLLINS GEM
1960s
a mine of information

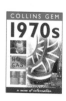

COLLINS GEM
1970s
NO GAS
a mine of information

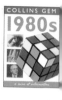

COLLINS GEM
1980s
a mine of information

COLLINS Jane's
CIVIL AIRCRAFT
a mine of information

COLLINS GEM
CLANS & Tartans
a mine of information

COLLINS GEM
Classic
TV SERIES
a mine of information

COLLINS Jane's
COMBAT AIRCRAFT
a mine of information

COLLINS GEM
FIRSTS
a mine of information

COLLINS GEM
GOLF
a mine of information

COLLINS GEM
HILLWALKER'S
Survival Guide
a mine of information

COLLINS GEM
HOME
EMERGENCY GUIDE
a mine of information

COLLINS GEM
Collecting
STAMPS
a mine of information

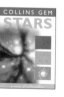

COLLINS GEM
STARS
a mine of information

COLLINS GEM
SUPERSTITIONS
a mine of information

COLLINS GEM
Using Your
SOFTWARE
a mine of information